Sarcopenia: Age-Related Muscle Wasting and Weakness (Mechanisms and Treatments)

Sarcopenia: Age-Related Muscle Wasting and Weakness (Mechanisms and Treatments)

Editor: Ryann Heckman

FOSTER ACADEMICS
www.fosteracademics.com

www.fosteracademics.com

FOSTER ACADEMICS

Cataloging-in-Publication Data

Sarcopenia : age-related muscle wasting and weakness (mechanisms and treatments) / edited by Ryann Heckman.
p. cm.
Includes bibliographical references and index.
ISBN 978-1-64646-583-5
1. Musculoskeletal diseases in old age. 2. Muscles--Diseases. 3. Older people--Diseases--Treatment.
4. Aging--Physiological aspects. 5. Geriatrics. 6. Older people--Health and hygiene. I. Heckman, Ryann.
RC925.53 .S27 2023
618.976 7--dc23

Foster Academics,
118-35 Queens Blvd., Suite 400,
Forest Hills, NY 11375, USA

ISBN 978-1-64646-583-5 (Hardback)

Contents

Preface

I am honored to present to you this unique book which encompasses the most up-to-date data in the field. I was extremely pleased to get this opportunity of editing the work of experts from across the globe. I have also written papers in this field and researched the various aspects revolving around the progress of the discipline. I have tried to unify my knowledge along with that of stalwarts from every corner of the world, to produce a text which not only benefits the readers but also facilitates the growth of the field.

Sarcopenia refers to the aging-related muscle wasting and weakness which involves a degenerative loss of skeletal muscle mass, quality and strength. It is a condition characterized by muscular atrophy. Exercise level, nutrition, and co-morbidities all influence the rate of muscle loss. Changes in muscle synthesis signaling pathways are linked to the loss of muscle. Sarcopenia can impair a person's capacity to perform daily tasks such as walking, climbing stairs and lifting objects. It is linked to severe comorbidities, including obesity, osteoporosis, type 2 diabetes and insulin resistance. Sarcopenia can be prevented and delayed by leading an active lifestyle and engaging in physical activity. This book is compiled in such a manner, that it will provide in-depth knowledge on the impact of age-related muscle wasting and weakness associated with sarcopenia. It aims to shed light on some of the unexplored aspects of this disease. A number of latest researches have been included to keep the readers up-to-date with the global concepts in this medical condition.

Finally, I would like to thank all the contributing authors for their valuable time and contributions. This book would not have been possible without their efforts. I would also like to thank my friends and family for their constant support.

Editor

1

Mitochondrial involvement and impact in aging skeletal muscle

Russell T. Hepple*

Department of Kinesiology, McGill University Health Center, McGill University, Montreal, QC, Canada

Correspondence:
Russell T. Hepple, Department of Critical Care Medicine, Royal Victoria Hospital, 675 Pine Avenue West, Montreal, QC H3A1A1, Canada
e-mail: russell.hepple@mcgill.ca

Atrophy is a defining feature of aging skeletal muscle that contributes to progressive weakness and an increased risk of mobility impairment, falls, and physical frailty in very advanced age. Amongst the most frequently implicated mechanisms of aging muscle atrophy is mitochondrial dysfunction. Recent studies employing methods that are well-suited to interrogating intrinsic mitochondrial function find that mitochondrial respiration and reactive oxygen species emission changes are inconsistent between aging rat muscles undergoing atrophy and appear normal in human skeletal muscle from septuagenarian physically active subjects. On the other hand, a sensitization to permeability transition seems to be a general property of atrophying muscle with aging and this effect is even seen in atrophying muscle from physically active septuagenarian subjects. In addition to this intrinsic alteration in mitochondrial function, factors extrinsic to the mitochondria may also modulate mitochondrial function in aging muscle. In particular, recent evidence implicates oxidative stress in the aging *milieu* as a factor that depresses respiratory function *in vivo* (an effect that is not present *ex vivo*). Furthermore, in very advanced age, not only does muscle atrophy become more severe and clinically relevant in terms of its impact, but also there is evidence that this is driven by an accumulation of severely atrophied denervated myofibers. As denervation can itself modulate mitochondrial function and recruit mitochondrial-mediated atrophy pathways, future investigations need to address the degree to which skeletal muscle mitochondrial alterations in very advanced age are a consequence of denervation, rather than a primary organelle defect, to refine our understanding of the relevance of mitochondria as a therapeutic target at this more advanced age.

Keywords: sarcopenia, bioenergetics, mitochondria, skeletal muscle, reactive oxygen species, permeability transition, oxidative stress, muscle atrophy

INTRODUCTION

Progressive atrophy is a defining feature of aging skeletal muscle and when it becomes severe in very advanced age (≥80 years of age), it can lead to weakness that precipitates mobility impairment, an increased risk of falls, and physically frailty (Cruz-Jentoft et al., 2010). For this reason, understanding the mechanisms underlying aging muscle atrophy so that suitable therapeutic targets can be identified is key to promoting health and mobility in the elderly. Whilst many possible targets have been suggested, the most effective therapeutic targets will be those that serve as a nexus point for modulating a wide range of cellular functions that are affected with aging; a concept that brings to mind the role of the mitochondrion.

Mitochondria serve a central role as an integrator of a variety of signals within the cell, and accordingly vary their function to modulate energy supply, reactive oxygen species (ROS) signaling, and intrinsic pathways of apoptosis (**Figure 1**). For this reason, mitochondria have been frequently studied as a target for combating cellular aging. This is also true of muscle cells where one of the first studies to suggest impaired mitochondrial function may be involved in muscle aging was performed in flies and poignantly found that mitochondrial dysfunction was associated with loss of the wings (Rockstein and Brandt, 1963)! A great many studies have followed and although a substantial number have found evidence for impaired mitochondrial function in aging muscle (Rumsey et al., 1987; Trounce et al., 1989; Cooper et al., 1992; Conley et al., 2000; Gouspillou et al., 2010, 2014a,b; Picard et al., 2011a), others have not (Kent-Braun and Ng, 2000; Rasmussen et al., 2003; Lanza et al., 2005), underscoring the complexity of understanding in this area. The purpose of this review, therefore, is to address the basis for these complexities, identify relevant mechanisms therein, and finally to provide some suggestions for future investigation.

ADDRESSING THE QUESTION OF MITOCHONDRIAL DYSFUNCTION IN AGING MUSCLE

There are numerous issues that need to be considered when evaluating the involvement of mitochondria in aging of skeletal muscle. The first issue to consider is the means by which the mitochondrial function is interrogated. For example, direct interrogation of mitochondrial function frequently employs mechanical isolation of mitochondria, a method that itself can induce alterations in the intrinsic function of the organelle (Picard et al., 2011c). Indeed, mechanical isolation of mitochondria not only exaggerates the magnitude of age-related impairment in various aspects of mitochondrial function but also induces changes not seen in a preparation where mitochondrial structure is preserved (Picard et al., 2010).

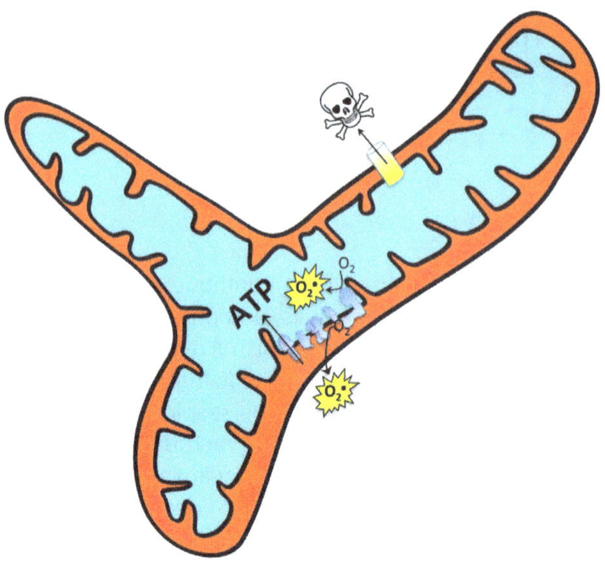

FIGURE 1 | Mitochondria respond to a wide array of intracellular signals and accordingly modulate their function [ATP production, reactive oxygen species (ROS) production, and sensitivity to permeability transition] across a large dynamic range to meet the cellular needs. It is thus important to understand whether alterations observed in aging muscle represent a primary organelle defect versus a secondary (potentially adaptive) response to a changing cellular environment.

A second issue to consider is which functional outputs are quantified as it relates to the different roles that mitochondria serve in skeletal muscle, including energy provision (respiration), signaling (ROS emission), and regulation of apoptosis (e.g., through permeability transition and release of mitochondrial-derived apoptotic factors) (Picard et al., 2011a). Further to this point, it is also essential to account for the fact that some mitochondrial functional properties vary between fast twitch and slow twitch muscles (Picard et al., 2012). For example, slow twitch muscles generally exhibit lower mitochondrial ROS emission (Anderson and Neufer, 2006; Picard et al., 2008) and a lower capacity for calcium retention before permeability transition occurs (Picard et al., 2008) when compared to fast twitch muscles. Thus, in situations where muscle exhibits a shift in fiber type with aging, the impact of this shift on the mitochondrial function properties needs to be considered.

The third issue to consider is the age studied and in this respect, it is important to address mitochondrial function across the aging continuum, including study of ages that are most affected by the consequences of aging muscle atrophy. As noted in the section "Introduction," this is typically ≥80 years of age (Cruz-Jentoft et al., 2010) and thus far there is very little known about muscle mitochondrial alterations in this age group from human studies, although several studies in the animal literature exist (Chabi et al., 2008; Ljubicic et al., 2009; Joseph et al., 2010; Picard et al., 2011a). Related to this point, when using an animal model system the age studied should represent points along the trajectory of muscle aging that are relevant for human muscle.

A fourth issue to consider is that of physical activity because it is well-established that skeletal muscle mitochondrial content is highly adaptable and not only increases in response to elevated metabolic demand but also decreases in response to reduced metabolic demand, with the latter being the typical situation in aging (Martin et al., 2014). As such, understanding the degree to which mitochondrial content and functional alterations are an obligatory consequence of aging versus being wholly or partially avoidable through a physically active lifestyle, is of critical importance.

Finally, since mitochondria serve as central integrators of a wide variety of cellular signals and thus exhibit a wide range of what should be considered physiological (rather than pathological) function (Picard et al., 2011b), it is essential to consider the involvement of cellular alterations that are extrinsic to the mitochondria as modulating factors in their function before concluding that a primary mitochondrial defect exists. For example, aging in muscle has long been known to induce neurological alterations such as neuromuscular junction instability leading to denervation (Tomonaga, 1977; Oda, 1984; Edstrom et al., 2007; Rudolf et al., 2014), and these changes may themselves exert an impact on the cellular environment that modulates mitochondrial function (Csukly et al., 2006; Muller et al., 2007; Bhattacharya et al., 2009). The suitability of the mitochondrion as a primary therapeutic target in this scenario needs to be carefully considered as reversing mitochondrial alterations that are secondary to denervation [e.g., those that result in activation of atrophy pathways (Romanello et al., 2010; Rowan et al., 2012)] could make the situation worse rather than better by preventing atrophy of denervated fibers and thereby increasing the burden on the remaining muscle fibers. These issues will be addressed in detail in the sections that follow to inform our current understanding of the role played by mitochondrial dysfunction in aging muscle atrophy and the resulting implications for intervening at this level.

METHODS FOR EVALUATING MITOCHONDRIAL FUNCTION

Many different methodological approaches have been taken to evaluate mitochondrial function in aging muscle, including direct measures (e.g., isolated mitochondria, permeabilized myofibers) and indirect measures [e.g., phosphocreatine (PCr) recovery kinetics following muscle contractions, enzyme assays, protein content, etc.]. Similarly, a variety of functional outputs of mitochondria have been examined, with indices related to mitochondrial respiration being by far the most frequent and measures of ROS emission second most frequent, whereas to date there are relatively few studies examining mitochondrial sensitivity to an apoptotic challenge, particularly in the human literature. Importantly, the impact of aging on the different aspects of mitochondrial function is often quite variable from one function to the next and this has implications for understanding the involvement of mitochondria in aging muscle. For example, a reduced respiratory capacity could impact muscle fatigue by limiting energy provision to the myocyte (Stary et al., 2004; Chabi et al., 2008), an increase in ROS emission could induce cellular and organelle oxidative stress and thereby increase the requirement for removal of resulting damage (Fulle et al., 2004; Mansouri et al., 2006), and an increased susceptibility to permeability transition could increase the release of mitochondrial-localized apoptotic factors thereby contributing to nuclear loss and myocyte atrophy (Marzetti et al., 2010; Gouspillou et al., 2014b).

MITOCHONDRIAL ENZYME ACTIVITIES

By far the most common approach to gaining insights about mitochondrial function in aging muscle is the use of enzymatic assays of representative mitochondrial enzymes, such as citrate synthase and electron transport chain complexes, and these measures provide indirect insights into the energy producing (respiratory) capacity of the mitochondria. Most of the studies performed to date indicate a marked decline in mitochondrial enzyme activities from aging muscle (Bass et al., 1975; Lezza et al., 1994; Desai et al., 1996; Hagen et al., 2004), although some studies find this to be maintained (Orlander et al., 1978; Barrientos et al., 1996) and others report it to be highly variable from one muscle to the next (Houmard et al., 1998; Lyons et al., 2006). Importantly, individual enzyme activities do not provide unambiguous insights about the respiratory function of the intact mitochondrion because individual enzyme activities can become very disparately related to whole organelle function when the mitochondrion becomes defective. Thus, more direct and integrated measures of function are required to interpret aging impact.

MECHANICALLY ISOLATED MITOCHONDRIA VERSUS SAPONIN-PERMEABILIZED MYOCYTES

Amongst the most frequently used methodological approaches to directly interrogate mitochondrial function involves the mechanical isolation of mitochondria (Chance and Williams, 1956). Although this method has been very widely used in the aging literature (Trounce et al., 1989; Boffoli et al., 1994; Capel et al., 2005; Chabi et al., 2008; Gouspillou et al., 2010), as we have recently reviewed (Picard et al., 2011b), not only does mechanical isolation markedly disrupt the normal architecture of skeletal muscle mitochondria from an irregular tubular network into smaller, relatively homogenous, spherical structures, but it also profoundly potentiates both mitochondrial ROS emission and sensitivity to permeability transition (**Figure 2**). The importance of this to studies in aging is illustrated by the fact that when we compared the apparent effect of aging on mitochondrial function in mitochondria isolated from skeletal muscle versus saponin-permeabilized myofibers (where mitochondrial structure is preserved) in very old rat muscle (35% survival rate, which is a similar relative age to $\geq$80 years old humans), we found the isolated mitochondria profoundly exaggerated the impact of aging (Picard et al., 2010). Specifically, with aging the decline in maximal mitochondrial respiratory capacity was fourfold greater, the increase in ROS emission was twofold greater and the reduction in time to permeability transition was twofold greater when examined in isolated mitochondria versus saponin-permeabilized myofibers (**Figure 3**). Not only this, but there were significant alterations in mitochondrial enzyme activity stoichiometry (reduced ratio of cytochrome oxidase to citrate synthase activity) and stoichiometry of respiratory states (suggestive of a defect in complex I) in isolated mitochondria with aging that were not seen in saponin-permeabilized myofibers. We have suggested that these latter observations may be indicative of a lesser ability of aged mitochondria to reseal during isolation procedures, since isolation induces transient disruption of tubular mitochondrial structures and subsequent reconstitution into the spherical organelles typical of isolates, resulting in greater contamination and/or loss of mitochondrial matrix

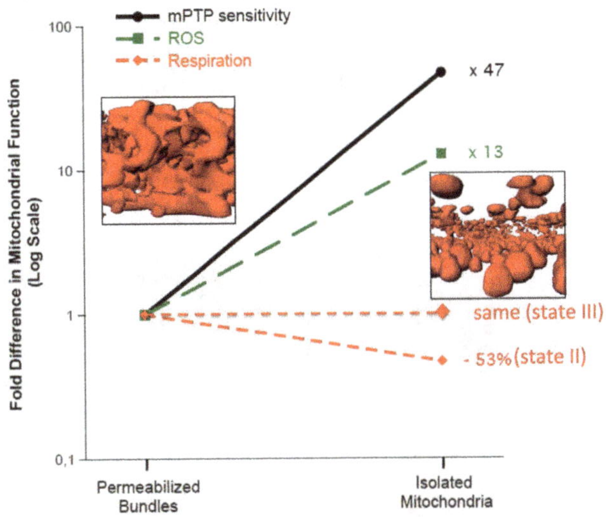

FIGURE 2 | Multiple features of mitochondrial structure and function are altered in mechanically isolated organelles compared to saponin-permeabilized myofibers (representing a preparation where all mitochondria are represented and their structure remains intact). In particular, the irregular tubular structure is lost following isolation, producing more homogenous spherical structures. Accompanying these structural changes is a marked potentiation of reactive oxygen species (ROS) emission and sensitization to mitochondrial permeability transition pore (mPTP) opening. Data are re-plotted from Picard et al. (2011c).

constituents in isolates prepared from aged muscles (Picard et al., 2010) (**Figure 4**). Collectively, therefore, our data show that the method used to interrogate mitochondrial function can have a profound influence on the degree to which mitochondrial function appears to be altered in aging muscle and that generally speaking, the degree to which mitochondrial function is altered in aging muscle is considerably less severe than has often been considered. This notion is consistent with other studies that have used the saponin-permeabilized myofibers method, which have found relatively mild (Joseph et al., 2012) or in other cases no impairments in mitochondrial respiratory capacity in aging muscle (Tonkonogi et al., 2000; Hutter et al., 2007; Gouspillou et al., 2014b).

Notwithstanding the point about mitochondrial respiratory alterations in aging muscle being less severe than often considered, in a follow-up study where we compared indices of mitochondrial function in saponin-permeabilized myofibers prepared from four rat muscles that exhibited contrasting fiber type and contrasting atrophy susceptibility with aging, we did find mitochondrial alterations that we believe bear consideration as a contributing factor in atrophy of aging muscle (Picard et al., 2011a). Our comparison involved two fast twitch muscles [extensor digitorum longus (EDL), gastrocnemius (Gas)] and two slow twitch muscles [soleus (Sol), adductor longus (AL)], where the Gas exhibited the most severe atrophy with aging, the EDL and Sol were similarly affected, and most strikingly, the AL actually hypertrophied by nearly 50% and the mitochondrial function was largely preserved in this muscle. Although the factors accounting for this profoundly better adjustment to aging in the rat AL remain under study, the other muscles exhibited varying degrees of mitochondrial functional alteration with aging. In particular, the Sol was the only muscle to exhibit a reduction in muscle respiratory capacity (**Figure 5A**) and in this case it was secondary to reduced mitochondrial content. In contrast, although the muscle respiratory capacity was largely preserved in both of the fast muscles, these two muscles had higher levels of representative subunits of the mitochondrial electron transport complexes, suggesting that the intrinsic respiratory capacity of the mitochondrial electron transport system was impaired in these fast muscles with aging. Muscle ROS emission normalized for respiration (an index of the proportion of O_2 consumption lost to ROS leak) demonstrated a general trend to be elevated in all four muscles under state II and state III conditions, although after normalizing for mitochondrial content only the Sol demonstrated an increase, suggesting an increase in intrinsic mitochondrial ROS emission in aging muscle is not a general feature of aging muscle (**Figure 5A**). On the other hand, the sensitivity to permeability transition was increased in the fast twitch muscles, suggesting greater apoptotic potential. Although we did not observe a change in this property in the Sol muscle, despite its marked atrophy with aging, as noted in Section "Addressing the Question of Mitochondrial Dysfunction in Aging Muscle," the time to mitochondrial permeability transition pore (mPTP) opening (permeability transition) in response to a calcium challenge is typically lower in slow twitch muscle (and higher in fast twitch muscle). As the aged Sol is characterized by a striking increase in the fraction of fibers that express fast myosin heavy chain isoforms (Edstrom and Ulfhake, 2005; Snow et al., 2005; Carter et al., 2010), after taking this shift into account, the aged Sol should have a longer time to mPTP opening than observed, meaning it too exhibits a sensitization to permeability transition with aging. This is depicted in **Figure 5B** as a time to pore (mPTP) opening that falls below the line predicted by the relationship between time to mPTP opening and percentage of fibers positive for fast myosin heavy chain. Collectively, therefore, since all three muscles, which atrophied with aging (EDL, Gas, Sol) exhibited a reduced time to permeability transition, whereas the only muscle that did not atrophy (AL) was unaffected, our results reveal that a general property of aging muscles undergoing atrophy is an increased mitochondrial sensitivity to an apoptotic challenge. Taken in context with the abundance of evidence for elevated recruitment of

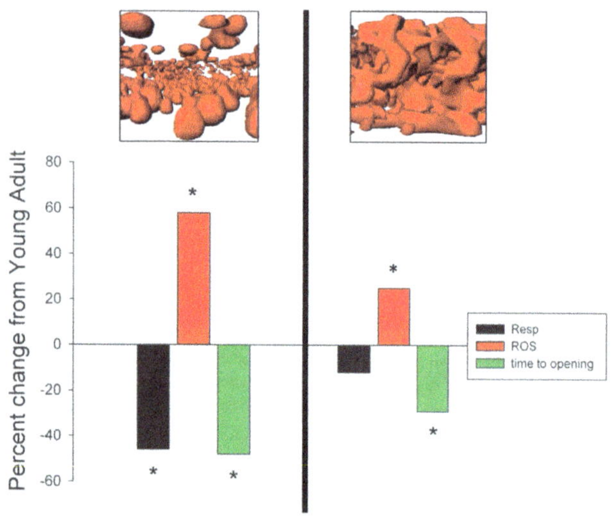

FIGURE 3 | Mechanical isolation (to the left of the vertical line) markedly exaggerates the apparent impact of aging on skeletal muscle mitochondria respiratory function, reactive oxygen species (ROS) emission, and sensitivity to mitochondrial permeability transition pore (mPTP) opening (permeability transition) compared to saponin-permeabilized myofibers (to the right of the vertical line). *$P < 0.05$ versus SEN. Data are re-plotted from Picard et al. (2010).

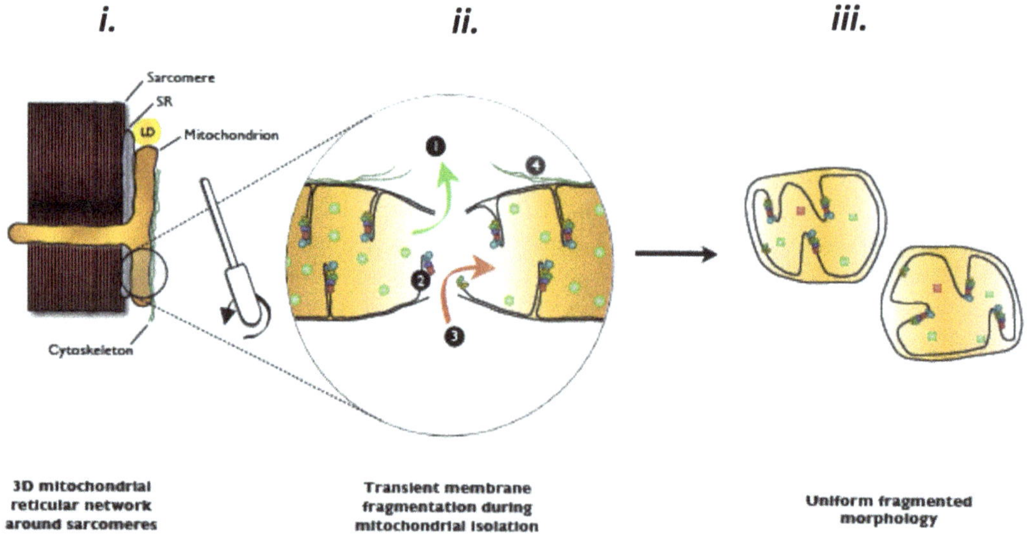

FIGURE 4 | Hypothesized contamination and/or matrix dilution occurring with the transient rupture of mitochondrial membranes during mitochondrial isolation procedures. Reproduced with permission from Picard et al. (2011b).

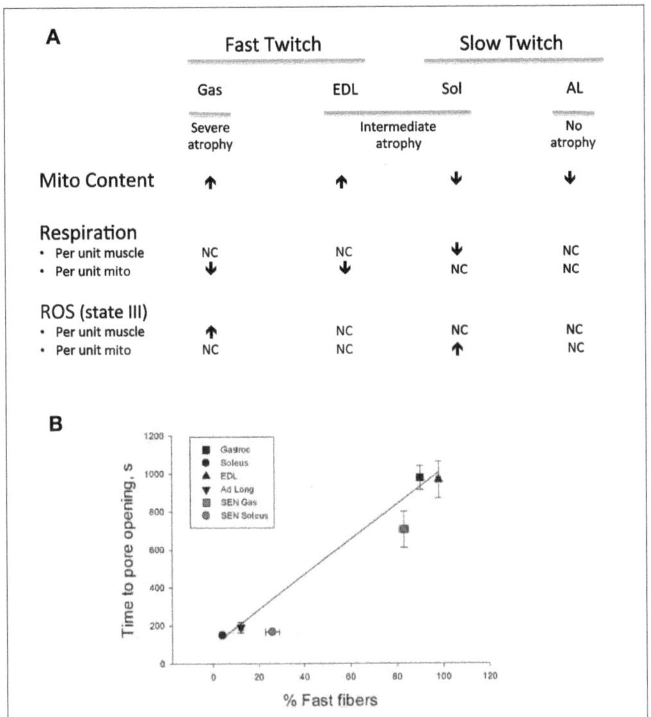

FIGURE 5 | Impact of aging on mitochondrial function in saponin-permeabilized myofibers prepared from rat muscles of contrasting fiber type and atrophy susceptibility is shown. Gas = gastrocnemius muscle, EDL = extensor digitorum longus muscle, Sol = soleus muscle, AL = adductor longus muscle. **(A)** Impact of aging on mitochondrial content, respiration, and reactive oxygen species (ROS) emission responses. **(B)** Sensitivity of mitochondria to permeability transition following a calcium challenge and how this varies as a function of fast twitch fiber abundance. Solid black symbols represent the responses of young adult muscles, whereas the solid red symbols represent responses of senescent muscles. After taking into account the shift in proportion of fibers positive for fast myosin heavy chain with aging in each muscle, both the soleus and gastrocnemius muscles exhibit a sensitization to permeability transition. Data for mitochondrial content, respiration, ROS, and time to pore opening are taken from Picard et al. (2011a). Data for proportion of fibers positive for fast myosin heavy chain are taken from Carter et al. (2010).

mitochondrial-mediated pathways of apoptosis in aging muscle (Dirks and Leeuwenburgh, 2002; Leeuwenburgh et al., 2005; Siu et al., 2005; Chabi et al., 2008; Marzetti et al., 2008; Gouspillou et al., 2014b), this change in mitochondrial function in aging muscle may be a key to induction of myofiber atrophy.

NON-INVASIVE SPECTROSCOPIC METHODS

The final methodological approach to be discussed in this review is the use of non-invasive spectroscopic techniques to interrogate mitochondrial function in aging muscle. Although the value of these measures is that they provide insights into the function of the organelle in its native environment, as will be discussed here, under some circumstances this can pose challenges in deciphering whether a primary mitochondrial defect exists.

The most common non-invasive spectroscopic approach for monitoring mitochondrial function *in vivo* involves ^{31}Phosphorous spectroscopy to determine PCr recovery time following muscle contractions, as the rate of PCr recovery is proportional to mitochondrial respiration and content (Mahler, 1985; Meyer, 1988; Prompers et al., 2014). While this is the only way currently available to gain insights into mitochondrial energy production *in vivo*; it is, however, important to note that the rate of PCr resynthesis following muscle contractions also depends upon oxygen supply (Haseler et al., 1999). Thus, if muscle blood flow is at all reduced in aging muscle during the recovery from contractions, noting that some studies have observed lower blood flow during dynamic exercise in the elderly (Lawrenson et al., 2003; Poole et al., 2003), the resulting lower muscle oxygen delivery with aging is a confounding factor in the interpretation of reduced mitochondrial energetic capacity in the elderly based upon slower PCr recovery kinetics alone.

Keeping this point in mind, although several studies report a reduced rate of PCr recovery following muscle contractions in aging human gastrocnemius (McCully et al., 1993) and vastus lateralis muscles (Conley et al., 2000), this was not seen in aging human tibialis anterior muscle of subjects matched for physical activity levels to the young comparison group (Kent-Braun and Ng, 2000; Lanza et al., 2005). Although differences in physical activity status may be part of the explanation for the different results between studies (Kent-Braun and Ng, 2000), it may also relate to the aforementioned impact of oxygen delivery and/or reflect differences in the impact of aging on mitochondrial function in different muscles, as we have shown that occurs in aged rodents (Picard et al., 2011a) (see Mechanically Isolated Mitochondria versus Saponin-Permeabilized Myocytes).

Non-invasive spectroscopic methods have also been used to evaluate mitochondrial coupling in skeletal muscle *in vivo*. In particular, several studies have now combined measures of PCr resynthesis (to derive what has been termed "ATPmax") with optical spectroscopic assessment of myoglobin and hemoglobin oxygen saturations (to derive intramuscular oxygen consumption) to yield a measure of coupling efficiency based upon the quotient of ATP turnover (derived from the PCr spectroscopy measures) and oxygen consumption (Amara et al., 2007). These studies have identified mild uncoupling of mitochondria in both mouse (Marcinek et al., 2005) and human (Amara et al., 2007) skeletal muscle. As discussed in the following section, mild uncoupling has also been reported in saponin-permeabilized myofibers from physically active septuagenarian humans (Gouspillou et al., 2014b). Since uncoupling of mitochondria has been argued as one strategy for reducing mitochondrial ROS emission and promoting healthy longevity (Speakman et al., 2004), the mild uncoupling observed in aged muscle may represent an adaptive response to keep ROS within physiological levels, rather than a defect *per se* (Amara et al., 2007).

MITOCHONDRIAL CONTENT AND FUNCTION IN RELATION TO AGE AND PHYSICAL ACTIVITY

Amongst the most controversial issues about mitochondrial impact in aging muscle is that of mitochondrial content. Whilst some studies have concluded that mitochondrial content is reduced in aging muscle (Kerner et al., 2001; Chabi et al., 2008), some find no change (Mathieu-Costello et al., 2005; Callahan et al., 2014; Gouspillou et al., 2014b; Konopka et al., 2014), and others find it to vary between muscles (Lyons et al., 2006; Picard et al., 2011a). As was the case with measuring mitochondrial function, many different approaches have been taken to characterize mitochondrial content in aging muscle, including mitochondrial marker enzymes (e.g., citrate synthase or cytochrome oxidase activities), select mitochondrial proteins (e.g., porin, electron transport system complex subunits), mitochondrial DNA (mtDNA) copy number, and the gold standard, electron microscopic quantitation of mitochondrial volume density. Although the wide variety of approaches to inferring mitochondrial content changes in aging muscle has no doubt contributed to the variability in interpretation herein, even in studies using the gold standard of electron microscopy significant variation has been observed. For example, in two studies examining aged rodent muscle (Mathieu-Costello et al., 2005) and aged human muscle (Callahan et al., 2014), there was no change in skeletal muscle mitochondrial content assessed by electron microscopy with aging, whereas another study in aged humans did observe a decrease with aging using the same method and examining the same muscle (*vastus lateralis* muscle) (Conley et al., 2000), underscoring the discrepancy on the question of how aging impacts muscle mitochondrial content. Amongst the factors that contribute to this variability between studies, as noted in Section "Addressing the Question of Mitochondrial Dysfunction in Aging Muscle," physical activity levels can play an important modulating role, where activity-matched subjects consistently show no decline in indices of mitochondrial content in aging muscle (Lanza et al., 2005; Gouspillou et al., 2014b). However, whether differences in physical activity status alone can explain the discordant results remains to be clarified.

Regardless of the controversy about the impact of aging on mitochondrial content, the capacity for generation of new mitochondria declines with aging at ages where the clinical consequences of aging in muscle are most relevant. Specifically, the ability of aged muscle to augment mitochondrial biogenesis in response to both endurance exercise training (Betik et al., 2009) and more severe muscle activity induced by chronic electrical stimulation (Ljubicic and Hood, 2009; Ljubicic et al., 2009) is severely compromised in rat muscle from animals at a similar relative age as humans ≥80 years of age. This impairment appears to be secondary to a failure to upregulate the machinery regulating mitochondrial biogenesis, including peroxisome proliferator activated receptor gamma coactivator-1 alpha (PGC-1α) (Betik et al., 2009), and an accelerated degradation of precursor proteins destined for import into mitochondria (Huang et al., 2010). To date, no therapeutic advances have been developed to restore the mitochondrial biogenesis response in very old muscle, designating this as an issue of high priority for future investigations.

Coming back to ages where muscle mitochondrial content remains adaptable (≤80 years of age), not only does physical activity level modulate mitochondrial content, but it can also modulate indices of mitochondrial function in aging muscle. In particular, previous studies have shown that when younger and older subjects are matched for physical activity levels, there is no reduction in muscle mitochondrial respiratory capacity with aging (Kent-Braun and Ng, 2000; Lanza et al., 2005; Safdar et al., 2010). We recently extended these results to show that, like respiratory capacity (**Figure 6A**), mitochondrial ROS emission is also not elevated with aging (**Figure 6B**) when comparing young adult and septuagenarian subjects with relatively high levels of recreational physical activity, although as seen in very old rodent muscle (see Mechanically Isolated Mitochondria versus Saponin-Permeabilized Myocytes; Picard et al., 2011a), we did observe a pronounced sensitization of the mitochondria to permeability transition (Gouspillou et al., 2014b) (**Figure 6C**). Indeed,

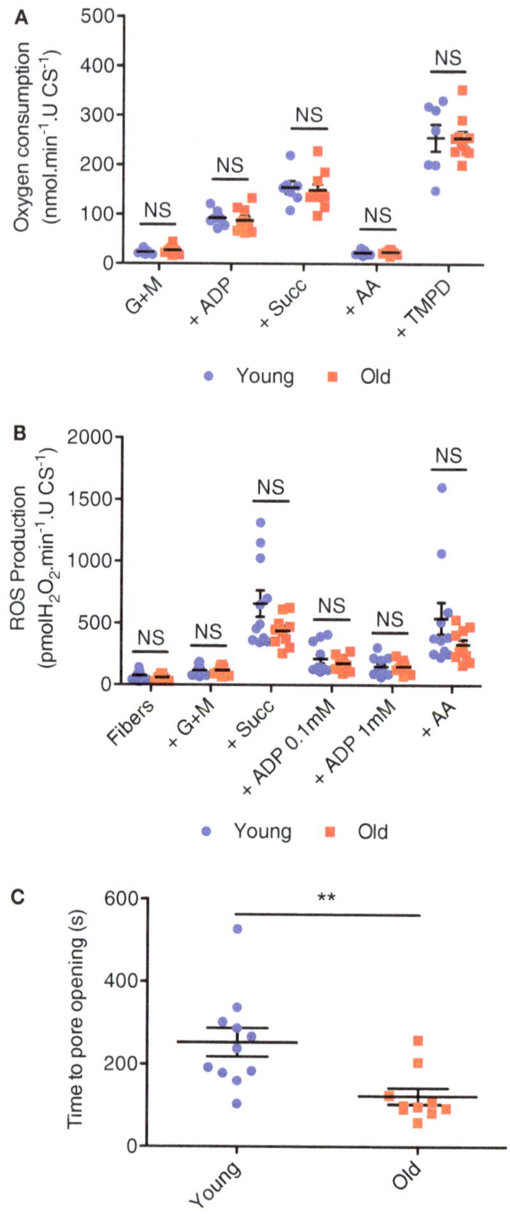

FIGURE 6 | Mitochondrial respiration (A), hydrogen peroxide emission (B), and sensitivity to permeability transition following a calcium challenge (C) in saponin-permeabilized myofibers prepared from vastus lateralis muscle biopsies obtained from recreationally active healthy young (24 ± 1 years; mean ± SE) and older (71 ± 2 years) men. Figures are reproduced with permission from Gouspillou et al. (2014b). G + M = glutamate + malate; Succ = succinate; AA = antimycin A, TMPD = artificial electron donor. ** $P < 0.05$ versus old.

the increased apoptotic sensitivity of aged mitochondria was also accompanied by a marked translocation of a mitochondrial-derived pro-apoptotic molecule, endonuclease G, to myonuclei in atrophied septuagenarian human muscle of recreationally active subjects, suggesting that this may be a key mechanism by which aged mitochondria contribute to aging muscle atrophy and one which cannot be circumvented through an active lifestyle (Gouspillou et al., 2014b). Potential mechanisms for this will be discussed in Section "Mechanisms of Primary Defects in Mitochondrial Function in Aging Muscle."

MECHANISMS OF PRIMARY DEFECTS IN MITOCHONDRIAL FUNCTION IN AGING MUSCLE

As noted above, a sensitization of mitochondria to permeability transition (Picard et al., 2011a) and release of mitochondrial-derived pro-apoptotic factors (Chabi et al., 2008; Marzetti et al., 2008) is evident in aged muscle, even in those who remain physically active (Gouspillou et al., 2014b). In accounting for the reasons for mitochondrial dysfunction in aging muscle, two primary hypotheses have been put forth to explain declining mitochondrial function with aging in general. The first hypothesis relates to the fact that mitochondria have their own genome, which, although only encoding for a small fraction of all mitochondrial proteins, is essential for production of normally functioning mitochondria. Since this genome accumulates damage progressively with aging (Richter et al., 1988; Katayama et al., 1991; Simonetti et al., 1992; Melov et al., 1995), it is posited that this leads to impaired synthesis of mitochondria and/or synthesis of mitochondria with aberrant function (Hiona and Leeuwenburgh, 2008). The second hypothesis relates to the fact that mitochondria must be regularly removed and replaced to preserve their fidelity (Schiavi and Ventura, 2014); it is posited that this process becomes impaired with aging, resulting in accumulation of damaged mitochondria with aberrant function (Terman et al., 2010; Joseph et al., 2013). The available evidence relating to these two hypotheses will be discussed in detail below.

SIGNIFICANCE OF mtDNA MUTATION TO MITOCHONDRIAL DYSFUNCTION AND AGING MUSCLE ATROPHY

The mtDNA molecule is a small circular genome (approximately 16 k base pairs in length) encoding 37 genes, of which 22 are for transfer RNAs, 2 are for ribosomal RNAs, and 13 are for polypeptide subunits of the respiratory chain and ATP synthase. In this last respect, the mtDNA encodes for 7 subunits of complex I, 1 subunit of complex III, 3 subunits of complex IV, and 2 subunits of the ATP synthase, and these components are essential to normal respiratory function. As evidence of the importance of mtDNA, there is marked mitochondrial dysfunction in patients with mtDNA mutations and when these mutations occur in skeletal muscle they can result in profound exercise intolerance (Taivassalo et al., 2003). As noted above, mtDNA mutations increase progressively with increasing age in multiple tissues, including skeletal muscle (Katayama et al., 1991; Melov et al., 1995; Bua et al., 2006). Furthermore, the focal accumulation of mtDNA mutations to high levels in skeletal myocytes with aging has been implicated in fiber atrophy, breakage, and loss (Lee et al., 1998; Wanagat et al., 2001; Bua et al., 2002). However, this latter aspect seems to be losing favor for several reasons. In particular, the proportion of fibers with severe mitochondrial dysfunction arising from mtDNA mutations is very low and these fibers do not seem to be consistently smaller than fibers with healthy mitochondria (Rowan et al., 2011). Further to this point, the proportion of fibers with focal atrophy at regions coinciding with high levels of mutant mtDNA and severe electron transport system dysfunction in human skeletal myocytes is also too low (in two subjects >65 years of age, only 5% of fibers with electron transport chain dysfunction exhibited focal atrophy; Bua et al., 2006) to be biologically meaningful compared to other causes of atrophy in aging muscle, particularly denervation, which is the primary cause of myofiber atrophy in very old rat muscle (Rowan et al., 2012).

Although focal accumulation of mtDNA mutations does not appear to be a primary cause of skeletal myocyte atrophy with aging, a mouse engineered with a faulty mtDNA proof-reading enzyme, the PolG mutant mouse, exhibits a dramatic increase in rate of mtDNA mutation, a markedly shortened lifespan, and numerous features that resemble premature aging (Trifunovic et al., 2004, 2005; Kujoth et al., 2005), including muscle atrophy (Hiona et al., 2010). Interestingly, the mitochondrial phenotypes observed in this so-called mtDNA mutator mouse differ in important ways from what is seen in normally aging muscle. In particular, whereas the PolG mutant mouse exhibits reduced levels of mitochondrial electron transport system complex subunits in skeletal muscle, as discussed in Sections "Mechanically Isolated Mitochondria versus Saponin-Permeabilized Myocytes" and "Mitochondrial Content and Function in Relation to Age and Physical Activity" this is not a consistent finding in aging rat (Picard et al., 2011a) or human muscle (Gouspillou et al., 2014b) where levels of mitochondrial electron transport system complex subunits are often higher in aged muscle. Similarly, whereas markers of mitochondrial fission and autophagy are higher in the PolG mouse muscle, normally aged mouse muscle exhibits higher levels of markers of mitochondrial fusion and lower levels of markers of autophagy (Joseph et al., 2013). On this basis, mtDNA mutations *per se* are unlikely to be the root cause of mitochondrial dysfunction in aging muscle.

IMPAIRED MITOCHONDRIAL AUTOPHAGY (MITOPHAGY) IN AGING MUSCLE

As mentioned above, mitochondria normally undergo degradation and replacement to ensure the fidelity of mitochondrial function. Indeed, impairment in mitochondrial autophagy (mitophagy) is implicated in a wide variety of neudegenerative disorders (Chu, 2010; Scheibye-Knudsen et al., 2014), in addition to normal aging (Schiavi and Ventura, 2014). Although in skeletal muscle the rate of mitochondrial turnover is unknown (nor it is understood if it differs between species), mitochondria have a half-life of approximately 2 days in mouse liver (Miwa et al., 2008), which when scaled up to the lifespan of an organism means that mitochondria undergo hundreds to thousands of cycles of turnover throughout the aging process. Clearly, therefore, if this rate of renewal were to decline, it seems a likely basis leading to accumulation of mitochondria with aberrant function in aging muscle.

Mitophagy is a tightly regulated process whereby dysfunctional/damaged mitochondria are targeted for removal by incorporation into autophagosomes for subsequent degradation by lysosomes. This targeting of dysfunctional mitochondria for removal depends upon several mechanisms that are likely relevant for aging. For example, mitophagy is elevated in response to mitochondrial fragmentation, reduced mitochondrial membrane potential (e.g., as occurs in mitochondria undergoing permeability transition), and increased mitochondrial ROS emission (Romanello et al., 2010; Twig and Shirihai, 2011; Schiavi and Ventura, 2014). Evidence that mitophagy is impaired in aging muscle is only now beginning to accumulate. Firstly, the fact that mitochondria with sensitization to permeability transition accumulate in aging muscle (Gouspillou et al., 2014b) is evidence that mitophagy of damaged mitochondria is impaired since permeability transition causes loss of mitochondrial membrane potential, a potent stimulus for mitophagy (Twig et al., 2008). In addition, two studies have now shown that Parkin, a mitochondrial-targeted ubiquitin ligase, which interacts with the autophagy protein LC3 to induce formation of autophagosomes around dysfunctional mitochondria, is reduced in skeletal muscle of both physically active septuagenarian men (Gouspillou et al., 2014b) and in physically inactive frail older women (Drummond et al., 2014). Furthermore, impairments in the signaling pathway that regulates mitochondrial quality control have also been reported in aging mouse muscle (Joseph et al., 2013) and aging human muscle (Koltai et al., 2012). Thus, whereas the significance of mtDNA mutations in mitochondrial dysfunction in aging muscle is less clear, impaired mitophagy appears a likely contributor to accumulation of dysfunctional mitochondria in aging muscle. Importantly, that this appears to also occur in physically active subjects (Gouspillou et al., 2014b) underscores that new therapeutic approaches will be required to address this problem.

Although their particular role in aging remains to be established, two promising new targets involved in regulating degradation of damaged mitochondria are the micro RNA miR137 and the AAA ATPase p97. miR137 has been identified to inhibit mitophagy occurring in response to hypoxia, through reducing the interaction of LC3 with two mitophagy receptors, FUNDC1 and NIX (Li et al., 2014). p97 is specifically involved in targeting and removal of carbonylated mitochondrial proteins for subsequent degradation by the ubiquitin proteasome (Hemion et al., 2014). If these pathways are disrupted in aging muscle, they are likely targets for improving removal of damaged mitochondria and thus, ameliorating aging impact.

EXTRINSIC FACTORS THAT COULD MODULATE MITOCHONDRIAL FUNCTION IN AGING MUSCLE

Although mitochondrial changes in aging muscle are most often considered as primary dysfunction suitable for therapeutic targeting, this view does not consider the influence of factors extrinsic to the mitochondrion that constitute the aging intracellular *milieu*. For example, age-related changes in the intracellular *milieu* could depress certain aspects of mitochondrial function independent of the intrinsic mitochondrial functional capacity *per se* and recent data support this idea. In addition, other changes impacting aging muscle, such as impaired neuromuscular junction stability and myofiber denervation, could also modulate mitochondrial function as a secondary consequence.

In addressing the potential involvement of the aging *milieu* as an inhibitory influence on mitochondrial function in aging muscle, Siegel et al. (2013) recently characterized mitochondrial function *in vivo* in distal hindlimb muscles of young (5 months old) and aged (27 months old) mice using optical and ^{31}Phosphorous magnetic resonance spectroscopy, finding a decrease in mitochondrial respiratory function (reduced maximal ATP production rate, reduced coupling, and reduced rate of PCr resynthesis). Strikingly, these age-related impairments in mitochondrial respiratory function were restored to youthful levels 1 h following the administration of a mitochondria-specific antioxidant peptide, SS-31 (**Figures 7A–E**), and this was also accompanied by an increased muscle fatigue resistance and running time to exhaustion in the aged mice but not younger mice. In stark contrast to these acute *in vivo* results, when mitochondrial respiratory function was examined in saponin-permeabilized myofibers there was no detectable impairment in mitochondrial respiratory function with aging and administration of SS-31 had no effect (**Figures 7F,G**), despite inducing a reduction in mitochondrial ROS emission. The implications of these results is that, independent of the intrinsic function of the organelle, mitochondrial function can be impeded *in vivo* by oxidative stress in the intracellular environment of aging muscle. Thus, these recent findings underscore the importance of considering aspects of the aging *milieu* as contributing factors to impairing mitochondrial function *in vivo*, and demand further study of how this may affect other aspects of mitochondrial function (e.g., ROS emission, sensitivity to permeability transition) with aging. Furthermore, these results also show that manipulation of the aging *milieu*, rather than the mitochondrion directly, can be an effective strategy for improving mitochondrial function in aging muscle.

As noted in the section "Introduction," mitochondria serve as cellular rheostats that integrate a wide variety of intracellular signals and modify aspects of their function as appropriate to those cellular conditions. Although intrinsic impairment in mitochondrial function involving an increased sensitivity to permeability transition in mitochondria from aged muscle has been demonstrated in both a sedentary rat model (Picard et al., 2011a) and in physically active aging humans (Gouspillou et al., 2014b), whether factors upstream of the mitochondrion can also modulate mitochondrial function is unclear. This question may be particularly relevant when aging muscle atrophy becomes severe and more likely to yield clinical impact because it is likely that additional mechanisms come into play in driving an acceleration of muscle atrophy. In this respect, as noted from the outset of this review, the age at which aging muscle atrophy is most likely to cause clinical consequences such as an increased risk of falls and physical frailty, is in individuals $\geq$80 years of age (Cruz-Jentoft et al., 2010). Significantly, in an aging rat model this corresponds to a period where muscle atrophy accelerates through the accumulation of small angular fibers characteristic of long-term denervation (Rowan et al., 2011).

Although evidence of an accumulation of denervated myofibers in skeletal muscle at very advanced age in humans thus far is based only upon the morphological appearance of small angular fibers

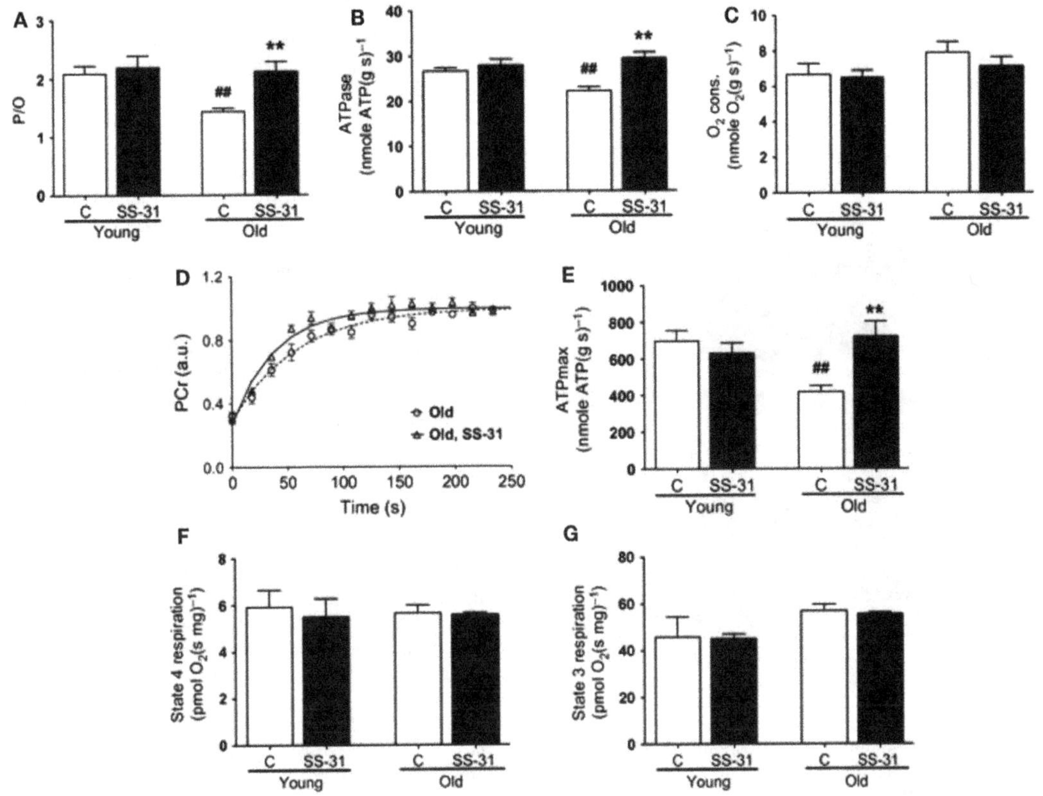

FIGURE 7 | Influence of the aging intracellular *milieu* on mitochondrial function *in vivo* in mouse skeletal muscle. **(A)** P/O ratio, **(B)** *in vivo* ATPase rate; **(C)** *in vivo* rate of oxygen consumption; **(D)** *in vivo* rate of phosphocreatine (PCr) resynthesis following muscle contractions; **(E)** *in vivo* maximal rate of ATP synthesis (ATPmax); **(F)** state 4 respiration in saponin-permeabilized myofibers; **(G)** state 3 respiration in saponin-permeabilized myofibers. Figures are reproduced with permission from Siegel et al. (2013).

(Scelsi et al., 1980) that are typical of neuropathologies such as amyotrophic lateral sclerosis and polyneurophathy (Baloh et al., 2007), the presence of denervated myofibers in very old mouse (Wang et al., 2005) and rat muscle (Rowan et al., 2012) has been confirmed by probing *in situ* for a sodium channel isoform typical of denervation in adult muscle, NAV1.5 (Kallen et al., 1990; Yang et al., 1991). Importantly, these denervated myofibers also demonstrate a marked up-regulation of the ubiquitin ligases muscle atrophy F-box (MAFbx) and muscle ring finger 1 (MuRF1) (Rowan et al., 2012), and the up-regulation of these proteins in response to denervation is dependent upon release of mitochondrial lipid hydroperoxides that can be detected in some ROS assays (Bhattacharya et al., 2009). Thus, denervation can also recruit mitochondrial-mediated proteolytic pathways, raising the likelihood that at least some of the alterations in mitochondria seen in skeletal muscle at very advanced age are a secondary event to denervation rather than a primary organelle defect. A schematic representation of how we hypothesize that denervation may modulate mitochondrial pathways of atrophy in aging muscle is provided in **Figure 8**. Since understanding this issue is key to advancing to new therapeutic targets, future study of how sporadic denervation may modulate mitochondrial function across the continuum of aging muscle atrophy is clearly warranted to better define when intervening at the level of the mitochondrion is most appropriate.

CONCLUSION

Our understanding of the impact of aging on mitochondrial function in aging skeletal muscle continues to evolve and has recently undergone significant revision. In particular, it now appears that mitochondrial functional alterations are more subtle than initially indicated, owing to an exaggeration of mitochondrial impact with aging when using isolated organelles (a common approach in early studies). Furthermore, whereas mitochondrial respiratory function and ROS emission changes are highly variable between muscles and are also largely attenuated by maintaining physical activity, a sensitization of the mitochondria to permeability transition seems to be a general property of aging muscles undergoing atrophy regardless of physical activity status. The mechanisms contributing to this mitochondrial functional alteration in aging muscle remains an area of intensive study. Presently, it seems that mtDNA-driven mechanisms are incompatible with the available evidence and instead impairment in mitophagy is appearing the more likely culprit based upon data from recent studies showing alterations in mitophagy signaling. In this respect, there is also emerging evidence that the aging *milieu* can itself depress mitochondrial respiratory function *in vivo*, even in the absence of an intrinsic organelle defect in mitochondria studied *ex vivo*. Furthermore, the likelihood that other extrinsic factors, such as denervation, may also be modulating mitochondrial function at

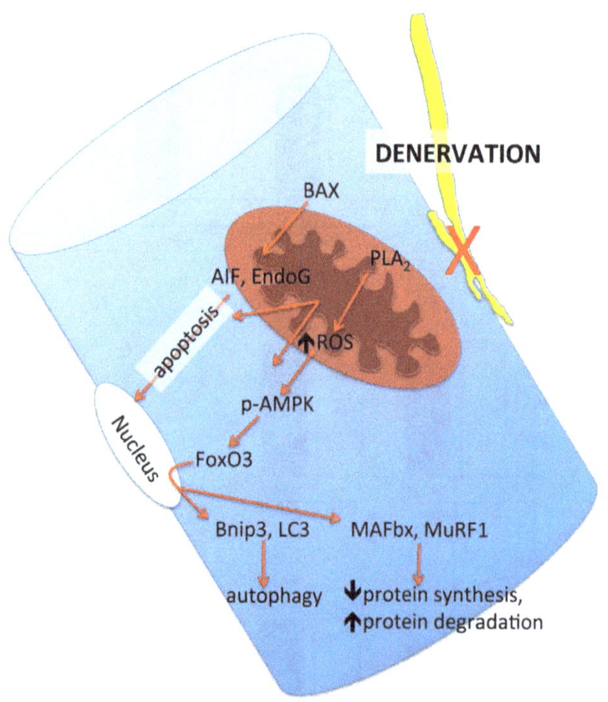

FIGURE 8 | Schematic representation of the mitochondrial-mediated atrophy pathways that have been observed to be up-regulated in aging muscle and their hypothesized link to the upstream influence of sporadic denervation in very advanced age where denervation becomes pronounced. BAX = Bcl2-associated X protein, PLA2 = cytoplasmic phospholipase A2, AIF = apoptosis inducing factor; EndoG = endonuclease G, p-AMPK = phosphorylated adenosine monophosphate kinase, FoxO3 = forkhead box O3, BNIP3 = BCl2/adenovirus E1B 19 kDa protein-interacting protein 3, LC3 = microtubule associated protein light chain 3, MAFbx = muscle atrophy F-box, MuRF1 = muscle ring finger 1.

very advanced and clinically relevant ages requires careful consideration of the most appropriate ages at which to target the mitochondrion in seeking more effective treatments for aging muscle. Based on current evidence, it is suggested that an increased susceptibility to permeability transition at ages preceding the most severe clinical impact of aging muscle atrophy ($\leq$75 years) is an appropriate therapeutic target and should be pursued. However, at clinically relevant ages where an increased falls risk, mobility impairment, and physical frailty are more likely to result from aging muscle impact, it remains to be determined whether mitochondrial alterations are now largely secondary to denervation, rendering the mitochondrion a less attractive therapeutic target for the $\geq$ 80 years age group.

REFERENCES

Amara, C. E., Shankland, E. G., Jubrias, S. A., Marcinek, D. J., Kushmerick, M. J., and Conley, K. E. (2007). Mild mitochondrial uncoupling impacts cellular aging in human muscles in vivo. *Proc. Natl. Acad. Sci. U.S.A.* 104, 1057–1062. doi:10.1073/pnas.0610131104

Anderson, E. J., and Neufer, P. D. (2006). Type II skeletal myofibers possess unique properties that potentiate mitochondrial H(2)O(2) generation. *Am. J. Physiol. Cell Physiol.* 290, C844–C851. doi:10.1152/ajpcell.00402.2005

Baloh, R. H., Rakowicz, W., Gardner, R., and Pestronk, A. (2007). Frequent atrophic groups with mixed-type myofibers is distinctive to motor neuron syndromes. *Muscle Nerve* 36, 107–110. doi:10.1002/mus.20755

Barrientos, A., Casademont, J., Rotig, A., Miro, O., Urbano-Marquez, A., Rustin, P., et al. (1996). Absence of relationship between the level of electron transport chain activities and aging in human skeletal muscle. *Biochem. Biophys. Res. Commun.* 229, 536–539. doi:10.1006/bbrc.1996.1839

Bass, A., Gutmann, E., and Hanzlikova, V. (1975). Biochemical and histochemical changes in energy supply enzyme pattern of muscles of the rat during old age. *Gerontologia* 21, 31–45. doi:10.1159/000212028

Betik, A. C., Thomas, M. M., Wright, K. J., Riel, C. D., and Hepple, R. T. (2009). Exercise training from late middle age until senescence does not attenuate the declines in skeletal muscle aerobic function. *Am. J. Physiol. Regul. Integr. Comp. Physiol.* 297, R744–R755. doi:10.1152/ajpregu.90959.2008

Bhattacharya, A., Muller, F. L., Liu, Y., Sabia, M., Liang, H., Song, W., et al. (2009). Denervation induces cytosolic phospholipase A2-mediated fatty acid hydroperoxide generation by muscle mitochondria. *J. Biol. Chem.* 284, 46–55. doi:10.1074/jbc.M806311200

Boffoli, D., Scacco, S. C., Vergari, R., Solarino, G., Santacroce, G., and Papa, S. (1994). Decline with age of the respiratory chain activity in human skeletal muscle. *Biochim. Biophys. Acta* 1226, 73–82. doi:10.1016/0925-4439(94)90061-2

Bua, E., Johnson, J., Herbst, A., Delong, B., McKenzie, D., Salamat, S., et al. (2006). Mitochondrial DNA-deletion mutations accumulate intracellularly to detrimental levels in aged human skeletal muscle fibers. *Am. J. Hum. Genet.* 79, 469–480. doi:10.1086/507132

Bua, E. A., McKiernan, S. H., Wanagat, J., McKenzie, D., and Aiken, J. M. (2002). Mitochondrial abnormalities are more frequent in muscles undergoing sarcopenia. *J. Appl. Physiol.* 92, 2617–2624. doi:10.1152/japplphysiol.01102.2001

Callahan, D. M., Bedrin, N. G., Subramanian, M., Berking, J., Ades, P. A., Toth, M. J., et al. (2014). Age-related structural alterations in human skeletal muscle fibers and mitochondria are sex specific: relationship to single-fiber function. *J. Appl. Physiol.* 116, 1582–1592. doi:10.1152/japplphysiol.01362.2013

Capel, F., Rimbert, V., Lioger, D., Diot, A., Rousset, P., Mirand, P. P., et al. (2005). Due to reverse electron transfer, mitochondrial H_2O_2 release increases with age in human vastus lateralis muscle although oxidative capacity is preserved. *Mech. Ageing Dev.* 126, 505–511. doi:10.1016/j.mad.2004.11.001

Carter, E. E., Thomas, M. M., Murynka, T., Rowan, S. L., Wright, K. J., Huba, E., et al. (2010). Slow twitch soleus muscle is not protected from sarcopenia in senescent rats. *Exp. Gerontol.* 45, 662–670. doi:10.1016/j.exger.2010.04.001

Chabi, B., Ljubicic, V., Menzies, K. J., Huang, J. H., Saleem, A., and Hood, D. A. (2008). Mitochondrial function and apoptotic susceptibility in aging skeletal muscle. *Aging Cell* 7, 2–12. doi:10.1111/j.1474-9726.2007.00347.x

Chance, B., and Williams, G. R. (1956). Respiratory enzymes in oxidative phosphorylation. VI. The effects of adenosine diphosphate on azide-treated mitochondria. *J. Biol. Chem.* 221, 477–489.

Chu, C. T. (2010). A pivotal role for PINK1 and autophagy in mitochondrial quality control: implications for Parkinson disease. *Hum. Mol. Genet.* 19, R28–R37. doi:10.1093/hmg/ddq143

Conley, K. E., Jubrias, S. A., and Esselman, P. C. (2000). Oxidative capacity and aging in human muscle. *J. Physiol.* 526, 203–210. doi:10.1111/j.1469-7793.2000.t01-1-00203.x

Cooper, J. M., Mann, V. M., and Schapira, A. H. (1992). Analyses of mitochondrial respiratory chain function and mitochondrial DNA deletion in human skeletal muscle: effect of ageing. *J. Neurol. Sci.* 113, 91–98. doi:10.1016/0022-510X(92)90270-U

Cruz-Jentoft, A. J., Landi, F., Topinkova, E., and Michel, J. P. (2010). Understanding sarcopenia as a geriatric syndrome. *Curr. Opin. Clin. Nutr. Metab. Care* 13, 1–7. doi:10.1097/MCO.0b013e328333c1c1

Csukly, K., Ascah, A., Matas, J., Gardiner, P. F., Fontaine, E., and Burelle, Y. (2006). Muscle denervation promotes opening of the permeability transition pore and increases the expression of cyclophilin D. *J. Physiol.* 574, 319–327. doi:10.1113/jphysiol.2006.109702

Desai, V. G., Weindruch, R., Hart, R. W., and Feuers, R. J. (1996). Influences of age and dietary restriction on gastrocnemius electron transport system activities in mice. *Arch. Biochem. Biophys.* 333, 145–151. doi:10.1006/abbi.1996.0375

Dirks, A., and Leeuwenburgh, C. (2002). Apoptosis in skeletal muscle with aging. *Am. J. Physiol. Regul. Integr. Comp. Physiol.* 282, R519–R527. doi:10.1152/ajpregu.00458.2001

Drummond, M. J., Addison, O., Brunker, L., Hopkins, P. N., McClain, D. A., LaStayo, P. C., et al. (2014). Downregulation of e3 ubiquitin ligases and mitophagy-related genes in skeletal muscle of physically inactive, frail older women: a cross-sectional comparison. *J. Gerontol. A Biol. Sci. Med. Sci.* 69, 1040–1048. doi:10.1093/gerona/glu004

Edstrom, E., Altun, M., Bergman, E., Johnson, H., Kullberg, S., Ramirez-Leon, V., et al. (2007). Factors contributing to neuromuscular impairment and sarcopenia during aging. *Physiol. Behav.* 92, 129–135. doi:10.1016/j.physbeh.2007.05.040

Edstrom, E., and Ulfhake, B. (2005). Sarcopenia is not due to lack of regenerative drive in senescent skeletal muscle. *Aging Cell* 4, 65–77. doi:10.1111/j.1474-9728.2005.00145.x

Fulle, S., Protasi, F., Di Tano, G., Pietrangelo, T., Beltramin, A., Boncompagni, S., et al. (2004). The contribution of reactive oxygen species to sarcopenia and muscle ageing. *Exp. Gerontol.* 39, 17–24. doi:10.1016/j.exger.2003.09.012

Gouspillou, G., Bourdel-Marchasson, I., Rouland, R., Calmettes, G., Biran, M., Deschodt-Arsac, V., et al. (2014a). Mitochondrial energetics is impaired in vivo in aged skeletal muscle. *Aging Cell* 13, 39–48. doi:10.1111/acel.12147

Gouspillou, G., Sgarioto, N., Kapchinsky, S., Purves-Smith, F., Norris, B., Pion, C. H., et al. (2014b). Increased sensitivity to mitochondrial permeability transition and myonuclear translocation of endonuclease G in atrophied muscle of physically active older humans. *FASEB J.* 28, 1621–1633. doi:10.1096/fj.13-242750

Gouspillou, G., Bourdel-Marchasson, I., Rouland, R., Calmettes, G., Franconi, J. M., Deschodt-Arsac, V., et al. (2010). Alteration of mitochondrial oxidative phosphorylation in aged skeletal muscle involves modification of adenine nucleotide translocator. *Biochim. Biophys. Acta* 1797, 143–151. doi:10.1016/j.bbabio.2009.09.004

Hagen, J. L., Krause, D. J., Baker, D. J., Fu, M., Tarnopolsky, M. A., and Hepple, R. T. (2004). Skeletal muscle aging in F344BN F1-hybrid rats: I. Mitochondrial dysfunction contributes to the age-associated reduction in VO_2max. *J. Gerontol. A Biol. Sci. Med. Sci.* 59A, 1099–1110. doi:10.1093/gerona/59.11.1099

Haseler, L. J., Hogan, M. C., and Richardson, R. S. (1999). Skeletal muscle phosphocreatine recovery in exercise-trained humans is dependent on O 2 availability. *J. Appl. Physiol.* 86, 2013–2018.

Hemion, C., Flammer, J., and Neutzner, A. (2014). Quality control of oxidatively-damaged mitochondrial proteins is mediated by p97 and the proteasome. *Free Radic. Biol. Med.* doi:10.1016/j.freeradbiomed.2014.07.016

Hiona, A., and Leeuwenburgh, C. (2008). The role of mitochondrial DNA mutations in aging and sarcopenia: implications for the mitochondrial vicious cycle theory of aging. *Exp. Gerontol.* 43, 24–33. doi:10.1016/j.exger.2007.10.001

Hiona, A., Sanz, A., Kujoth, G. C., Pamplona, R., Seo, A. Y., Hofer, T., et al. (2010). Mitochondrial DNA mutations induce mitochondrial dysfunction, apoptosis and sarcopenia in skeletal muscle of mitochondrial DNA mutator mice. *PLoS ONE* 5:e11468. doi:10.1371/journal.pone.0011468

Houmard, J. A., Weidner, M. L., Gavigan, K. E., Tyndall, G. L., Hickey, M. S., and Alshami, A. (1998). Fiber type and citrate synthase activity in the human gastrocnemius and vastus lateralis with aging. *J. Appl. Physiol.* 85, 1337–1341.

Huang, J. H., Joseph, A. M., Ljubicic, V., Iqbal, S., and Hood, D. A. (2010). Effect of age on the processing and import of matrix-destined mitochondrial proteins in skeletal muscle. *J. Gerontol. A Biol. Sci. Med. Sci.* 65, 138–146. doi:10.1093/gerona/glp201

Hutter, E., Skovbro, M., Lener, B., Prats, C., Rabol, R., Dela, F., et al. (2007). Oxidative stress and mitochondrial impairment can be separated from lipofuscin accumulation in aged human skeletal muscle. *Aging Cell* 6, 245–256. doi:10.1111/j.1474-9726.2007.00282.x

Joseph, A. M., Adhihetty, P. J., Buford, T. W., Wohlgemuth, S. E., Lees, H. A., Nguyen, L. M., et al. (2012). The impact of aging on mitochondrial function and biogenesis pathways in skeletal muscle of sedentary high- and low-functioning elderly individuals. *Aging Cell* 11, 801–809. doi:10.1111/j.1474-9726.2012.00844.x

Joseph, A. M., Adhihetty, P. J., Wawrzyniak, N. R., Wohlgemuth, S. E., Picca, A., Kujoth, G. C., et al. (2013). Dysregulation of mitochondrial quality control processes contribute to sarcopenia in a mouse model of premature aging. *PLoS ONE* 8:e69327. doi:10.1371/journal.pone.0069327

Joseph, A. M., Ljubicic, V., Adhihetty, P. J., and Hood, D. A. (2010). Biogenesis of the mitochondrial Tom40 channel in skeletal muscle from aged animals and its adaptability to chronic contractile activity. *Am. J. Physiol. Cell Physiol.* 298, C1308–C1314. doi:10.1152/ajpcell.00644.2008

Kallen, R. G., Sheng, Z. H., Yang, J., Chen, L. Q., Rogart, R. B., and Barchi, R. L. (1990). Primary structure and expression of a sodium channel characteristic of denervated and immature rat skeletal muscle. *Neuron* 4, 233–242. doi:10.1016/0896-6273(90)90098-Z

Katayama, M., Tanaka, M., Yamamoto, H., Ohbayashi, T., Nimura, Y., and Ozawa, T. (1991). Deleted mitochondrial DNA in the skeletal muscle of aged individuals. *Biochem. Int.* 25, 47–56.

Kent-Braun, J. A., and Ng, A. V. (2000). Skeletal muscle oxidative capacity in young and older women and men. *J. Appl. Physiol.* 89, 1072–1078.

Kerner, J., Turkaly, P. J., Minkler, P. E., and Hoppel, C. L. (2001). Aging skeletal muscle mitochondria in the rat: decreased uncoupling protein-3 content. *Am. J. Physiol. Endocrinol. Metab.* 281, E1054–E1062.

Koltai, E., Hart, N., Taylor, A. W., Goto, S., Ngo, J. K., Davies, K. J., et al. (2012). Age-associated declines in mitochondrial biogenesis and protein quality control factors are minimized by exercise training. *Am. J. Physiol. Regul. Integr. Comp. Physiol.* 303, R127–R134. doi:10.1152/ajpregu.00337.2011

Konopka, A. R., Suer, M. K., Wolff, C. A., and Harber, M. P. (2014). Markers of human skeletal muscle mitochondrial biogenesis and quality control: effects of age and aerobic exercise training. *J. Gerontol. A Biol. Sci. Med. Sci.* 69, 371–378. doi:10.1093/gerona/glt107

Kujoth, G. C., Hiona, A., Pugh, T. D., Someya, S., Panzer, K., Wohlgemuth, S. E., et al. (2005). Mitochondrial DNA mutations, oxidative stress, and apoptosis in mammalian aging. *Science* 309, 481–484. doi:10.1126/science.1112125

Lanza, I. R., Befroy, D. E., and Kent-Braun, J. A. (2005). Age-related changes in ATP-producing pathways in human skeletal muscle in vivo. *J. Appl. Physiol.* 99, 1736–1744. doi:10.1152/japplphysiol.00566.2005

Lawrenson, L., Poole, J. G., Kim, J., Brown, C., Patel, P., and Richardson, R. S. (2003). Vascular and metabolic response to isolated small muscle mass exercise: effect of age. *Am. J. Physiol. Heart Circ. Physiol.* 285, H1023–H1031. doi:10.1152/ajpheart.00135.2003

Lee, C. M., Lopez, M. E., Weindruch, R., and Aiken, J. M. (1998). Association of age-related mitochondrial abnormalities with skeletal muscle fiber atrophy. *Free Radic. Biol. Med.* 25, 964–972. doi:10.1016/S0891-5849(98)00185-3

Leeuwenburgh, C., Gurley, C. M., Strotman, B. A., and Dupont-Versteegden, E. E. (2005). Age-related differences in apoptosis with disuse atrophy in soleus muscle. *Am. J. Physiol. Regul. Integr. Comp. Physiol.* 288, R1288–R1296. doi:10.1152/ajpregu.00576.2004

Lezza, A. M., Boffoli, D., Scacco, S., Cantatore, P., and Gadaleta, M. N. (1994). Correlation between mitochondrial DNA 4977-bp deletion and respiratory chain enzyme activities in aging human skeletal muscles. *Biochem. Biophys. Res. Commun.* 205, 772–779. doi:10.1006/bbrc.1994.2732

Li, W., Zhang, X., Zhuang, H., Chen, H. G., Chen, Y., Tian, W., et al. (2014). MicroRNA-137 is a novel hypoxia-responsive microRNA that inhibits mitophagy via regulation of two mitophagy receptors FUNDC1 and NIX. *J. Biol. Chem.* 289, 10691–10701. doi:10.1074/jbc.M113.537050

Ljubicic, V., and Hood, D. A. (2009). Diminished contraction-induced intracellular signaling towards mitochondrial biogenesis in aged skeletal muscle. *Aging Cell* 8, 394–404. doi:10.1111/j.1474-9726.2009.00483.x

Ljubicic, V., Joseph, A. M., Adhihetty, P. J., Huang, J. H., Saleem, A., Uguccioni, G., et al. (2009). Molecular basis for an attenuated mitochondrial adaptive plasticity in aged skeletal muscle. *Aging (Albany NY)* 1, 818–830.

Lyons, C. N., Mathieu-Costello, O., and Moyes, C. D. (2006). Regulation of skeletal muscle mitochondrial content during aging. *J. Gerontol. A Biol. Sci. Med. Sci.* 61, 3–13. doi:10.1093/gerona/61.1.3

Mahler, M. (1985). First-order kinetics of muscle oxygen consumption, and an equivalent proportionality between QO 2 and phosphoryl-creatine level. *J. Gen. Physiol.* 86, 165.

Mansouri, A., Muller, F. L., Liu, Y., Ng, R., Faulkner, J., Hamilton, M., et al. (2006). Alterations in mitochondrial function, hydrogen peroxide release and oxidative damage in mouse hind-limb skeletal muscle during aging. *Mech. Ageing Dev.* 127, 298–306. doi:10.1016/j.mad.2005.11.004

Marcinek, D. J., Schenkman, K. A., Ciesielski, W. A., Lee, D., and Conley, K. E. (2005). Reduced mitochondrial coupling in vivo alters cellular energetics in aged mouse skeletal muscle. *J. Physiol.* 569, 467–473. doi:10.1113/jphysiol.2005.097782

Martin, K. R., Koster, A., Murphy, R. A., Van Domelen, D. R., Hung, M. Y., Brychta, R. J., et al. (2014). Changes in daily activity patterns with age in U.S. men and women: National Health and Nutrition Examination Survey 2003-04 and 2005-06. *J. Am. Geriatr. Soc.* 62, 1263–1271. doi:10.1111/jgs.12893

Marzetti, E., Hwang, J. C., Lees, H. A., Wohlgemuth, S. E., Dupont-Versteegden, E. E., Carter, C. S., et al. (2010). Mitochondrial death effectors: relevance to sarcopenia and disuse muscle atrophy. *Biochim. Biophys. Acta* 1800, 235–244. doi:10.1016/j.bbagen.2009.05.007

Marzetti, E., Wohlgemuth, S. E., Lees, H. A., Chung, H. Y., Giovannini, S., and Leeuwenburgh, C. (2008). Age-related activation of mitochondrial caspase-independent apoptotic signaling in rat gastrocnemius muscle. *Mech. Ageing Dev.* 129, 542–549. doi:10.1016/j.mad.2008.05.005

Mathieu-Costello, O., Ju, Y., Trejo-Morales, M., and Cui, L. (2005). Greater capillary-fiber interface per fiber mitochondrial volume in skeletal muscles of old rats. *J. Appl. Physiol.* 99, 281–289. doi:10.1152/japplphysiol.00750.2004

McCully, K. K., Fielding, R. A., Evans, W. J., Leigh, J. S. Jr., and Posner, J. D. (1993). Relationships between in vivo and in vitro measurements of metabolism in young and old human calf muscles. *J. Appl. Physiol.* 75, 813–819.

Melov, S., Shoffner, J. M., Kaufman, A., and Wallace, D. C. (1995). Marked increase in the number and variety of mitochondrial DNA rearrangements in aging human skeletal muscle. *Nucleic Acids Res.* 23, 4122–4126. doi:10.1093/nar/23.23.4938-a

Meyer, R. A. (1988). A linear model of muscle respiration explains monoexponential phosphocreatine changes. *Am. J. Physiol.* 254, C548–C553.

Miwa, S., Lawless, C., and von Zglinicki, T. (2008). Mitochondrial turnover in liver is fast in vivo and is accelerated by dietary restriction: application of a simple dynamic model. *Aging Cell* 7, 920–923. doi:10.1111/j.1474-9726.2008.00426.x

Muller, F. L., Song, W., Jang, Y. C., Liu, Y., Sabia, M., Richardson, A., et al. (2007). Denervation-induced skeletal muscle atrophy is associated with increased mitochondrial ROS production. *Am. J. Physiol. Regul. Integr. Comp. Physiol.* 293, R1159–R1168. doi:10.1152/ajpregu.00767.2006

Oda, K. (1984). Age changes of motor innervation and acetylcholine receptor distribution on human skeletal muscle fibres. *J. Neurol. Sci.* 66, 327–338. doi:10.1016/0022-510X(84)90021-2

Orlander, J., Kiessling, K. H., Larsson, L., Karlsson, J., and Aniansson, A. (1978). Skeletal muscle metabolism and ultrastructure in relation to age in sedentary men. *Acta Physiol. Scand.* 104, 249–261. doi:10.1111/j.1748-1716.1978.tb06277.x

Picard, M., Csukly, K., Robillard, M. E., Godin, R., Ascah, A., Bourcier-Lucas, C., et al. (2008). Resistance to Ca2+-induced opening of the permeability transition pore differs in mitochondria from glycolytic and oxidative muscles. *Am. J. Physiol. Regul. Integr. Comp. Physiol.* 295, R659–R668. doi:10.1152/ajpregu.90357.2008

Picard, M., Hepple, R. T., and Burelle, Y. (2012). Mitochondrial functional specialization in glycolytic and oxidative muscle fibers: tailoring the organelle for optimal function. *Am. J. Physiol. Cell Physiol.* 302, C629–C641. doi:10.1152/ajpcell.00368.2011

Picard, M., Ritchie, D., Thomas, M. M., Wright, K. J., and Hepple, R. T. (2011a). Alterations in intrinsic mitochondrial function with aging are fiber type-specific and do not explain differential atrophy between muscles. *Aging Cell* 10, 1047–1055. doi:10.1111/j.1474-9726.2011.00745.x

Picard, M., Taivassalo, T., Gouspillou, G., and Hepple, R. T. (2011b). Mitochondria: isolation, structure and function. *J. Physiol.* 589, 4413–4421. doi:10.1113/jphysiol.2011.212712

Picard, M., Taivassalo, T., Ritchie, D., Wright, K. J., Thomas, M. M., Romestaing, C., et al. (2011c). Mitochondrial structure and function are disrupted by standard isolation methods. *PLoS ONE* 6:e18317. doi:10.1371/journal.pone.0018317

Picard, M., Ritchie, D., Wright, K. J., Romestaing, C., Thomas, M. M., Rowan, S. L., et al. (2010). Mitochondrial functional impairment with aging is exaggerated in isolated mitochondria compared to permeabilized myofibers. *Aging Cell* 9, 1032–1046. doi:10.1111/j.1474-9726.2010.00628.x

Poole, J. G., Lawrenson, L., Kim, J., Brown, C., and Richardson, R. S. (2003). Vascular and metabolic response to cycle exercise in sedentary humans: effect of age. *Am. J. Physiol. Heart Circ. Physiol.* 284, H1251–H1259. doi:10.1152/ajpheart.00790.2002

Prompers, J. J., Wessels, B., Kemp, G. J., and Nicolay, K. (2014). MITOCHONDRIA: investigation of in vivo muscle mitochondrial function by 31P magnetic resonance spectroscopy. *Int. J. Biochem. Cell Biol.* 50, 67–72. doi:10.1016/j.biocel.2014.02.014

Rasmussen, U. F., Krustrup, P., Kjaer, M., and Rasmussen, H. N. (2003). Human skeletal muscle mitochondrial metabolism in youth and senescence: no signs of functional changes of ATP formation and mitochondrial capacity. *Pflugers Arch.* 446, 270–278. doi:10.1007/s00424-003-1022-2

Richter, C., Park, J. W., and Ames, B. N. (1988). Normal oxidative damage to mitochondrial and nuclear DNA is extensive. *Proc. Natl. Acad. Sci. U.S.A.* 85, 6465–6467. doi:10.1073/pnas.85.17.6465

Rockstein, M., and Brandt, K. F. (1963). Enzyme changes in flight muscle correlated with aging and flight ability in the male housefly. *Science* 139, 1049–1051. doi:10.1126/science.139.3559.1049

Romanello, V., Guadagnin, E., Gomes, L., Roder, I., Sandri, C., Petersen, Y., et al. (2010). Mitochondrial fission and remodelling contributes to muscle atrophy. *EMBO J.* 29, 1774–1785. doi:10.1038/emboj.2010.60

Rowan, S. L., Purves-Smith, F. M., Solbak, N. M., and Hepple, R. T. (2011). Accumulation of severely atrophic myofibers marks the acceleration of sarcopenia in slow and fast twitch muscles. *Exp. Gerontol.* 46, 660–669. doi:10.1016/j.exger.2011.03.005

Rowan, S. L., Rygiel, K., Purves-Smith, F. M., Solbak, N. M., Turnbull, D. M., and Hepple, R. T. (2012). Denervation causes fiber atrophy and Myosin heavy chain co-expression in senescent skeletal muscle. *PLoS ONE* 7:e29082. doi:10.1371/journal.pone.0029082

Rudolf, R., Khan, M. M., Labeit, S., and Deschenes, M. R. (2014). Degeneration of neuromuscular junction in age and dystrophy. *Front. Aging Neurosci.* 6:99. doi:10.3389/fnagi.2014.00099

Rumsey, W. L., Kendrick, Z. V., and Starnes, J. W. (1987). Bioenergetics in the aging Fischer 344 rat: effects of exercise and food restriction. *Exp. Gerontol.* 22, 271–287. doi:10.1016/0531-5565(87)90006-4

Safdar, A., Hamadeh, M. J., Kaczor, J. J., Raha, S., Debeer, J., and Tarnopolsky, M. A. (2010). Aberrant mitochondrial homeostasis in the skeletal muscle of sedentary older adults. *PLoS ONE* 5:e10778. doi:10.1371/journal.pone.0010778

Scelsi, R., Marchetti, C., and Poggi, P. (1980). Histochemical and ultrastructural aspects of m. vastus lateralis in sedentary old people (aged 65-89 years). *Acta Neuropathol.* 51, 99–105. doi:10.1007/BF00690450

Scheibye-Knudsen, M., Fang, E. F., Croteau, D. L., and Bohr, V. A. (2014). Contribution of defective mitophagy to the neurodegeneration in DNA repair-deficient disorders. *Autophagy* 10, doi:10.4161/auto.29321

Schiavi, A., and Ventura, N. (2014). The interplay between mitochondria and autophagy and its role in the aging process. *Exp. Gerontol.* 56, 147–153. doi:10.1016/j.exger.2014.02.015

Siegel, M. P., Kruse, S. E., Percival, J. M., Goh, J., White, C. C., Hopkins, H. C., et al. (2013). Mitochondrial-targeted peptide rapidly improves mitochondrial energetics and skeletal muscle performance in aged mice. *Aging Cell* 12, 763–771. doi:10.1111/acel.12102

Simonetti, S., Chen, X., DiMauro, S., and Schon, E. A. (1992). Accumulation of deletions in human mitochondrial DNA during normal aging: analysis by quantitative PCR. *Biochim. Biophys. Acta* 1180, 113–122. doi:10.1016/0925-4439(92)90059-V

Siu, P. M., Pistilli, E. E., and Alway, S. E. (2005). Apoptotic responses to hindlimb suspension in gastrocnemius muscles from young adult and aged rats. *Am. J. Physiol. Regul. Integr. Comp. Physiol.* 289, R1015–R1026. doi:10.1152/ajpregu.00198.2005

Snow, L. M., McLoon, L. K., and Thompson, L. V. (2005). Adult and developmental myosin heavy chain isoforms in soleus muscle of aging Fischer Brown Norway rat. *Anat. Rec. A Discov. Mol. Cell. Evol. Biol.* 286, 866–873. doi:10.1002/ar.a.20218

Speakman, J. R., Talbot, D. A., Selman, C., Snart, S., McLaren, J. S., Redman, P., et al. (2004). Uncoupled and surviving: individual mice with high metabolism have greater mitochondrial uncoupling and live longer. *Aging Cell* 3, 87–95. doi:10.1111/j.1474-9728.2004.00097.x

Stary, C. M., Mathieu-Costello, O., and Hogan, M. C. (2004). Resistance to fatigue of individual Xenopus single skeletal muscle fibres is correlated with mitochondrial volume density. *Exp. Physiol.* 89, 617–621. doi:10.1113/expphysiol.2004.027763

Taivassalo, T., Jensen, T. D., Kennaway, N., DiMauro, S., Vissing, J., and Haller, R. G. (2003). The spectrum of exercise tolerance in mitochondrial myopathies: a study of 40 patients. *Brain* 126, 413–423. doi:10.1093/brain/awg028

Terman, A., Kurz, T., Navratil, M., Arriaga, E. A., and Brunk, U. T. (2010). Mitochondrial turnover and aging of long-lived postmitotic cells: the mitochondrial-lysosomal axis theory of aging. *Antioxid. Redox Signal.* 12, 503–535. doi:10.1089/ars.2009.2598

Tomonaga, M. (1977). Histochemical and ultrastructural changes in senile human skeletal muscle. *J. Am. Geriatr. Soc.* 25, 125–131.

Tonkonogi, M., Walsh, B., Svensson, M., and Sahlin, K. (2000). Mitochondrial function and antioxidative defence in human muscle: effects of endurance training and oxidative stress. *J. Physiol.* 528, 379–388. doi:10.1111/j.1469-7793.2000.00379.x

Trifunovic, A., Hansson, A., Wredenberg, A., Rovio, A. T., Dufour, E., Khvorostov, I., et al. (2005). From the cover: somatic mtDNA mutations cause aging phenotypes without affecting reactive oxygen species production. *Proc. Natl. Acad. Sci. U.S.A.* 102, 17993–17998. doi:10.1073/pnas.0508886102

Trifunovic, A., Wredenberg, A., Falkenberg, M., Spelbrink, J. N., Rovio, A. T., Bruder, C. E., et al. (2004). Premature ageing in mice expressing defective mitochondrial DNA polymerase. *Nature* 429, 417–423. doi:10.1038/nature02517

Trounce, I., Byrne, E., and Marzuki, S. (1989). Decline in skeletal muscle mitochondrial respiratory chain function: possible factor in ageing. *Lancet* 1, 637–639. doi:10.1016/S0140-6736(89)92143-0

Twig, G., Elorza, A., Molina, A. J., Mohamed, H., Wikstrom, J. D., Walzer, G., et al. (2008). Fission and selective fusion govern mitochondrial segregation and elimination by autophagy. *EMBO J.* 27, 433–446. doi:10.1038/sj.emboj.7601963

Twig, G., and Shirihai, O. S. (2011). The interplay between mitochondrial dynamics and mitophagy. *Antioxid. Redox Signal.* 14, 1939–1951. doi:10.1089/ars.2010.3779

Wanagat, J., Cao, Z., Pathare, P., and Aiken, J. M. (2001). Mitochondrial DNA deletion mutations colocalize with segmental electron transport system abnormalities, muscle fiber atrophy, fiber splitting, and oxidative damage in sarcopenia. *FASEB J.* 15, 322–332. doi:10.1096/fj.00-0320com

Wang, Z. M., Zheng, Z., Messi, M. L., and Delbono, O. (2005). Extension and magnitude of denervation in skeletal muscle from ageing mice. *J. Physiol. (Lond.)* 565, 757–764. doi:10.1113/jphysiol.2005.087601

Yang, J. S., Sladky, J. T., Kallen, R. G., and Barchi, R. L. (1991). TTX-sensitive and TTX-insensitive sodium channel mRNA transcripts are independently regulated in adult skeletal muscle after denervation. *Neuron* 7, 421–427. doi:10.1016/0896-6273(91)90294-A

2

Nutritional status evaluation in patients affected by Bethlem myopathy and Ullrich congenital muscular dystrophy

Silvia Toni*[1], *Riccardo Morandi*[1], *Marcello Busacchi*[1], *Lucia Tardini*[1], *Luciano Merlini*[2], *Nino Carlo Battistini*[1] and *Massimo Pellegrini*[1]

[1] *Laboratory of Nutrition and Lifestyle, Department of Diagnostic, Clinical and Public Health Medicine, Modena, Italy*
[2] *Laboratory of Musculoskeletal Cell Biology, Istituto Ortopedico Rizzoli, Bologna, Italy*

***Correspondence:**
Massimo Pellegrini, University of Modena and Reggio Emilia, Italy
e-mail: massimo.pellegrini@unimore.it

Collagen VI mutations lead to disabling myopathies like Bethlem myopathy (BM) and Ullrich congenital muscular dystrophy (UCMD). We have investigated the nutritional and metabolic status of one UCMD and seven BM patients (five female, three male, mean age 31 ± 9 years) in order to find a potential metabolic target for nutritional intervention. For this study, we used standard anthropometric tools, such as BMI evaluation and body circumference measurements. All results were compared to dual-energy X-ray absorptiometry (DXA), considered the "gold standard" method. Energy intake of each patient was evaluated through longitudinal methods (7-day food diary) while resting energy expenditure (REE) was predicted using specific equations and measured by indirect calorimetry. Clinical evaluation included general and nutritional blood and urine laboratory analyses and quantitative muscle strength measurement by hand-held dynamometry. BM and UCMD patients showed an altered body composition, characterized by low free fat mass (FFM) and high fat mass (FM), allowing us to classify them as sarcopenic, and all but one as sarcopenic-obese. Another main result was the negative correlation between REE/FFM ratio (basal energy expenditure per kilograms of fat-free mass) and the severity of the disease, as defined by the muscle megascore (correlation coefficient −0.955, *P*-value <0.001). We postulate that the increase of the REE/FFM ratio in relation to the severity of the disease may be due to an altered and pathophysiological loss of energetic efficiency at the expense of skeletal muscle. We show that a specific metabolic disequilibrium is related to the severity of the disease, which may represent a target for a nutritional intervention in these patients.

Keywords: collagen VI, muscular dystrophies, nutritional assessment, body composition, basal energy expenditure

INTRODUCTION

Mutations in the genes COL6A1, COL6A2, and COL6A3, coding for three α chains of collagen type VI, cause COL6-related myopathies (COL6-RM), including the severe Ullrich congenital muscular dystrophy (UCMD), the milder Bethlem myopathy (BM) (Bertini and Pepe, 2002; Allamand et al., 2010), and the Myosclerosis Myopathy in a single family (Merlini et al., 2008a,b).

The prevalence of UCMD and BM has been calculated as 0.13 per 100,000 and 0.77 per 100,000, respectively (Norwood et al., 2009). BM (MIM #158810) (Merlini et al., 1994) is characterized by axial and proximal muscle wasting and weakness with finger flexion contractures. BM is usually mild, sometimes slowly progressive (Pepe et al., 2002). BM has both dominant and recessive inheritance (Gualandi et al., 2009). Immunohistochemistry shows normal or mildly reduced levels of ColVI in the endomysium of most BM patients (Allamand et al., 2010). UCMD (MIM #254090) (Mercuri et al., 2005) is a severe congenital muscular dystrophy, characterized by early onset, generalized and rapidly progressive muscle wasting and weakness, proximal joint contractures, and distal joint hypermobility. Walking ability is rarely achieved or preserved during adolescence, and the rapid progression of the clinical symptoms usually leads to early death, due to respiratory failure (Mercuri et al., 2005). UCMD is caused both by recessive and *de novo* dominant mutations (Mercuri et al., 2005). ColVI appears to be strongly reduced or absent in muscle biopsies from UCMD patients.

A dystrophic mouse model, where collagen VI synthesis was prevented by targeted inactivation of the Col6a1 gene, allowed the investigation of the pathogenesis, revealing the existence of a Ca(2+)-mediated dysfunction of the mitochondria and sarcoplasmic reticulum and defective autophagy (Bernardi and Bonaldo, 2013). Similar defects contribute to the disease pathogenesis in patients, irrespective of the genetic lesion causing the collagen VI defect (Irwin et al., 2003; Grumati et al., 2010). These studies indicate that permeability transition pore opening and defective autophagy represent key elements of skeletal muscle fiber death, and provide a rationale for the use of cyclosporin A (Merlini et al., 2008a,b) and of nutritional interventions to correct defective autophagy (Merlini et al., 2014) in patients affected by COL6-RM, a strategy that holds great promise for treatment.

In the last decade, several studies have demonstrated that nutritional status and body composition are strictly related to clinical outcomes and that nutritional intervention can be effective in the prevention and treatment of many diseases related to metabolism, bioenergetics, and even cancer.

According to a three-compartment model of body composition (Moon et al., 2008), total body weight is the sum of lean mass (LM), fat mass (FM), and bone mineral content (BMC). The LM, which includes the mass of the internal organs and that of the muscles, together with the BMC, form the fat-free mass (FFM), which represents the more metabolically active component of the human body. A "pathological" ratio between FFM and FM and/or an abnormal distribution of these components in the body, mainly trunk versus appendages, is found in many pathological conditions and correlates with the severity of the metabolic or energy status alteration; moreover, modifications of body composition *per se* may represent an independent health risk factor (Wohlfahrt et al., 2014). Augmented FM leads to a higher cardiometabolic risk and to a higher incidence of hypertension, diabetes (Rohan et al., 2013), and cardiovascular diseases.

Muscular dystrophies (MD) are characterized by progressive deterioration of muscle mass, muscle strength, and function. Resting energy expenditure (REE), which comprises 70% of daily energy needs, is determined by the amount and composition of the metabolically active fat-free mass (FFM). The reduced muscle mass and muscular activity, characteristic of MDs, could result in a significant parallel decrease in REE. Surprisingly, it was found that that patients with Emery-Dreifuss MD (Vaisman et al., 2004) and Duchenne and Becker MD (Zanardi et al., 2003a; Gonzalez-Bermejo et al., 2005; Hogan, 2008; Elliott et al., 2012) may have increased energy expenditure. If not met with increased caloric intake, this greater energy expenditure may partially contribute to further deterioration in their muscle mass and function.

It has already been shown that patients with COL6-RM have reduced muscle mass, muscle strength, and muscle function (Miscione et al., 2013). To date, no data are available on the energy expenditure in COL6-RM. The aim of this study is to investigate the relationship between REE, body composition, and muscle strength in COL6-RM.

MATERIALS AND METHODS

PATIENTS

We analyzed eight adult patients (five women, three men, mean age 31 ± 9 years) with COL6-RM: seven had BM and one UCMD. The UCMD patient was never able to walk and was on nocturnal non-invasive mechanical ventilation. This study was approved by the institutional ethical committee of the Istituto Ortopedico Rizzoli (ClinicalTrials.gov identifier: NCT01438788). All subjects were fully informed about the study and gave their written informed consent.

BODY COMPOSITION

Nutritional status was evaluated throughout the study by both non-invasive and invasive techniques (El Ghoch et al., 2014). Body composition was obtained by DXA (Hologic 4500 W; software version 11.2; Hologic, Inc., Waltham, MA, USA) software, which provides regional and whole-body estimation of LM, FM, and BMC, according to the three-compartment model of body composition. FFM was calculated as the sum of LM and BMC, and has been provided for each body part (i.e., trunk and limbs) (Scaglioni et al., 2013). From these whole-body measures, the following derivative values were calculated: FMI (FM/height2), LM/height2, appendicular lean mass/height2 (ALMI). Appendicular lean mass (ALM) was the sum of bone-free and fat-free tissue masses in the arms and legs. Sarcopenic obesity was defined, according to Baumgartner et al. (2004), as ALM divided by stature squared (ALMI) less than 7.26 kg/m^2 in men and 5.45 kg/m^2 in women and percentage body fat, derived by DXA, greater than 28% in men and 40% in women (Baumgartner et al., 2004).

Anthropometric measurements included: body weight (Wt), height (Ht), and circumferences [waist, hip, waist-hip ratio (WHR)]. All measurements were determined by the same operator following the Anthropometric Standardization Reference Manual recommendations (Lohman et al., 1988). Body mass index (BMI) was calculated as Wt [Kg/Ht(m^2)]. We used BMI to categorized participants as obese (BMI $\geq$30), overweight ($25 \leq \text{BMI} < 30$), normal weight ($18.5 < \text{BMI} < 25$), or underweight $\leq$18.5.

ENERGY AND NITROGEN BALANCE

Resting energy expenditure was estimated by indirect calorimetry using a metabolic measurement cart with a canopy hood (CareFusion Vmax Encore, San Diego, CA, USA). Subjects were instructed to fast for 12 h and abstain from exercise for 24 h before the test (Mifflin et al., 1990). Before measuring REE, all subjects were asked to rest quietly in the supine position for approximately 30–40 min in an isolated room, with a temperature between 21° and 24°C. The criterion for a valid REE was 15 min of steady state, determined as <5% variation in respiratory quotient (RQ)/minute and oxygen consumption/minute. Oxygen consumption and carbon dioxide production were used to calculate REE, in accordance with the Weir equation (Turell and Alexander, 1964). REE were also calculated with the equations based on weight, height, age, and sex [Harris-Benedict and Schofield (Energy and protein requirements. Report of a joint FAO/WHO/UNU expert consultation, 1985; Roza and Shizgal, 1984)] using the free fat mass (FFM)-based predictive equations of Mifflin and Katch and McArdle (McArdle et al., 1986; Mifflin et al., 1990).

Food intake was evaluated by a 7-day food diary and a dietitian interview (O'Connor et al., 2014). Nitrogen balance, an important tool for estimating adequate protein intake (Tarnopolsky et al., 1988), was calculated as the difference between nitrogen input (24 h dietary protein intake) and nitrogen output (24 h urinary urea nitrogen).

General and nutritional blood and urine laboratory analyses (albumin: transferrin; creatinine; uric acid; glucose; triglycerides: total, HDL, and LDL cholesterol; urinary creatinine; and nitrogen) were taken to assess the metabolic status of the patients. The 24-h urinary creatinine excretion value was used as an index of protein nutrition; the creatinine height index (CHI) and lean body mass was estimated from this value.

MUSCLE STRENGTH

A composite score (megascore) was calculated by summing the maximal force of eight physical tests (Bryan et al., 2003; Merlini et al., 2003) using a hand-held dynamometer (Type CT 3001, Citec, C.I.T. Technics BV, Groningen, The Netherlands) (Van der Ploeg et al., 1991; Beenakker et al., 2001). Four muscle groups were examined bilaterally: hand grip, elbow flexors, knee extensors, and knee flexors (Merlini et al., 2002, 2003, 2004). Each individual muscle group was tested for at least 3 s using a "make" test (Merlini et al., 2004). The maximum force from three attempts was used in the analysis.

STATISTIC ANALYSIS

Pearson correlation coefficients were calculated to study the association between different parameters. Statistical significance was set at 0.05. All analyses were conducted using the STATA software package for Windows 13.1 (Stata Corp, College Station, TX, USA). Measurable variables are presented as mean ± SD and categorical data as number and percentage.

RESULTS

ANTHROPOMETRIC EVALUATION

Anthropometric analysis showed that UCMD and BM patients have average BMI values in the range of normality, comparable with a healthy population (Janssen et al., 2002). Body circumference measurements do not show any significant variations from normality (Janssen et al., 2002) (**Table 1**).

BODY COMPOSITION ANALYSIS

Body composition analysis showed quantitative changes in all the partitions of the body. All the patients had a loss of muscle mass, as shown by a marked reduction of FFM, FFMI, and ALMI, and augmented FM, as indicated by % FM and FMI.

In particular, all patients were sarcopenic, based on ALMI, and seven were sarcopenic-obese, based on ALMI and % FM (**Tables 2** and **3**).

Table 1 | Anthropometric analysis.

	M ($n = 3$)	W ($n = 5$)
Body weight (Kg)	67.40 (±11.39)	61.24 (±12.34)
Body height (m)	1.72 (±0.01)	1.63 (±0.05)
BMI (Kg/m^2)	22.73 (±3.72) (N.V. 18.5–24.9)	23.05 (±4.25) (N.V. 18.5–24.9)
Waist circumference (cm)	83.83 (±8.78) (N.V. <94)	74.85 (±7.19) (N.V. <80)
Hip circumference (cm)	96.83 (±6.25)	103.13 (±13.24)
waist-hip ratio (WHR)	0.86 (±0.05) (N.V. <1)	0.72 (±0.05) (N.V. <0.85)

The table shows the values obtained from the standard anthropometric analysis. For each parameter, the mean values ± SD are presented. When possible, normal values (N.V.) were reported (M, men and W, women).

Moreover, from the DXA data (trunk-to-limb FM ratio) and anthropometric parameters (waist circumference and waist/hip ratio index), we can deduce that, in the two compartments, the increased fat tissue was equally distributed (DXA) compensating for the loss of muscle mass (circumferences).

Bone mineral content, the other component of the FFM, is also strongly reduced in these patients, especially in men. The data are confirmed by T-score calculations in our male patients (Male T-score −1.87). T-score is a diagnostic for osteopenia (Kanis et al., 2013) (**Tables 2** and **3**).

BLOOD, URINE BIOCHEMICAL ANALYSIS, AND NITROGEN BALANCE

Blood and urine analysis do not show any specific pathological modification. In particular, although seven out of eight patients were obese, according to % fat determined by DXA, none had high levels of blood triglycerides, total cholesterol, HDL, or LDL (Jukema and Simoons, 1999). Blood creatinine levels were

Table 2 | Dual-energy X-ray absorptiometry.

	M ($n = 3$)	W ($n = 5$)
Fat-free mass (FFM) (%)	62.03 (±18.19)	48.36 (±6.55)
Fat-free mass (FFM) (Kg)	42.39 (±4.08)	29.22 (±3.53)
FFMI (FFM/height^2) (Kg/m^2)	14.43 (±1.27)	10.90 (±0.85)
Fat mass (FM) (%)	34.63 (±14.21)	51.64 (±6.55)
Fat mass (FM) (Kg)	23.86 (±12.05)	31.93 (±9.76)
FMI (FM/height^2) (Kg/m^2)	8.18 (±4.20)	12.07 (±3.71)
Bone mineral content (BMC) (%)	3.16 (±0.61)	3.06 (±0.84)
Bone mineral content (BMC) (Kg)	2.08 (±0.04)	1.82 (±0.36)
T-score	−1.87 (±0.49)	−0.23 (±0.86)
Trunk-to-limb fat mass ratio	1.10 (±0.03)	0.82 (±0.06)
ALMI (Kg/m^2)	5.68 (±0.57)	4.25 (±1.43)
ALM (Kg)	9.79 (±1.01)	6.92 (±2.35)
Trunk lean mass (Kg)	21.35 (±2.24)	14.66 (±1.12)
Trunk fat mass (Kg)	11.85 (±6.13)	13.70 (±5.11)

The table shows DXA body composition values. Mean values ± SD are presented (M, men and W, Women).

Table 3 | Body composition values obtained by anthropometric and DXA analyses, in BM and UCMD patients, compared to a healthy population.

ID	Sex	Age (years)	BMI (Kg/m²)	Fat %	FFM%	BFMI (Kg/m²)	Trunk to limbs FM ratio	ALMI (Kg/m²)
Pt. 1	W	48	20.9 N.V. (18.5–24.9)	49.90↑ N.V. (39.8–40.8)	50.1↓ N.V. (59.2–60.2)	10.10↓ N.V. (10.72–11.20)	0.88↓ N.V. (0.92–0.947)	3.60↓ N.V. (6.93–6.9)
Pt. 2	W	19	22.10 N.V. (18.5–24.9)	53.50↑ N.V. (35.1)	46.5↓ N.V. (64.8)	11.80↑ N.V. (8.48)	0.83↑ N.V. (0.745)	3.48↓ N.V. (6.81)
Pt. 3	W	42	18.19 N.V. (18.5–24.9)	41.30↑ N.V. (38.9–39.8)	58.7↓ N.V. (60.2–62.1)	7.53↓ N.V. (10.27–10.72)	0.80↓ N.V. (0.897–0.920)	3.81↓ N.V. (6.95–6.93)
Pt. 4	W	29	24.60 N.V. (18.5–24.9)	55.00↑ N.V. (36–37)	45↓ N.V. (63–64)	13.50↑ N.V. (8.9–9.35)	0.86↑ N.V. (0.796–0.841)	4.94↓ N.V. (6.86–6.9)
Pt. 5	W	22	29.44 N.V. (18.5–24.9)	58.50↑ N.V. (35.1–36)	41.5↓ N.V. (64–64.9)	17.40↑ N.V. (8.48–8.9)	0.73↓ N.V. (0.745–0.796)	4.93↓ N.V. (6.81–6.86)
Pt. 6	M	36	23.29 N.V. (18.5–24.9)	44.20↑ N.V. (26.6–27.5)	45.8↓ N.V. (72.5–73.4)	10.30↑ N.V. (7.19–7.57)	1.14↑ N.V. (1.125–1.183)	5.05↓ N.V. (9.09–9.12)
Pt. 7	M	27	18.76 N.V. (18.5–24.9)	18.30↓ N.V. (24.60–25.70)	81.7↑ N.V. (74.3–75.4)	3.34↓ N.V. (6.37–6.78)	1.15↑ N.V. (0.995–1.063)	6.35↓ N.V. (8.94–9.02)
Pt. 8	M	28	26.13 N.V. (18.5–24.9)	41.40↑ N.V. (24.60–25.70)	58.6↓ N.V. (74.3–75.4)	10.90↑ N.V. (6.37–6.78)	1.08↑ N.V. (0.995–1.063)	5.81↓ N.V. (8.94–9.02)

The table shows the body composition values of our subjects (M, men and F, women) compared to healthy values reported in the literature (Kelly et al., 2009; Wang et al., 2010). We used: "↑" when the values were increased; "↓" when the values were low.

moderately decreased (Ballesteros et al., 1994), particularly in women. Urinary creatine levels were generally low, particularly in men. Consequently, calculated CHI, an index of muscle mass (Rosenfalck et al., 1994), was greatly reduced in UCMD and BM patients.

Nitrogen balance was in the normal range.

Moreover, megascore values in our patients reflect the low strength condition typical of MDs (**Table 4**).

RESTING ENERGY EXPENDITURE AND RESPIRATORY QUOTIENT

Resting energy expenditure was measured by indirect calorimetry and estimated by specific predictive equations. The REEs estimated by the equations based on weight, height, age, and sex accurately predicted the same values measured with indirect calorimetry [Harris-Benedict and Schofield ("Energy and protein requirements. Report of a joint FAO/WHO/UNU Expert Consultation," 1985; Roza and Shizgal, 1984)]. REE was instead severely underestimated using the FFM-based predictive equations of Mifflin and Katch and McArdle (McArdle et al., 1986; Mifflin et al., 1990). Hence, considering that these patients are characterized by a reduced FFM in kilograms, we can deduce that there is a relative hypermetabolic state (Müller, 2007) with a higher ratio of REE (kcal)/FFM (kg) (**Figure 1**).

Measured RQs values are indicative of a mixed nutrient-based metabolism. However, there was a sex difference concerning the type of substrates utilized. While male patients had a higher carbohydrate-based metabolism (57.67 ± 14.57% carbohydrates), women showed a higher lipid-based metabolism (56.00 ± 16.39% lipids) (**Table 5**) (**Figure 2**). There was a strong positive correlation between the quantity of FFM in kg and the percentage of carbohydrates metabolized during REE. This correlation, however, was negative for the percentage of lipids metabolized. No correlation was found between the percentage of proteins used as a metabolic substrate and FFM.

All in all, patients are characterized by an augmented REE per kilogram of FFM; additionally, subjects with higher FFM values metabolize more carbohydrates and less lipids then the ones with minor FFM levels (**Figure 3**).

MUSCLE STRENGTH

Megascores expressed as the sum of the muscle strength of eight different tests, were 1093.33 (±306.37) Newton in men and 572.60 (±233.11) in women. These values were markedly reduced, as muscle strength was low in all muscle groups, compared with the normative values (Van der Ploeg et al., 1991; Beenakker et al., 2001).

There was a strong correlation between muscle strength, expressed as Megascore, and the various indices of muscle mass, but no correlation with the indices of body fat. A strong correlation was found between Megascore and blood creatinine. This correlation was even stronger with urinary creatinine and the derived index "CHI" (**Figure 6**). UCMD and BM patients who had a higher FFM showed a better performance in the muscle strength tests. The Megascore was directly proportional to FFM in kilograms and inversely proportional to the REE/FFM ratio (**Figure 4**).

This trend is maintained in the correlation between the Megascore and both trunk and limbs FFM. However, the linear correlation coefficient was higher between Megascore and appendicular FFM than Megascore and Trunk FFM (**Figure 5**). FFM% also correlated with Megascore, but the correlation was weaker.

Table 4 | Clinical and laboratory data.

	Men ($n=3$)	Women ($n=5$)
Creatinine (mg/dL)	0.64 (±0.30) N.V. (0.8–1.3)	0.26 (±0.07) N.V. (0.6–1.1)
Urinary creatinine (mg/24 h)	893.33 (±347.04) N.V. (500–2000)	394.00 (±107.84) N.V. (500–2000)
Creatinine height index (CHI) (%)	57.63 (±22.45) N.V. (109)	39.19 (±10.83) N.V. (110)
Dietary CHO intake (g)	342.56 (±48.17)	197.62 (±62.38)
Dietary lipid intake (g)	89.05 (±27.47)0	63.62 (±27.55)
Dietary protein intake (g)	83.58 (±8.90)	68.12 (±26.02)
Nitrogen intake (g)	13.37 (±1.42)	10.90 (±4.16)
Urinary urea nitrogen (g)	13.04 (±1.08)	11.99 (±3.48)
Nitrogen balance	−0.67 (±1.67) N.V. (0.00)	−1.84 (±1.30 N.V. (0.00)
Megascore	1093.33 (±306.37)	572.60 (±233.11)

The table shows the biochemical values obtained from blood and urine analysis and Megascore (Merlini et al., 2002, 2004). For each parameter, the mean values ± SD are presented. When possible, normal values (N.V.) were reported (M, men and W, women).

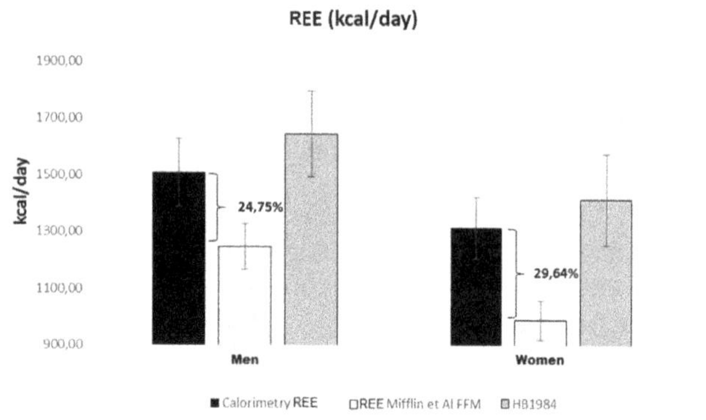

FIGURE 1 | Predicted and measured REE in UCMD and BM patients grouped by sex. Mean REE measured with indirect calorimetry (black rectangles); REE estimated with FFM-based Mifflin equation (Mifflin et al., 1990) (white rectangles) or Harris-Benedict) revised equation (Roza and Shizgal, 1984) (gray rectangles).

No correlation was found any between the Megascore and the indices of fat mas, FM in kilograms, FM percentage, or REE/FM ratio.

Table 5 | Energy balance.

	M ($n=3$)	W ($n=5$)
REE indirect calorimetry (Kcal)	1508.33 (±120.03)	1315.02 (±107.55)
REE Mifflin et Al (Kcal)	1248.09 (±80.28)	988.67 (±69.62)
REE Katch and McArdle (Kcal)	1285.63 (±88.02)	1001.19 (±76.34)
REE FAO Schofield et al. (Kcal)	1708.48 (±175.28)	1392.91 (±173.51)
REE Harris-Benedict 1984 (Kcal)	1645.34 (±152.67)	1412.83 (±159.62)
Mifflin FFM/REE Indirect calorimetry %	76.25 (±8.28)	70.36 (±5.20)
FAO/REE indirect calorimetry %	113.15 (±4.14)	106.35 (±15.14)
Harris-Benedict 1984/REE Indirect calorimetry %	109.01 (±1.71)	107.88 (±14.32)
Respiratory quotient (RQ)	0.90 (±0.06)	0.80 (±0.03)
RQ proteins (%)	19.67 (±2.89)	20.00 (±9.89)
RQ lipids (%)	22.33 (±17.95)	56.00 (±16.39)
RQ carbohydrates (%)	57.67 (±14.57)	23.75 (±7.45)
REE/FFM (Kcal/Kg)	35.77 (±3.92)	45.46 (±6.13)
REE/FM (Kcal/Kg)	80.61 (±51.94)	44.54 (±13.75)

In this table, values of indirect calorimetry and predictive equations analysis are presented. For each parameter, the mean values ± SD are presented (M, men and W, women).

DISCUSSION

In this study, we have investigated the relationship between body composition, energetic metabolism, and muscle strength in a cohort of patients with COL6-RM.

According to body composition, evaluated by DXA, all patients could be defined as sarcopenic and all but one as sarcopenic-obese. The patients showed a marked increment of the amount of FM and a severe loss of FFM without important modifications in the BMI, which ranged from underweight to overweight, or in waist circumferences measures, which were within a normal range. This peculiar modification in body composition can be explained by the process of fatty infiltration of the muscle in MD (Tuffery-Giraud et al., 2004; Jarraya et al., 2012; Willis et al., 2014).

Since FFM is the major determinant of energy expenditure in normal subjects, we integrated body composition analysis with the analysis of energy status and of muscle strength in accordance

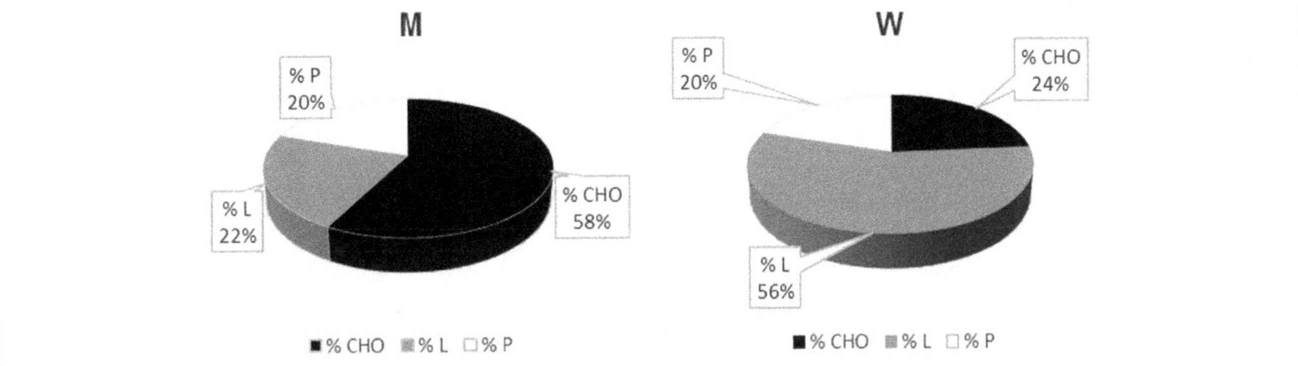

FIGURE 2 | UCMD and BM patients' metabolism. Percentage of Carbohydrates (CHO), Lipids (L) and Proteins (P) utilized during indirect calorimetry examination. These values were calculated from respiratory quotients and urine nitrogen measurement (Livesey and Elia, 1988) Mean values in men (left) and women (right) are reported.

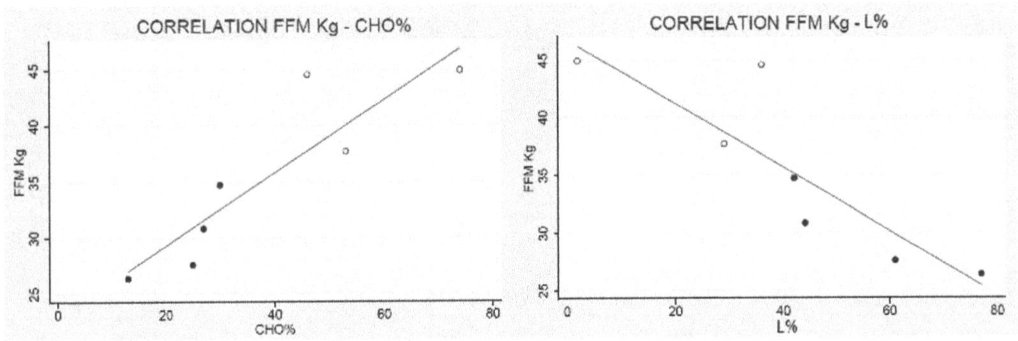

FIGURE 3 | Collagen VI myopathies: FFM metabolism. (Left) Linear correlation between FFM in kg and percentage of carbohydrates used as metabolic substrate (correlation coefficient $R = 0.89$ e $P < 0.01$), and (right) correlation between FFM and percentage of lipids used as metabolic substrate (correlation coefficient $R = -0.87$ e $P = 0.01$). White dots represent men and black dots represent women. The percentage of substrate utilized was calculated using the respiratory quotient and urinary urea nitrogen (Livesey and Elia, 1988). Data from one BM were missing.

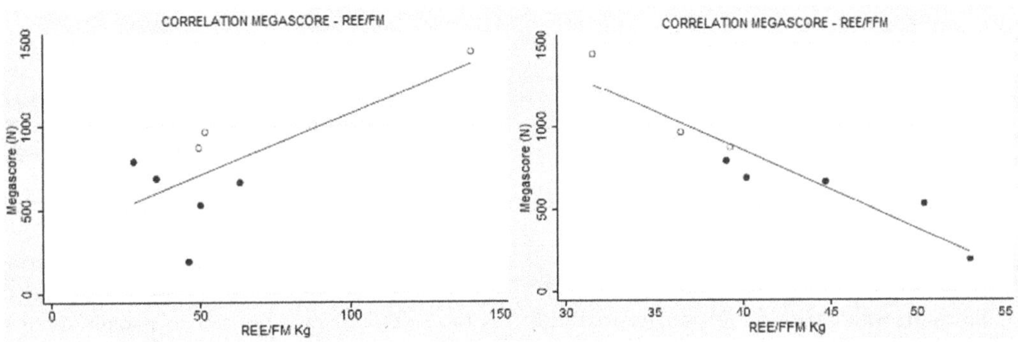

FIGURE 4 | Muscle strength and functional body composition. As expected there was no correlation between Megascore and REE/FM, but instead a strong correlation between Megascore and the REE/FFM ratio ($R = -0.94$, $P < 0.001$) (right).

with the new concept of functional body composition (Müller et al., 2009).

COL6-RM patients showed a REE, analyzed by indirect calorimetry, in the range of normality, despite the severe reduction of the FFM. Predictive formulas estimate REE values in line with what we actually have found by indirect calorimetry. Applying the concept of functional body composition and relating FFM to energy expenditure, we found a clear deviation from normality

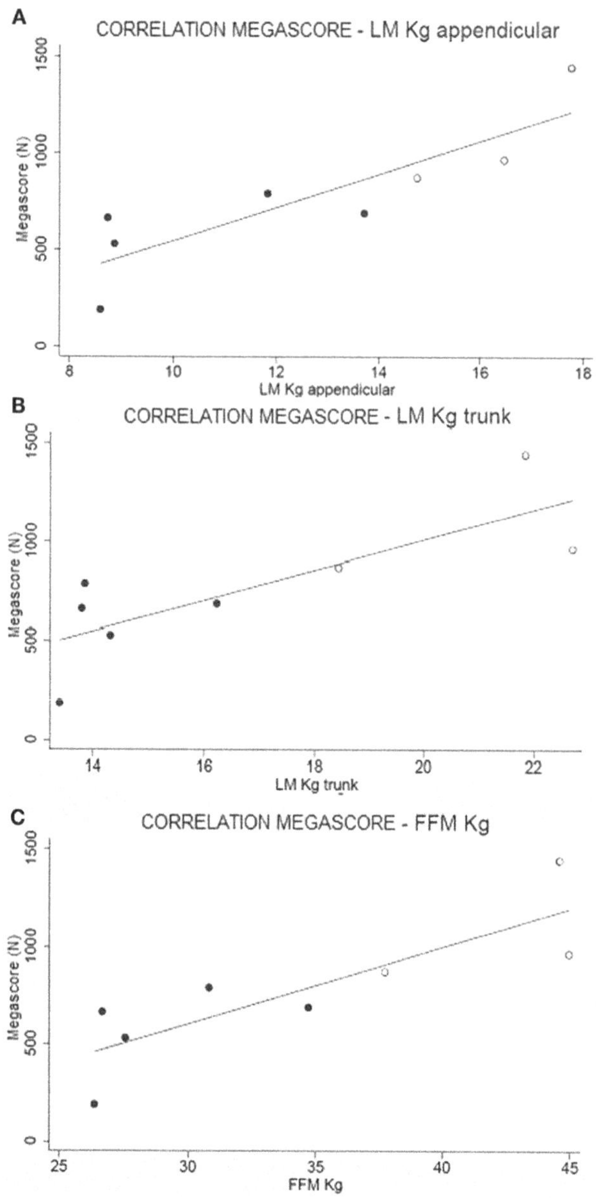

FIGURE 5 | Muscle strength and body composition. Correlation between appendicular LM **(A)** and Trunk LM **(B)** with the Megascore [respectively for limbs and trunk, $R = 0.87$ ($P < 0.01$) and $R = 0.80$ ($P < 0.05$)]. **(C)** Correlation between total FFM in kg and Megascore ($R = 0.84$, $P < 0.01$).

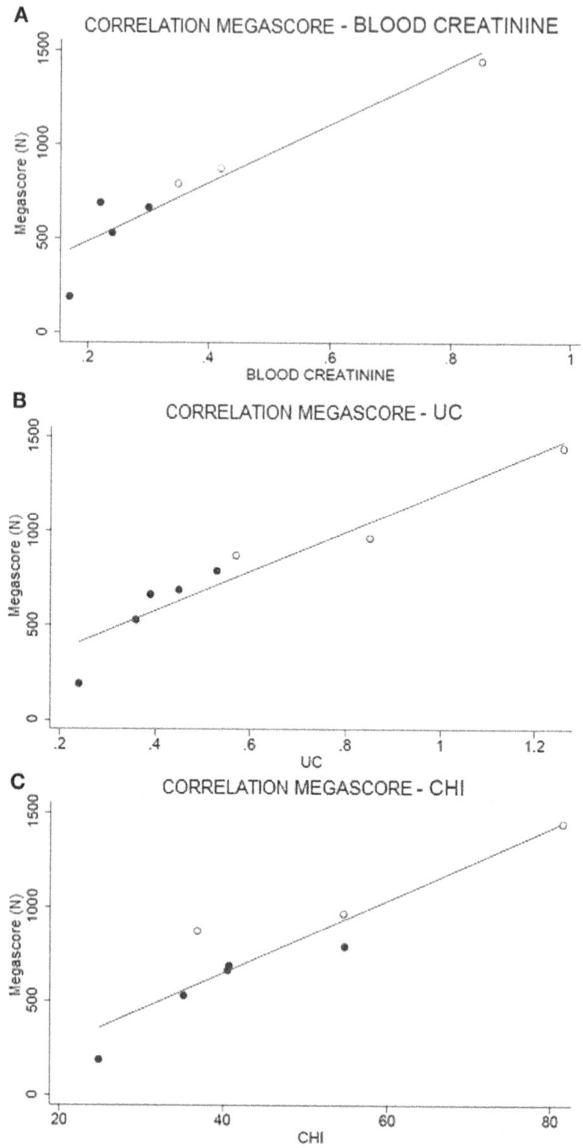

FIGURE 6 | Muscle strength and creatinine. **(A)** Correlation between Megascore and blood creatinine ($R = 0.94$, $P = 0.001$), or **(B)** urine creatinine (UC) ($R = 0.95$, $P < 0.001$). **(C)** Correlation between Megascore and CHI (Rosenfalck et al., 1994) ($R = 0.93$, $P = 0.001$).

(metabolic disequilibrium) with a considerably augmented REE per kilogram of FFM. Our assumptions are supported by the fact that REE, estimated through FFM-based equations, clearly underestimate the effective metabolism of these patients by 25–30% (**Figure 1**).

If we compare the metabolism predicted by FFM-based-formulas with the values of REE, adjusted for body composition, we find that the FFM of these patients is overworking or in a hypermetabolic state (Müller, 2007). A similar metabolic alteration has been reported by Zanardi et al. in Duchenne patients (Zanardi et al., 2003b). It has been considered an enduring enigma: why is the ratio of REE to metabolically active tissue mass, expressed as the REE/FFM ratio, greater in magnitude in subjects with a small FFM than in subjects with a large FFM? (Heymsfield et al., 2002).

In COL6-RM patients, FFM requires more energy than in healthy subjects, and because FFM is made up of muscle and internal organs, we can only speculate as to which of these two components presents a hypermetabolic state. In particular, the augmented REE/FFM ratio could be due to a non-physiological increase in visceral organ metabolism, or to an altered energy expenditure of muscle cells. However, even if our study cannot completely answer this question, all evidence suggests that the second hypothesis is the right one.

If we consider the pathological alteration of muscle structures, underlined in mouse model studies (De Palma et al., 2013), with the loss of muscular protein stability leads to a loss of efficiency, and additional energy is necessary to maintain muscle cell homeostasis. Even if this theory has been demonstrated in other studies no one had ever pointed out that this behavior is strictly correlated with the severity of the disease. Our hypothesis is that, in a dystrophic environment, the energy that the muscle has to spend in order to maintain its function is inversely proportional to the total muscular mass. Moreover, if the augmented REE/FFM were due to an increased metabolism of the visceral organs, we should have found some alterations in bio-humoral parameters (Gelfand et al., 1987; Izamis et al., 2012). On the contrary COL6-RM subjects do not show any important variation in blood or urine biochemical assays.

Additionally, there was no correlation between the REE/FM and the clinical status portrayed by Megascore analysis (**Figure 4**). Therefore, we can exclude increased adipocytes energy expenditure as a source of the hypermetabolic state.

Finally, recent discoveries about mitochondrial metabolism (Bernardi and Bonaldo, 2008; Shaham et al., 2010) offer a possible biochemical explanation of the increased REE/FFM ratio. In particular, Bernardi et al. have found important alterations in mitochondrial membrane permeability due to the ColA6 mutation. The lack of Collagen VI causes increased transient openings of the Permeability Transition Pore ion channel in the mitochondrial inner membrane, with consequent mitochondrial depolarization and energy dissipation. This leads to a switch of the ATP synthase into an ATP hydrolase with a progressive impairment of respiration which may be responsible for the augmented REE spent by the muscular mass. This pathophysiology mechanism may explain our findings.

We also discovered that the metabolic substrates consumed by these patients are strictly related to their FFM (**Figures 2** and **3**). In particular, patients with higher FFM have a carbohydrate-based metabolism, while the ones with lower FFM prevalently use fatty acids as metabolic substrates. These findings suggest that patients with a relatively greater FFM have more muscular mass, and consequently an increased glycogen reserve to be used, compared to patients with lower FFM (Tsujino et al., 2000). On the other hand, the fat-based metabolism is explained by the increasing fat infiltration with disease progression; the depletion of muscular mass and the correlated decrement in glycogen storage lead to a metabolic shift toward burning fatty acids, whose reserves increase and infiltrate muscular tissue (Tagliavini et al., 2014). These evidences suggest that the worsening of the pathology is closely correlated to important changes in muscle metabolism.

Another significant result is the correlation between FFM and muscle strength, summarized by the Megascore (**Figure 5**). Other studies have previously demonstrated that Megascore is a good indicator of patients' muscular efficiency, paralleling muscle function (Merlini et al., 2002, 2004). Hence, the correlation between muscle Megascore and FFM is more a portrait of the muscular mass and its efficiency, rather than of visceral organ activity. The strong correlations between Megascore and appendicular LM, where the non-muscle component of FFM is minimal, support this hypothesis.

This is a perfect expression of the concept of functional body composition: in COL6-RM, a pure body composition parameter like appendicular LM is directly correlated to muscular strength (Megascore) and contributes to the diagnosis of sarcopenia, a condition in which the loss of skeletal muscle mass is associated with lower muscle strength and function (Abellan Baumgartner et al., 1998; van Kan et al., 2012)

Creatinine is derived from the metabolism of creatine, which is transformed into phosphocreatine and used by muscles as an energetic substrate (Hoagland et al., 1945). A higher production of creatinine is linked to a higher use of phosphocreatine and, consequently, to greater muscular efficiency. In order to confirm this hypothesis, and to exclude any artifact due to individual body composition, we have analyzed the CHI, which evaluates urinary creatinine levels by normalizing the individual differences among subjects (Rosenfalck et al., 1994). Even in this case, the CHI scores perfectly correlate to the muscle strength, as evaluated by Megascore (**Figure 6**).

Hence, even if Franciotta et al. (2003) declare that urinary creatinine is not a good predictive indicator of skeletal muscular mass in Duchenne dystrophy; our results suggest that it is a good indicator of muscular performance.

Another important correlation is the one between blood creatinine and Megascore. Even if we have to consider renal filtration, blood creatinine gives an instant picture of the muscle metabolism (Baxmann et al., 2008). The probability of finding circulating creatinine is directly proportional to the quantity of phosphocreatine produced and used by muscle cells. Considering our results about urinary creatinine and CHI, this finding confirms the previous ones.

All in all, in this study, we have pointed out the importance of a nutritional approach to genetically based pathologies, such as UCMD and BM diseases. Additionally, we have underlined the necessity of a functional body composition analysis, which could be a powerful clinical tool for patients' follow-up and prognosis.

The main limit of our study is represented by the scant number of recruited patients, caused by the rarity of these pathologies; hence, our conclusions should be confirmed by the analysis of a wider sample of subjects.

Our results confirm and complete what has been reported in the literature about collagen VI myopathies, further supporting the rationale for nutritional interventions aimed at correcting the metabolic imbalance and maintaining the patient's muscular mass.

AUTHOR CONTRIBUTIONS

Silvia Toni made substantial contributions to acquisition of the data, carried out the nutritional evaluation, and performed the statistical analysis. Riccardo Morandi and Marcello Busacchi substantially contributed by discussing the data, writing the manuscript, and performing statistical analysis. Lucia Tardini contributed to the acquisition of data and carried out the anthropometric evaluation. Luciano Merlini conceived the study and participated in its design and coordination. Nino Carlo Battistini evaluated the body composition data. Massimo Pellegrini participated in the design of the study, contributed to the statistical analysis, and has contributed substantially in the interpretation of data.

ACKNOWLEDGMENTS

This study was supported by Grant no. GUP11007 (Luciano Merlini) from Telethon, Italy.

REFERENCES

Allamand, V., Merlini, L., Bushby, K., and Consortium for Collagen VI-Related Myopathies. (2010). 166th ENMC international workshop on collagen type VI-related myopathies, 22-24 May 2009, naarden, The Netherlands. *Neuromuscul. Disord.* 20, 346–354. doi:10.1016/j.nmd.2010.02.012

Ballesteros, M., Cortes, A., Arleaga, C. I., Puerto, R., and Bojac, B. (1994). [The usefulness of serum creatinine levels in identifying hospital malnutrition]. *Nutr. Hosp.* 9, 186–196.

Baumgartner, R. N., Koehler, K. M., Gallagher, D., Romero, L., Heymsfield, S. B., Ross, R. R., et al. (1998). Epidemiology of sarcopenia among the elderly in New Mexico. *Am. J. Epidemiol.* 147, 755–763. doi:10.1093/oxfordjournals.aje.a009520

Baumgartner, R. N., Wayne, S. J., Waters, D. L., Janssen, I., Gallagher, D., and Morley, J. E. (2004). Sarcopenic obesity predicts instrumental activities of daily living disability in the elderly. *Obes. Res.* 12, 1995–2004.

Baxmann, A. C., Ahmed, M. S., Marques, N. C., Menon, V. B., Pereira, A. B., Kirsztajn, G. M., et al. (2008). Influence of muscle mass and physical activity on serum and urinary creatinine and serum cystatin C. *Clin. J. Am. Soc. Nephrol.* 3, 348–354. doi:10.2215/CJN.02870707

Beenakker, E. A., van der Hoeven, J. H., Fock, J. M., and Maurits, N. M. (2001). Reference values of maximum isometric muscle force obtained in 270 children aged 4-16 years by hand-held dynamometry. *Neuromuscul. Disord.* 11, 441–446. doi:10.1016/S0960-8966(01)00193-6

Bernardi, P., and Bonaldo, P. (2008). Dysfunction of mitochondria and sarcoplasmic reticulum in the pathogenesis of collagen VI muscular dystrophies. *Ann. N. Y. Acad. Sci.* 1147, 303–311. doi:10.1196/annals.1427.009

Bernardi, P., and Bonaldo, P. (2013). Mitochondrial dysfunction and defective autophagy in the pathogenesis of collagen VI muscular dystrophies. *Cold Spring Harb. Perspect. Biol.* 5, a011387. doi:10.1101/cshperspect.a011387

Bertini, E., and Pepe, G. (2002). Collagen type VI and related disorders: Bethlem myopathy and Ullrich scleroatonic muscular dystrophy. *Eur. J. Paediatr. Neurol.* 6, 193–198. doi:10.1053/ejpn.2002.0593

Bryan, W. W., Hoagland, R. J., Murphy, J., Armon, C., Barohn, R. J., Goodpasture, J. C., et al. (2003). Can we eliminate placebo in ALS clinical trials? *Amyotroph. Lateral Scler. Other Motor Neuron Disord.* 4, 11–15. doi:10.1080/14660820310006661

De Palma, S., Leone, R., Grumati, P., Vasso, M., Polishchuk, R., Capitanio, D., et al. (2013). Changes in muscle cell metabolism and mechanotransduction are associated with myopathic phenotype in a mouse model of collagen VI deficiency. *PLoS ONE* 8:e56716. doi:10.1371/journal.pone.0056716

El Ghoch, M., Milanese, C., Calugi, S., Pellegrini, M., Battistini, N. C., and Dalle Grave, R. (2014). Body composition, eating disorder psychopathology, and psychological distress in anorexia nervosa: a longitudinal study. *Am. J. Clin. Nutr.* 99, 771–778. doi:10.3945/ajcn.113.078816

Elliott, S. A., Davidson, Z. E., Davies, P. S. W., and Truby, H. (2012). Predicting resting energy expenditure in boys with Duchenne muscular dystrophy. *Eur. J. Paediatr. Neurol.* 16, 631–635. doi:10.1016/j.ejpn.2012.02.011

Franciotta, D., Zanardi, M. C., Albertotti, L., Orcesi, S., Berardinelli, A., Pichiecchio, A., et al. (2003). Measurement of skeletal muscle mass in Duchenne muscular dystrophy: use of 24-h creatinine excretion. *Acta Diabetol.* 40(Suppl. 1), S290–S292. doi:10.1007/s00592-003-0089-8

Gelfand, R. A., Hutchinson-Williams, K. A., Bonde, A. A., Castellino, P., and Sherwin, R. S. (1987). Catabolic effects of thyroid hormone excess: the contribution of adrenergic activity to hypermetabolism and protein breakdown. *Metab. Clin. Exp.* 36, 562–569. doi:10.1016/0026-0495(87)90168-5

Gonzalez-Bermejo, J., Lofaso, F., Falaize, L., Lejaille, M., Raphaël, J.-C., Similowski, T., et al. (2005). Resting energy expenditure in Duchenne patients using home mechanical ventilation. *Eur. Respir. J.* 25, 682–687. doi:10.1183/09031936.05.00031304

Grumati, P., Coletto, L., Sabatelli, P., Cescon, M., Angelin, A., Bertaggia, E., et al. (2010). Autophagy is defective in collagen VI muscular dystrophies, and its reactivation rescues myofiber degeneration. *Nat. Med.* 16, 1313–1320. doi:10.1038/nm.2247

Gualandi, F., Urciuolo, A., Martoni, E., Sabatelli, P., Squarzoni, S., Bovolenta, M., et al. (2009). Autosomal recessive Bethlem myopathy. *Neurology* 73, 1883–1891. doi:10.1212/WNL.0b013e3181c3fd2a

Heymsfield, S. B., Gallagher, D., Kotler, D. P., Wang, Z., Allison, D. B., and Heshka, S. (2002). Body-size dependence of resting energy expenditure can be attributed to nonenergetic homogeneity of fat-free mass. *Am. J. Physiol. Endocrinol. Metab.* 282, E132–E138.

Hoagland, C. L., Gilder, H., and Shank, R. E. (1945). The synthesis, storage, and excretion of creatine, creatinine, and glycocyamine in progressive muscular dystrophy and the effects of certain hormones on these processes. *J. Exp. Med.* 81, 423–438. doi:10.1084/jem.81.5.423

Hogan, S. E. (2008). Body composition and resting energy expenditure of individuals with Duchenne and Becker muscular dystrophy. *Can. J. Diet. Pract. Res.* 69, 208–212. doi:10.3148/69.4.2008.208

Irwin, W. A., Bergamin, N., Sabatelli, P., Reggiani, C., Megighian, A., Merlini, L., et al. (2003). Mitochondrial dysfunction and apoptosis in myopathic mice with collagen VI deficiency. *Nat. Genet.* 35, 367–371. doi:10.1038/ng1270

Izamis, M.-L., Uygun, K., Sharma, N. S., Uygun, B., Yarmush, M. L., and Berthiaume, F. (2012). Development of metabolic indicators of burn injury: very low density lipoprotein (vldl) and acetoacetate are highly correlated to severity of burn injury in rats. *Metabolites* 2, 458–478. doi:10.3390/metabo2030458

Janssen, I., Katzmarzyk, P. T., and Ross, R. (2002). Body mass index, waist circumference, and health risk: evidence in support of current National Institutes of Health guidelines. *Arch. Intern. Med.* 162, 2074–2079. doi:10.1001/archinte.162.18.2074

Jarraya, M., Quijano-Roy, S., Monnier, N., Béhin, A., Avila-Smirnov, D., Romero, N. B., et al. (2012). Whole-body muscle MRI in a series of patients with congenital myopathy related to TPM2 gene mutations. *Neuromuscul. Disord.* 22(Suppl. 2), S137–S147. doi:10.1016/j.nmd.2012.06.347

Jukema, J. W., and Simoons, M. L. (1999). Treatment and prevention of coronary heart disease by lowering serum cholesterol levels; from the pioneer work of C.D. de Langen to the third "Dutch consensus on cholesterol.". *Acta Cardiol.* 54, 163–168.

Kanis, J. A., McCloskey, E. V., Johansson, H., Cooper, C., Rizzoli, R., and Reginster, J.-Y. (2013). European guidance for the diagnosis and management of osteoporosis in postmenopausal women. *Osteoporos. Int.* 24, 23–57. doi:10.1007/s00198-012-2074-y

Kelly, T. L., Wilson, K. E., and Heymsfield, S. B. (2009). Dual energy X-ray absorptiometry body composition reference values from NHANES. *PLoS ONE* 4:e7038. doi:10.1371/journal.pone.0007038

Livesey, G., and Elia, M. (1988). Estimation of energy expenditure, net carbohydrate utilization, and net fat oxidation and synthesis by indirect calorimetry: evaluation of errors with special reference to the detailed composition of fuels. *Am. J. Clin. Nutr.* 47, 608–628.

Lohman, T. G., Martorell, R., and Roche, A. F. (1988). *Anthropometric Standardization Reference Manual.* Champaign IL: Human Kinetics Books.

McArdle, W. D., Katch, F. I., and Katch, V. L. (1986). *Exercise Physiology Energy, Nutrition, and Human Performance.* Philadelphia: Lea & Febiger.

Mercuri, E., Lampe, A., Allsop, J., Knight, R., Pane, M., Kinali, M., et al. (2005). Muscle MRI in Ullrich congenital muscular dystrophy and Bethlem myopathy. *Neuromuscul. Disord.* 15, 303–310. doi:10.1016/j.nmd.2005.01.004

Merlini, L., Angelin, A., Tiepolo, T., Braghetta, P., Sabatelli, P., Zamparelli, A., et al. (2008a). Cyclosporin A corrects mitochondrial dysfunction and muscle apoptosis in patients with collagen VI myopathies. *Proc. Natl. Acad. Sci. U. S. A.* 105, 5225–5229. doi:10.1073/pnas.0800962105

Merlini, L., Martoni, E., Grumati, P., Sabatelli, P., Squarzoni, S., Urciuolo, A., et al. (2008b). Autosomal recessive myosclerosis myopathy is a collagen VI disorder. *Neurology* 71, 1245–1253. doi:10.1212/01.wnl.0000327611.01687.5e

Merlini, L., Bertini, E., Minetti, C., Mongini, T., Morandi, L., Angelini, C., et al. (2004). Motor function-muscle strength relationship in spinal muscular atrophy. *Muscle Nerve* 29, 548–552. doi:10.1002/mus.20018

Merlini, L., Mazzone, E. S., Solari, A., and Morandi, L. (2002). Reliability of hand-held dynamometry in spinal muscular atrophy. *Muscle Nerve* 26, 64–70. doi:10.1002/mus.10166

Merlini, L., Morandi, L., Granata, C., and Ballestrazzi, A. (1994). Bethlem myopathy: early-onset benign autosomal dominant myopathy with contractures. Description of two new families. *Neuromuscul. Disord.* 4, 503–511. doi:10.1016/0960-8966(94)90091-4

Merlini, L., Nishino, I., and Consortium for Autophagy in Muscular Dystrophies. (2014). 201st ENMC international workshop: autophagy in muscular dystrophies – translational approach, 1-3 november 2013, Bussum, The Netherlands. *Neuromuscul. Disord.* 24, 546–561. doi:10.1016/j.nmd.2014.03.009

Merlini, L., Solari, A., Vita, G., Bertini, E., Minetti, C., Mongini, T., et al. (2003). Role of gabapentin in spinal muscular atrophy: results of a multi-center, randomized Italian study. *J. Child Neurol.* 18, 537–541. doi:10.1177/08830738030180080501

Mifflin, M. D., St Jeor, S. T., Hill, L. A., Scott, B. J., Daugherty, S. A., and Koh, Y. O. (1990). A new predictive equation for resting energy expenditure in healthy individuals. *Am. J. Clin. Nutr.* 51, 241–247.

Miscione, M. T., Bruno, F., Ripamonti, C., Nervuti, G., Orsini, R., Faldini, C., et al. (2013). Body composition, muscle strength, and physical function of patients with Bethlem myopathy and Ullrich congenital muscular dystrophy. *Scientific World Journal* 2013:152684. doi:10.1155/2013/152684

Moon, J. R., Tobkin, S. E., Smith, A. E., Roberts, M. D., Ryan, E. D., Dalbo, V. J., et al. (2008). Percent body fat estimations in college men using field and laboratory methods: a three-compartment model approach. *Dyn. Med.* 7, 7. doi:10.1186/1476-5918-7-7

Müller, M. J. (2007). Malnutrition and hypermetabolism in patients with liver cirrhosis. *Am. J. Clin. Nutr.* 85, 1167–1168.

Müller, M. J., Bosy-Westphal, A., Later, W., Haas, V., and Heller, M. (2009). Functional body composition: insights into the regulation of energy metabolism and some clinical applications. *Eur. J. Clin. Nutr.* 63, 1045–1056. doi:10.1038/ejcn.2009.55

Norwood, F. L. M., Harling, C., Chinnery, P. F., Eagle, M., Bushby, K., and Straub, V. (2009). Prevalence of genetic muscle disease in Northern England: in-depth analysis of a muscle clinic population. *Brain* 132, 3175–3186. doi:10.1093/brain/awp236

O'Connor, L. M., Lentjes, M. A. H., Luben, R. N., Khaw, K.-T., Wareham, N. J., and Forouhi, N. G. (2014). Dietary dairy product intake and incident type 2 diabetes: a prospective study using dietary data from a 7-day food diary. *Diabetologia* 57, 909–917. doi:10.1007/s00125-014-3176-1

Pepe, G., de Visser, M., Bertini, E., Bushby, K., Vanegas, O. C., Chu, M. L., et al. (2002). Bethlem myopathy (BETHLEM) 86th ENMC international workshop, 10-11 November 2000, Naarden, The Netherlands. *Neuromuscul. Disord.* 12, 296–305. doi:10.1016/S0960-8966(01)00275-9

Rohan, T. E., Heo, M., Choi, L., Datta, M., Freudenheim, J. L., Kamensky, V., et al. (2013). Body fat and breast cancer risk in postmenopausal women: a longitudinal study. *J. Cancer Epidemiol.* 2013, 754815. doi:10.1155/2013/754815

Rosenfalck, A. M., Snorgaard, O., Almdal, T., and Binder, C. (1994). Creatinine height index and lean body mass in adult patients with insulin-dependent diabetes mellitus followed for 7 years from onset. *JPEN J. Parenter. Enteral Nutr.* 18, 50–54. doi:10.1177/014860719401800150

Roza, A. M., and Shizgal, H. M. (1984). The Harris Benedict equation reevaluated: resting energy requirements and the body cell mass. *Am. J. Clin. Nutr.* 40, 168–182.

Scaglioni, F., Marino, M., Ciccia, S., Procaccini, A., Busacchi, M., Loria, P., et al. (2013). Short-term multidisciplinary non-pharmacological intervention is effective in reducing liver fat content assessed non-invasively in patients with nonalcoholic fatty liver disease (NAFLD). *Clin. Res. Hepatol. Gastroenterol.* 37, 353–358. doi:10.1016/j.clinre.2012.10.009

Shaham, O., Slate, N. G., Goldberger, O., Xu, Q., Ramanathan, A., Souza, A. L., et al. (2010). A plasma signature of human mitochondrial disease revealed through metabolic profiling of spent media from cultured muscle cells. *Proc. Natl. Acad. Sci. U. S. A.* 107, 1571–1575. doi:10.1073/pnas.0906039107

Tagliavini, F., Sardone, F., Squarzoni, S., Maraldi, N. M., Merlini, L., Faldini, C., et al. (2014). Ultrastructural changes in muscle cells of patients with collagen VI-related myopathies. *Muscles Ligaments Tendons J.* 3, 281–286.

Tarnopolsky, M. A., MacDougall, J. D., and Atkinson, S. A. (1988). Influence of protein intake and training status on nitrogen balance and lean body mass. *J. Appl. Physiol.* 1985, 187–193.

Tsujino, S., Nonaka, I., and DiMauro, S. (2000). Glycogen storage myopathies. *Neurol. Clin.* 18, 125–150. doi:10.1016/S0733-8619(05)70181-X

Tuffery-Giraud, S., Saquet, C., Chambert, S., Echenne, B., Marie Cuisset, J., Rivier, F., et al. (2004). The role of muscle biopsy in analysis of the dystrophin gene in Duchenne muscular dystrophy: experience of a national referral centre. *Neuromuscul. Disord.* 14, 650–658. doi:10.1016/j.nmd.2004.05.002

Turell, D. J., and Alexander, J. K. (1964). Experimental evaluation of weir's formula for estimating metabolic rate in man. *J. Appl. Physiol.* 19, 946–948.

Vaisman, N., Katzenellenbogen, S., and Nevo, Y. (2004). Increased resting energy expenditure in subjects with Emery-Dreifuss muscular dystrophy. *Neuromuscul. Disord.* 14, 142–146. doi:10.1016/j.nmd.2003.10.012

Van der Ploeg, R. J., Fidler, V., and Oosterhuis, H. J. (1991). Hand-held myometry: reference values. *J. Neurol. Neurosurg. Psychiatry* 54, 244–247. doi:10.1136/jnnp.54.3.244

van Kan, G., Houles, M., and Vellas, B. (2012). Identifying sarcopenia. *Curr. Opin. Clin. Nutr. Metab. Care* 15, 436–441. doi:10.1097/MCO.0b013e328356bbf4

Wang, Z., Heymsfield, S. B., Chen, Z., Zhu, S., and Pierson, R. N. (2010). Estimation of percentage body fat by dual-energy x-ray absorptiometry: evaluation by in vivo human elemental composition. *Phys. Med. Biol.* 55, 2619–2635. doi:10.1088/0031-9155/55/9/013

Willis, T. A., Hollingsworth, K. G., Coombs, A., Sveen, M.-L., Andersen, S., Stojkovic, T., et al. (2014). Quantitative magnetic resonance imaging in limb-girdle muscular dystrophy 2I: a multinational cross-sectional study. *PLoS ONE* 9:e90377. doi:10.1371/journal.pone.0090377

Wohlfahrt, P., Somers, V. K., Sochor, O., Kullo, I., Jean, N., and Lopez-Jimenez, F. (2014). Influence of body fatness distribution and total lean mass on aortic stiffness in nonobese individuals. *Am. J. Hypertens* doi:10.1093/ajh/hpu153

Energy and protein requirements. Report of a joint FAO/WHO/UNU expert consultation. (1985). *World Health Organ. Tech. Rep. Ser* 724, 1–206.

Zanardi, M. C., Tagliabue, A., Orcesi, S., Berardinelli, A., Uggetti, C., and Pichiecchio, A. (2003a). Body composition and energy expenditure in Duchenne muscular dystrophy. *Eur. J. Clin. Nutr.* 57, 273–278. doi:10.1038/sj.ejcn.1601524

Zanardi, M. C., Tagliabue, A., Orcesi, S., Berardinelli, A., Uggetti, C., and Pichiecchio, A. (2003b). Body composition and energy expenditure in Duchenne muscular dystrophy. *Eur. J. Clin. Nutr.* 57, 273–278. doi:10.1038/sj.ejcn.1601524

3

Qualitative alteration of peripheral motor system begins prior to appearance of typical sarcopenia syndrome in middle-aged rats

Tetsuro Tamaki[1,2]*, Maki Hirata[1,2,3] and Yoshiyasu Uchiyama[1,3]

[1] *Muscle Physiology and Cell Biology Unit, Tokai University School of Medicine, Isehara, Japan*
[2] *Division of Basic Clinical Science, Department of Regenerative Medicine, Tokai University School of Medicine, Isehara, Japan*
[3] *Division of Surgery, Department of Orthopedics, Tokai University School of Medicine, Isehara, Japan*

Correspondence:
Tetsuro Tamaki, Muscle Physiology and Cell Biology Unit, Division of Basic Clinical Science, Department of Regenerative Medicine, Tokai University School of Medicine, 143-Shimokasuya, Isehara, Kanagawa 259-1143, Japan
e-mail: tamaki@is.icc.u-tokai.ac.jp

Qualitative changes in the peripheral motor system were examined using young, adult, middle-aged, and old-aged rats in order to assess before and after the appearance of sarcopenia symptoms. Significant loss of muscle mass and strength, and slow-type fiber grouping with a loss of innervated nerve fibers were used as typical markers of sarcopenia. Dynamic twitch and tetanus tension and evoked electromyogram (EEMG) were measured via electrical stimulation through the sciatic nerve under anesthesia using our force-distance transducer system before and after sciatectomy. Digital and analog data sampling was performed and shortening and relaxing velocity of serial twitches was calculated with tension force. Muscle tenderness in passive stretching was also measured as stretch absorption ability, associated with histological quantitation of muscle connective tissues. The results indicated the validity of the present model, in which old-aged rats clearly showed the typical signs of sarcopenia, specifically in the fast-type plantaris muscles, while the slow-type soleus showed relatively mild syndromes. These observations suggest the following qualitative alterations as the pathophysiological mechanism of sarcopenia: (1) reduction of shortening and relaxing velocity of twitch; (2) decline of muscle tenderness following an increase in the connective tissue component; (3) impaired recruitment of motor units (MUs) (sudden depression of tetanic force and EEMG) in higher stimulation frequencies over 50–60 Hz; and (4) easy fatigability in the neuromuscular junctions. These findings are likely to be closely related to significant losses in fast-type MUs, muscle strength and contraction velocity, which could be a causative factor in falls in the elderly. Importantly, some of these symptoms began in middle-aged rats that showed no other signs of sarcopenia. Thus, prevention should be started in middle age that could be retained relatively higher movement ability.

Keywords: muscle shortening-relaxation velocity, demyelination, axon loss, synaptic depression, neuromuscular junction, motor neuron pool, stretch-reflex

INTRODUCTION

Sarcopenia is defined as the loss of muscle mass and strength that occurs with aging, leading to increased frailty, impaired mobility and loss of independence with general disability (Morley et al., 2001; Cruz-Jentoft et al., 2010; Mitchell et al., 2012). An increase in the associated loss of independence is a great burden for both affected individuals, and for caregivers and society (Lang et al., 2010); therefore, the precise mechanisms underpinning sarcopenia have been investigated vigorously for many years in order to prevent of these syndromes. Through numerous reports, it is likely that the loss of muscle mass is induced by an age-related decline in muscle fiber number and size, and this wholly depends on the age-related loss of spinal motor neurons (MNs), as defined by both animal and human data (Tomlinson and Irving, 1977; Edstrom and Larsson, 1987; Einsiedel and Luff, 1992; Deschenes, 2004). Consequently, reduced maximal muscle strength, power and rate of force development are induced, and this translates into impaired daily physical activities, such as walking, stair climbing and rising from a seated position, leading to an increase in fall risk (Thelen et al., 2000; Madigan and Lloyd, 2005; Maki and McIlroy, 2006; Zietz et al., 2011). To consider the physiological causes combined with falls, it has been reported that the ability to recover from a fall depends largely on maximum stepping speed (Thelen et al., 1997; Wojcik et al., 1999), except when there are specific pathological reasons via other sensory systems and/or the central nervous system. An age-related reduction in stepping speed could potentially be caused by a reduction in joint-movement velocity in each localized individual joint of the body, and this further depends on the strength and velocity of each muscle. Furthermore, the strength and velocity of the muscle depends a great deal on the state of motor unit (MU) recruitment, particularly the high-threshold fast-twitch MUs (FF type). In this regard, age-related quantitative reductions specific to Type II muscle fibers (Lexell, 1995; Larkin et al., 2003; Deschenes, 2004) are considered to be a supportive reason for accidental falls after a stumble. These quantitative declines following aging, associated with reduced Type II muscle fibers, have been widely reported. However, qualitative changes, such as the recruitment state of MUs, the contraction and relaxing velocities during twitch contraction, and the muscle tenderness have not been well-documented in relation to aging and sarcopenia. In addition, there has been little information to directly connect the quantitative and qualitative data in relation to before and after the appearance of sarcopenia.

In this study, therefore, we used young, adult, middle-aged, and old-aged rats in order to assess before and after the appearance of sarcopenia. On that basis, apparent muscle atrophy (decreased muscle mass) and appearance of slow-type fiber groupings with loss of innervated nerve axons were used as markers of sarcopenia, and we then measured muscle shortening and relaxation velocity during serial twitch contractions as the markers for myosin head oscillation and ATP-dependent Ca^{++} pump functions. To clarify the changes in peripheral motor nervous system, we also recorded evoked electromyogram (EEMG) and contractility in response to stimulation frequencies from 10 to 140 Hz associated with tension output of twitch and tetanus. These measurements were performed under *in situ* electrical stimulation via the sciatic nerve on fast-type plantaris (PLT) and slow-type soleus (SOL) muscles. Muscle tenderness of extensor digitorum longus (EDL) muscles during isokinetic stretching were also measured. The results indicated that functional deterioration preceded the appearance of sarcopenia syndromes, and further suggested that habitual recruitment of FF-MUs during middle age may be an important factor in preventing the earlier appearance of sarcopenia syndromes.

MATERIALS AND METHODS

ANIMALS

Male Wistar rats aged 3 weeks were used as the Young group ($n = 10$), rats aged 12–17 weeks were used as the adult group ($n = 28$), rats aged 1.2–1.4 years were used as the middle-aged group ($n = 11$), and rats aged more than 2.5 years were used as the old-aged group ($n = 17$). Animals were housed in standard cages at a temperature of 23 ± 1°C and a 12-h light/dark cycle was used throughout the experiment. All experimental procedures were conducted in accordance with the Japanese Physiological Society Guide for the Care and Use of Laboratory Animals, and were approved by the Tokai University School of Medicine Committee on Animal Care and Use.

EVALUATION OF SARCOPENIA

First evaluation of sarcopenia was performed based on the standard relationship between body and plantaris (PLT) muscle mass, as reported previously (Tamaki and Uchiyama, 1995). Basically, growth of the body and PLT muscle mass shows a proportional relationship equation curve, and hypertrophied and/or atrophied muscle is seen as a change in this equation curve ($n = 528$, aged 2–60 week-old, refer to **Figure 2**).

FUNCTIONAL MEASUREMENT

The twitch and tetanic tension outputs of the right plantaris (PLA) and left soleus (SOL) muscles were measured and compared among the adult ($n = 27$), middle-aged ($n = 6$), and old-aged ($n = 11$) groups. Measurements were performed *in situ* under inhalation anesthesia (Isoflurane; Abbot, Osaka, Japan), and body (rectal) temperature was maintained at 36 ± 1°C with a radiant heat light throughout the measurement. The reference muscles and sciatic nerves (about 15 mm) on both sides were carefully exposed, and tissues were coated with mineral oil to prevent tissue drying and to minimize electric-noise interference. A bipolar silver (Ag/Ag) electrode (inter-electrode distance: 2 mm) was placed under the sciatic nerve and a stainless steel hook was attached to the distal tendon of each reference muscles using silk ligature. The animal was transferred to a custom-made operating table that allowed stabilization of the head and limbs in a prone position using surgical tape. A stainless steel hook was attached to a force-distance transducer (FD-Pickup, TB-611T; Nihon Kohden, Tokyo, Japan) connected to a carrier amplifier (AP-621G; Nihon Kohden). A bipolar silver electrode (inter-electrode distance: 5/1 mm diameter) was also attached to the surface of the reference muscle in order to obtain an evoked electrical myogram (EEMG). Care was taken to avoid interference with the normal blood supply of the reference muscles. Twitches were then elicited using single pulse (1 ms duration, 0.5 Hz) electrical stimulation via the sciatic nerve, at a voltage above the threshold for maximum response (1.5–3.0 V). Serial twitch responses (10 times) were recorded on a personal computer after analog/digital (A/D) conversion (sampling rate was set at 5–10 kHz). Subsequently, the peak tetanic tension was determined using stimulation frequencies of 10, 20, 40, 60, 80, 100, 120, and 140 Hz at 10-s intervals. The frequency that produced the highest tetanic tension was considered to be the optimal stimulation for tetanus. All mechanical and electrical measurements were recorded on a Linearcorder (Mark VII, WR3101; Graphtec, Tokyo, Japan) as analog raw data. Digital data was stored on the personal computer using an A/D converter (MacADIOS II; GW Instruments, Somerville, MA) and was analyzed by SuperScript II software (GW Instruments). Importantly, in the present functional measurement, we used a force-distance transducer that was able to add a variable spring load at 0–500 g to maintain a linear and proportional relationship with 0–6.0 mm displacement. Using this force/distance transducer, we detected shortening and relaxation velocity during dynamic twitch contractions (10 twitches), and calculated these as 10% changes. Calibration of the force/distance transducer in the range used in twitch analysis is presented in **Supplementary Figure S1**.

MEASUREMENT OF MUSCLE TENDERNESS

Muscle tenderness (isokinetic stretch-absorption) was also measured using the force/distance transducer above (TB-611T; Nihon Kohden, **Figure 1A**). In this measurement, EDL muscles were used because of their characteristics, as follows; (1) muscle-tendon junctions are easily detectable, and are on the distal and proximal ends; and (2) it is a multijoint muscle that spans the knee and ankle, thus receiving growth effects from crural bone length in the hindlimb. EDL muscles were obtained from the

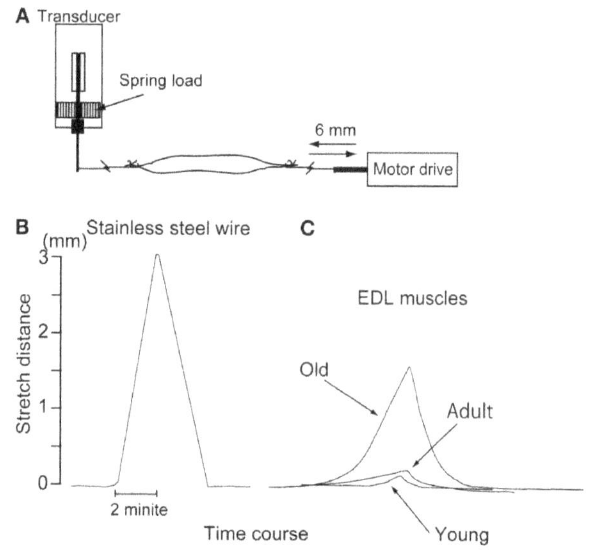

FIGURE 1 | Schematic drawing of the muscle tenderness measurement method (A) and representative raw data for stainless steel wire (B) and three types of muscle (C). Muscle stretch/return speed was strictly regulated by electric motor drive micrometer at 1.5 mm/min. Stainless wire showed a symmetric response as it was a non-elastic substance **(B)**, but the muscles showed apparently different responses as they are elastic substances **(C)**. This measurement could be established by using a force/distance transducer, which would have the ability to vary with both the force and distance (see **Supplementary Figure S1**).

young ($n = 4$), adult ($n = 5$), and old-aged ($n = 4$) rats under overdose with sodium pentobarbital (60 mg/kg, i.p.). Stainless steel hooks were attached to both the distal and proximal ends. The proximal end was connected with the force/distance transducer, and the distal end was connected to the electric motor drive micrometer (EMDM). The muscle was then stretched in isokinetic mode (stable speed: 1.5 mm/min) using EMDM both absolutely (6 mm each) and relatively (14% of entire *in situ* EDL length), and return and displacement curves were recorded using Linearcorder (Graphtec). The outline of this method, and typical measurements are presented in **Figure 1A**. In this case, if the material had no elasticity, such as stainless steel wire, linear changes with absolute stretch length (3 mm) were recorded as symmetrical with the stretch-return phase (see **Figure 1B**). However, if the materials had elasticity and/or tenderness, stretch effects were absorbed and changes were reduced according to the stretch-absorbed capacity (see **Figure 1C**). Note that linearly increased spring load was equally added to the reference muscles during the 6-mm stretch and return phase. Values were presented as the absolute and relative muscle tenderness calculated as % absorption when stretched 6 mm each and/or 14% of the entire EDL muscle length *in situ*.

HISTOCHEMICAL AND IMMUNOHISTOCHEMICAL STAINING

Animals were anesthetized by overdose with sodium pentobarbital (60 mg/kg, i.p.), blood removal was performed through cardiac puncture, and plantaris (PLT) muscles were excised and weighed. In this analysis, adult ($n = 6$–10), middle-aged ($n = 4$–6), and old-aged ($n = 4$–10) rats were used. Muscles were then quick frozen in isopentane pre-cooled with liquid nitrogen, and were stored at −80°C until use. Subsequently, several 7-μm cross-sections were obtained. In order to detect the nerve fiber degeneration and/or decline in PLT muscle, localization of nerve fibers (axons) was detected using rabbit polyclonal anti-Neurofilament 200 (N-200, 1:1000, room temperature for 1 h; Sigma, Saint Louis, MO). Similarly, the presence of myelination was also detected by rabbit polyclonal anti-myelin basic protein (MBP; 1:200, room temperature for 2 h; Millipore, Billerica, MA). Rabbit polyclonal anti-collagen I (ab34714; 1:100, room temperature for 1 h; Abcam, Tokyo, Japan) was used to evaluate the increase in connective tissue content in the muscle following aging. In addition, myosin ATPase (mATPase) after acid preincubation (pH 4.3 and 4.6) was used to characterize the fiber type in the muscle. After staining of collagen and ATPase, we calculated the percentage of collagen Type I area, and the percentage distribution of Type-I, Type-IIa, and Type-IIb fibers per unit area using a Stereo-investigator system (mbf Bioscience; Micro Bright Field Inc., Williston, VT) and Photoshop (Adobe). Analysis was performed in 4–5 sections per sample, and 6–9 unit areas were selected in each section (refer to representative analysis in **Figure 11**).

STATISTICAL ANALYSIS

All data are expressed mean's ± *SE*. Differences between controls and experimental groups were determined using Dunnet *post-hoc* multi-comparison method, and Tukey–Kramer *post-hoc* multi-comparison was used for all individual differences. Differences between selected groups were determined by Student's *t*-test. Standard regression analysis and Pearson's product correlation procedures were used to determine the relationship between body and muscle mass, and calibration of the transducer. Differences were considered to be statistically significant at either the $P < 0.05$ (in the figures) or $P < 0.01$ (in the table) level.

RESULTS

CONFIRMATION OF SARCOPENIA

First, occurrence of sarcopenia in the muscles in old-aged rats was confirmed using standard indices for body and PLT muscle mass (**Figure 2**). This index was based on 528 rats, between 2 and 60 weeks of age, and weighing between 25 and 650 g. A very high correlation coefficient was observed between body and PLT muscle mass ($R^2 = 0.9735$). However, the old-aged rats showed lower relative muscle masses from the established standard range, indicating that age-dependent muscle atrophy (sarcopenia) occurred. In addition, apparent increases in Type-I fibers with aggregated fiber-type grouping, which is a typical characteristic of sarcopenia (Lexell and Downham, 1991; Saini et al., 2009; Kung et al., 2014), was evident in the histochemical ATPase staining in PLT muscles in old-aged rats (**Figures 3C–F**), whereas uniform distribution was observed in adult rats (**Figure 3A**). Increases in Type-I fibers in basically fast PLT muscles of normal adult rats were also usually observed after 6 weeks of chronic stretch stimulation following surgical ablation of synergistic SOL and gastrocnemius muscles. However, in such cases, increases in Type-I fibers showed a relatively uniform trend, as was seen in normal controls

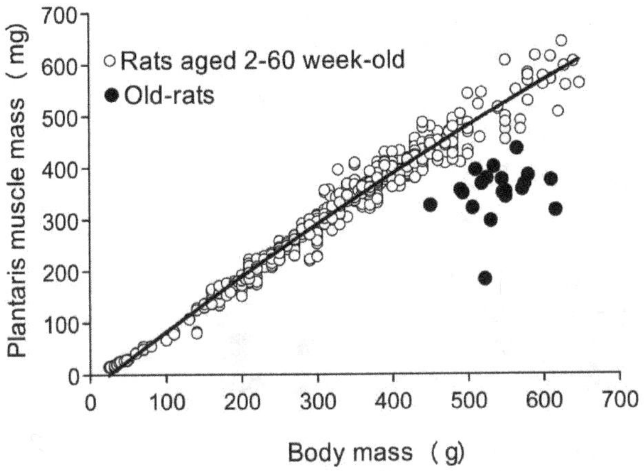

FIGURE 2 | The standard index for body and PLT muscle mass based on over 500 rats. The equation for the correlation coefficient curve is $y = -8E-10x^3 + 6E-07x^2 + 0.0009x - 0.0161$, and $R^2=0.9735$. Old-aged rats (closed circle) were clearly showed far below the standard curve, indicating muscle atrophy.

(**Figure 3B**), as a result of physiological stimulation (chronic stretch). Therefore, the appearance of fiber-type groupings in the present old-aged rats was considered to be due to type S MU remodeling following degradation of type F (FF, FR) units, which was also a typical trend in sarcopenia. The above trends were also supported by the results of axons and myelin staining for the dominant nerves in PLT muscles in the old-aged, middle-aged, and adult rats (**Figure 4A**). Both types of staining were sparse in the old-aged rats, suggesting a relative decrease in the number of axons (red reactions of N200) and myelin (red reactions of MBP) in the old-aged rats, whereas the middle-aged and adult rats showed similar results. When there were calculated, the old-aged rats showed significantly lower values in the number of axons and myelin compared to both adult and middle-aged (**Figure 4B**). This also indicates age-dependent decreases in the number of MUs in the present old-aged rats. Note that apparent differences between the adult and middle-aged rats were not detected in this analysis.

ASSESSMENT OF MUSCLE TENSION OUTPUT

Using the above groups of rats, we measured *in situ* muscle contraction characteristics via electrical stimulation through the sciatic nerve and performed analyses based on body and muscle mass. The stats for PLT muscle functions are summarized in **Figure 5**. In this analysis, the older two groups showed significantly higher body mass than adults, with the highest levels seen in the middle-aged group. However, for PLT muscle mass, the same trend as for body mass was observed between the adult and middle-aged groups, but significantly lower values were observed in the old-aged group. Consequently, the muscle/body mass index (relative muscle mass) was largely the same in the adult and middle-aged groups, but the old-aged group showed significantly lower values, as was seen in **Figure 2**. For the functions, age-dependent significant decreases in absolute twitches and tetanus were observed among the three groups, and a similar trend was also seen in relative tensions/body mass. However, significant differences between the middle- and old-aged disappeared when they were compared by relative tension/muscle mass, while a significantly higher value was observed in the adult group. These results indicate two important points: (1) in the middle-aged rat PLT muscles, muscle atrophy was not seen, but functional decreases were already significant, and the assumed body-supportive effects were also significantly diminished; and (2) in the old-aged rat PLT muscle, three sarcopenia factors, functional deterioration and decreased body-supportive effects were apparent, but tension/muscle mass did not differ from the middle-aged group.

The stats for SOL muscle function are summarized in **Figure 6**. The trend was apparently different from PLT muscles. The same trend for mean body mass was observed, but significant differences were seen only between the adult and middle-aged groups. However, the adult and middle-aged groups showed similar absolute muscle mass, and the old-aged group showed a significantly lower value than the other two groups. Age dependent significant decreases were seen in muscle mass index. In functional examinations, as a whole, the adult group showed higher values than the two older groups; however, significant differences were observed only in the twitch/body mass and absolute tetanus. Interestingly, functions in the old-aged group were comparatively similar or rather higher than in the middle-aged group, both absolutely and relatively. Taken together, volumetric decreases following aging were also evident in slow-type SOL muscle, but the functional decreases were less than in the fast PLT muscle.

MUSCLE SHORTENING AND RELAXING VELOCITY DURING TWITCH CONTRACTION

Muscle shortening and relaxing velocity was also compared among the three groups at 10% divisions during twitch (**Figure 7**). In the PLT muscle, the older two groups showed significantly lower values when compared with the adult group in all division stages through the shortening and relaxing phase (**Figure 7A**). This group difference trend was similar to the results for tension output (as shown in **Figure 5**). In a comparison between the middle-aged and old-aged groups, significant decreases in the old-aged group could be seen in the 20–70% range during the shortening phase and in the 10–0% range in the relaxing phase. In this regard, it is likely that the myosin head oscillation was easily affected by aging in the fast-type PLT muscles. However, comparatively lower values were seen in the old-aged group when compared with the middle-aged throughout the shortening-relaxing phase (**A**).

In the SOL muscle (**Figure 7B**), comparative functional decreases were seen throughout the shortening-relaxing phase in the two older groups when compared with the adult group, but significant differences were detected during the 70–30% range in the relaxing phase (**B**), in contrast to the PLT muscle (**A**). Thus, it is likely that the aging effects are smaller in the slow-type SOL muscle than in the fast-type PLT muscle (compare **A** and **B**), and the influence was apparent in the relaxing phase, which was assumed to be due to the ATP-dependent Ca^{++} pump functions of the sarcoplasmic reticulum. However, there were no differences

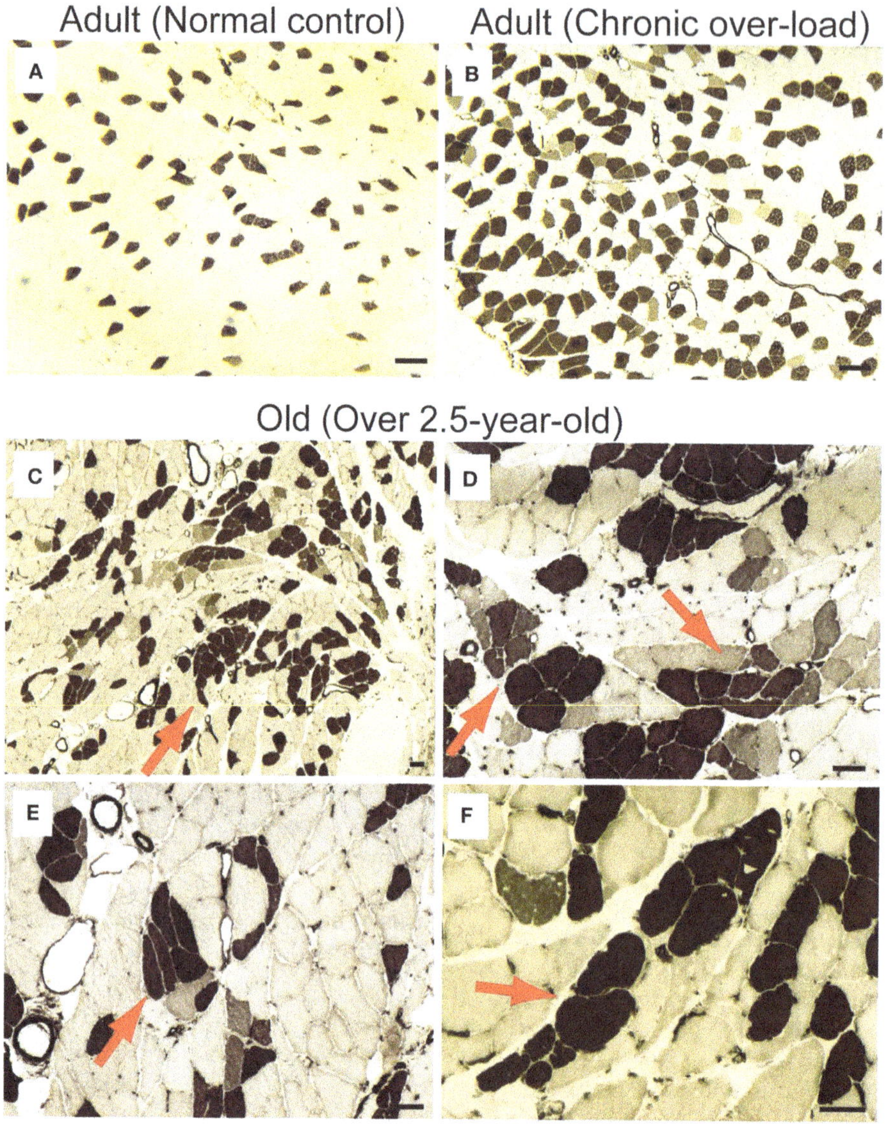

FIGURE 3 | ATPase staining for adult (A, 15-week-old) and old-aged (C–F, 136–139-week-old) rat PLT muscles. ATPase staining was performed after incubation at pH 4.3; thus, Type I fibers were stained dark. Note that **(B)** is a comparative positive control for ATPase staining using compensatory hypertrophied PLT muscle after 6 weeks of surgical ablation of synergistic gastrocnemius and soleus muscles (16-week-old rats). This demonstrated that the shift to slow fibers occurred after chronic stretch stimulation. However, slow-type fiber grouping was evident in the old-aged PLT muscle **(C)**, suggesting remodeling of S-type motor units in the process of sarcopenia (red arrows in **C–F**). Panels **(D–F)** shows higher magnification of **(C)**. Bars in **(A,B)** = 100 μm, **(C–F)** = 50 μm.

between the two older groups throughout the shortening-relaxing phase. These data also indicate that the functional declines in shortening-relaxing velocity of slow-type SOL muscle already occurred in the middle-aged group and did not develop until to old age.

EVALUATION OF MUSCLE FIBER TYPE DISTRIBUTION IN ADULT vs. MIDDLE-AGED GROUPS

With regard to the decline in shortening-relaxing velocity in the middle-aged group without an apparent decrease in muscle mass, we further examined muscle fiber type distribution in PLT muscles (**Figure 8**). For this analysis, the old-aged group was eliminated because they showed significant decreases in muscle mass and increases in Type I fibers with typical grouping (**Figure 3**), and this corresponded to the literature (Kung et al., 2014). Therefore, advanced analysis was performed between the adult and middle-aged groups. In the ATPase (pH 4.6) staining of whole cross-sections, dark-brown Type I fibers were impressively higher in middle-aged than in adult rats, whereas Type IIa (relative white in **C**) and IIb (light-brown in **C**) fibers were similar (**Figures 8A** vs. **B**). However, when these distributions were calculated, there were significant increases in Type I and decreases in Type IIb fibers, and non-significant changes in Type IIa fibers were observed in the middle-aged group (**Figure 8D**).

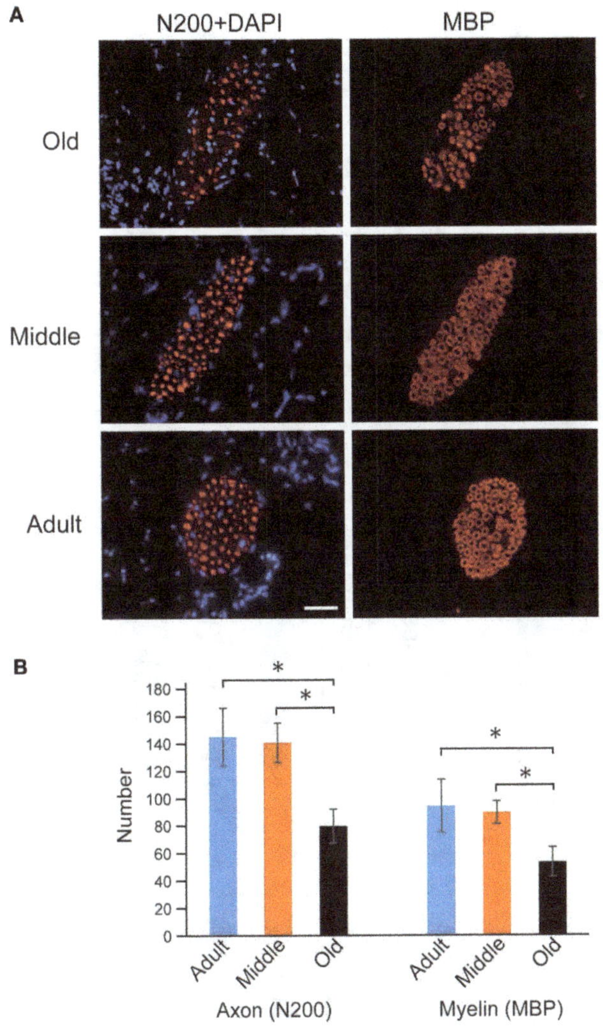

FIGURE 4 | Axon (N-200) and myelin (MBP) immunostaining for dominant nerve in PLT muscles (A), and their statistics (B). Reactions were relatively sparse in the old-aged group when compared to middle-aged and adult rats **(A)**. The number of axons and myelin were 80 ± 12 and 53 ± 11 in old-aged, 141 ± 14 and 90 ± 8 in middle-aged, and 145 ± 21 and 95 ± 19 in adult, thus showing that significant decrease was occurred in the old-aged rats. Blue nuclear staining is DAPI. Bar = 50 μm and all photographs were at the same magnification. *$P < 0.05$.

Thus, the shift from Type IIb to Type I fibers appears to begin in middle-aged rats, corresponding to the results of twitch-shortening and -relaxing velocity (**Figure 7A**), while muscle mass was maintained (**Figure 5**).

FORCE DEPRESSIONS DURING TETANIC STIMULATIONS

In addition to the declines in muscle contractile ability (as in **Figures 5–7**), we also detected force depressions in the older two groups during *in situ* tetanic stimulations. Typical measurement of force depressions in the old-aged rats are shown in **Figure 9**. Sudden force depression was detected at over 50 Hz stimulation following depression of EEMG (surface electrode), whereas normal discharges and tetanus was seen at 40 Hz (**A**). However, this trend disappeared when stimulation returned to 40 Hz. This phenomenon was confirmed in several repetitions, and means that force depressions were caused by the cut-off of electrical discharge. Subsequently, we cut the sciatic nerve (sciatectomy) at the upper portion of the stimulation site in order to confirm whether electrical depression occurred in the MN pool of the ventral horn of the spinal cord or neuromuscular junctions. We then obtained complete tetanus at 40- to 100-Hz stimulation without any force, and EEMG depression following a gradual increase in tension outputs (**B**). Therefore, this test clearly indicated that the cause of electrical cut off occurred in the spinal cord. An increase in tension output was also evident after sciatectomy (compare **A** to **B**). This also showed that recruitment of the MU, which was responsible for higher stimulation frequency, occurred after sciatectomy, and further suggested that the high threshold large MNs were affected under *in situ* physiological conditions before sciatectomy. Interestingly, the same and/or similar trends were observed in 73% (8/11) of PLT and 13% (1/8) of SOL muscles in old-aged rats, and 1/6 of middle-aged PLT and SOL muscles.

Furthermore, the two above cases in the old-aged rats (2/8) continued to show abnormalities after sciatectomy. Thus, these two cases also had abnormalities in the neuromuscular junction. A typical symptom in these two cases was depressed transmission that was enhanced after fatigue. A typical pattern of abnormal neuromuscular transmission is shown in **Figure 10**. When tetanic stimulation was repeatedly added, the trends on EEMG and tension depression gradually became heavier following repetitions (arrows in **Figure 10**). Tension output appeared to completely disappear when the EEMG amplitude decreased to less than 0.4 mV, and then discharge wholly disappeared also at around 50 repetitions.

COMPARISON OF MUSCLE TENDERNESS AND CONNECTIVE TISSUE CONTENT

With regard to the force depression in the older two groups during *in situ* tetanic stimulation, we believe that the muscle stiffness is closely related, and tenderness of the EDL muscle was compared among very young (age, 3-weeks; positive control), adult, and old-aged rats (**Table 1**). It is natural that EDL muscle length is significantly shorter in young rats when compared with the other two groups, but there were no significant differences between the adult and old-aged groups. However, significant differences were seen in both absolute and relative tenderness between all three groups. Young rats showed the highest absorption of stretching effects, even under the unfavorable conditions of this measurement, because of the shortest muscle length. In this regard, the condition of adult and old-aged rats was same, but the old-aged group showed substantial and significant losses in tenderness when compared with adults. Thus, age (sarcopenia)-dependent increases in massive muscle stiffness occurred in old-aged rats.

In order to confirm whether a similar event occurred in PLT muscles, we performed the immunohistochemical analysis of the connective tissues (collagen Type-I) in the adult, middle-aged, and old-aged groups (**Figures 11A–C**). As expected, the old-aged group showed significantly higher contents than the other two groups (**C** and **E**). However, there were no differences in the connective tissue contents between the adult and middle-aged groups

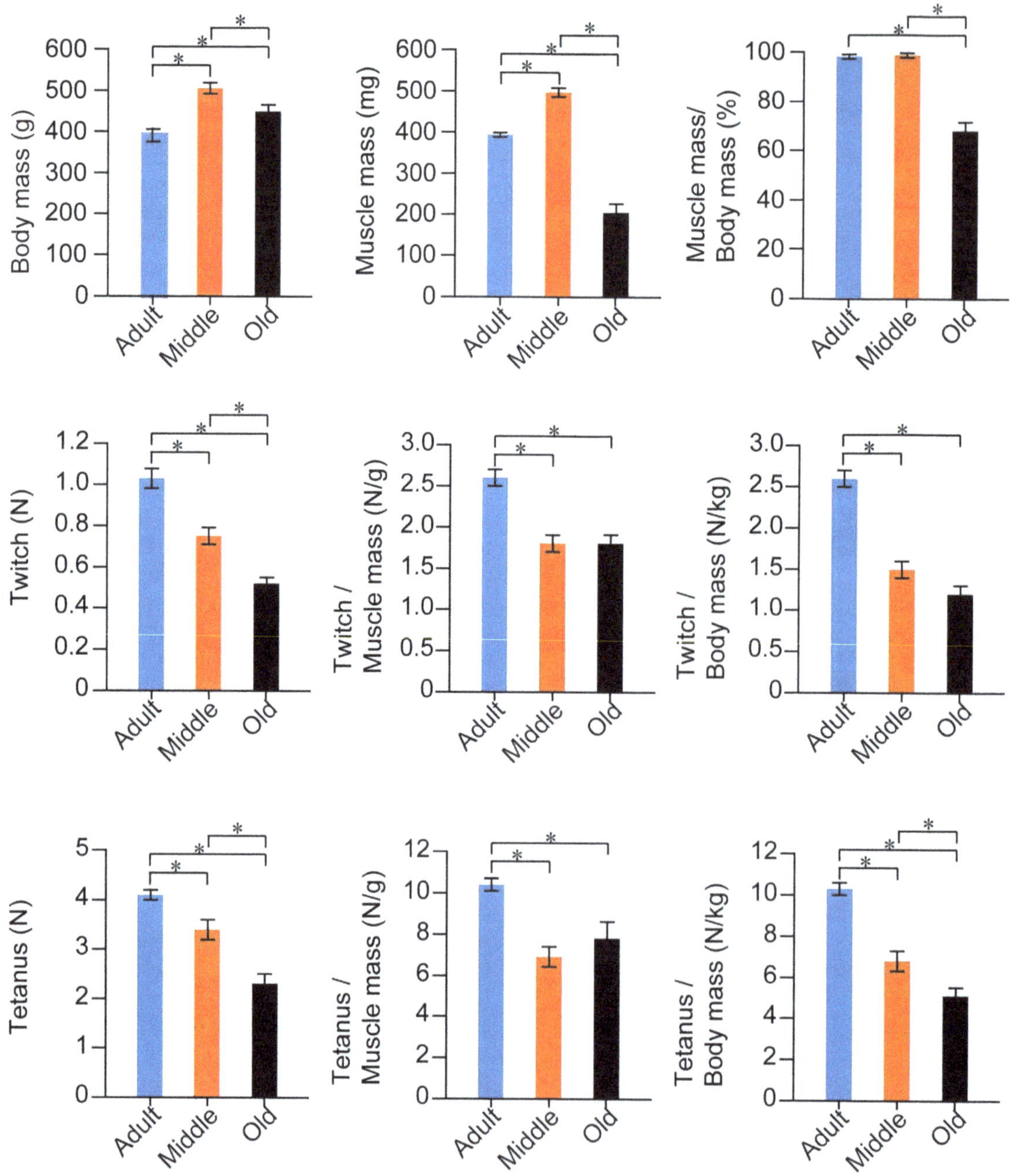

FIGURE 5 | Stats for PLT muscle functions in the three groups. Muscle twitches and tetanus are expressed in terms of Newtons (N), and are evaluated as absolute and relative (per muscle and body mass) values. There were numerous significant differences among the three groups in all items in fast-type PLT muscles. $^{*}p < 0.05$.

(**B** and **E**); thus, it appears that the increase in muscle stiffness did not occur in the middle-aged group. These data suggest that muscle stiffness may also be higher in the old-aged PLT muscles, because of the increased connective tissue contents, and further suggest that this affects the functional aspects of the PLT muscle.

DISCUSSION

In the present study, the old-aged rats clearly showed the typical characteristics of sarcopenia, such as loss of muscle mass and strength, and slow-type fiber grouping associated with a significant reduction in the number of innervated nerve axons and myelin, specifically in fast-type PLT muscles, while the slow-type SOL muscle showed relatively mild syndromes. This is consistent with sarcopenia syndromes in humans and the experimental animals (Tomlinson and Irving, 1977; Edstrom and Larsson, 1987; Einsiedel and Luff, 1992; Deschenes, 2004). Therefore, the present old-aged rats represent a suitable sarcopenia model. In this regard, the present qualitative findings in the peripheral motor system

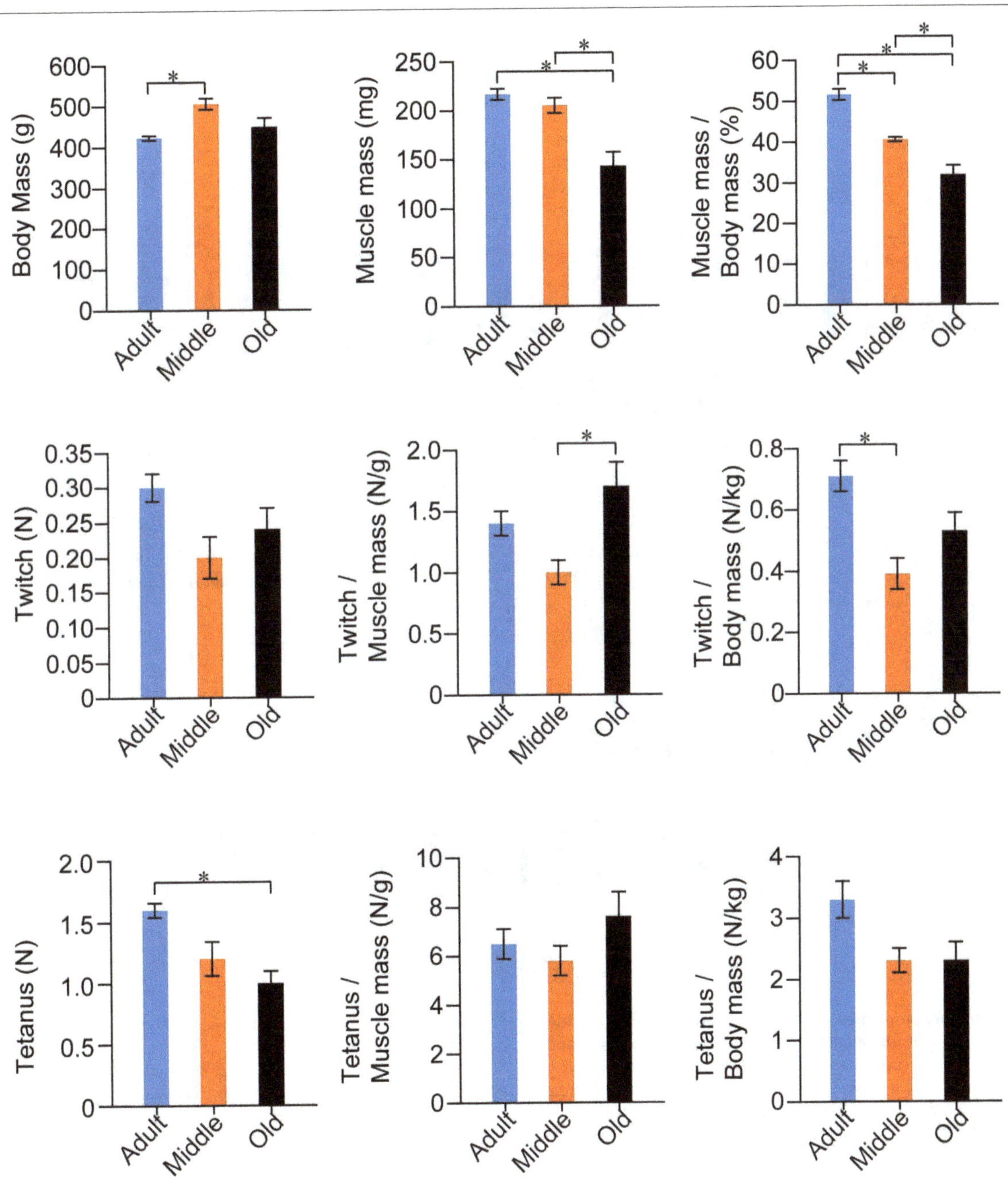

FIGURE 6 | Stats for SOL muscle functions in the three groups. Muscle twitches and tetanus are expressed in terms of Newtons (N), and are evaluated as absolute and relative (per muscle and body mass) values. Overall significant differences among the three groups were apparently lower in slow-type SOL when compared with fast-type PLT muscles (see previous **Figure 5**), thus suggesting that functional decreases were more apparent in fast-type muscle with aging. $*p < 0.05$.

could be also considered in the etiology and/or pathogenesis of sarcopenia: (1) reduction of shortening and relaxing velocity during serial twitch contractions; (2) decline of muscle tenderness (increased muscle stiffness following the increase in the connective tissue component); (3) impaired recruitment of MUs (sudden depression of tetanic force and EEMG) appearing during higher stimulation frequencies (over 50–60 Hz); and (4) easy fatigability in neuromuscular junctions. To our knowledge, there have been few reports describing such observations and their interrelationships in relation to sarcopenia. Concurrently, these data support several typical behaviors seen in elderly humans.

The present impaired recruitment of MUs during higher frequencies suggests the poor recruitment of high threshold fast-type MUs, and this would lead to lower muscle power output, as is observed by muscle weakness in the elderly. It is also plausible that a lower discharge rate during maximal contractions in

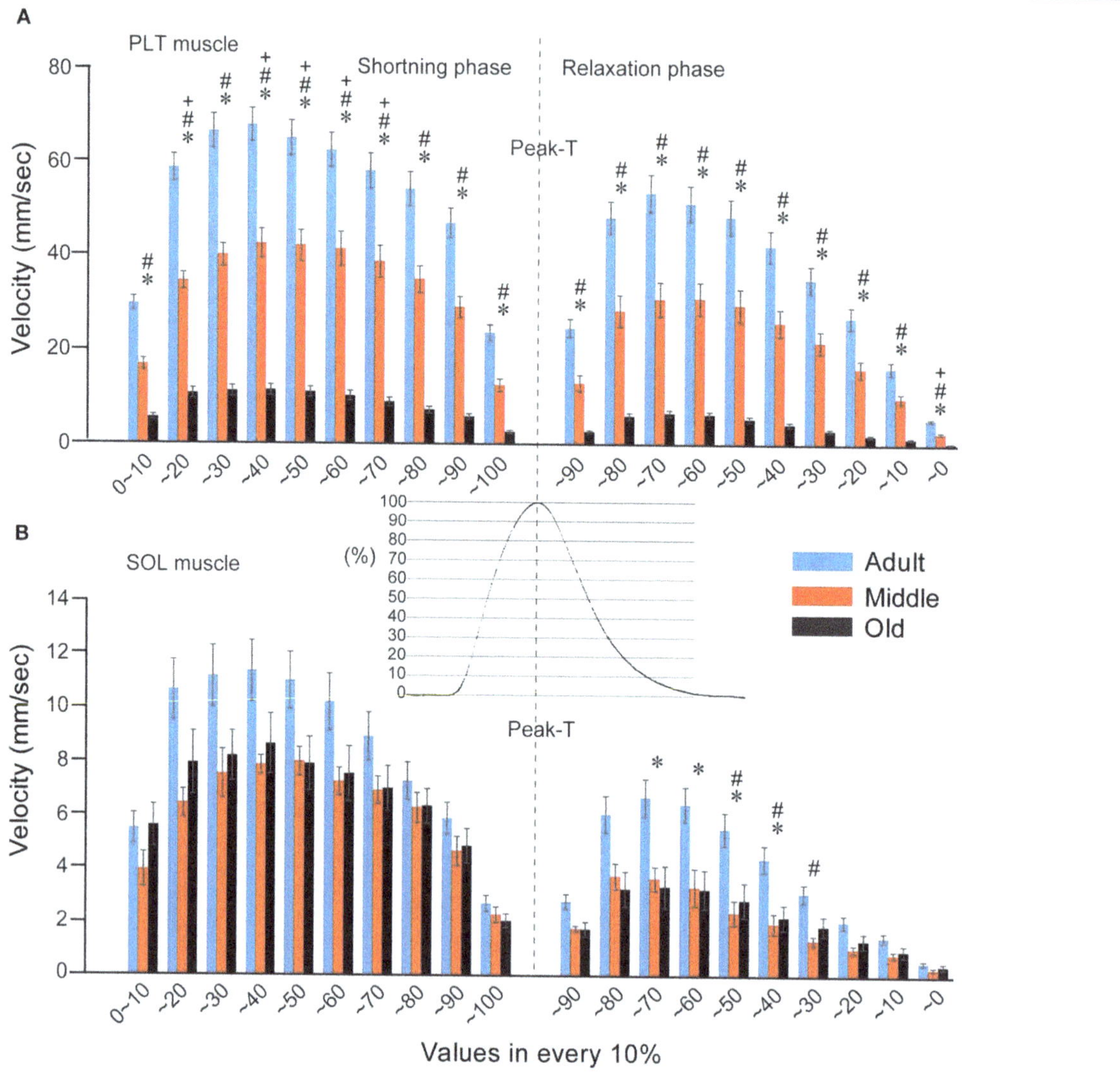

FIGURE 7 | Comparison of muscle shortening and relaxing velocity in both PLT (A) and SOL (B) muscles among adult, middle-aged, and old-aged rats. Gradual decreases in both velocities in the three age groups were evident in the fast-type PLT muscle **(A)**. Similarly, decreases were observed between the adult and middle-aged groups, but there were no significant differences between the middle-aged and old-aged groups in slow-type SOL **(B)**. Typical raw data for twitch tension curves in PLT muscle are shown out in central area. Velocity was averaged in 10% divisions from 10 serial twitches and is presented as group values (mean's ± *SE*). $^{*}P < 0.05$, $^{\#}P < 0.05$, $^{+}P < 0.05$.

the muscles of human lower-extremity has been reported (Kamen et al., 1995; Klass et al., 2007). Age-related decreases in MU discharge rate and force control during isometric planter flection have also been reported, even in submaximal contractions (Kallio et al., 2012). These decreases in MU discharge rate are closely related to the higher amplitude of force fluctuations in the old-age than that of the young (Enoka et al., 2003; Kallio et al., 2012). It has also been suggested that the decreased MU discharge rate is an adaptation to the increased twitch duration to optimize force generation, because twitch duration increases with age, tetanus could theoretically be achieved with lower discharge rate (Roos et al., 1997, 1999). Therefore, the present significant declines in shortening and relaxing velocity during twitch in old-aged rats (**Figure 7**) reasonably supported this notion.

Importantly, the present results demonstrate that the cause of these phenomena exists in the spinal cord complex, as was clearly confirmed by the higher tensions of complete tetanus at 50- to 100-Hz stimulation after sciatectomy in the old-aged rats (**Figure 9**). This result also demonstrated the important fact that neural alterations preceded reductions in peripheral muscle substance itself. Therefore, neural qualitative changes preceded quantitative changes following sarcopenia. We believe that the significant increase in connective tissues in the old-aged rats (**Figure 11**) may play a key role for the alteration of the spinal cord reflex arc. There are several possibilities regarding the related mechanisms: (1) the poor recruitment of high threshold fast-type MUs was caused by pre-synaptic inhibition in the MN pool of the ventral horn; (2) the strong firing of Golgi tendon organs (GTO)

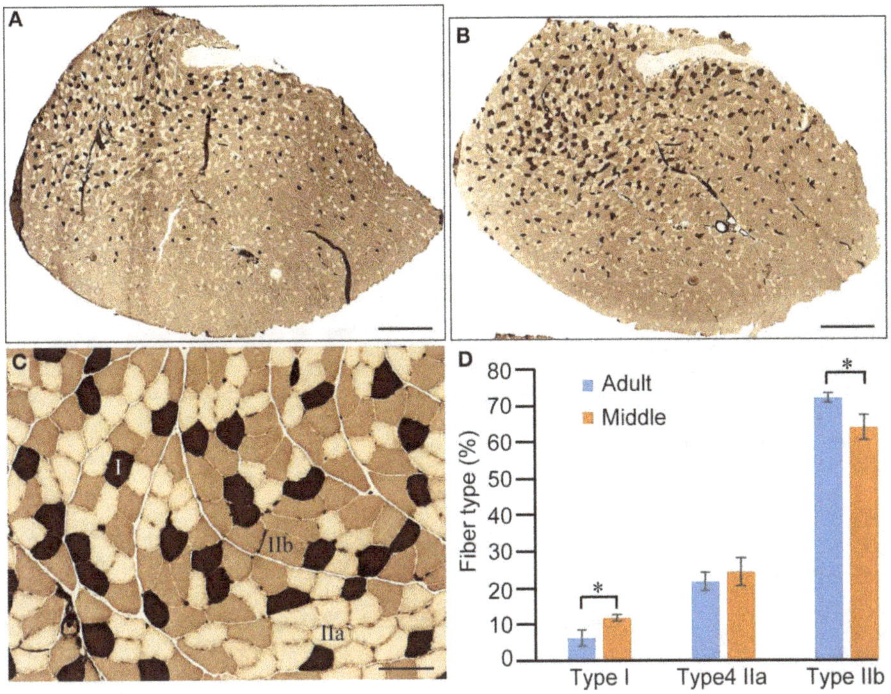

FIGURE 8 | Comparison of fiber-type components in PLT muscle between adult and middle-aged rats. Whole PLT sections were stained for ATPase (preincubation, 4.6); thus, the darkest staining represents Type I, medium Type IIb, and light Type IIa **(C)**. This is likely to give the impression that the distribution of Type I fibers is slightly higher in middle-aged rats **(B)** than in adult rats **(A)**. Differences were significant when calculated per unit area (section) for Type I and Type IIb **(D)**, thus confirming the histochemical changes from fast- to slow-type fibers. Bars in **(A,B)** = 1 mm, **(C)** = 100 μm. $^*P < 0.05$.

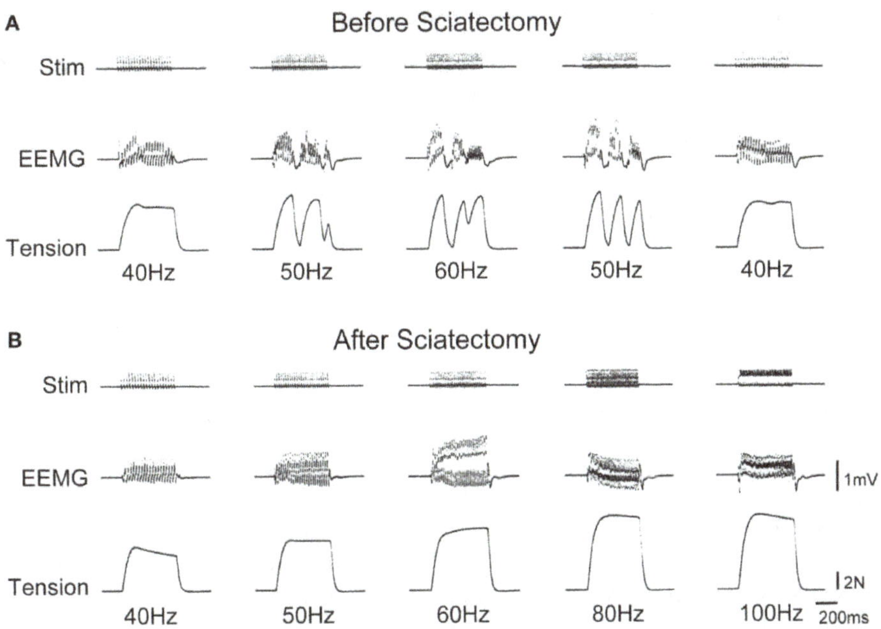

FIGURE 9 | Typical depressions of EEMG and tension force in old-aged rats *in vivo* before (A) and after (B) sciatectomy. Sudden depression of EEMG and tension force occurred after 50-Hz stimulation, but this recovered when stimulation returned to 40 Hz **(A)**. However, there were no abnormalities observed after sciatectomy in the proximal portion from stimuli, even through 100 Hz **(B)**, thus suggesting that the cause of the decrease originated in the spinal cord. Stim, stimulation; EEMG, evoked electro-myogram; N, newton.

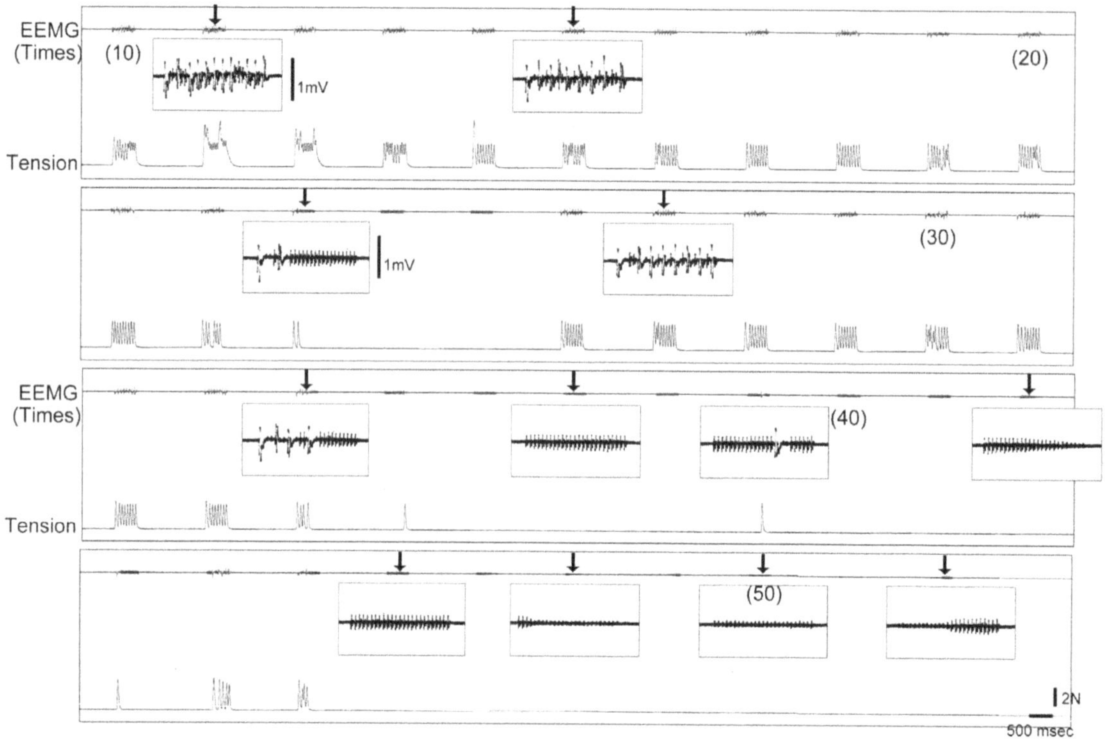

FIGURE 10 | Typical pattern of failure transmission in neuromuscular junction of old-aged rats after sciatectomy. Gradual decrease in electrical activity associated with tension outputs could be seen following repetitive tetanic stimulation (50 Hz), and this wholly disappeared around 50 times. EEMG, evoked electro-myogram; N, newton.

Table 1 | Comparison of muscle tenderness among 3-week-old, adult, and old-aged rats.

	EDL muscle length *in situ* (mm)	Absolute tenderness (absorbed % when stretched 6 mm)	Relative tenderness (absorbed % when stretched 14% of *in situ* muscle length)
3 week-old ($n = 4$)	16.6 ± 0.3	97.9 ± 0.6	99.1 ± 0.4
Adult ($n = 5$)	38.6 ± 0.8	94.1 ± 0.9	94.7 ± 0.8
Old ($n = 4$)	42.3 ± 3.6	78.2 ± 2.1	78.2 ± 2.1
3 week vs. adult	$^{**}P \leq 0.01$	$^{**}P \leq 0.01$	$^{**}P \leq 0.01$
3 week vs. old	$^{**}P \leq 0.01$	$^{**}P \leq 0.01$	$^{**}P \leq 0.01$
Adult vs. old	ns	$^{**}P \leq 0.01$	$^{**}P \leq 0.01$

may frequently occur *in vivo* by the increase in muscle stiffness (decreased tenderness) in the old-aged rats in daily life; (3) this trend raises the sensitivity of GTO and may have resulted in facilitating the autogenetic inhibition by type Ib afferent fibers; and (4) autogenetic inhibition may be induced under the submaximal voluntary contraction (SMVC), such as the force output at 50-Hz stimulation, whereas the peripheral muscle itself retained the ability to follow 100-Hz stimuli. It is also likely that there is a mechanism for increasing the sensitivity of the recurrent inhibition of Renshaw cells, but this was not confirmed.

With the regard to ease of falling in the elderly, increased muscle stiffness through the increase in interstitial connective tissues probably also affects the sensitivity of muscle spindles. Lower sensitivity in isolated spindle afferents from the medial gastrocnemius muscle of older rats in both dynamic and static states has been reported (Miwa et al., 1995). The rationale is that increased stiffness in the spindle capsule due to the presence of more intracapsular collagen decreases dynamic sensitivity, and reduces the opening of sensory spirals. This mechanism may largely blunt the stretch-reflex *in vivo*, which is mainly related to FF-type motor units (FF-MUs), and results in insufficient exertion of instant muscle power to postural maintenance. This mechanism may also be closely related to the ability to recover from a fall, particularly in the quick response to sudden, unanticipated body imbalance, and this depends largely on maximum stepping speed (Thelen et al., 1997, 2000; Wojcik et al., 1999). For this reason, decreased recruitment and/or use of FF-MUs in daily life also facilitates the disuse depending on decreases in FF-MUs,

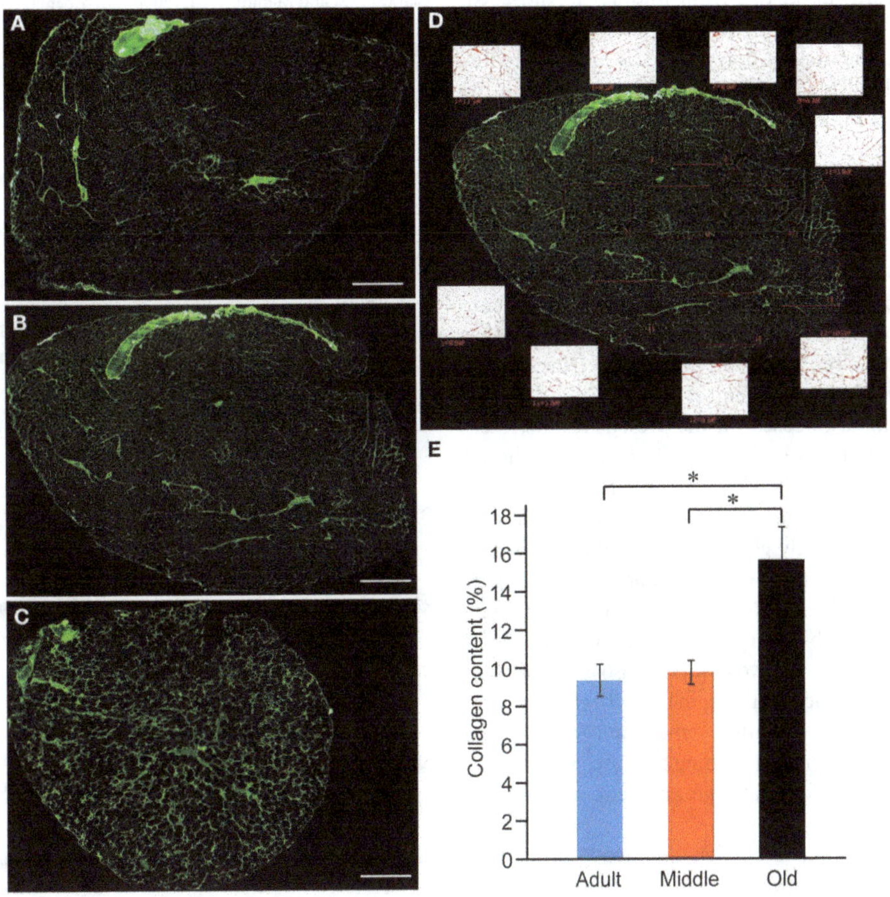

FIGURE 11 | Immunohistochemical detection of connective tissues (anti-collagen type-I) in adult (A), middle-aged (B), and old-aged (C) rat PLT muscles. A large volume of connective tissues could be seen in old-aged rats (**A,B** vs. **C**). These were calculated in terms of percent (%) content/sections, and significant increases were evident in old-aged rats **(E)**. Panel **(D)** shows typical analysis method for middle-aged muscle. Bars in **(A–C)** = 1 mm. $^*p < 0.05$.

as defined by remodeling of MU with slow-type fiber grouping in the present old-aged rats.

For the easy fatigability of neuromuscular junctions in old-aged rats (**Figure 10**), this may be the result of a decline in synaptic metabolic rate, because of evidence that the height of EEMG decreased and disappeared even after 20–30 repetitions of tetanus. Generally, such symptoms are not observed in normal adults over 100 repetitions. Thus, impaired uptake and/or metabolism of acetylcholine in the synaptic vesicles may be a mechanism in this case. However, this sign was observed in 2 of 8 abnormal old-aged rats; thus, it was considered to be a more progressive stage symptom of sarcopenia.

More importantly, the present study showed that a significant decrease in muscle shortening and relaxing velocity during serial twitch contractions with a shift from Type-IIb to Type-I fibers without any muscle atrophy could be detected in PLT muscle from middle-aged rats. These results indicate that qualitative decreases had begun, even in middle-aged rats, which showed no typical sarcopenia symptoms. This notion was well supported by the observation that a significant decrease in tension output both in the absolute and relative twitch and tetanus was also evident in the middle-aged rats when compared with adults (**Figure 7**). This state was considered to be the early stage of "dynapenia," which consists of age-associated loss of muscle strength and power (Clark and Manini, 2012). The contributors to dynapenia are compartmentalized into two factors; (1) neurologic, and (2) skeletal muscle properties. As these factors control muscle force production (Clark and Manini, 2008; Clark, 2009), muscle size plays a relatively minor role. In this regard, the present neural and mechanical data demonstrated the potential antecedent mechanisms to dynapenia. In addition, in the analysis of shortening and relaxing velocity during twitch, a deeper influence of aging could be observed in the shortening phase of PLT and in the relaxing phase of SOL muscle. The former mainly depended on the ability of myosin head oscillation, and the latter mainly depended on ATP-dependent Ca^{++} pump functions in the sarcoplasmic reticulum (**Figures 7A,B**). Thus, this was also assumed to be the potential antecedent mechanisms for dynapenia on fast (PLT) and slow (SOL)-type muscles. Interestingly, similar functional decrease in the slow-type SOL muscles compared to the adult were observed both in the middle- and old-aged rats, in contrast to the age-related gradual decrease in the fast-type PLA, through the functional assessments of present study. It was supposed that this trend may represent the minimal physical/functional requirement of standard life in rats from middle- to old-aged. In other words, standard life in middle- to old-aged rats may be mainly covered by the functions of slow type MUs such as remaining in the SOL muscles. This is why; progressive decrease in the function could be seen in fast-type PLT, while the ceasing to fall at minimal requirements were observed in slow-type SOL muscle. Taken together, it is possible that dynapenia precedes sarcopenia, and/or the pathogenesis of dynapenia is the start of sarcopenia. Therefore, the present data suggests that preventing the loss of muscle tenderness and high-threshold fast-type MUs during middle age is important for the relief of subsequent sarcopenia syndrome. This notion is also supported by the observation that 1/6 of middle-aged rats already showed impaired recruitment of the MUs at higher stimulation frequency.

Considering human cases based on the present results, exercise with the preferential use of F-type (FF, FR) MUs should be performed habitually in daily life to prevent their decline of them, particularly in middle age (age, 40–60 years), that can be expecting the retain of relatively good motor abilities. This may be a good contributor to the relief of sarcopenia syndrome, particularly for falls in the elderly. Preventing the loss of muscle tenderness (ability of stretch-absorption), which is induced by increases in excess muscle connective tissues, is also an important factor, because of its influence in the spinal-cord reflex system. However, specific ideas for prevention remain uncertain in the present study, although moderate stretching of muscles with optimal nutrition may a provide foundation for prevention of muscle tenderness.

In conclusion, we demonstrated that qualitative alterations in the peripheral motor system, such as the impaired recruitment of high-threshold fast-type MUs, impaired transmission of neuromuscular junction following fatigue, loss of muscle tenderness (significantly increased muscle stiffness due to the increase in muscle connective tissues), and significant decreases of shortening-relaxing velocity during serial twitch contractions occurred as typical symptoms of dynapenia/sarcopenia syndrome. These factors may be closely related to the spinal-cord reflexes, such as the stretch and the autogenetic inhibition reflex, and decreases in these abilities can make the elderly more prone to falls.

ACKNOWLEDGMENTS

This work was supported by a Grant-in-aid for Scientific Research (C-249590303) from the Ministry of Education, Science and Culture of Japan.

SUPPLEMENTARY MATERIAL

Supplementary Figure S1 | Calibration of the force-distance transducer. High linearity was confirmed both in relation to the distance and force following quite similar equations.

REFERENCES

Clark, B. C. (2009). *In vivo* alterations in skeletal muscle form and function after disuse atrophy. *Med. Sci. Sports Exerc.* 41, 1869–1875. doi: 10.1249/MSS.0b013e3181a645a6

Clark, B. C., and Manini, T. M. (2008). Sarcopenia =/= dynapenia. *J. Gerontol. A Biol. Sci. Med. Sci.* 63, 829–834. doi: 10.1093/gerona/63.8.829

Clark, B. C., and Manini, T. M. (2012). What is dynapenia? *Nutrition* 28, 495–503. doi: 10.1016/j.nut.2011.12.002

Cruz-Jentoft, A. J., Baeyens, J. P., Bauer, J. M., Boirie, Y., Cederholm, T., Landi, F., et al. (2010). Sarcopenia: European consensus on definition and diagnosis: report of the European working group on Sarcopenia in older people. *Age Ageing* 39, 412–423. doi: 10.1093/ageing/afq034

Deschenes, M. R. (2004). Effects of aging on muscle fibre type and size. *Sports Med.* 34, 809–824. doi: 10.2165/00007256-200434120-00002

Edstrom, L., and Larsson, L. (1987). Effects of age on contractile and enzyme-histochemical properties of fast- and slow-twitch single motor units in the rat. *J. Physiol.* 392, 129–145.

Einsiedel, L. J., and Luff, A. R. (1992). Alterations in the contractile properties of motor units within the ageing rat medial gastrocnemius. *J. Neurol. Sci.* 112, 170–177. doi: 10.1016/0022-510X(92)90147-D

Enoka, R. M., Christou, E. A., Hunter, S. K., Kornatz, K. W., Semmler, J. G., Taylor, A. M., et al. (2003). Mechanisms that contribute to differences in motor performance between young and old adults. *J. Electromyogr. Kinesiol.* 13, 1–12. doi: 10.1016/S1050-6411(02)00084-6

Kallio, J., Sogaard, K., Avela, J., Komi, P., Selanne, H., and Linnamo, V. (2012). Age-related decreases in motor unit discharge rate and force control during isometric plantar flexion. *J. Electromyogr. Kinesiol.* 22, 983–989. doi: 10.1016/j.jelekin.2012.05.009

Kamen, G., Sison, S. V., Du, C. C., and Patten, C. (1995). Motor unit discharge behavior in older adults during maximal-effort contractions. *J. Appl. Physiol. (1985)* 79, 1908–1913.

Klass, M., Baudry, S., and Duchateau, J. (2007). Voluntary activation during maximal contraction with advancing age: a brief review. *Eur. J. Appl. Physiol.* 100, 543–551. doi: 10.1007/s00421-006-0205-x

Kung, T. A., Cederna, P. S., Van Der Meulen, J. H., Urbanchek, M. G., Kuzon, W. M., and Faulkner, J. A. Jr. (2014). Motor unit changes seen with skeletal muscle sarcopenia in oldest old rats. *J. Gerontol. A Biol. Sci. Med. Sci.* 69, 657–665. doi: 10.1093/gerona/glt135

Lang, T., Streeper, T., Cawthon, P., Baldwin, K., Taaffe, D. R., and Harris, T. B. (2010). Sarcopenia: etiology, clinical consequences, intervention, and assessment. *Osteoporos. Int.* 21, 543–559. doi: 10.1007/s00198-009-1059-y

Larkin, L. M., Kuzon, W. M., and Halter, J. B. (2003). Effects of age and nerve-repair grafts on reinnervation and fiber type distribution of rat medial gastrocnemius muscles. *Mech. Ageing Dev.* 124, 653–661. doi: 10.1016/S0047-6374(02)00190-2

Lexell, J. (1995). Human aging, muscle mass, and fiber type composition. *J. Gerontol. A Biol. Sci. Med. Sci.* 50(Spec. No), 11–16.

Lexell, J., and Downham, D. Y. (1991). The occurrence of fibre-type grouping in healthy human muscle: a quantitative study of cross-sections of whole vastus lateralis from men between 15 and 83 years. *Acta Neuropathol.* 81, 377–381. doi: 10.1007/BF00293457

Madigan, M. L., and Lloyd, E. M. (2005). Age and stepping limb performance differences during a single-step recovery from a forward fall. *J. Gerontol. A Biol. Sci. Med. Sci.* 60, 481–485. doi: 10.1093/gerona/60.4.481

Maki, B. E., and McIlroy, W. E. (2006). Control of rapid limb movements for balance recovery: age-related changes and implications for fall prevention. *Age Ageing* 35(Suppl. 2), ii12–ii18. doi: 10.1093/ageing/afl078

Mitchell, W. K., Williams, J., Atherton, P., Larvin, M., Lund, J., and Narici, M. (2012). Sarcopenia, dynapenia, and the impact of advancing age on human skeletal muscle size and strength; a quantitative review. *Front. Physiol.* 3:260. doi: 10.3389/fphys.2012.00260

Miwa, T., Miwa, Y., and Kanda, K. (1995). Dynamic and static sensitivities of muscle spindle primary endings in aged rats to ramp stretch. *Neurosci. Lett.* 201, 179–182. doi: 10.1016/0304-3940(95)12165-X

Morley, J. E., Baumgartner, R. N., Roubenoff, R., Mayer, J., and Nair, K. S. (2001). Sarcopenia. *J. Lab. Clin. Med.* 137, 231–243. doi: 10.1067/mlc.2001.113504

Roos, M. R., Rice, C. L., Connelly, D. M., and Vandervoort, A. A. (1999). Quadriceps muscle strength, contractile properties, and motor unit firing rates in young and old men. *Muscle Nerve* 22, 1094–1103.

Roos, M. R., Rice, C. L., and Vandervoort, A. A. (1997). Age-related changes in motor unit function. *Muscle Nerve* 20, 679–690.

Saini, A., Faulkner, S., Al-Shanti, N., and Stewart, C. (2009). Powerful signals for weak muscles. *Ageing Res. Rev.* 8, 251–267. doi: 10.1016/j.arr.2009.02.001

Tamaki, T., and Uchiyama, S. (1995). Absolute and relative growth of rat skeletal muscle. *Physiol. Behav.* 57, 913–919. doi: 10.1016/0031-9384(94)00359-D

Thelen, D. G., Muriuki, M., James, J., Schultz, A. B., Ashton-Miller, J. A., and Alexander, N. B. (2000). Muscle activities used by young and old adults when stepping to regain balance during a forward fall. *J. Electromyogr. Kinesiol.* 10, 93–101. doi: 10.1016/S1050-6411(99)00028-0

Thelen, D. G., Wojcik, L. A., Schultz, A. B., Ashton-Miller, J. A., and Alexander, N. B. (1997). Age differences in using a rapid step to regain balance during a forward fall. *J. Gerontol. A Biol. Sci. Med. Sci.* 52, M8–M13. doi: 10.1093/gerona/52A.1.M8

Tomlinson, B. E., and Irving, D. (1977). The numbers of limb motor neurons in the human lumbosacral cord throughout life. *J. Neurol. Sci.* 34, 213–219. doi: 10.1016/0022-510X(77)90069-7

Wojcik, L. A., Thelen, D. G., Schultz, A. B., Ashton-Miller, J. A., and Alexander, N. B. (1999). Age and gender differences in single-step recovery from a forward fall. *J. Gerontol. A Biol. Sci. Med. Sci.* 54, M44–M50. doi: 10.1093/gerona/54.1.M44

Zietz, D., Johannsen, L., and Hollands, M. (2011). Stepping characteristics and centre of mass control during stair descent: effects of age, fall risk and visual factors. *Gait Posture* 34, 279–284. doi: 10.1016/j.gaitpost.2011.05.017

4

Insights into muscle degeneration from heritable inclusion body myopathies

Sabine Krause*

Laboratory for Molecular Myology, Department of Neurology, Friedrich Baur Institute, Ludwig Maximilians University, Munich, Germany

Correspondence:
Sabine Krause, Laboratory for Molecular Myology, Department of Neurology, Friedrich Baur Institute, Ludwig Maximilians University, Marchioninistr. 17, Munich 81377, Germany
e-mail: sabine.krause@med.uni-muenchen.de

Muscle mass and function are gradually lost in age-related, degenerative neuromuscular disorders, which also reflect the clinical hallmarks of sarcopenia. The consensus definition of sarcopenia includes a condition of age-related loss of muscle mass, quality, and strength. The most common acquired muscle disease affecting adults aged over 50 years is sporadic inclusion body myositis (sIBM). Besides inflammatory effects and immune-mediated muscle injury, degenerative myofiber changes are characteristic features of the disease. Although the earliest triggering events in sIBM remain elusive, a plethora of downstream mechanisms are implicated in the pathophysiology of muscle wasting. Although it remains controversial whether hereditary forms of inclusion body myopathy (IBM) may be considered as degenerative sIBM disease models, partial pathophysiological aspects can mimic the much more frequent sporadic condition, in particular the occurrence of inclusion bodies in skeletal muscle. Various clinical aspects in genetically determined skeletal muscle disorders reflect age-related alterations observed in sarcopenia. Several intriguing clues from monogenic defects in heritable IBMs contributing to the molecular basis of muscle loss will be discussed with special emphasis on inclusion body myopathy with Paget's disease of bone and frontotemporal dementia (IBMPFD) and GNE myopathy. Finally, also the recently identified dominant multisystem proteinopathy will be considered, which may rarely present as IBM.

Keywords: VCP/p97, IBMPFD, GNE myopathy, multisystem proteinopathy, HNRNPA1

INTRODUCTION

Pathogenic mutations in genes involved in diverse cellular pathways as VCP/p97, also called valosin-containing protein [resulting in autosomal-dominant inclusion body myopathy (IBM) associated with Paget's disease of bone and frontotemporal dementia, IBMPFD] and *GNE*, also referred to as UDP-*N*-acetyl-D-glucosamine 2-epimerase/*N*-acetylmannosamine kinase (GNE) (resulting in biallelic GNE myopathy) can elicit a pathophysiological phenotype in skeletal muscle that partially overlaps with histopathology findings in sporadic inclusion body myositis (sIBM), in particular the detection of inclusion bodies in skeletal muscle. While formal proof is lacking, it remains a hypothesis that genetically determined IBM syndromes may share some aspects of the pathogenetic cascade.

However, immune-mediated, inflammatory changes are a hallmark of sIBM and only a very rare exception in GNE myopathy (Krause et al., 2003; Yabe et al., 2003). Furthermore, the typical clinical presentation of sIBM features progressive muscle weakness in the knee extensors and the long finger flexors (Rose and ENMC IBM Working Group, 2013). By contrast, in GNE myopathy the quadriceps muscles are remarkably spared from muscle weakness (reviewed in Nishino et al., 2014). IBMPFD patients present clinically with a variable pattern of slowly progressive proximal and distal pareses (reviewed in Weihl et al., 2009). Scapular winging in IBMPFD may be as prominent as in neuromuscular shoulder girdle or limb girdle syndromes (Kimonis et al., 2008; Stojkovic et al., 2009).

VCP/p97 acts as an ubiquitin-selective multitasking switchboard in regulating basic cellular proteostasis including autophagy and myosin assembly in skeletal muscle (reviewed by Pokrzywa and Hoppe, 2013; Meyer and Weihl, 2014). GNE, the key enzyme of sialic acid biosynthesis, can regulate muscle glycoprotein sialylation and might contribute to additional cellular signaling pathways (reviewed by Nishino et al., 2014). *HNRNPA1*, the ubiquitously expressed gene for the heterogeneous nuclear ribonucleoprotein A1 is the causative gene for the rare multisystem proteinopathy, which may be associated with IBM was identified only very recently (Kim et al., 2013a).

In the adult-onset, heritable degenerative neuromuscular disorders, muscle mass and function are gradually lost and reflect the clinical hallmarks of sarcopenia. The consensus definition of sarcopenia includes a condition of age-related loss of muscle mass, quality, and strength (Cruz-Jentoft et al., 2010; Fielding et al., 2011). Key findings potentially related to sarcopenia at multiple levels of muscle metabolism in hereditary IBMs like IBMPFD and GNE myopathy as well as the HNRNPA1-associated multisystem proteinopathy presenting as IBM will be highlighted.

IBMPFD ASSOCIATED WITH VCP/p97 MUTATIONS

The multifaceted role of the AAA-family ATPase VCP/p97 in the pathophysiology of IBMPFD involves numerous essential signaling pathways governing cellular homeostasis and depends on the cellular context. To exploit the therapeutic potential of VCP/p97, it is important to understand how its activity is regulated and how specific organs and cells can be targeted to regulate the versatile enzyme. The specificity of VCP/p97 depends significantly on cofactors, which confer precise catalytic function. The majority of pathogenic mutations in VCP/p97 resulting in neuromuscular disorders are localized in the cofactor binding domain (Tang et al., 2010) and abrogate binding to a distinct subset of cofactors (Fernandez-Saiz and Buchberger, 2010).

Myosin filament assembly is disturbed in myogenic cells from IBMPFD patients *in vitro* (Janiesch et al., 2007). Functional development of striated muscle depends on the accurate organization of regulatory, structural, and motor proteins into basic contractile elements called the sarcomeres. VCP/p97 acts in a ternary complex together with the cofactors CHIP and UFD2a to tightly regulate the level of the myosin-directed chaperone Unc45 within confined limits, which allow proper myosin filament assembly and sarcomere formation (Janiesch et al., 2007). CHIP is also called carboxyl terminus of Hsp70-interacting protein. UFD2a is the human homolog of yeast UFD2a, also known as ubiquitination factor E4B (UBE4B) and human Unc45 is the homolog of the *C. elegans* Unc45 chaperone, which is essential to regulate myosin-directed functions from fungi to vertebrates (reviewed in Hellerschmied and Clausen, 2014). Defective myosin assembly may contribute to myofiber fragility and reduced mechanical stability. Inclusion bodies might develop secondary and due high amounts of accumulated, unassembled myosin in the sarcoplasm. Similarly, in another form of familial IBM (IBM 3), dominantly inherited mutations in the head domain of MYH2 (adult skeletal muscle myosin heavy chain 2, fast myosin IIa) render MYH2 filament proteins to aggregate (Martinsson et al., 2000; Tajsharghi et al., 2005). Deregulated, elevated levels of Unc45 in skeletal muscle of affected IBMPFD patients suggest a related, relevant myosin biosynthesis defect *in vivo*.

Furthermore, deregulation of major protein degradation pathways has been implicated in VCP/p97-related disorders (Ju et al., 2009a,b; Tresse et al., 2010). An imbalance in protein turnover contributes also to muscle loss in sarcopenia (Barns et al., 2014).

Primary human myoblasts containing disease-related VCP/p97 mutations revealed increased apoptosis and defective maturation to myotubes *in vitro* (Vesa et al., 2009). This suggests that IBMPFD satellite cells have a reduced regeneration capability, and may generate defective myotubes thus contributing to muscle degeneration.

Furthermore, VCP/p97 is essential for mitochondrial quality control by PINK1/Parkin (PTEN induced putative kinase 1), which is associated with autosomal-recessive early-onset Parkinson disease. PINK1 prevents stress-induced mitochondrial dysfunction. This important protective capacity is impaired by disease-related VCP/p97 mutations (Kim et al., 2013b). Mutant VCP/p97 malfunction involves recruitment to and clearance of damaged mitochondria. These processes are paralleled in part by the mitochondrial theory of aging, which predicts the accumulation of damage by reactive oxygen species (ROS) over time to lead to age-associated mitochondrial impairment (Cesari et al., 2012; Johnson et al., 2013).

Epigenetic changes have been implicated in sarcopenia; however, detailed evidence is limited (Ong and Holbrook, 2014). For efficient gene expression, dynamic cycles of monoubiquitylation and de-ubiquitylation are indispensable (Wyce et al., 2007). In a collaborative project, we defined a novel regulatory role of VCP/p97 in histone H2B metabolism, which is conserved from yeast to man. Moreover, in IBMPFD cells carrying a point mutation at the highly conserved residue R155H that does not affect the ATPase activity, H2B de-ubiquitylation was significantly delayed 48 h after induction of differentiation *in vitro*. Our findings further extend the functional spectrum of VCP/p97 and suggest an additional molecular pathomechanism for IBMPFD at the level of chromatin remodeling and transcription control (Bonizec et al., 2015).

GNE MYOPATHY

GNE myopathy is an inherited autosomal-recessive IBM. The causative gene was identified more than a decade ago (Eisenberg et al., 2001). The bi-functional enzyme UDP-*N*-acetyl-D-glucosamine 2-epimerase/*N*-acetylmannosamine kinase GNE is the key enzyme of the sialic acid biosynthesis pathway (Hinderlich et al., 1997; Stasche et al., 1997). Sialic acid deficiency and hyposialylation of glycoproteins and glycolipids appear to be a major underlying defect in GNE myopathy. Consistent with this hypothesis, a murine disease model for GNE myopathy shows clinical improvement of muscle strength and function upon metabolite supplementation of sialic acid or its precursor *N*-acetylmannosamine (ManNAc) (Malicdan et al., 2009). Notably in this context, monomeric sialic acids are decreased in quadriceps muscle of normal elder males (Marini et al., 2014). Although GNE myopathy patients can benefit from metabolic precursor supplementation (reviewed by Nishino et al., 2014), it cannot be excluded that GNE myopathy is caused by additional pathomechanisms (Krause et al., 2005; Wang et al., 2006; Amsili et al., 2008).

In a GNE myopathy patient myoblast culture model, a primary defect in response to apoptotic stimuli was observed, in particular an extended stabilization of pAkt expression (Amsili et al., 2007). Moreover, in age-related muscle deterioration a critical role for Akt has also been demonstrated (reviewed by Glass, 2003; Schiaffino and Mammucari, 2011).

Disturbance of apoptotic signaling was further supported by proteomic profiling of GNE myopathy muscle biopsy (Sela et al., 2011). In line with the hypothesis that alterations in mitochondrial metabolism might be a primary event in the pathogenetic cascade of GNE myopathy, mitochondrial deregulation was suggested at the transcriptome and morphological level (Eisenberg et al., 2008). It is well established that mitochondria are important regulators of apoptotic signaling and mitochondrial dysfunction can contribute to sarcopenia (reviewed in Marzetti et al., 2012; Marzetti et al., 2013). Although the data sets of individual proteins regulated in aging skeletal muscle differ substantially between individual proteomic surveys (Gelfi et al., 2006; Doran et al., 2007; O'Connell et al., 2007, 2008), the main trends of differentially expressed proteins involved in the cytoskeleton architecture, energy metabolism, contraction, cellular signaling and the stress response agree between various studies. These processes refer to general disturbances in skeletal muscle common to many myopathies and muscular dystrophies. In search of upstream events more specific to GNE myopathy, previously established transcriptomic data from 10 patients' muscle biopsies (Eisenberg et al., 2008; Table S1 in Supplementary Material) were revisited. Differentially *upregulated* genes in GNE myopathy (vs. control samples with $p \leq 0.002$) were reassessed utilizing the DAVID bioinformatics enrichment tool (Huang da et al., 2009a,b). Interestingly, a significant upregulation of *HNRNPA2B1* (1.3-fold; $p \leq 0.002$) was revealed along with additional RNA processing and transcription regulators including small nuclear ribonucleoprotein polypeptide G (*SNRNPG*), arginine/serine-rich-splicing factor 14 (*SUGP2/SFRS14*), TAR DNA binding protein (*TARDBP*), and heterogeneous nuclear ribonucleoprotein A3 (*HNRNPA3*). Although the upregulation of these RNA regulatory factors was comparably small, their impact on myocellular metabolism might be pathophysiologically meaningful.

Moreover, Activin A receptor, type II (*ACVR2*) was among the most significantly downregulated genes (−0.88-fold; $p \leq 0.002$) in GNE myopathy (Eisenberg et al., 2008; Table S1 in Supplementary Material). Activins are the most efficient negative regulators of muscle mass (Chen et al., 2014). It remains to be determined whether reduced *ACVR2* expression might represent a compensatory mechanism in GNE myopathy to escape or decrease loss of muscle mass.

Finally, re-evaluation by functional annotation clustering of *downregulated* genes in GNE myopathy (Eisenberg et al., 2008) with the DAVID bioinformatics resources revealed slightly reduced expression of nuclear or steroid hormone receptors including hepatocyte nuclear factor 4-gamma (*HNF4G*), nuclear receptor subfamily 1, group I, member 3 (*NR1I3*), and nuclear receptor subfamily 1, group H, member 2 (*NR1H2*). Also, vitamin D receptor (VDR) belongs to the large family of steroid hormone receptors. Intriguingly, VDR signaling has been implicated in the regulation of calcium homeostasis, myoblast proliferation, and differentiation and might be a future approach for treatment of sarcopenia (reviewed in Wagatsuma and Sakuma, 2014). It cannot be excluded that deregulation of other components of the nuclear or steroid hormone pathway can contribute to muscle weakness and wasting in GNE myopathy.

MULTISYSTEM PROTEINOPATHY ASSOCIATED WITH hnRNPA1 AND hnRNPA2B1 MUTATIONS

Autosomal-dominant mutations in the genes for the heterogeneous nuclear ribonucleoproteins *HNRNPA1* or *HNRNPA2B1* are rare causes for multisystem proteinopathy (Kim et al., 2013a). HnRNPA1 and hnRNPA2B1 are multifunctional RNA-binding proteins involved in the regulation of RNA biogenesis. The clinical phenotype may present as IBM and may be initially indistinguishable from the VCP/p97-related neuromuscular syndromes. The identified missense mutations are predicted to generate hyperstable multimers by their so-called "prion-like" domains (PrLDs), facilitate recruitment to stress granules, and drive cytoplasmic aggregate formation (Shorter and Taylor, 2013). Interestingly, also in sporadic IBM and VCP-associated myopathy, the subcellular distribution of wild type HNRNPs is altered in skeletal muscle suggesting disturbances in RNA metabolism (Pinkus et al., 2014) that might be a secondary event downstream of inflammation or protein dyshomeostasis. In multisystem proteinopathy, it remains to be determined whether hnRNPA1 or hnRNPA2B1 mutants (i) may form immediately cytotoxic oligomers, (ii) overload the proteolytic capacity of the cell, or (iii) sequester other essential proteins in cytoplasmic and nuclear aggregates. At the molecular level, also additional disease mechanisms are conceivable that may be reminiscent of sarcopenia and relate to age-dependent alterations in skeletal muscle. A well-established biomarker for cellular aging is the length of the protective caps at the physical ends of eukaryotic chromosomes, called telomeres, which shorten with each cell division cycle and with increasing chronological age. Telomerase activity is inhibited by large non-coding RNA referred to as telomeric repeat containing RNA (TERRA), which is transcribed from telomeres. Recent evidence suggests that balanced levels of hnRNPA1 and TERRA are required to regulate telomerase activity (Redon et al., 2013). This finding supports the idea that hnRNPA1 mutants might also disturb telomere formation and maintenance thereby contributing to premature aging and possibly sarcopenia.

Cellular senescence was initially defined as permanent growth arrest of primary human cells after repeated serial passaging *in vitro* (Hayflick and Moorhead, 1961). Cellular senescence is not only a safeguard against cancer but also of multifunctional physiological relevance in embryonic development, tissue repair, and aging. Novel discoveries support the hypothesis that senescence can be a highly dynamic, multi-step process (reviewed by van Deursen, 2014). Recent evidence demonstrated a close link between cellular senescence and age-dependent tissue deterioration (Baker et al., 2008). Aging increases CCN1/CYR61 expression leading to muscle senescence (Du et al., 2014). CCN1/CYR61 depends on exon skipping to provide functional protein (Hirschfeld et al., 2009). The matricellular protein CCN1/CYR61 contains several possible binding motifs (YAGR) in the exon 3–intron 3–exon 4 system for the transcription factor hnRNPA1. Disturbed or lacking HNRNPA1 due to sequestration in aggregates as suggested in multisystem proteinopathy might promote exon 3 inclusion, resulting in non-functional protein that might compromise muscle angiogenesis and endothelial cell survival (Leu et al., 2002).

CORRELATION WITH GENETIC SUSCEPTIBILITY OF SARCOPENIA AND AGE-RELATED GENE EXPRESSION IN SKELETAL MUSCLE

Hereditary IBM syndromes might involve cellular mechanisms previously related to sarcopenia and aging. Therefore, several representative susceptibility genes for sarcopenia (reviewed in Garatachea and Lucia, 2013) were evaluated to elucidate potential genetic correlations with hereditary IBMs.

A certain polymorphism in the *ACTN3* gene (R577X, rs1815739) is a well-established marker of a muscular endurance phenotype in humans. The precise localization of α-actinin 1 and GNE in the myofibrillar apparatus centered on the *Z* line remains elusive (Amsili et al., 2008). It is conceivable that physiological interaction by GNE with other resident components of the sarcomeric *Z*-disk might modulate cytoskeletal architecture and functions. Interestingly, GNE showed predominant protein expression in type II fibers in transversal muscle sections (Krause et al., 2007) and α-actinin 3 is also exclusively detected in fast-twitch (type II) fibers (Mills et al., 2001).

The myostatin phenotype is among the most favorable candidates to clarify variance among muscle phenotypes in the elder population (Garatachea and Lucia, 2013). Accordingly, also the downregulation of myostatin receptors can modulate myostatin signaling. As suggested in GNE myopathy, this mechanism could prevent muscle degeneration and might be considered an adaptive muscular response.

Epigenetic studies revealed that the differentially methylated regions related to aging are significantly enriched for muscle biogenesis (Ong and Holbrook, 2014). Similarly, VCP/p97 can regulate dynamics and chromatin organization by monoubiquitylation of histone H2B (Bonizec et al., 2015) and might contribute to pathogenic gene expression in IBMPFD.

CONCLUSION

In conclusion, it will be essential to continue studying fundamental cellular pathways underlying muscular hypertrophy and atrophy to advance the discovery of promising targets for the development of causative and safe therapies for skeletal muscle disorders.

An encouraging approach is a novel strategy to promote muscle maintenance and delay muscular atrophy by utilizing an antibody, which modulates the activin type II receptor (ActRII) response (Lach-Trifilieff et al., 2014). The wide therapeutic spectrum holds promise to treat a variety of progressive neuromuscular conditions regardless of the underlying molecular defect. Another example of a non-disease specific treatment option is the molecular chaperone 4-phenylbutyrate (4-PBA), an FDA-approved substance to treat children suffering from urea cycle disorders. 4-PBA acts as an ER stress inhibitor by aiding in protein folding and preventing misfolded protein accumulation and aggregation. Recently, convincing evidence was provided that 4-PBA might be also functional to resolve protein aggregates *in vitro* and *in vivo* and to improve grip strength in a mouse model for plectinopathy, a hereditary protein aggregate myopathy (Winter et al., 2014).

In summary, recent history of gene identification in hereditary inclusion body myopathies has fostered enthusiasm to facilitate detailed understanding of molecular disease mechanisms in these familial disorders. However, the involved genes show an unprecedented functional diversity.

Therefore, a plethora of key mechanisms underlying disease onset in hereditary IBMs remain to be elucidated at the molecular and physiological level, some of which may be also relevant for the etiology of sarcopenia. Neglected aspects that may be specific to the discussed hIBMs include regulation of RNA transcription and processing, cellular senescence, angiogenesis, and *Z*-disk architecture.

Understanding the deleterious combination of disease mechanisms in detail will be an important goal for future research to establish targeted intervention strategies and to prevent sarcopenia in those at risk to develop disease-associated or age-related muscle loss. Additionally and regardless of the underlying defect, it will be important for affected patients to immediately translate current broad understanding of muscle wasting and general advances to improve muscle function into safe, approved therapy. Clinically, meaningful improvements for patients suffering from sarcopenia, hereditary, or degenerative myopathies will be the challenging goal for the immediate future.

ACKNOWLEDGMENTS

This work was funded in part by intramural research grants from the Faculty of Medicine, Ludwig Maximilians University of Munich, Germany (FöFoLe 60/2012 and FöFoLe 41/2014) to SK.

REFERENCES

Amsili, S., Shlomai, Z., Levitzki, R., Krause, S., Lochmuller, H., Ben-Bassat, H., et al. (2007). Characterization of hereditary inclusion body myopathy myoblasts: possible primary impairment of apoptotic events. *Cell Death Differ.* 14, 1916–1924. doi:10.1038/sj.cdd.4402208

Amsili, S., Zer, H., Hinderlich, S., Krause, S., Becker-Cohen, M., Macarthur, D. G., et al. (2008). UDP-*N*-acetylglucosamine 2-epimerase/*N*-acetylmannosamine kinase (GNE) binds to alpha-actinin 1: novel pathways in skeletal muscle? *PLoS One* 3:e2477. doi:10.1371/journal.pone.0002477

Baker, D. J., Perez-Terzic, C., Jin, F., Pitel, K. S., Niederlander, N. J., Jeganathan, K., et al. (2008). Opposing roles for p16Ink4a and p19Arf in senescence and ageing caused by BubR1 insufficiency. *Nat. Cell Biol.* 10, 825–836. doi:10.1038/ncb1744

Barns, M., Gondro, C., Tellam, R. L., Radley-Crabb, H. G., Grounds, M. D., and Shavlakadze, T. (2014). Molecular analyses provide insight into mechanisms underlying sarcopenia and myofibre denervation in old skeletal muscles of mice. *Int. J. Biochem. Cell Biol.* 53, 174–185. doi:10.1016/j.biocel.2014.04.025

Bonizec, M., Herissant, L., Pokrzywa, W., Geng, F., Wenzel, S., Howard, G. C., et al. (2015). The ubiquitin-selective chaperone Cdc48/p97 associates with Ubx3 to modulate monoubiquitylation of histone H2B. *Nucleic Acids Res.* 42, 10975–10986. doi:10.1093/nar/gku786

Cesari, M., Fielding, R. A., Pahor, M., Goodpaster, B., Hellerstein, M., Van Kan, G. A., et al. (2012). Biomarkers of sarcopenia in clinical trials-recommendations from the International Working Group on Sarcopenia. *J. Cachexia Sarcopenia Muscle* 3, 181–190. doi:10.1007/s13539-012-0078-2

Chen, J. L., Walton, K. L., Winbanks, C. E., Murphy, K. T., Thomson, R. E., Makanji, Y., et al. (2014). Elevated expression of activins promotes muscle wasting and cachexia. *FASEB J.* 28, 1711–1723. doi:10.1096/fj.13-245894

Cruz-Jentoft, A. J., Baeyens, J. P., Bauer, J. M., Boirie, Y., Cederholm, T., Landi, F., et al. (2010). Sarcopenia: European consensus on definition and diagnosis: report of the European Working Group on Sarcopenia in older people. *Age Ageing* 39, 412–423. doi:10.1093/ageing/afq034

Doran, P., Gannon, J., O'Connell, K., and Ohlendieck, K. (2007). Aging skeletal muscle shows a drastic increase in the small heat shock proteins alphaB-crystallin/HspB5 and cvHsp/HspB7. *Eur. J. Cell Biol.* 86, 629–640. doi:10.1016/j.ejcb.2007.07.003

Du, J., Klein, J. D., Hassounah, F., Zhang, J., Zhang, C., and Wang, X. H. (2014). Aging increases CCN1 expression leading to muscle senescence. *Am. J. Physiol. Cell Physiol.* 306, C28–C36. doi:10.1152/ajpcell.00066.2013

Eisenberg, I., Avidan, N., Potikha, T., Hochner, H., Chen, M., Olender, T., et al. (2001). The UDP-*N*-acetylglucosamine 2-epimerase/*N*-acetylmannosamine kinase gene is mutated in recessive hereditary inclusion body myopathy. *Nat. Genet.* 29, 83–87. doi:10.1038/ng718

Eisenberg, I., Novershtern, N., Itzhaki, Z., Becker-Cohen, M., Sadeh, M., Willems, P. H., et al. (2008). Mitochondrial processes are impaired in hereditary inclusion body myopathy. *Hum. Mol. Genet.* 17, 3663–3674. doi:10.1093/hmg/ddn261

Fernandez-Saiz, V., and Buchberger, A. (2010). Imbalances in p97 co-factor interactions in human proteinopathy. *EMBO Rep.* 11, 479–485. doi:10.1038/embor.2010.49

Fielding, R. A., Vellas, B., Evans, W. J., Bhasin, S., Morley, J. E., Newman, A. B., et al. (2011). Sarcopenia: an undiagnosed condition in older adults. Current consensus definition: prevalence, etiology, and consequences. International working group on sarcopenia. *J. Am. Med. Dir. Assoc.* 12, 249–256. doi:10.1016/j.jamda.2011.01.003

Garatachea, N., and Lucia, A. (2013). Genes and the ageing muscle: a review on genetic association studies. *Age (Dordr)* 35, 207–233. doi:10.1007/s11357-011-9327-0

Gelfi, C., Vigano, A., Ripamonti, M., Pontoglio, A., Begum, S., Pellegrino, M. A., et al. (2006). The human muscle proteome in aging. *J. Proteome Res.* 5, 1344–1353. doi:10.1021/pr050414x

Glass, D. J. (2003). Signalling pathways that mediate skeletal muscle hypertrophy and atrophy. *Nat. Cell Biol.* 5, 87–90. doi:10.1038/ncb0203-87

Hayflick, L., and Moorhead, P. S. (1961). The serial cultivation of human diploid cell strains. *Exp. Cell Res.* 25, 585–621. doi:10.1016/0014-4827(61)90192-6

Hellerschmied, D., and Clausen, T. (2014). Myosin chaperones. *Curr. Opin. Struct. Biol.* 25, 9–15. doi:10.1016/j.sbi.2013.11.002

Hinderlich, S., Stasche, R., Zeitler, R., and Reutter, W. (1997). A bifunctional enzyme catalyzes the first two steps in *N*-acetylneuraminic acid biosynthesis of rat liver. Purification and characterization of UDP-*N*-acetylglucosamine 2-epimerase/*N*-acetylmannosamine kinase. *J. Biol. Chem.* 272, 24313–24318. doi:10.1074/jbc.272.39.24313

Hirschfeld, M., Zur Hausen, A., Bettendorf, H., Jager, M., and Stickeler, E. (2009). Alternative splicing of Cyr61 is regulated by hypoxia and significantly changed in breast cancer. *Cancer Res.* 69, 2082–2090. doi:10.1158/0008-5472.CAN-08-1997

Huang da, W., Sherman, B. T., and Lempicki, R. A. (2009a). Bioinformatics enrichment tools: paths toward the comprehensive functional analysis of large gene lists. *Nucleic Acids Res.* 37, 1–13. doi:10.1093/nar/gkn923

Huang da, W., Sherman, B. T., and Lempicki, R. A. (2009b). Systematic and integrative analysis of large gene lists using DAVID bioinformatics resources. *Nat. Protoc.* 4, 44–57. doi:10.1038/nprot.2008.211

Janiesch, P. C., Kim, J., Mouysset, J., Barikbin, R., Lochmuller, H., Cassata, G., et al. (2007). The ubiquitin-selective chaperone CDC-48/p97 links myosin assembly to human myopathy. *Nat. Cell Biol.* 9, 379–390. doi:10.1038/ncb1554

Johnson, M. L., Robinson, M. M., and Nair, K. S. (2013). Skeletal muscle aging and the mitochondrion. *Trends Endocrinol. Metab.* 24, 247–256. doi:10.1016/j.tem.2012.12.003

Ju, J. S., Fuentealba, R. A., Miller, S. E., Jackson, E., Piwnica-Worms, D., Baloh, R. H., et al. (2009a). Valosin-containing protein (VCP) is required for autophagy and is disrupted in VCP disease. *J. Cell Biol.* 187, 875–888. doi:10.1083/jcb.200908115

Ju, J. S., Miller, S. E., Jackson, E., Cadwell, K., Piwnica-Worms, D., and Weihl, C. C. (2009b). Quantitation of selective autophagic protein aggregate degradation in vitro and in vivo using luciferase reporters. *Autophagy* 5, 511–519. doi:10.4161/auto.5.4.7761

Kim, H. J., Kim, N. C., Wang, Y. D., Scarborough, E. A., Moore, J., Diaz, Z., et al. (2013a). Mutations in prion-like domains in hnRNPA2B1 and hnRNPA1 cause multisystem proteinopathy and ALS. *Nature* 495, 467–473. doi:10.1038/nature11922

Kim, N. C., Tresse, E., Kolaitis, R. M., Molliex, A., Thomas, R. E., Alami, N. H., et al. (2013b). VCP is essential for mitochondrial quality control by PINK1/Parkin and this function is impaired by VCP mutations. *Neuron* 78, 65–80. doi:10.1016/j.neuron.2013.02.029

Kimonis, V. E., Mehta, S. G., Fulchiero, E. C., Thomasova, D., Pasquali, M., Boycott, K., et al. (2008). Clinical studies in familial VCP myopathy associated with Paget disease of bone and frontotemporal dementia. *Am. J. Med. Genet. A* 146A, 745–757. doi:10.1002/ajmg.a.31862

Krause, S., Aleo, A., Hinderlich, S., Merlini, L., Tournev, I., Walter, M. C., et al. (2007). GNE protein expression and subcellular distribution are unaltered in HIBM. *Neurology* 69, 655–659. doi:10.1212/01.wnl.0000267426.97138.fd

Krause, S., Hinderlich, S., Amsili, S., Horstkorte, R., Wiendl, H., Argov, Z., et al. (2005). Localization of UDP-GlcNAc 2-epimerase/ManAc kinase (GNE) in the golgi complex and the nucleus of mammalian cells. *Exp. Cell Res.* 304, 365–379. doi:10.1016/j.yexcr.2004.11.010

Krause, S., Schlotter-Weigel, B., Walter, M. C., Najmabadi, H., Wiendl, H., Muller-Hocker, J., et al. (2003). A novel homozygous missense mutation in the GNE gene of a patient with quadriceps-sparing hereditary inclusion body myopathy associated with muscle inflammation. *Neuromuscul. Disord.* 13, 830–834. doi:10.1016/S0960-8966(03)00140-8

Lach-Trifilieff, E., Minetti, G. C., Sheppard, K., Ibebunjo, C., Feige, J. N., Hartmann, S., et al. (2014). An antibody blocking activin type II receptors induces strong skeletal muscle hypertrophy and protects from atrophy. *Mol. Cell. Biol.* 34, 606–618. doi:10.1128/MCB.01307-13

Leu, S. J., Lam, S. C., and Lau, L. F. (2002). Pro-angiogenic activities of CYR61 (CCN1) mediated through integrins alphavbeta3 and alpha6beta1 in human umbilical vein endothelial cells. *J. Biol. Chem.* 277, 46248–46255. doi:10.1074/jbc.M209288200

Malicdan, M. C., Noguchi, S., Hayashi, Y. K., Nonaka, I., and Nishino, I. (2009). Prophylactic treatment with sialic acid metabolites precludes the development of the myopathic phenotype in the DMRV-hIBM mouse model. *Nat. Med.* 15, 690–695. doi:10.1038/nm.1956

Marini, M., Ambrosini, S., Sarchielli, E., Thyrion, G. D., Bonaccini, L., Vannelli, G. B., et al. (2014). Expression of sialic acids in human adult skeletal muscle tissue. *Acta Histochem.* 116, 926–935. doi:10.1016/j.acthis.2014.03.005

Martinsson, T., Oldfors, A., Darin, N., Berg, K., Tajsharghi, H., Kyllerman, M., et al. (2000). Autosomal dominant myopathy: missense mutation (Glu-706 – > Lys) in the myosin heavy chain IIa gene. *Proc. Natl. Acad. Sci. U.S.A.* 97, 14614–14619. doi:10.1073/pnas.250289597

Marzetti, E., Calvani, R., Bernabei, R., and Leeuwenburgh, C. (2012). Apoptosis in skeletal myocytes: a potential target for interventions against sarcopenia and physical frailty – a mini-review. *Gerontology* 58, 99–106. doi:10.1159/000330064

Marzetti, E., Calvani, R., Cesari, M., Buford, T. W., Lorenzi, M., Behnke, B. J., et al. (2013). Mitochondrial dysfunction and sarcopenia of aging: from signaling pathways to clinical trials. *Int. J. Biochem. Cell Biol.* 45, 2288–2301. doi:10.1016/j.biocel.2013.06.024

Meyer, H., and Weihl, C. C. (2014). The VCP/p97 system at a glance: connecting cellular function to disease pathogenesis. *J. Cell. Sci.* 127, 3877–3883. doi:10.1242/jcs.093831

Mills, M., Yang, N., Weinberger, R., Vander Woude, D. L., Beggs, A. H., Easteal, S., et al. (2001). Differential expression of the actin-binding proteins, alpha-actinin-2 and -3, in different species: implications for the evolution of functional redundancy. *Hum. Mol. Genet.* 10, 1335–1346. doi:10.1093/hmg/10.13.1335

Nishino, I., Carrillo-Carrasco, N., and Argov, Z. (2014). GNE myopathy: current update and future therapy. *J. Neurol. Neurosurg. Psychiatr.* doi:10.1136/jnnp-2013-307051

O'Connell, K., Doran, P., Gannon, J., and Ohlendieck, K. (2008). Lectin-based proteomic profiling of aged skeletal muscle: decreased pyruvate kinase isozyme M1 exhibits drastically increased levels of N-glycosylation. *Eur. J. Cell Biol.* 87, 793–805. doi:10.1016/j.ejcb.2008.04.003

O'Connell, K., Gannon, J., Doran, P., and Ohlendieck, K. (2007). Proteomic profiling reveals a severely perturbed protein expression pattern in aged skeletal muscle. *Int. J. Mol. Med.* 20, 145–153. doi:10.3892/ijmm.20.2.145

Ong, M. L., and Holbrook, J. D. (2014). Novel region discovery method for Infinium 450K DNA methylation data reveals changes associated with aging in muscle and neuronal pathways. *Aging Cell* 13, 142–155. doi:10.1111/acel.12159

Pinkus, J. L., Amato, A. A., Taylor, J. P., and Greenberg, S. A. (2014). Abnormal distribution of heterogeneous nuclear ribonucleoproteins in sporadic inclusion body myositis. *Neuromuscul. Disord.* 24, 611–616. doi:10.1016/j.nmd.2014.04.012

Pokrzywa, W., and Hoppe, T. (2013). Chaperoning myosin assembly in muscle formation and aging. *Worm* 2, e25644. doi:10.4161/worm.25644

Redon, S., Zemp, I., and Lingner, J. (2013). A three-state model for the regulation of telomerase by TERRA and hnRNPA1. *Nucleic Acids Res.* 41, 9117–9128. doi:10.1093/nar/gkt695

Rose, M. R., and ENMC IBM Working Group. (2013). 188th ENMC International Workshop: inclusion body myositis, 2-4 December 2011, Naarden, The Netherlands. *Neuromuscul. Disord.* 23, 1044–1055. doi:10.1016/j.nmd.2013.08.007

Schiaffino, S., and Mammucari, C. (2011). Regulation of skeletal muscle growth by the IGF1-Akt/PKB pathway: insights from genetic models. *Skelet. Muscle* 1, 4. doi:10.1186/2044-5040-1-4

Sela, I., Milman Krentsis, I., Shlomai, Z., Sadeh, M., Dabby, R., Argov, Z., et al. (2011). The proteomic profile of hereditary inclusion body myopathy. *PLoS One* 6:e16334. doi:10.1371/journal.pone.0016334

Shorter, J., and Taylor, J. P. (2013). Disease mutations in the prion-like domains of hnRNPA1 and hnRNPA2/B1 introduce potent steric zippers that drive excess RNP granule assembly. *Rare Dis.* 1, e25200. doi:10.4161/rdis.25200

Stasche, R., Hinderlich, S., Weise, C., Effertz, K., Lucka, L., Moormann, P., et al. (1997). A bifunctional enzyme catalyzes the first two steps in *N*-acetylneuraminic acid biosynthesis of rat liver. Molecular cloning and functional expression of UDP-*N*-acetyl-glucosamine 2-epimerase/*N*-acetylmannosamine kinase. *J. Biol. Chem.* 272, 24319–24324. doi:10.1074/jbc.272.39.24319

Stojkovic, T., Hammouda El, H., Richard, P., Lopez De Munain, A., Ruiz-Martinez, J., Camano, P., et al. (2009). Clinical outcome in 19 French and Spanish patients with valosin-containing protein myopathy associated with Paget's disease of bone and frontotemporal dementia. *Neuromuscul. Disord.* 19, 316–323. doi:10.1016/j.nmd.2009.02.012

Tajsharghi, H., Darin, N., Rekabdar, E., Kyllerman, M., Wahlstrom, J., Martinsson, T., et al. (2005). Mutations and sequence variation in the human myosin heavy chain IIa gene (MYH2). *Eur. J. Hum. Genet.* 13, 617–622. doi:10.1038/sj.ejhg.5201375

Tang, W. K., Li, D., Li, C. C., Esser, L., Dai, R., Guo, L., et al. (2010). A novel ATP-dependent conformation in p97 N-D1 fragment revealed by crystal structures of disease-related mutants. *EMBO J.* 29, 2217–2229. doi:10.1038/emboj.2010.104

Tresse, E., Salomons, F. A., Vesa, J., Bott, L. C., Kimonis, V., Yao, T. P., et al. (2010). VCP/p97 is essential for maturation of ubiquitin-containing autophagosomes and this function is impaired by mutations that cause IBMPFD. *Autophagy* 6, 217–227. doi:10.4161/auto.6.2.11014

van Deursen, J. M. (2014). The role of senescent cells in ageing. *Nature* 509, 439–446. doi:10.1038/nature13193

Vesa, J., Su, H., Watts, G. D., Krause, S., Walter, M. C., Martin, B., et al. (2009). Valosin containing protein associated inclusion body myopathy: abnormal vacuolization, autophagy and cell fusion in myoblasts. *Neuromuscul. Disord.* 19, 766–772. doi:10.1016/j.nmd.2009.08.003

Wagatsuma, A., and Sakuma, K. (2014). Vitamin D signaling in myogenesis: potential for treatment of sarcopenia. *Biomed Res. Int.* 2014:121254. doi:10.1155/2014/121254

Wang, Z., Sun, Z., Li, A. V., and Yarema, K. J. (2006). Roles for UDP-GlcNAc 2-epimerase/ManNAc 6-kinase outside of sialic acid biosynthesis: modulation of sialyltransferase and BiP expression, GM3 and GD3 biosynthesis, proliferation, and apoptosis, and ERK1/2 phosphorylation. *J. Biol. Chem.* 281, 27016–27028. doi:10.1074/jbc.M604903200

Weihl, C. C., Pestronk, A., and Kimonis, V. E. (2009). Valosin-containing protein disease: inclusion body myopathy with Paget's disease of the bone and fronto-temporal dementia. *Neuromuscul. Disord.* 19, 308–315. doi:10.1016/j.nmd.2009.01.009

Winter, L., Staszewska, I., Mihailovska, E., Fischer, I., Goldmann, W. H., Schroder, R., et al. (2014). Chemical chaperone ameliorates pathological protein aggregation in plectin-deficient muscle. *J. Clin. Invest.* 124, 1144–1157. doi:10.1172/JCI71919

Wyce, A., Xiao, T., Whelan, K. A., Kosman, C., Walter, W., Eick, D., et al. (2007). H2B ubiquitylation acts as a barrier to Ctk1 nucleosomal recruitment prior to removal by Ubp8 within a SAGA-related complex. *Mol. Cell* 27, 275–288. doi:10.1016/j.molcel.2007.01.035

Yabe, I., Higashi, T., Kikuchi, S., Sasaki, H., Fukazawa, T., Yoshida, K., et al. (2003). GNE mutations causing distal myopathy with rimmed vacuoles with inflammation. *Neurology* 61, 384–386. doi:10.1212/01.WNL.0000061520.63546.8F

5

Myogenic potential of canine craniofacial satellite cells

Rita Maria Laura La Rovere[1,2,3], Mattia Quattrocelli[2,4], Tiziana Pietrangelo[1,2,3], Ester Sara Di Filippo[1,2,3], Lisa Maccatrozzo[2,5], Marco Cassano[6], Francesco Mascarello[2,7], Inès Barthélémy[8], Stephane Blot[8], Maurilio Sampaolesi[2,4,9]* and Stefania Fulle[1,2,3]*

[1] Department of Neuroscience and Imaging, University "G. d'Annunzio" Chieti-Pescara, Chieti, Italy
[2] Interuniversity Institute of Myology (IIM), University "G. d'Annunzio" Chieti-Pescara, Chieti, Italy
[3] Center for Excellence on Ageing (CeSI), G d'Annunzio Foundation, Chieti, Italy
[4] Translational Cardiomyology Laboratory, Stem Cell Biology and Embryology, Department of Development and Regeneration, KU Leuven, Leuven, Belgium
[5] Department of Experimental Veterinary Sciences, Faculty of Veterinary Medicine, University of Padua, Padua, Italy
[6] School of Life Sciences, Ecole Polytechnique Fédérale de Lausanne, Lausanne, Switzerland
[7] Department of Comparative Biomedicine and Food Safety, University of Padua, Padua, Italy
[8] Laboratoire de Neurobiologie, Ecole Nationale Vétérinaire d'Alfort, Maisons-Alfort, France
[9] Department of Public Health, Experimental and Forensic Medicine, Division of Human Anatomy, University of Pavia, Pavia, Italy

***Correspondence:**
Maurilio Sampaolesi, Translational Cardiomyology Laboratory, Stem Cell Biology and Embryology, Department of Development and Regeneration, KU Leuven, Herestraat 49, Leuven B-3000, Belgium
e-mail: maurilio.sampaolesi@med.kuleuven.be;
Stefania Fulle, Physiology Lab, Department of Neuroscience and Imaging, University of "G. d'Annunzio" Via dei Vestini 29, Chieti 66013, Italy
e-mail: s.fulle@phobos.unich.it

The skeletal fibers have different embryological origin; the extraocular and jaw-closer muscles develop from prechordal mesoderm while the limb and trunk muscles from somites. These different origins characterize also the adult muscle stem cells, known as satellite cells (SCs) and responsible for the fiber growth and regeneration. The physiological properties of presomitic SCs and their epigenetics are poorly studied despite their peculiar characteristics to preserve muscle integrity during chronic muscle degeneration. Here, we isolated SCs from canine somitic [somite-derived muscle (SDM): vastus lateralis, rectus abdominis, gluteus superficialis, biceps femoris, psoas] and presomitic [pre-somite-derived muscle (PSDM): lateral rectus, temporalis, and retractor bulbi] muscles as myogenic progenitor cells from young and old animals. In addition, SDM and PSDM-SCs were obtained also from golden retrievers affected by muscular dystrophy (GRMD). We characterized the lifespan, the myogenic potential and functions, and oxidative stress of both somitic and presomitic SCs with the aim to reveal differences with aging and between healthy and dystrophic animals. The different proliferation rate was consistent with higher telomerase activity in PSDM-SCs compared to SDM-SCs, although restricted at early passages. SDM-SCs express early (Pax7, MyoD) and late (myosin heavy chain, myogenin) myogenic markers differently from PSDM-SCs resulting in a more efficient and faster cell differentiation. Taken together, our results showed that PSDM-SCs elicit a stronger stem cell phenotype compared to SDM ones. Finally, myomiR expression profile reveals a unique epigenetic signature in GRMD SCs and miR-206, highly expressed in dystrophic SCs, seems to play a critical role in muscle degeneration. Thus, miR-206 could represent a potential target for novel therapeutic approaches.

Keywords: presomitic and somitic satellite cells, differentiation, dystrophic muscle, microRNA

INTRODUCTION

Satellite cells (SCs) are quiescent adult stem cells and they are located between the basal lamina and sarcolemma of myofibers (Mauro, 1961). Since SCs function to repair skeletal muscle damaged by injury or disease, they are responsible for muscle preservation and growth.

Satellite cells exhibit limited gene expression and protein synthesis due to extremely low cellular turnover (Rando, 2006) and upon activation they leave the quiescent state and move outside of the basal lamina, enter the cell cycle and proliferate. The proliferating SCs, known as myogenic progenitor cells, co-express Pax7 and MyoD, and undergo multiple rounds of division (Chargé and Rudnicki, 2004). Subsequently, SCs withdraw from the cell cycle down-regulating Pax7 and expressing myogenin in order to differentiate into multinucleated myofibers. A limited number of SCs maintain Pax7 for self-renewing and enter again a quiescent state. The fact that activated SCs can loose the expression of myogenic markers or eventually leave the cell cycle shows that they are a heterogeneous mixture of stem cells and committed progenitors. The myogenic commitment of SCs is finely regulated by the expression of a temporal class of myogenic transcription factors (MRFs), which are important for the renewal of SCs (Porter et al., 2006; McLoon et al., 2007) or for determining their differentiation. However, the signaling pathways that maintain or suppress SCs at different functional states are largely unknown and recent studies have emphasized the role of microRNAs (miRNAs) as novel post-transcriptional modulators of myogenic gene expression (Drummond et al., 2010). miRNAs are small non-coding RNAs that negatively regulate gene expression by binding mRNA target and interfering with protein synthesis, also by reducing the accumulation of target messengers. A recent analysis found that between 74 and 92% of the transcriptome is potentially regulated by miRNAs (Miranda et al., 2006).

Emerging evidence has demonstrated that miRNAs are essential for several biological functions including homeostasis, apoptosis (Huang et al., 2012), and deleterious changes in miRNA expression are associated with human diseases (Chen et al., 2008). Several muscle-specific miRNAs in heart and skeletal muscle (myomiRs) including miR-1, miR-26a, miR-125b, miR-133, miR-206, miR-208, etc. (McCarthy and Esser, 2007; Small et al., 2010) are considered important for myoblast differentiation, proliferation, and muscle remodeling. Among the various myomiRs, miR-1 and miR-133 are involved in the modulation of muscle growth and differentiation, while miR-206 specifically promotes muscle myogenesis. The regulation of these myomiRs is controlled by MRFs, as MyoD and myogenin (Rao et al., 2006). SC regenerative potential is impaired in Duchenne muscular dystrophies (DMD), a recessive X-linked form of muscular degeneration, and in age-related loss of muscle mass, i.e., a condition known as sarcopenia (Snijders et al., 2009). In DMD patients, the SC-mediated regenerative process is not sufficient to rescue the phenotype, resulting in a general tissue inflammation. This culminates in continuous cycles of degeneration/regeneration that finally deplete the pool of skeletal muscle stem cells. However, masseter (Mas), extraocular, laryngeal, and pharyngeal muscles are less affected during sarcopenic and dystrophic degeneration. These muscles present peculiar isoforms of myosin heavy chain (MyHC) proteins, as MyHC 2B, EO, alpha-cardiac, and M. For this peculiarity, some authors refer to cranial facial muscles as "special muscles" (Sciote et al., 1994; Toniolo et al., 2008; Schiaffino and Reggiani, 2011). The embryonic origin of these special muscles is the presomitic mesoderm while trunk, leg, and arm muscles derive from somites. As described by Biressi and Rando (2010), signaling pathways responsible for myogenic differentiation of SCs isolated from trunk and special muscles are different. Interestingly, eye extrinsic muscles responsible for complex and highly coordinated movements do not show signs of sarcopenia and are not affected by DMD (McLoon et al., 2007).

The muscular dystrophy golden retriever (GRMD) dog is the closest pathological counterpart of DMD patients (Collins and Morgan, 2003). In addition, sarcopenia is an emerging syndrome of importance in dogs (Freeman, 2012). Here, we report for the first time the characterization of SCs isolated from presomitic muscles of young, old, and GRMD dogs. We focus on stem cell properties during aging and in the dystrophic context, highlighting the epigenetic signature of SC-myotube transition.

Table 1 | Summary of canine muscle biopsies.

Group	Dog	Muscle biopsies	Age	Embryonic origin
HEALTHY YOUNG DOGS				
	#1	*Rectus abdominis*	1 year	Somites
	#2	*Gluteus superficialis*	3 years	Somites
		Rectus abdominis		Somites
	#3	*Rectus abdominis*	10 months	Somites
	#4	*Biceps femoris*	8 months	Somites
	#5	*Extraocular*	1 year	Presomitic cranial mesoderm
		Vastus lateralis		Somites
	#6	*Extraocular*	5 months	Presomitic cranial mesoderm
		Vastus lateralis		Somites
	#7	*Extraocular*	1 year	Presomitic cranial mesoderm
		Vastus lateralis		Somites
	#8	*Rectus abdominis*	1 year	Somites
		Vastus lateralis		Somites
HEALTHY AGED DOGS				
	#9	*Psoas*	9 years	Presomitic cranial mesoderm
		Temporalis, M fiber		Presomitic cranial mesoderm
		Rectus lateralis		Presomitic cranial mesoderm
	#10	*Masseter*	18 years	Presomitic cranial mesoderm
		Rectus lateralis		Presomitic cranial mesoderm
		Retractor bulbi		Presomitic cranial mesoderm
	#11	*Rectus abdominis*	13 years	Somites
		Vastus lateralis		Somites
GRMD				
	#12	*Extraocular*	1 year	Presomitic cranial mesoderm
		Vastus lateralis		Somites
	#13	*Extraocular*	1 year	Presomitic cranial mesoderm
		Vastus lateralis		Somites

MATERIALS AND METHODS

SAMPLING OF CANINE BIOPSIES

Muscle biopsies were collected from different institutions involved in this study: (1) Veterinary University Clinics in Padua; (2) Veterinary School of Maison-Alfort, Paris. In Padua, the samples were obtained from dogs that had been euthanized in the Veterinary University Clinics. Those dogs were diagnosed as terminally ill following accidents. The muscle tissues were collected during the normal surgical procedures. Biopsies from GRMD were obtained from the Veterinary School of Maison-Alfort (Paris, France). All GRMD dogs considered in this study (see **Table 1**) were maintained until natural death, and underwent necropsy only upon decease. The muscle sampling was done according to Institutional Animal Care and Use Committee recommendations and according to the local ethical rules and the Declaration of Helsinki. The muscles were divided according to their embryonic origin, MyHC isoform composition, and the anatomical location (**Table 1**). Trunk and limb muscles: *vastus lateralis* (VL), *psoas*, *rectus abdominis* (RA), *gluteus superficialis* (GS), *biceps femoris* (BF) as somite-derived muscles (SDM). Head muscles: *rectus lateralis* (RL), *retractor bulbi* (RB), *temporalis-M fiber* (MT), *Mas* as pre-somite-derived muscle (PSDM). GRMD SCs were collected only from young dog, while samples from wild-type (WT) dogs were collected from dogs of different ages.

ISOLATION AND CULTURE OF CANINE SCs

Satellite cells were isolated from muscle tissues stored in liquid nitrogen in FBS (# ECS0100187, Euroclone, Milan, Italy) + 10% of DMSO (#D5879, Sigma-Aldrich, Milan, Italy). Frozen dissected muscle biopsies were thawed at 37°C and washed with PBS. Under sterile condition, few drops of enzymatic solution of 0.4 mg/ml collagenase type V (#C9263, Sigma-Aldrich, Milan, Italy), 0.6 mg/ml pancreatin (#P3292, Sigma-Aldrich, Milan, Italy) dissolved in PBS (# ECB4004L, Euroclone, Milan, Italy), filtered using a sterile syringe filter of 0.2 μm pore size, stored at 4°C until use. The solution was added and the muscles were minced to fine slurry using a scalpel. After transferring the minced tissue into 50 ml tubes, 10 ml of enzymatic solution was added and incubated at 37°C in a shaking incubator for 30 min. After gravity sedimentation, the supernatant was collected into new falcon tube, through filtration by 100 μm cell strainer; the digestion was stopped by adding an equal volume of filtered FBS. The cell suspension was centrifuged at 1200 rpm for 5 min, the supernatant was discarded and the cells were resuspended in growth medium (GM). GM contains (% vol/vol): DMEM high glucose (# ECB7501L, Euroclone, Milan, Italy), 0.1 gentamicin (# ECM0011B, Euroclone, Milan, Italy), 20 FBS, 1 MEM NEAA 100× (#11140, GIBCO, Life Technology, Carlsbad, CA, USA), 1 sodium pyruvate 100 mM (#11360, GIBCO, Life Technology, Carlsbad, CA, USA), 1 penicillin/streptomycin 100× (# ECB3001D, Euroclone, Milan, Italy), 1 L-glutamine 100× (#25030-024, GIBCO, Life Technology, Carlsbad, CA, USA), 2 chicken embryo extract (#2850145, MP, Santa Ana, CA, USA), 2 heat-inactivated HS (# ECS0091L, Euroclone, Milan, Italy) (56°C, 36 min) plus 5 ng/ml bFGF (# PHG0026, GIBCO, Life Technology, Carlsbad, CA, USA) in PBS. Canine cells were pre-plated for 1 h on uncoated petri dishes to permit the attachment of fibroblasts. Unattached cells were transferred to collagen I-coated 60 mm cell culture dish. Five days later, small round and poorly adhering cells appeared on collagen coated-plates and were allowed to proliferate in GM until reaching 70–80% confluence. The cells were either cryoconserved or expanded for further analysis. To generate batches, 70–80% confluent SCs were frozen for long-term storage at density of 10^6 cells/ml in liquid nitrogen. To expand the culture, SCs were plated again until reaching 80% confluence and then again detached (passage). The population doubling level (PDL) was calculated at each passage with the following equation: $\log 10(N/n)/\ln 2$ with N as the number of cells at the time of the passage and n as the number of cells initially plated. At first passage, all SC populations were considered to be as 1 PDL and we evaluated the maximal PDL reached by the cultures.

SC PROLIFERATION ANALYSIS BY EDU (5-ETHYNYL-2′-DEOXYURIDINE) FLOW CYTOMETRY

Cells were plated in six well at density of 5×10^4/well; after 24 h the cells were treated with 100 μM H_2O_2 (Sigma). The flow cytometry method was performed at 24 and 48 h after treatment with hydrogen peroxide. Briefly, 10 μM Edu was added to the culture medium for 2 h; after the cells were harvested and washed twice with 1% BSA in PBS. The cells were fixed with 2% paraformaldehyde in PBS for 15 min at RT. After wash, the cell pellet was resuspended with permeabilization solution and incubated with FxCycle Violet for DNA stain. After an incubation period of 15 min at 37°C in the dark, cells were transferred on ice until analysis with FACS Calibur™ (BD, USA).

CELL DIFFERENTIATION

Skeletal muscle differentiation was induced by culturing 5,000 cells/cm^2 in differentiative medium (DM) for 7 days in the same medium. DM contains (% vol/vol): DMEM high glucose, 0.1 gentamicin, 5 heat-inactivated HS (56°C, 36 min), 10 μg/ml insulin, 100 μg/ml apo-transferrin (#T-2036, Sigma-Aldrich, Milan, Italy), 1 MEM NEAA 100×, 1 sodium pyruvate 100 mM, 1 penicillin/streptomycin 100×, 1 L-glutamine 100×. The fusion index (FI) was calculated as the ratio of the number of nuclei inside myotubes to the number of total nuclei in 10–20 fields for each sample. We considered myotubes exclusively the cells positive for MyHC with two or more nuclei.

TELOMERASE ACTIVITY

Telomerase activity was assessed by TraPEZE RT Telomerase Detection Kit (#S7710, Millipore, Merck KGaA, Darmstadt, Germany), according to the recommendations of the manufacturer. Briefly, cell pellets of the samples were resuspended in CHAPS lysis buffer and protein concentrations were measured by the Bradford Assay (#500-0205, Bio-Rad, Bio-Rad Laboratories s.r.l., Segrate, Milan, Italy). The quantification of telomerase activity was obtained from the standard curve of TRS8 template. TRS8 template is an oligonucleotide with a sequence identical to the oligonucleotide substrate primer extended with eight telomeric repeats AG(GGTTAG). The kit provided cell pellets as positive controls. According to the manufacturer's instructions, we also performed a negative control for each sample. Negative controls were obtained incubating samples at 85°C for 10 min prior to the TRAP assay to inactivate telomerase. For each sample, 100 ng of total proteins were adjusted to a volume of 2 μl by CHAPS lysis buffer and used for the telomerase activity assay. The quantitative real-time polymerase chain reactions were performed in 96-well optical reaction plates (Applied BioSystems, Life Technologies, Molecular Device, Sunnyvale, CA, USA) using the ABI PRISM 7700 Sequence Detection System. Reactions were carried out in triplicates using the recommended Titanium Taq Polymerase (BD Clontech, #639208). The experiments were performed according to the manufacturer's instructions. We tested telomerase activity in SC samples collected at early (II–III) and late (VIII–X) passages and expressed as log copy number calculated using threshold cycle values and the standard curve for each sample.

IMMUNOFLUORESCENCE ASSAY

Satellite cells were fixed for immunocytochemistry and immunofluorescence analysis to reveal myogenic markers (MF-20 for MyHC and Pax7 Abs DSHB, USA; MyoD Abs, Dako, USA) and Ki67 (Dako, USA). Cells were washed twice with PBS and incubated with 2% PFA (#P6148, Sigma-Aldrich, Milan, Italy) for 10 min at RT. Membrane permeabilization was obtained at RT in 0.2% of Triton X-100 (#93443, Sigma-Aldrich, Milan, Italy),

1% BSA (#A9647, Sigma-Aldrich, Milan, Italy) in PBS and non-specific binding of secondary antibodies was blocked with PBS containing 5% serum from the species in which the secondary antibody was produced. Without washing, the cells were incubated for 1 h with primary antibody diluted in 1% BSA–PBS. Then, cells were washed twice with PBS and incubated in the dark for 30 min at RT with the secondary antibody, diluted 1:500 in 1% BSA + PBS. Nuclei were stained with DAPI (#D1306, Invitrogen, Life Technologies, Molecular Device, Sunnyvale, CA, USA). Unbound antibodies were washed out with PBS and samples were mounted and analyzed with a fluorescence Nikon inverted microscope Eclipse Ti-U equipped with a Qicam Fast1354 camera using Pro-Plus software (Media Cybernetics).

IMMUNOCYTOCHEMISTRY

Immunocytochemistry to reveal desmin protein was performed using LSAB + System-AP Universal kit (#K0678, Dako, Dakocytomation, Glostrup, Denmark) according to manufacturer's protocols.

ISOLATION AND QUANTIFICATION OF microRNA

Small RNA extraction from both SDM and PSDM samples was performed using the PureLink miRNA isolation kit (#K1570-01, Invitrogen, Life Technologies, Molecular Device, Sunnyvale, CA, USA) following manufacturer's instructions. Briefly, 10^6 cells were resuspended in 300 μl binding buffer and 300 μl of 70% alcohol was added to the cell lysate. Cell lysate was added to a spin cartridge and centrifuged for 1 min at 12,000 × *g*. Seven hundred microliters of 100% alcohol was added to the supernatant and centrifuged in a new spin cartridge for 1 min at 12,000 × *g*. The filtrate was discarded, then 500 μl wash buffer was added and centrifuged for 1 min at 12000 × *g*. This procedure was repeated twice. Sterile RNase-free water (30 μl) was added to the spin cartridge and incubated for 1 min at RT before centrifugation at maximum speed for 1 min to elute the RNA. The RNA concentration was quantified using NanoDrop™ spectrophotometer readings of A260, A260/280, and A260/230 ratios. RNA-free nuclease water was used as blank.

RT REAL-TIME PCR FOR microRNAs SINGLE ASSAY EXPRESSION

RT-stem-loop real-time PCR was performed to evaluate miRNAs relative expression. Assays for miRNA profile analysis were carried out according to Applied Biosystems protocols (TaqMan miRNA assay Kit). Briefly, RT reactions containing 20 ng of small RNA preparation, specific stem-loop primers for each miRNA, 1× buffer, dNTPs reverse transcriptase, and RNAse inhibitor were incubated in Thermocycler for 30 min at 16°C, 30 min at 42°C, 5 min at 85°C, and then held at 4°C. Then, real-time PCR for miRNA expression levels was performed using miRNA specific TaqMan probes and TaqMan universal master mix in a Eppendorf Mastercycler® ep realplex system in 96-well plates, in triplicate. Expression quantification was normalized vs. *miR-16* levels. Taqman-based qPCR were conducted using miRNA-specific probes (Applied Biosystems) as: has-miR-1 (UGGAAUGUAAAGAAGUAUGUAU; #002222); has-miR-206 (UGGAAUGUAAGGAAGUGUGUGG; #000510); hsamiR-133a (UUUGGUCCCCUUCAACCAGCUG; #002246); has-miR-133b (UUUGGUCCCCUUCAACCAGCUA; #002247); has-miR-16-5p (UAGCAGCACGUAAAUAUUGGCG; #000391).

The quantitative real-time polymerase chain reactions were performed in 96-well optical reaction plates (Applied BioSystems) using the ABI PRISM 7700 Sequence Detection System. Reactions were carried out in triplicates using the recommended Titanium Taq Polymerase (#639208, BD Clontech, BD Bioscience, Clontech Laboratories Inc., San Jose, CA, USA). The relative quantification of target gene expression was evaluated using the arithmetical formula $2^{-\Delta\Delta Ct}$, according to the comparative C_t method, which represents the amount of target, as normalized to the miR-16 endogenous control. The samples were analyzed as means of the log base-10 of the ratios, $\log_2$ differentiated/undifferentiated. The data were reported as Log_{10} RQ, in which upregulated miRNAs have positive values and downregulated miRNAs have negative values.

RELATIVE QUANTIFICATION OF MYOGENIC FACTOR GENES BY RT REAL-TIME PCR

Total RNA from isolated canine SCs was extracted using the Trizol reagent (Invitrogen, Paisley, UK), according to the manufacturer's protocol, from about 10^6 cells. To assess the integrity and the amount of the RNA extracted, denaturing agarose gel electrophoresis and spectrophotometric A260/280 readings were performed. Two micrograms of total RNA was reverse transcribed into cDNA with the Superscript III kit (Invitrogen) after treatment with DNAse I (Invitrogen) to remove contaminating genomic DNA. Real-time PCR reactions were achieved using an ABI 7500 real-time PCR System (Applied Biosystems, Foster City, CA, USA) with the following conditions: 1× PowerSybrGreen Master mix (containing buffer, dNTPs, SybrGreen I dye and AmpliTaq Gold® DNA Polymerase), 300 nM forward and reverse primers each, 1 μl cDNA in 20 μl total volume. PCR primers for the specific target genes and for the housekeeping gene (β-actin) were designed using the Primer Express 3.0 software (Applied Biosystems). All the primer sequences (**Table 2**) were designed to span introns in the genomic DNA in order to minimize non-specific fluorescence signals due to contaminating genomic DNA. Relative quantifications were calculated using the $\Delta\Delta C_t$ method, normalized to the reference gene (beta actin) and expressed in arbitrary units as fold change as compared to the calibrator sample (1 unit).

MEASUREMENT OF INTRACELLULAR REACTIVE OXYGEN SPECIES

Cellular reactive oxygen species (ROS) were quantified by the 2,7-dichlorofluorescein diacetate (DCFH-DA, #D6883, Sigma) assay using a microplate reader (Fluorometer SPECTRAmax Gemini XS, Molecular Devices), using excitation and emission wavelengths of 480 and 530 nm, respectively and analyzed by SOFTmax Pro software, according to Menghini et al. method (Menghini et al., 2011).

NBT ASSAY

The NBT assay is based on the reduction of NBT (Nitro blue tetrazolium chloride, #N6639, Sigma) in formazan by O_2^-. Reduced formazan is then quantified at the spectrophotometer. In the presence of potentially antioxidant substances, the superoxide is detoxified (scavenger action) and decreases the amount of NBT

Table 2 | Primer sequences for RT real-time PCR.

Gene	Forward sequence	Reverse sequence
Myf5	5′-CTGTCTGGTCCCGAAAGAAC-3′	5′-TGATTCGATCCAC TATGCTG-3′
Myogenin	5′-AGTGACTGCAGCTCCCACAG-3′	5′-GACGTGAGAGA GTGCAGGTT-3′
MSTN	5′-CCCGTCAAGACTCCTACAACAG-3′	5′-AATGCTCTGC CAAATACCAGT-3′
MyHC 1	5′-CACCAACCTGTCCAAGTTCC-3′	5′-CCGGGCAGAT CAAGAGAAGATA-3′
β-actin	5′-CCATCTACGAGGGGTACGCCC-3′	5′-TGCTCGAAGTCC AGGGCGACGTA-3′

reduced, hence lower levels of reduced formazan are detected. Cells (10^6 cells) were detached, centrifuged 5 min at 170 × *g* and resuspended in 1 mg/ml of NBT with 1 ml 0.9% NaCl. Then, the cells were left for 3 h at 37°C (incubator), centrifuged 10 min at 100 × *g* in microfuge, resuspended in 1 ml DMSO and left for 20 min at 37°C. For the assay, cells were plated in a 96-well plate (2×10^5 cell/well) and assayed at the spectrophotometer at 550 nm on a scanning multi-well reader (Microplate spectrometer SPECTRAmax 190, Molecular Devices, Sunnyvale, CA, USA) according to Sozio et al. (2013).

CALCIUM IMAGING

Satellite cells were plated at a confluence of 6,000 cells/cm^2 in 96-well plates (Corning, Tewksbury, MA, USA). The measurements were performed using Fura-2 AM (#F1221, Invitrogen) as Ca^{2+} indicator. Myoblasts and myotubes were loaded with 5 μM Fura-2 AM in normal external solution (NES) supplemented with 10 mg/ml of BSA for 40 min at 37°C and 5% CO_2. NES is composed of 10 mM glucose (#454337, Carlo Erba), 140 mM NaCl (#S7653, Sigma), 2.8 mM KCl (#471177, Carlo Erba), 2 mM $CaCl_2$, 2 mM $MgCl_2$ (Sigma), and 10 mM HEPES (#101926, ICN, Biomedicals Inc.), pH 7.4, 290–300 mOsM. After loading, the cells were rinsed and maintained in NES for 10 min at room temperature (RT), to allow the de-esterification of the probe. Myoblasts and myotubes of similar size were selected for measurement and the region of interest (ROI) was drawn around the cells. Then, living cells were sequentially excited at 340 or 380 nm with a high-speed wavelength switcher Polychrome II (Till Photonics, Germany). Fluorescence images were collected using a 40× oil objective lens, acquired using an intensified CCD camera (Hamamatsu Photonics, Hamamatsu), stored on a PC, and analyzed off-line. The acquisition time for each fluorescence emission was 0.5 s and the background fluorescence was subtracted from the signal in the ROI. The 340 and 380 traces and 340/380-ratio were recorded and analyzed using Aquacosmos software (Hamamatsu).

STATISTICAL ANALYSIS

Unpaired *t*-test with Welch's correction and ANOVA as mentioned in the figure legends, were performed using Prism5 GraphPad software (Abacus Concepts, GraphPad Software, San Diego, CA, USA). A p-value <0.05 was considered to indicate statistical significance.

RESULTS

CANINE SATELLITE CELL CHARACTERIZATION

Following canine muscle biopsies dissociation with enzymatic solution (as described in Materials and Methods), SCs gave rise to myogenic progenitor cells in culture. To avoid confusion, we used SCs throughout the manuscript to indicate also myogenic progenitor cells, and the list of canine biopsies used to isolate SCs in our study is reported in **Table 1**. WT SCs isolated from somitic (SDM) and presomitic (PSDM) muscles were morphologically similar (**Figure 1A**) and were organized in small clones derived from single cell divisions (**Figure 1B**). We cultured the cells at very low density in order to identify single cells. We plated 500 cells (SDM and PSDM) on 100 mm collagen I-coated Petri dishes and marked those separate cells with a number. By counting the number of cells per clone, we evaluated the clonogenic ability of primary cell culture isolated from trunk and head muscles of young and old dogs. The ability of a single cell to proliferate independently to form a colony was similar in samples at comparable ages (data not shown).

Satellite cells in culture were expanded until replicative senescence was reached and the PDL was calculated. The growth curves of young (age ranging between 5 and 36 months) and old (age ranging between 9 and 18 years) showed higher rate of doubling level in PSDM-SCs with respect to SDM-derived SCs (**Figures 1C,D**). This difference was marked in SCs derived from old dogs (**Figure 1D**) where SDM-SCs stopped their proliferation at 25 days, after only 20 PDL. Differently, PSDM-SCs could proliferate longer (until 40 days) and undergo to senescence after about 30 PDL. No significant differences were observed between old and young SCS derived from comparable muscles. **Figure 1E** shows the growth curve of 1-year-old GRMD SCs isolated from SDM and PSDM samples. PSDM-SCs from GRMD samples (**Figure 1E**) showed a higher doublings activity in respect to SDM-SCs. This is probably due to the fact that head muscles are less affected in dystrophic dogs, and SCs were not exhausted by multiple attempts to regenerate lost tissue as occurred in more active muscles.

We tested the telomerase activity in SC samples collected at early (2, 3 p) and late (8–10 p) passages and expressed as log copy number calculated using threshold cycle values and the standard curve for each sample. As shown in **Figure 1F**, in PSDM-SCs there was a trend toward a higher telomerase activity (9.0 ± 0.6) compared with SDM-SCs (8.0 ± 1.0) at early passages. At late passages, the telomerase activities were similar among all analyzed samples. Immunofluorescence analysis showed that 10% of PSDM-SCs still express Ki67 after 30 days in culture, while SDM-SCs were completely negative (Figure S1 in Supplementary Material). Although we cannot exclude that SDM-SCs enter in a quiescent status, the results suggest that PSDM-SCs can still proliferate after 30 days while SDM-SCs cannot. In addition, large nuclei in SDM-SCs are further indicating senescent cells (De Cecco et al., 2011) as indicated in Figure S1 in Supplementary Material, inset and right panels.

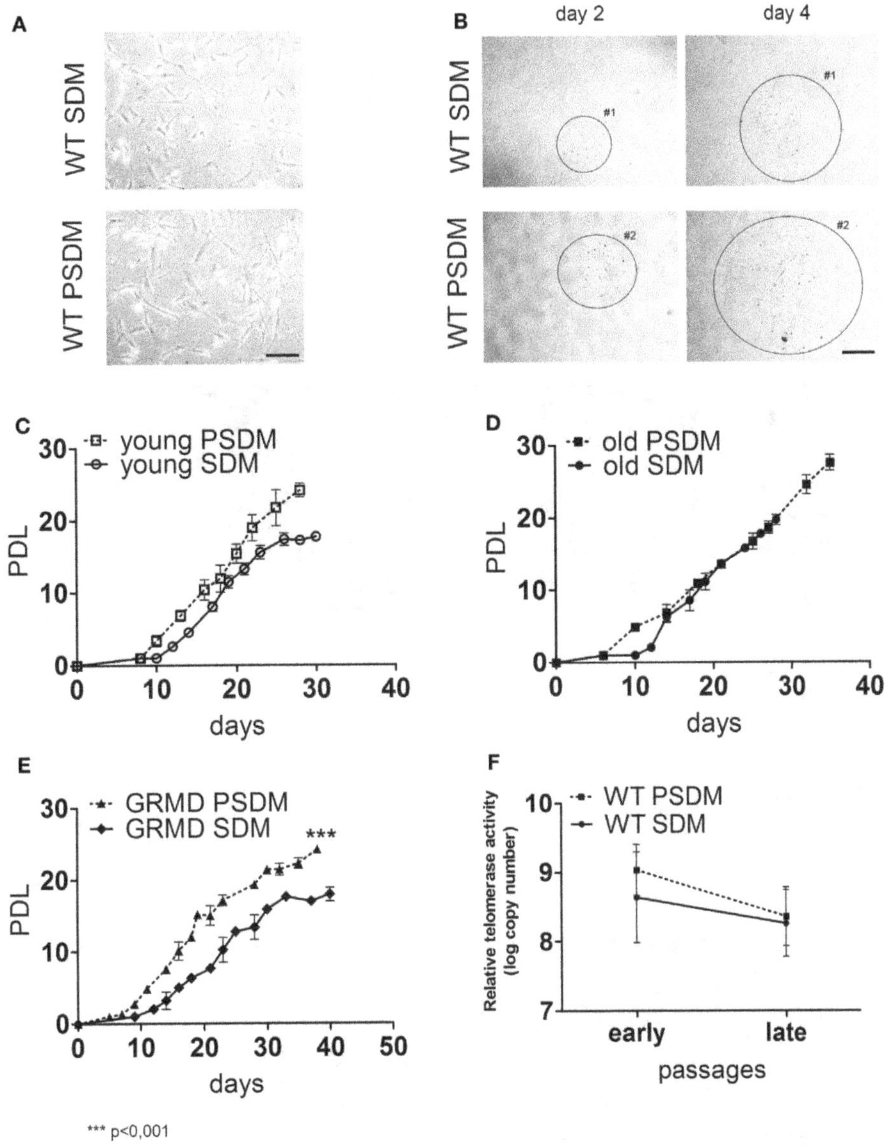

FIGURE 1 | Characterization of canine satellite cells (SCs). **(A,B)** Phase contrast morphology of freshly isolated SCs **(A)** from somitic (SDM) and presomitic (PSDM) muscles biopsies; bar = 50 μm. SCs were cultured at low density to generate clones **(B)** and cells were maintained in culture until they stop to divide; bar = 250 μm. Growth curves of **(C)** SDM- and PSDM-SCs from young donors; **(D)** SDM- and PSDM-SCs from old donors; **(E)** SDM and PSDM-SCs from dystrophic dogs. Telomerase activity **(F)** in SCs collected at early and late passages from SDM and PSDM. Data are represented as mean ± SD.

EXPRESSION OF MYOGENIC REGULATORY FACTORS IN CANINE SCs

Taken into account the SC heterogeneity due to the adopted enzymatic digestion method, the myogenic index (MI) was estimated as a percentage of desmin (an early myogenic marker) positive ($Desm^+$) cells and revealed by immunocytochemistry (**Figure 2A**). SCs are capable to spontaneously differentiate when they reach 80–90% of confluence, however in all experiments we differentiate SCs into myotubes by serum starvation in differentiation medium containing 2% horse serum. In general, PSDM biopsies have a lower content of myogenic cells compared to SDM samples. Age-independent differences have been found both in WT (**Figure 2B**, 79.1% in SDM vs. 56.5% in PSDM of young dogs, and 91.1% in SDM vs. 54.2% in PSDM of old dogs) and GRMD (72.0% in SDM vs. 47.8% in PSDM) dogs. By immunofluorescence assay (**Figures 2C,D**), SDM-SCs isolated from WT dog showed an higher content of $Pax7^+$ (49.1 vs. 32.5%) and $MyoD^+$ (65.5 vs. 29.0%) cells compared with PSDM-SCs (**Figure 2E**); while GRMD SCs displayed an opposite result: lower content of both $Pax7^+$ (5.5 vs. 25.0%) and $MyoD^+$ (8.0 vs. 54.7%) SDM vs. PSDM-SCs (**Figure 2F**). In addition, myogenin expression resulted upregulated during differentiation in SCs isolated from SDM and PSDM and its expression was not affected with aging (**Figure 2G**). However, in GRMD dogs myogenin was upregulated only in PSDM-SCs during differentiation,

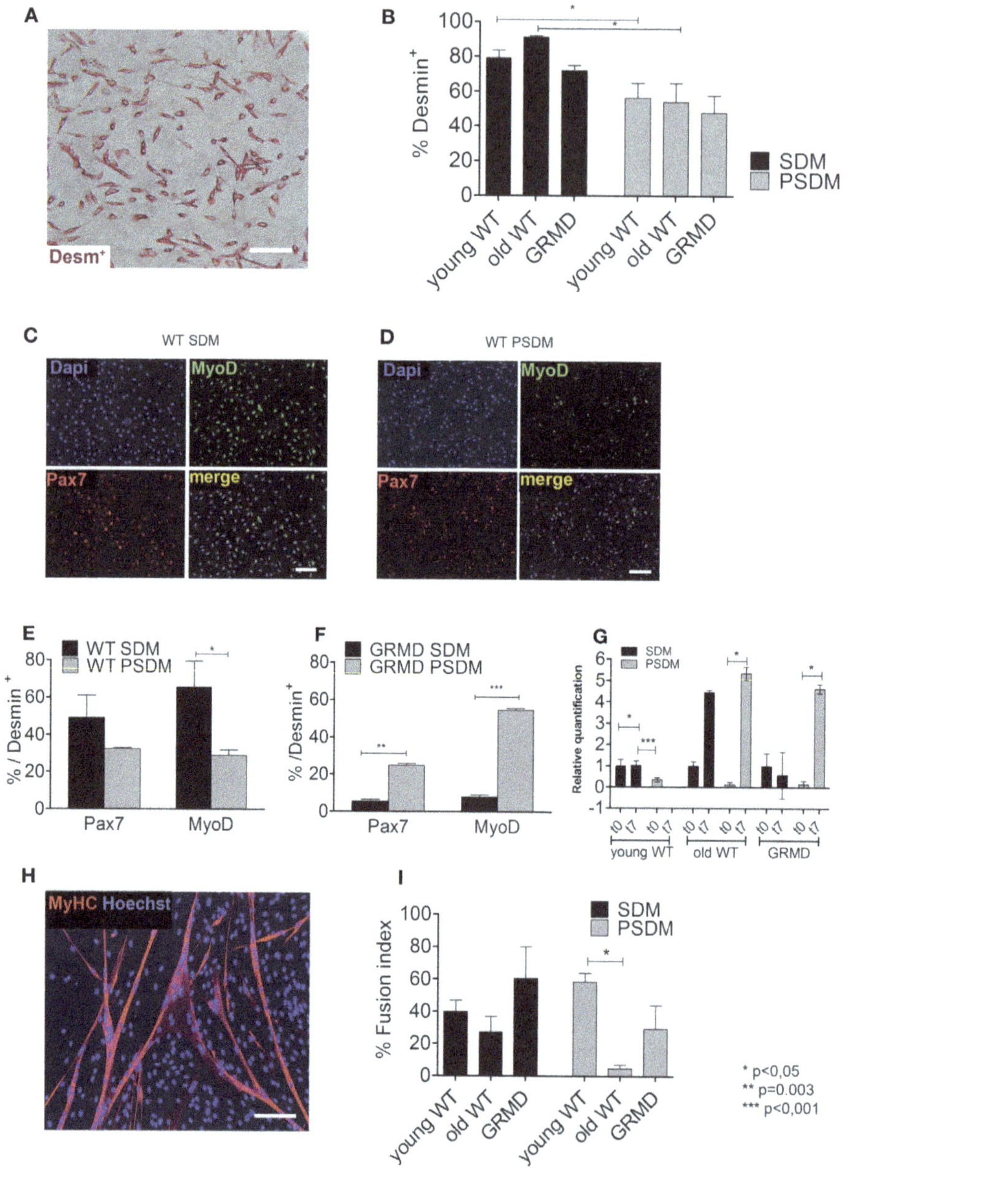

FIGURE 2 | Expression of myogenic markers in canine SCs. **(A)** Desmin positive (Desm+) SCs were quantified **(B)** for WT young SCs isolated from SDM and PSDM muscle biopsies; for WT old SCs isolated from SDM and PSDM; similarly the percentage of Desm+ SCs in SDM and PSDM isolated from GRMD dogs. **(C,D)** Examples of immunofluorescence analysis for Pax7 and MyoD of WT SDM-SCs **(C)** and PSDM-SCs **(D)**. Quantifications of Pax7 and MyoD positive SCs **(E)** normalized to percentage of Des+ from WT SDM and PSDM are shown; in **(F)** are reported SCs from dystrophic dogs SDM and PSDM. Myogenin expression in SCs during differentiation was measured by quantitative real-time PCR **(G)**. Myogenin is upregulated after 7 days of differentiation in all samples expect in GRDM SDM-SCs. Three independent experiments were performed in triplicates and statistically analyzed using Dunn's Multiple Comparison Test. MyHC staining **(H)** was used to quantify the FI **(I)** of SCs isolated from SDM and PSDM of WT young; from SDM and PSDM of WT old and of GRMD SCs isolated from SDM and PSDM. Data are represented as mean ± SD and statistically analyzed using *t*-test; $*p < 0.05$. Bar = 50 μm.

while SDM-SCs failed to increase the expression of myogenin at day 7 (**Figure 2G**).

Then, we examined the ability of SCs to fuse into multinucleated myotubes after 7 days in culture with low serum (2% HS). **Figure 2H** shows an example of MyHC positive canine myotubes used for the FI analysis. Young PSDM-SCs presented a higher FI compared with SDM-SCs (**Figure 2I**, 58.5 vs. 39.8% in PSDM vs. SDM, respectively). Interestingly, FI was drastically lower in PSDM-SCs compared to SDM-SCs isolated from old dogs (4.7 vs. 27.4%, respectively). The same trend was found in GRMD where SDM-SCs differentiate more efficiently than PSDM-SCs (60.5 vs. 29.5%). These results suggest that SCs isolated from GRMD dogs act similarly as old WT SCs.

OXIDANT LEVELS IN CANINE SCs

Oxidants such as ROS/RNS are known to affect cell function, including the ability to differentiate. It has been proposed that several factors, including ROS, are able to regulate skeletal muscle gene expression. However, when the levels of oxidants consistently remain high and are not reduced by endogenous scavenger systems, as occurring in elderly skeletal muscle (Musarò et al., 2010), the cell undergoes oxidative stress, which may affect its ability to differentiate (Beccafico et al., 2007). For this reason, we analyzed the oxidant levels present in SCs isolated from muscle biopsies (**Figure 3**). After an oxidant insult represented by H_2O_2, old SCs were less capable to reduce ROS levels (SDM = 148.0 ± 26%; PSDM = 136.0 ± 9%) present in cells, demonstrating a poor antioxidant capacity (**Figures 3A,B**). Furthermore, the levels of superoxide anion (**Figure 3C**) were lower in all SDM-SCs as compared to PSDM-SCs, but in old SCs these values were very high (SDM = 0.34 ± 0.01; PSDM = 0.47 ± 0.04) as compared to young (SDM = 0.15 ± 0.01; PSDM = 0.18 ± 0.01) and GRMD (SDM = 0.11 ± 0.01; PSDM = 0.24 ± 0.01) SCs.

To address whether SCs from PSDM or SDM were still able to proliferate under stress conditions, we evaluated the effect of 100 nM H_2O_2 on PSDM- and SDM-SCs by Edu (5-ethynyl-2'-deoxyuridine) flow cytometry analysis (Figure S2 in Supplementary Material). The nucleoside analog EdU for thymidine substitution in cell proliferation assays has recently been proposed in FACS analysis studies (Diermeier-Daucher et al., 2009). As reported in Figure S2A in Supplementary Material, PSDM and SDM-SC did not show any alterations of proliferative capability. However, a higher number of cells in S phase were observed in PSDM-SCs compared to SDM-SCs (28 vs. 16% after 24 h and 19 vs. 9% after 48 h). In addition, cell viability revealed marginal differences among the analyzed samples and the minimal viability rate was observed in SDM-SCs at 24 h post treatment (approximately 93%, Figure S2B in Supplementary Material).

The ability to fuse under stress condition was evaluated by immunostaining. The H_2O_2 treatment was sufficient to dramatically reduce myogenic differentiation in SDM-SCs while PSDM-SCs were not affected. This suggests that, differently from SDM-SCs, PSDM-SCs are resistant to oxidative stress.

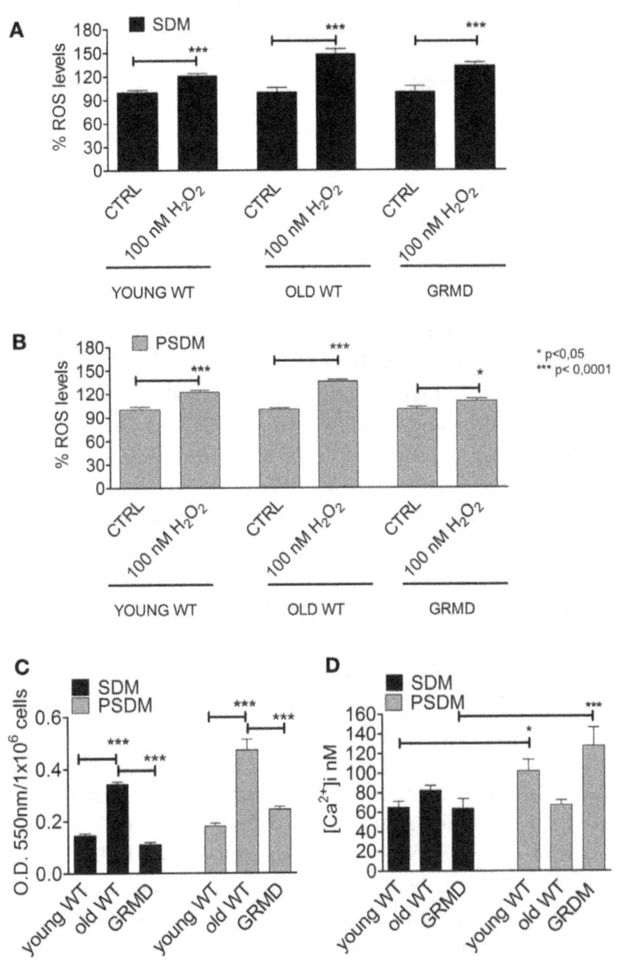

FIGURE 3 | Oxidant and calcium levels. Quantification of intracellular ROS levels by DCFH-DA assay expressed as a percentage respect to CTRL in SCs isolated from SDM **(A,B)** PSDM. **(C)** Quantification of O_2^- by rate reduction of NBT. The OD 550 nm represents the quantity of formazan revealed spectrophotometrically. **(D)** Basal levels of $[Ca2^+]_i$ expressed in nanomole measured on undifferentiated living cells by video-imaging technique. Data are represented as mean ± SD and statistically analyzed using *t*-test; $*p < 0.05$; $**p < 0.0001$.

RESTING CYTOPLASMIC $[CA^{2+}]_I$

Myogenesis is a strictly Ca^{2+}-dependent process and according to Bijlenga et al. (2000) the biophysical properties of specific ionic channels are important actors in the fusion process. We measured the resting $[Ca^{2+}]_i$ in myoblasts derived from somitic and presomitic, young, old, and GRMD muscles. The findings for PSDM GRMD SCs showed an increasing resting intracellular calcium concentration (127.0 ± 18 nM, $n = 24$) as compared to the somitic ones (SDM GRMD SCs; 63.5 ± 10 nM, $n = 50$) (**Figure 3D**). On the contrary, SDM GRMD and SDM WT young had similar content in cytoplasmic calcium at resting condition (63.5 ± 10 nM, $n = 24$; 65.0 ± 6 nM, $n = 27$) (**Figure 3D**). Likewise, the old SDM-SCs presented a higher level of resting $[Ca^{2+}]_i$ as compared to young and GRDM, but differently from those that did not show an increase of Ca^{2+} level in PSDM.

CA^{2+} TRANSIENT INDUCED BY EXTRACELLULAR STIMULI

To verify the presence of functional receptors, Ca^{2+} imaging experiments were performed on single myoblasts isolated from somitic and presomitic muscles, young, old, and GRMD. The physiological agents used on living cells were: (1) 100 μM ATP, which mainly causes a release of Ca^{2+} via IP_3/PKC (protein kinase) pathway in muscle cells; (2) 400 μM nicotine, which acts on nicotine receptors, a typical channel of neuromuscular junction; (3) 40 mM KCl, which induces a chemical depolarization of external membranes on myotube.

As shown in **Table 3**, all samples analyzed were responsive to 100 μM ATP with no significant differences, demonstrating that

Table 3 | Small molecule responsiveness of undifferentiated SCs; values are expressed as a percentage.

	Young		Old		GRMD	
	SDM	PSDM	SDM	PSDM	SDM	PSDM
Nicotine	0	90	3	80	50	65
KCl	6	0	3	35	4	66
ATP	100	65	93	65	100	56

the release of calcium via IP_3 pathway was unaffected by aging, or disease, or embryonic origin of SCs.

Surprisingly, a high percentage of stimulated cells of young (90%), old (80%), and GRMD (65%) from PSDM were responsive to 400 μM nicotine, revealing the presence of cholinergic receptors on the external membrane of undifferentiated cells. Furthermore, PSDM-SCs from old (35%) and GRDM (65.0%) dogs were also shown to respond to depolarizing stimulus (40 mM KCl).

MUSCLE-SPECIFIC miRNAs IN WT CANINE SCs

Some miRNAs are involved in post-transcriptional regulation of gene expression during skeletal muscle development. Therefore, we examined the expression of miR-1, miR-206, miR-133a, miR-133b (**Figures 4–6**), collectively known as myo-miRNAs and using miR-16 ubiquitously expressed as internal control. The results reported in **Figures 4A,B** showed no differences in miR-133a and miR-133b expression after 7 days of differentiation (t7) in isolated SCs from young SDM. However, we found that miR-133a and miR-133b were highly expressed in PSDM-SCs upon differentiation. The myogenic miR-1 was slightly upregulated at t7 only in PSDM-SCs from young donors (**Figure 4C**). miR-206 was similarly expressed in young PSDM- and to SDM-SCs (**Figure 4D**). With aging, the expression levels of miR-133a (**Figure 5A**) and miR-133b (**Figure 5B**) resulted affected and old PSDM-SCs did not positively regulate those miRNAs, whereas the expression of miR-1 was not modified in PSDM-SCs from old dogs (**Figure 5C**). Also, miR-206 in PSDM-SCs from old donors was found downregulated as compared to values from young donors and not modified during myogenic differentiation (**Figure 5D**). In summary, the expressions of myomiRs appeared to be modulated in SCs isolated from PSDM and this phenomenon seems to be age-dependent.

MUSCLE-SPECIFIC miRNAs IN GRMD SCs

Recent studies have shown that changes in miRNA expressions are associated with various skeletal muscle disorders, including muscular dystrophy (Eisenberg et al., 2009; Williams et al., 2009). However, the contradictory literature motivated the investigation for the expression profile of myomiRs during myogenic differentiation of dystrophic SCs. In fact, some authors referred to myo-miRNAs as markers of muscle regeneration while others support their critical role to sustain muscle degeneration. As for WT SCs, we studied the expression of myogenic miRNAs in SCs isolated from SDM and PSDM of GRMD dogs. As shown in **Figure 6**, miR-133a and miR-133b were upregulated at day 7 in SCs isolated from GRMD PSDM (**Figures 6A,B**). This result was consistent with WT expression. In addition, similarly to WT cells, miR-133a and miR-133b were not upregulated in SDM-SCs upon differentiation (**Figures 6A,B**). Likewise, miR-1 and miR-206 were markedly upregulated in PSDM-SCs after 7 days of differentiation in GRMD dogs (**Figures 6C,D**) and not in GRDM SDM-SCs (**Figures 6C,D**). The expression profile of myomiRs appeared to be affected by the dystrophic niche and miR-206 miR-1 seem to be primarily involved since they are highly expressed in differentiated SCs from both SDM and PSDM of GRMD samples.

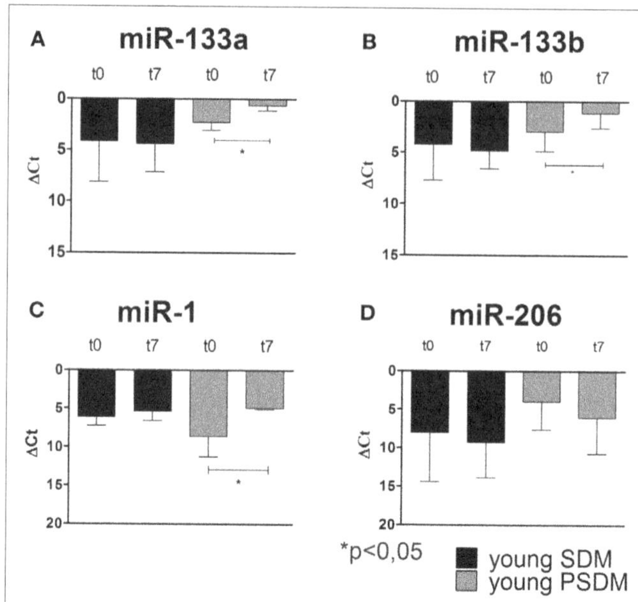

FIGURE 4 | Relative miR-133a, miR-133b, miR-1, and miR-206, expression in canine SCs measured by quantitative real-time PCR. SCs were isolated from SDM and PSDM of young dogs. Note that miR-133a **(A)** and miR-133b **(B)** are upregulated only in PSDM-SCs after 7 days of differentiation (t7). miR-1 is upregulated only in PSDM-SCs **(C)** after 7 days of differentiation. At variance, miR-206 is highly expressed in PSDM-SCs during proliferation **(D)**. The ubiquitously produced miR-16 was used as an internal control. Three independent experiments were performed in triplicates and statistically analyzed using ANOVA. Data are presented as mean ± SD; $*p < 0.05$.

DISCUSSION

In the last decades, SCs have been shown as muscle stem cells responsible for tissue regeneration in adulthood (Scharner and Zammit, 2011). Most of clinically relevant protocols for testing potential therapeutic approaches have been performed in small animal models, meaning mice and rats (Blau, 2008; Kuang and Rudnicki, 2008). However, large animal models have been considered essential to better mimic human diseases, to validate outcome measures, and to obtain reliable protocols for novel pharmaceutical, gene, and cell therapies. Thus, GRMD dogs represent a valuable large animal model to perform preclinical studies (Kornegay et al., 1988; Sharp et al., 1992). However, our knowledge on biological behavior of muscle regeneration in canine tissues remains primitive and requires further investigations.

In this work, extensive analysis for the biological properties of WT (young and old) and GRMD SCs isolated from somitic (SDM) and presomitic (PSDM) muscles are carried out. Although

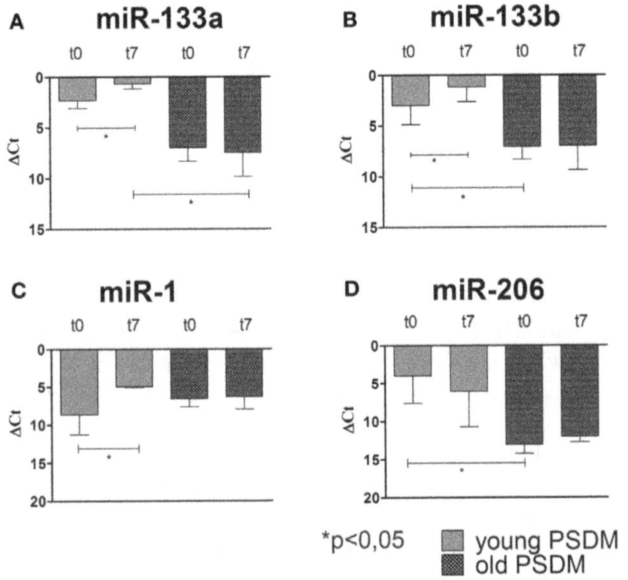

FIGURE 5 | Relative miR-133a, miR-133b, miR-1, and miR-206, expression in old canine PSDM-SCs measured by quantitative real-time PCR. In old PSDM-SCs, miR-133a **(A)** and miR-133b **(B)** are downregulated in both proliferating and differentiating cells. miR-1 and miR-206 regulations seem age-dependent, since old PSDM-SCs did not upregulate miR-1 during differentiation **(C)**, while miR-206 is not highly expressed during proliferation **(D)**. The ubiquitously produced miR-16 was used as an internal control. Three independent experiments were performed in triplicates and statistically analyzed using ANOVA; Data are presented as mean ± SD; $*p < 0.05$.

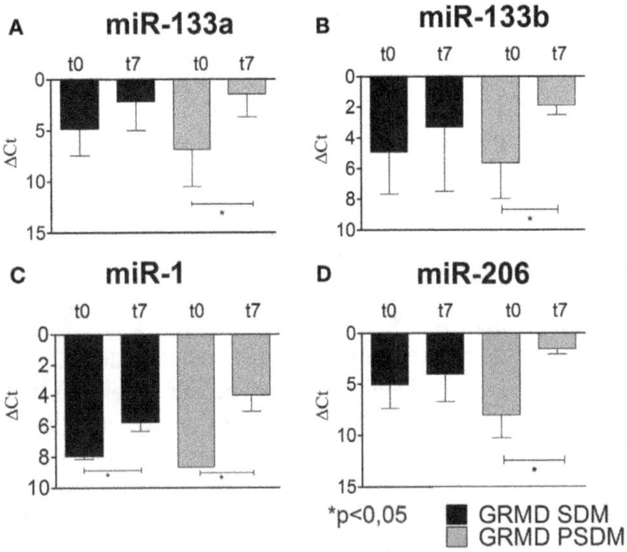

FIGURE 6 | Relative miR-133a, miR-133b, miR-1, and miR-206 expression in GRMD SCs measured by quantitative real-time PCR. SCs were isolated from SDM and PSDM of GRMD dogs. Consistent with data obtained with WT canine SCs, miR-133a and miR-133b are highly expressed after 7 days of differentiation in PSDM-SCs. At variance, miR-133a and miR-133b are upregulated in SDM-SCs after 7 days of differentiation **(A,B)**. Intriguingly, miR-1 and miR-206 are highly upregulated after 7 days of differentiation in PSDM-SCs **(C,D)**. Three independent experiments were performed in triplicates and statistically analyzed using ANOVA; miR-16 was used as an internal control. Data are presented as mean ± SD; $*p < 0.05$.

the gross morphology is quite similar in these muscles, several studies revealed unexpected molecular and cellular differences depicting peculiar biological characteristics in proliferation, lifespan, and differentiation potential of SDM and PSDM-SCs (Ono et al., 2010). With enzymatic dissociation it was possible to isolate SCs in all biopsies obtained by different research centers including Ecole de Veterinaire Maison-Alfort, Veterinary and University Clinics of Padua. In general, there were no observed differences in terms of SC quality, among the samples obtained by fresh or frozen biopsies. The proliferative lifespans of SCs derived from SDM and PSDM in both WT and GRMD dogs at different ages was also considered and compared. While the proliferative ability of SCs isolated from young SDM was approximately 20 population doublings before replicative senescence, SCs from young PSDM had 25 divisions *in vitro*. These differences were remarkable in WT old muscle as SCs isolated from PSDM stop to proliferate after 28 divisions while the cells derived from SDM had only 18 divisions. At later stage although SDM-SCs isolated from GRMD biopsies were phenotypically indistinguishable from WT SCs in *ex vivo* cultures, the cells showed a slower proliferative rate compared to the young WT SCs. Indeed, after 40 days they reached about 18 divisions compared to 30 days necessary to SDM-SCs isolated from WT samples. These findings suggest that SDM-SCs in GRMD dogs were exhausted by multiple attempts to regenerate lost tissues resulting in a limited proliferative ability. Nevertheless, they were prone to differentiate into myotubes much faster when compared to their WT counterparts. It is possible that when cultured *in vitro* they recapitulate their *in vivo* needs, i.e., to faster replace damaged myofibers. In this view, several articles recently showed a potential cell memory in reprogrammed cells (Kim et al., 2010; Polo et al., 2010; Quattrocelli et al., 2011). Our group also previously proposed that the SC pool is affected by the same lifestyle or pathological condition of the muscle in which they reside (Fulle et al., 2004). Similarly, SCs generated from degeneration/regeneration cycles appear to adapt to their biological behavior to better counteract the following degenerative processes (La Rovere et al., unpublished observation).

After isolation SCs are characterized by a period of rapid growth upon serial passages, until their proliferation rate gradually slows down and ultimately enters a non-dividing state called replicative senescence (Allsopp et al., 1995). Each cell division is characterized by a decrease of telomerase length and that has been proposed as a mitotic clock that regulates proliferative capacity of somatic cells *in vitro* (Di Donna et al., 2000). Thus, the higher telomerase activity observed in PSDM-SCs supports the hypothesis that those cells preserve a better proliferation capability compared to SDM-SCs, and consistently their lifespan is prolonged.

In our study, desmin expression was used as internal standard for normalization to avoid misinterpretation of comparative evaluations. Generally, low content of myogenic cells were obtained from head muscles compared to somite muscles and this difference was independent of sample age and between WT and GRMD. The FI and skeletal muscle differentiation potential of WT and GRMD

SCs was evaluated and analyzed. Our data show that WT limb muscles (SDM) contained a higher percentage of activated SCs compared to PSDM, as indicated by Pax7 and MyoD expression analysis. Conversely, SDM-SCs from GRMD dogs showed a lower percentage of Pax7 and MyoD positive cells, whereas craniofacial muscle (PSDM) contained significantly higher numbers of Pax7 and MyoD positive SCs. Overall, our analyses strongly support the idea that PSDM-SCs retain a higher myogenic potential compared to the SDM-SCs isolated from GRMD muscles. Despite a higher number of MyoD positive cells in PSDM-SCs isolated from GRDM dogs, they show less differentiation capacity compared to the WT counterparts.

To verify if PSDM-SCs have an intrinsic capability to resist to toxic insults, or whether their invulnerable behavior can be justified from specific niche characteristics, the response of both PSDM-SCs and SDM-SCs to hydrogen peroxide treatment has been assessed. Notwithstanding that the proliferation ability of SCs from PSDM and SDM samples were not affected, 100 nM H_2O_2 treatment impaired the myogenic differentiation exclusively in SDM-SCs.

To fully investigate if this reduced differentiative capability was due to high oxidant levels, ROS contents have been evaluated. Although for a long time the ROS formation has been believed harmful, evidences are accumulating showing the key role of ROS presence and production in cell signaling. In addition, changes in ROS content seem to be modulated during myogenic processes (Musarò et al., 2010). It was previously observed that human SC derived from old subjects showed to have a high oxidative stress with respect to young samples (Fulle et al., 2004; Beccafico et al., 2007; Pietrangelo et al., 2009). This was associated to higher $[Ca^{2+}]_i$, probably due to alteration of calcium homeostasis regulatory proteins functionality. Here, it is confirmed that elderly SDM and PSDM canine SCs showed high ROS levels, however, dystrophic SCs displayed ROS levels similarly to young WT samples. In all PSDM-SCs, high responsiveness to nicotine determined the characteristic calcium transients and revealed the presence of nicotinic receptors on undifferentiated cells (Krause et al., 1995). SCs express low levels of functional nicotinic acetylcholine receptors (nAChR) before myosin becomes detectable (Grassi et al., 2004) and considered to be an early marker of myogenic differentiation. Thus, this opens up new cues to examine presomitic aged and dystrophic SCs that showed to still remain functional and able to fuse with existing fibers.

To date, the crucial miRNAs involved in skeletal muscle differentiation are miR-1, miR-206, miR-133a, miR-133b and are collectively known as myomiRs. miR-1 and miR-206 are key myo-miRNAs for Mef2c-dependent terminal myogenic differentiation. miR-1 and miR-206 act as positive controls for the progression of differentiation via Notch 3 and utrophin inhibition (Rosenberg et al., 2006; Gagan et al., 2012). Several studies have shown that changes in miRNA expressions are associated with various skeletal muscle disorders, including muscular dystrophy (Eisenberg et al., 2009; Williams et al., 2009). Thus, we examined the expression of myomiRs during proliferation (day 0) and differentiation (day 7) of SCs isolated from WT and GRMD samples. Our data showed that miR-133a and miR-133b, involved in early myogenic differentiation, were upregulated after 7 days of differentiation in WT PSDM. However, this upregulation disappeared with aging and the PSDM-SCs acted similarly to SDM-SCs. miR-1 is also upregulated at day 7 in WT PSDM-SCs and again aging affected negatively its modulation. miR-206 is highly expressed in young WT PSDM samples while in aged samples it is much less expressed. Overall from the collected results, myomiRs are clearly modulated in PSDM-SCs of WT canine muscles and this regulation is lost with aging. In the GRMD, a similar modulation for miR-133a, miR-133b, and miR-1 was found in the PSDM-SCs. In addition, miR-206 was strongly upregulated at day 7 of differentiation. Intriguingly, myomiR upregulation was observed in SDM-SCs of GRMD dogs that feature worse locomotion ability. In this view, myomiR overexpression could sustain the muscle chronic degeneration of GRMD dogs by affecting the expression of myomiR target genes.

Emerging literature confirmed that the expression of miR-206 is essentially confined to skeletal muscle (Baskerville and Bartel, 2005; Liang et al., 2007) and involved in muscle differentiation by repressing the expression of DNA polymerase A, connexin 43, follistatin-like 1, and utrophin. Intriguingly, miR-206 was found highly expressed in the diaphragm of *mdx* mouse, the murine counterpart of GRMD dogs, and not in the hindlimb muscles (McCarthy et al., 2007). This result is significant because the diaphragm of the *mdx* mouse displays DMD phenotype differently from hindlimb muscles. McCarthy et al. (2007) proposed that increased miR-206 expression may contribute to the chronic pathology of *mdx* diaphragm. In fact, miR-206 represses the expression of genes, including utrophin, that otherwise would serve as compensatory function. Utrophin is indeed a verified target of miR-206, and this observation explains at least in part the higher expression of utrophin protein in the *mdx* hindlimb musculature where miR-206 is barely detectable. Conversely, Eisenberg et al. (2007) showed recently the expression profiling of 10 different human dystrophies, including DMD, in which miR-206 expression was similar to one observed in control muscles. One possible explanation for this discrepancy is again the different muscles used to evaluate miRNA expressions. In conclusion, the expression profile of MRFs and myomiRs reveals a unique molecular signature in canine SCs. In addition, miR-206 seems to be primarily involved in GRMD SC impairment, although its precise role needs to be carefully considered in the light of discordant literature.

ACKNOWLEDGMENTS

Maurilio Sampaolesi is supported by CARE-MI FP7, AFM, CARIPLO, FWO, GOA, UIAP, and OT grants. Maurilio Sampaolesi and Mattia Quattrocelli would like to thank Christina Vochten and Vicky Raets for professional secretarial service and Paolo Luban and Rondoufonds voor Duchenne Onderzoek for kind donations. We also thank Raymon Floyd Principe for generous editing of the manuscript. Tiziana Pietrangelo would like to thank Dr. F. Jamali and Dr. A. Di Domizio for their invaluable availability. Tiziana Pietrangelo and Stefania Fulle are supported by University "G. d'Annunzio" of Chieti-Pescara local research grants. Stefania Fulle is supported by research grants from MIUR (Ministero Istruzione Università e Ricerca).

SUPPLEMENTARY MATERIAL

Figure S1 | Immunofluorescence analysis for Ki67 expression in early and late passages of SC cultures. Examples of Ki67 staining indicating that up to 30% of SCs are proliferating in both SDM and PSDM samples. Consistent with growth curve data at late stage (30 days) while up to 10% of PSDM-SCs (22 PDL) are still positive for Ki67, SDM-SCs (20 PDL) stopped proliferation and the majority of cells present large nuclei (red arrow heads). Ki67 positive nuclei (green arrow heads) are much smaller compared to negative ones (right lower panel). Bar = 100 μm.

Figure S2 | Effect of hydrogen peroxide on SC differentiation. SCs were isolated from SDM and PSDM of WT dogs and harvested after 24 and 48 h of treatment with 100 nM hydrogen peroxide. SCs did not show any differences under this condition. However, a higher number of cells in S phase were observed in PSDM-SCs compared to SDM-SCs (28 vs. 16% after 24 h and 19 vs. 9% after 48 h) **(A)**. Cell viability was assessed using Countess Automated Cell Counter (Life Technologies) after trypan blue staining **(B)**. The H_2O_2 treatment was sufficient to dramatically reduce myogenic differentiation in SDM-SCs while PSDM-SCs were not affected **(C)**. Bar = 100 μm.

REFERENCES

Allsopp, R. C., Chang, E., Kashefi-Aazam, M., Rogaev, E. I., Piatyszek, M. A., Shay, J. W., et al. (1995). Telomere shortening is associated with cell division in vitro and in vivo. *Exp. Cell Res.* 220, 194–200. doi:10.1006/excr.1995.1306

Baskerville, S., and Bartel, D. P. (2005). Microarray profiling of microRNAs reveals frequent coexpression with neighboring miRNAs and host genes. *RNA* 11, 241–247. doi:10.1261/rna.7240905

Beccafico, S., Puglielli, C., Pietrangelo, T., Bellomo, R., Fanò, G., and Fulle, S. (2007). Age-dependent effects on functional aspects in human satellite cells. *Ann. N. Y. Acad. Sci.* 1100, 345–352. doi:10.1196/annals.1395.037

Bijlenga, P., Liu, J. H., Espinos, E., Haenggeli, C. A., Fischer-Lougheed, J., Bader, C. R., et al. (2000). T-type alpha 1H Ca2+ channels are involved in Ca2+ signaling during terminal differentiation (fusion) of human myoblasts. *Proc. Natl. Acad. Sci. U.S.A.* 97, 7627–7632. doi:10.1073/pnas.97.13.7627

Biressi, S., and Rando, T. A. (2010). Heterogeneity in the muscle satellite cell population. *Semin. Cell Dev. Biol.* 21, 845–854. doi:10.1016/j.semcdb.2010.09.003

Blau, H. M. (2008). Cell therapies for muscular dystrophy. *N. Engl. J. Med.* 359, 1403–1405. doi:10.1056/NEJMcibr0805708

Chargé, S. B. P., and Rudnicki, M. A. (2004). Cellular and molecular regulation of muscle regeneration. *Physiol. Rev.* 84, 209–238. doi:10.1152/physrev.00019.2003

Chen, J.-F., Callis, T. E., and Wang, D.-Z. (2008). microRNAs and muscle disorders. *J. Cell. Sci.* 122, 13–20. doi:10.1242/jcs.041723

Collins, C. A., and Morgan, J. E. (2003). Duchenne's muscular dystrophy: animal models used to investigate pathogenesis and develop therapeutic strategies. *Int. J. Exp. Pathol.* 84, 165–172. doi:10.1046/j.1365-2613.2003.00354.x

De Cecco, M., Jeyapalan, J., Zhao, X., Tamamori-Adachi, M., and Sedivy, J. M. (2011). Nuclear protein accumulation in cellular senescence and organismal aging revealed with a novel single-cell resolution fluorescence microscopy assay. *Aging (Albany NY)* 3, 955–967.

Di Donna, S., Renault, V., Forestier, C., Piron-Hamelin, G., Thiesson, D., Cooper, R. N., et al. (2000). Regenerative capacity of human satellite cells: the mitotic clock in cell transplantation. *Neurol. Sci.* 21, S943–S951.

Diermeier-Daucher, S., Clarke, S. T., Hill, D., Vollmann-Zwerenz, A., Bradford, J. A., and Brockhoff, G. (2009). Cell type specific applicability of 5-ethynyl-2'-deoxyuridine (EdU) for dynamic proliferation assessment in flow cytometry. *Cytometry A* 75, 535–546. doi:10.1002/cyto.a.20712

Drummond, M. J., McCarthy, J. J., Sinha, M., Spratt, H. M., Volpi, E., Esser, K. A., et al. (2010). Ageing and microRNA expression in human skeletal muscle: a microarray and bioinformatics analysis. *Physiol. Genomics* 43, 595–603. doi:10.1152/physiolgenomics.00148.2010

Eisenberg, I., Alexander, M. S., and Kunkel, L. M. (2009). miRNAs in normal and diseased skeletal muscle. *J. Cell. Mol. Med.* 13, 2–11. doi:10.1111/j.1582-4934.2008.00524.x

Eisenberg, I., Eran, A., Nishino, I., Moggio, M., Lamperti, C., Amato, A. A., et al. (2007). Distinctive patterns of microRNA expression in primary muscular disorders. *Proc. Natl. Acad. Sci. U.S.A.* 104, 17016–17021. doi:10.1073/pnas.0708115104

Freeman, L. M. (2012). Cachexia and sarcopenia: emerging syndromes of importance in dogs and cats. *J. Vet. Intern. Med.* 26, 3–17. doi:10.1111/j.1939-1676.2011.00838.x

Fulle, S., Protasi, F., Di Tano, G., Pietrangelo, T., Beltramin, A., Boncompagni, S., et al. (2004). The contribution of reactive oxygen species to sarcopenia and muscle ageing. *Exp. Gerontol.* 39, 17–24. doi:10.1016/j.exger.2003.09.012

Gagan, J., Dey, B. K., Layer, R., Yan, Z., and Dutta, A. (2012). Notch3 and Mef2c proteins are mutually antagonistic via Mkp1 protein and miR-1/206 microRNAs in differentiating myoblasts. *J. Biol. Chem.* 287, 40360–40370. doi:10.1074/jbc.M112.378414

Grassi, F., Pagani, F., Spinelli, G., De Angelis, L., Cossu, G., and Eusebi, F. (2004). Fusion-independent expression of functional ACh receptors in mouse mesoangioblast stem cells contacting muscle cells. *J. Physiol.* 560, 479–489. doi:10.1113/jphysiol.2004.070607

Huang, Z.-P., Espinoza-Lewis, R., and Wang, D.-Z. (2012). Determination of miRNA targets in skeletal muscle cells. *Methods Mol. Biol.* 798, 475–490. doi:10.1007/978-1-61779-343-1_28

Kim, K., Doi, A., Wen, B., Ng, K., Zhao, R., Cahan, P., et al. (2010). Epigenetic memory in induced pluripotent stem cells. *Nature* 467, 285–290. doi:10.1038/nature09342

Kornegay, J. N., Tuler, S. M., Miller, D. M., and Levesque, D. C. (1988). Muscular dystrophy in a litter of golden retriever dogs. *Muscle Nerve* 11, 1056–1064. doi:10.1002/mus.880111008

Krause, R. M., Hamann, M., Bader, C. R., Liu, J. H., Baroffio, A., and Bernheim, L. (1995). Activation of nicotinic acetylcholine receptors increases the rate of fusion of cultured human myoblasts. *J. Physiol.* 489(Pt 3), 779–790.

Kuang, S., and Rudnicki, M. A. (2008). The emerging biology of satellite cells and their therapeutic potential. *Trends Mol. Med.* 14, 82–91. doi:10.1016/j.molmed.2007.12.004

Liang, Y., Ridzon, D., Wong, L., and Chen, C. (2007). Characterization of microRNA expression profiles in normal human tissues. *BMC Genomics* 8:166. doi:10.1186/1471-2164-8-166

Mauro, A. (1961). Satellite cell of skeletal muscle fibres. *J. Biophys. Biochem. Cytol.* 9, 493–495. doi:10.1083/jcb.9.2.493

McCarthy, J. J., and Esser, K. A. (2007). MicroRNA-1 and microRNA-133a expression are decreased during skeletal muscle hypertrophy. *J. Appl. Physiol.* 102, 306–313. doi:10.1152/japplphysiol.00932.2006

McCarthy, J. J., Esser, K. A., and Andrade, F. H. (2007). MicroRNA-206 is overexpressed in the diaphragm but not the hindlimb muscle of mdx mouse. *Am. J. Physiol. Cell Physiol.* 293, C451–C457. doi:10.1152/ajpcell.00077.2007

McLoon, L. K., Thorstenson, K. M., Solomon, A., and Lewis, M. P. (2007). Myogenic precursor cells in craniofacial muscles. *Oral Dis.* 13, 134–140. doi:10.1111/j.1601-0825.2006.01353.x

Menghini, L., Leporini, L., Scanu, N., Pintore, G., La Rovere, R., Di Filippo, E. S., et al. (2011). Effect of phytochemical concentrations on biological activities of cranberry extracts. *J. Biol. Regul. Homeost. Agents* 25, 27–35.

Miranda, K. C., Huynh, T., Tay, Y., Ang, Y.-S., Tam, W.-L., Thomson, A. M., et al. (2006). A pattern-based method for the identification of MicroRNA binding sites and their corresponding heteroduplexes. *Cell* 126, 1203–1217. doi:10.1016/j.cell.2006.07.031

Musarò, A., Fulle, S., and Fanò, G. (2010). Oxidative stress and muscle homeostasis. *Curr. Opin. Clin. Nutr. Metab. Care* 13, 236–242. doi:10.1097/MCO.0b013e3283368188

Ono, Y., Boldrin, L., Knopp, P., Morgan, J. E., and Zammit, P. S. (2010). Muscle satellite cells are a functionally heterogeneous population in both somite-derived and branchiomeric muscles. *Dev. Biol.* 337, 29–41. doi:10.1016/j.ydbio.2009.10.005

Pietrangelo, T., Puglielli, C., Mancinelli, R., Beccafico, S., Fanò, G., and Fulle, S. (2009). Molecular basis of the myogenic profile of aged human skeletal muscle satellite cells during differentiation. *Exp. Gerontol.* 44, 523–531. doi:10.1016/j.exger.2009.05.002

Polo, J. M., Liu, S., Figueroa, M. E., Kulalert, W., Eminli, S., Tan, K. Y., et al. (2010). Cell type of origin influences the molecular and functional properties of mouse induced pluripotent stem cells. *Nat. Biotechnol.* 28, 848–855. doi:10.1038/nbt.1667

Porter, J. D., Israel, S., Gong, B., Merriam, A. P., Feuerman, J., Khanna, S., et al. (2006). Distinctive morphological and gene/protein expression signatures during myogenesis in novel cell lines from extraocular and hindlimb muscle. *Physiol. Genomics* 24, 264–275. doi:10.1152/physiolgenomics.00234.2004

Quattrocelli, M., Palazzolo, G., Floris, G., Schöffski, P., Anastasia, L., Orlacchio, A., et al. (2011). Intrinsic cell memory reinforces myogenic commitment of pericyte-derived iPSCs. *J. Pathol.* 223, 593–603. doi:10.1002/path.2845

Rando, T. A. (2006). Stem cells, ageing and the quest for immortality. *Nature* 441, 1080–1086. doi:10.1038/nature04958

Rao, P. K., Kumar, R. M., Farkhondeh, M., Baskerville, S., and Lodish, H. F. (2006). Myogenic factors that regulate expression of muscle-specific microRNAs. *Proc. Natl. Acad. Sci. U.S.A.* 103, 8721–8726. doi:10.1073/pnas.0602831103

Rosenberg, M. I., Georges, S. A., Asawachaicharn, A., Analau, E., and Tapscott, S. J. (2006). MyoD inhibits Fstl1 and Utrn expression by inducing transcription of miR-206. *J. Cell Biol.* 175, 77–85. doi:10.1083/jcb.200603039

Scharner, J., and Zammit, P. S. (2011). The muscle satellite cell at 50: the formative years. *Skelet. Muscle* 1, 28–28. doi:10.1186/2044-5040-1-28

Schiaffino, S., and Reggiani, C. (2011). Fibre types in mammalian skeletal muscles. *Physiol. Rev.* 91, 1447–1531. doi:10.1152/physrev.00031.2010

Sciote, J. J., Rowlerson, A. M., Hopper, C., and Hunt, N. P. (1994). Fibre type classification and myosin isoforms in the human masseter muscle. *J. Neurol. Sci.* 126, 15–24. doi:10.1016/0022-510X(94)90089-2

Sharp, N. J., Kornegay, J. N., Van Camp, S. D., Herbstreith, M. H., Secore, S. L., Kettle, S., et al. (1992). An error in dystrophin mRNA processing in golden retriever muscular dystrophy, an animal homologue of Duchenne muscular dystrophy. *Genomics* 13, 115–121. doi:10.1016/0888-7543(92)90210-J

Small, E. M., O'Rourke, J. R., Moresi, V., Sutherland, L. B., McAnally, J., Gerard, R. D., et al. (2010). Regulation of PI3-kinase/Akt signaling by muscle-enriched microRNA-486. *Proc. Natl. Acad. Sci. U.S.A.* 107, 4218–4223. doi:10.1073/pnas.1000300107

Snijders, T., Verdijk, L. B., and van Loon, L. J. C. (2009). The impact of sarcopenia and exercise training on skeletal muscle satellite cells. *Ageing Res. Rev.* 8, 328–338. doi:10.1016/j.arr.2009.05.003

Sozio, P., Cerasa, L. S., Laserra, S., Cacciatore, I., Cornacchia, C., Di Filippo, E. S., et al. (2013). Memantine-sulfur containing antioxidant conjugates as potential prodrugs to improve the treatment of Alzheimer's disease. *Eur. J. Pharm. Sci.* 49, 187–198. doi:10.1016/j.ejps.2013.02.013

Toniolo, L., Cancellara, P., Maccatrozzo, L., Patruno, M., Mascarello, F., and Reggiani, C. (2008). Masticatory myosin unveiled: first determination of contractile parameters of muscle fibres from carnivore jaw muscles. *Am. J. Physiol. Cell Physiol.* 295, C1535–C1542. doi:10.1152/ajpcell.00093.2008

Williams, A. H., Liu, N., van Rooij, E., and Olson, E. N. (2009). MicroRNA control of muscle development and disease. *Curr. Opin. Cell Biol.* 21, 461–469. doi:10.1016/j.ceb.2009.01.029

6

Sarcopenia and sarcopenic obesity in patients with muscular dystrophy

Luciano Merlini[1]*, Alessandro Vagheggini[2] and Daniela Cocchi[2]

[1] *Laboratory of Musculoskeletal Cell Biology, Istituto Ortopedico Rizzoli, Bologna, Italy*
[2] *Department of Statistical Sciences, University of Bologna, Bologna, Italy*

Correspondence:
Luciano Merlini, Laboratory of Musculoskeletal Cell Biology, Istituto Ortopedico Rizzoli, Via Di Barbiano 1/10, Bologna 40136, Italy
e-mail: luciano.merlini@ior.it

Aging sarcopenia and muscular dystrophy (MD) are two conditions characterized by lower skeletal muscle quantity, lower muscle strength, and lower physical performance. Aging is associated with a peculiar alteration in body composition called "sarcopenic obesity" characterized by a decrease in lean body mass and increase in fat mass. To evaluate the presence of sarcopenia and obesity in a cohort of adult patients with MD, we have used the measurement techniques considered golden standard for sarcopenia that is for muscle mass dual-energy X-ray absorptiometry (DXA), for muscle strength hand-held dynamometry (HHD), and for physical performance gait speed. The study involved 14 adult patients with different types of MD. We were able to demonstrate that all patients were sarcopenic obese. We showed, in fact, that all were sarcopenic based on appendicular lean, fat and bone free, mass index (ALMI). In addition, all resulted obese according to the percentage of body fat determined by DXA in contrast to their body mass index ranging from underweight to obese. Skeletal muscle mass determined by DXA was markedly reduced in all patients and correlated with residual muscle strength determined by HHD, and physical performances determined by gait speed and respiratory function. Finally, we showed that ALMI was the best linear explicator of muscle strength and physical function. Altogether, our study suggests the relevance of a proper evaluation of body composition in MD and we propose to use, both in research and practice, the measurement techniques that has already been demonstrated effective in aging sarcopenia.

Keywords: muscular dystrophy, sarcopenia, sarcopenic obesity, body composition, muscle strength, physical performance

INTRODUCTION

Muscular dystrophies (MDs) are a clinically and genetically heterogeneous group of inherited diseases characterized by progressive muscle wasting and weakness (Emery, 2002). In the dystrophic muscle, there is a progressive loss of muscle fibers that are substituted by fat and connective tissue. The dystrophic muscle weakness reflects the loss of muscle tissue and compromises physical performance. In summary, MD can specifically be defined as a condition characterized by lower skeletal muscle quantity, lower muscle strength, and lower physical performance. The other condition that combines these three characteristics is sarcopenia.

Sarcopenia is defined according to European consensus group (Cruz-Jentoft et al., 2010) as a condition that involves a loss of muscle mass and declining strength and/or physical performance. In particular, "severe sarcopenia" is the stage identified when all three criteria of the definition are met (low muscle mass, low muscle strength, and low physical performance) (Cruz-Jentoft et al., 2010). With aging, skeletal muscle atrophy in human beings appears to be inevitable. A gradual loss of muscle fibers begins at approximately 50 years of age and continues such that by 80 years of age, approximately 50% of the fibers are lost from the limb muscles that have been studied (Faulkner et al., 2007). Although primarily a disease of the elderly, sarcopenia can be observed at any age resulting associated with conditions like disuse, malnutrition, and neuromuscular diseases (Muscaritoli et al., 2010).

Body composition changes with aging. Cross-sectional and longitudinal data have shown that aging is associated with a peculiar alteration in body composition – a decrease in lean body mass and increase in fat mass (FM). Baumgartner et al. (2004) have proposed criteria for this new condition that combines sarcopenia and obesity, which has been called sarcopenic/obesity (Baumgartner et al., 2004). High body mass index (BMI), low muscle mass, and the combination of excess FM with low muscle mass have been associated with increased risk for physical disability in older adults (Fielding et al., 2011). It is, therefore, recognized that sarcopenic/obesity has an important impact on physical capacity in older individuals as the prevalence of this condition is <10% of the elderly population (Baumgartner et al., 2004; Batsis et al., 2013), whereas the prevalence of sarcopenia is 13–36% and circa 30% of older Americans are obese (Jankowski et al., 2008).

The aim of this study was to evaluate the presence and severity of sarcopenia and of sarcopenic obesity in a cohort of adult patients with MD. In order to conduct a valid and reliable diagnosis of these conditions in patients with MD, we have measured muscle mass, muscle strength, and physical performance. The measurement techniques were the ones suggested by the European Working Group, recognized useful both in research and practice that is for muscle mass dual-energy X-ray absorptiometry (DXA), for muscle strength hand-held dynamometry (HHD), and for physical performance gait speed (Mijnarends et al., 2013).

MATERIALS AND METHODS

PATIENTS

We included in the study, adult patients with a clinical and molecular diagnosis of MD and clinical and body composition evaluations performed within 1 month and with the same equipment. Data of 14 adult patients (7 were women) with a clinical/laboratory phenotype compatible with the diagnosis of MD were collected. The mean age of women was 35.6 (range 19–56) years and of men 29.5 (range 18–64) years; this difference was not significant ($p = 0.47$). All the patients had a definite molecular diagnosis. There were six patients with Bethlem myopathy (BM) and one with Ullrich congenital muscular dystrophy (UCMD) with recognition of a pathogenetic mutation/s in one of the three *COL6* genes (Pepe et al., 1999; Lucioli et al., 2005; Merlini et al., 2008b; Gualandi et al., 2009, 2011; Martoni et al., 2009; Sabatelli et al., 2011, 2012). Two patients had a rigid spine syndrome due to a mutation of the FHL1 gene. One patient had a limb girdle MD type 2D (LGMD2D) due to a homozygous mutation in the alpha-sarcoglycan gene. Three patients had a Duchenne MD (DMD) and one a Becker MD (BMD) with mutations in the *DMD* gene. Three patients were non-ambulatory: the UCMD patient was never able to walk and was on nocturnal non-invasive ventilation, the patient with LGMD2D and one with rigid spine lost ambulation at 15 and 21 years of age, respectively. The study protocol was approved for patients with MD by the institutional ethical committee in 1994 and specifically for patients with COL6 related myopathies in 2011 (ClinicalTrials.gov identifier: NCT01438788). All subjects were fully informed and gave their written informed consent.

BODY COMPOSITION

Body composition was obtained by DXA (Hologic 4500 W; software version 11.2; Hologic, Inc., Waltham, MA). According to the tree-compartment model of body composition, the Hologic software provided regional and whole body estimation of lean mass (LM), FM, and bone mineral content (BMC). BMC and LM were added to obtain fat-free mass (FFM). Appendicular lean mass (ALM) was the sum of bone-free and fat-free tissue mass in the arms and legs. Body mass, FM, LM, FFM, and ALM were normalized to height^2 to control for skeletal size. ALM/height^2, appendicular lean mass index (ALMI), was considered the sarcopenia index. ALMI two standard deviations (Baumgartner et al., 1998) or more (Tanko et al., 2002; Newman et al., 2003) lower than a mean derived from young male and female reference groups was defined as the gender-specific cut point for sarcopenia (Baumgartner et al., 1998; Tanko et al., 2002; Newman et al., 2003). BMI, an index of obesity, was derived from body mass measured by DXA to the nearest gram and height measured to the nearest 0.1 cm. We used BMI to categorized participants as obese ($BMI \geq 30$), overweight ($25 \leq BMI < 30$), normal weight ($18.5 < BMI < 25$), or underweight (≤ 18.5) (WHO, 2000). Sarcopenic obesity was defined according to Baumgartner et al. (2004) as ALMI < 7.26 kg/m^2 in men and 5.45 kg/m^2 in women and percentage body fat greater than 28% in men and 40% in women (Baumgartner et al., 2004).

MUSCLE STRENGTH AND PHYSICAL PERFORMANCES

Maximal isometric strength was assessed using a hand-held dynamometer (Type CT 3001, Citec, C.I.T. Technics BV, Groningen, The Netherlands) (van der Ploeg et al., 1991). Two muscle groups were examined bilaterally: handgrip (HG) and knee extensor (KE) (Merlini et al., 2002, 2003, 2004). The maximum force from three attempts was used in analysis. Patients were considered to have low muscle strength if HG strength was <20 kg in women and <30 kg in men (Bohannon et al., 2006; Cruz-Jentoft et al., 2010). This is also the diagnostic threshold in handgrip strength that best discriminates subjects with mobility limitations to be used in clinical practice (Fried et al., 2001; Lauretani et al., 2003). A ratio of maximal muscular strength of knee extensors to body weight was calculated by dividing the muscular strength (N) by body weight (kg). In older adults (81–89 years), muscular strength thresholds to perform activities of daily living (ADL) independently were 2.8 N/kg for knee extensors (Hasegawa et al., 2008). Ploutz-Snyder et al. (2002) have found similar figures: ambulatory tasks (chair rise, gait speed, and stair ascent and descent) were compromised in individuals with a ratio of isometric leg extension peak torque to body weight (STR/WT) <3.0 N m/kg (Ploutz-Snyder et al., 2002).

Forced vital capacity (FVC) was determined with an electronic spirometer, and percent-predicted values were calculated based on normal published values. A value between 50 and 70% was considered moderately reduced; a value less than 50% was considered severely reduced (van der Kooi et al., 2006). Timed test included the time to walk 10 m. Patients were considered to have a low mobility based on the walking speed threshold of 1.22 m/s proposed by Langlois et al. (1997), evaluating the ability to cross the street in the time typically allotted at signalized intersections (Langlois et al., 1997).

STATISTICAL ANALYSIS

In order to determine the separate relative contributions of the various indices to the strength variables, we used the linear regression models. Due to the limited sample size, we chose to estimate the linear regression model without intercept, $y_i = bx_i + e_i$, via ordinary least squares. Each b coefficient is the slope of the regression line and represents the increment/decrement of the dependent variable for a unit increment of each explanatory variable. Linear correlation coefficients have, therefore, been computed for various couples of variables with the aim of choosing the variables for simple linear models without intercept. High values of the linear correlation coefficients helped in the choice of identifying the body mass and muscularity as explanatory variables to the dependent variables muscle strength, gait speed, and pulmonary function. The strength of each simple linear relationship was investigated via the adjusted R^2, which represents a well-known goodness of fit measure. Measurable variables are presented as mean (x) ± SD and their range of variation is presented in parentheses.

RESULTS

BODY COMPOSITION

Six participants were normal weight, four overweight, three underweight, and one obese based on BMI (**Table 1**). All were sarcopenic based on ALMI, which was well below of the cut off for the

Table 1 | Body mass, adiposity, and muscularity.

	Women ($n=7$)	Men ($n=7$)	p-value
Total mass (kg)	60.90 ± 13.09 (45.47–76.38)	61.05 ± 16.80 (40.01–79.63)	0.99
BMI (kg/m^2)	22.41 ± 4.61 (16.10–29.20)	23.99 ± 4.79 (17.40–31.70)	0.54
Total fat (%)	50.66 ± 6.02 (41.30–58.50)	42.93 ± 8.61 (29.70–58.80)	0.08
FMI (kg/m^2)	11.54 ± 3.58 (7.10–17.10)	10.53 ± 4.04 (5.70–18.60)	0.63
FFMI (kg/m^2)	10.86 ± 1.23 (9.00–12.70)	13.30 ± 2.01 (9.60–15.40)	0.02
LMI (kg/m^2)	10.20 ± 1.19 (8.50–12.10)	12.76 ± 1.87 (9.40–14.70)	0.01
ALMI (kg/m^2)	3.84 ± 0.69 (3.14–4.78)	4.82 ± 0.81 (3.67–5.55)	0.03

Kg, kilogram; BMI, body mass index; m^2, square meter; FMI, fat mass index; FFMI, fat-free mass index; LMI, lean mass index; ALMI, appendicular lean mass index.
Summaries of individual data grouped according to sex. p-Value of the two sample t-test for the mean.

sarcopenia index of 7.26 kg/m^2 for men and 5.45 for women, and all were sarcopenic obese based on ALMI and % FM that was greater than 28% in men and 40% in women. In addition, ALMI was significantly different ($p \approx 0.00$) between walkers and non-walkers (4.6 ± 0.8 vs. 3.4 ± 0.3). FFMI was well below the fifth percentile for all the patients as compared to the normal age-related Italian population and also to the 70–80–year olds (17 kg/m^2 in men and 13.4 kg/m^2 in women) (Coin et al., 2008). Gender differences in body composition were significant for the indices of muscularity (FFMI, LMI, and ALMI) but not for total mass, BMI, and FMI.

MUSCLE STRENGTH AND PHYSICAL FUNCTION

Muscle strength was markedly reduced comparing with the normative values (van der Ploeg et al., 1991; Beenakker et al., 2001) (**Table 2**). Knee extension strength (KES) with a mean value of 60 N (range 15–132 N) was very weak comparing with healthy subjects in which it exceeded in both genders 250 N (van der Ploeg et al., 1991; Beenakker et al., 2001). Non-walkers had a significant lower ($p \approx 0.00$) KES mean value as compared with walkers (22.5 N vs. 69.2 N). HGS was also very weak, and in all well below the T-score value less than −2 (20 kg in women and 30 kg in men). Again, there was a significant difference ($p = 0.011$) between mean HGS of non-walkers and walkers (2.9 kg vs. 13.0 kg), confirming that HGS is a good indicator of global muscle strength. The ratio between KES and body weight was in all well below (range 0.3–1.7 N/kg) the threshold (2.8 N/kg) in which performance on ambulatory tasks is compromised. Walking speed was below the threshold of 1.22 m/s, indicating a low mobility, in 10 patients (range 0–1, 11 m/s), and above it in 4 (range 1.25–1.72 m/s). % FVC was moderately (<70%) reduced in four, and severely reduced (<50%) in three patients (range 13–41%); non-walkers had a significantly lower ($p = 0.03$) % FVC as compared with walkers (39 vs. 72). Gender differences were significant only for FVC and % FVC.

Table 2 | Muscle strength and measured physical function.

	Women ($n=7$)	Men ($n=7$)	p-value
HGS (kg)	9.69 ± 5.98 (1.00–18.50)	11.91 ± 6.35 (4.50–22.50)	0.51
KES (N)	62.86 ± 41.22 (15.00–131.00)	56.29 ± 40.67 (18.00–132.00)	0.77
KES/body weight (N/kg)	1.00 ± 0.57 (0.30–1.80)	0.90 ± 0.57 (0.40–1.70)	0.75
Gait speed (m/s)	1.01 ± 0.73 (0.00–1.72)	0.81 ± 0.40 (0.00–1.25)	0.55
FVC (L)	1.74 ± 0.97 (0.46–2.77)	3.06 ± 0.62 (2.09–3.93)	0.01
% FVC	49.71 ± 29.12 (13.00–90.00)	79.43 ± 14.63 (53.00–90.00)	0.04

HGS, handgrip strength; kg, kilogram; KES, knee extension strength; N, Newton; m, meter; s, second; FVC, forced vital capacity; L, liter.
Summaries of individual data grouped according to sex. p-value of the two sample t-test for the equality of the means.

Table 3 | Linear correlation coefficients between muscle strength (lines) and physical function (columns) variables.

	Gait speed (m/s)	FVC (L)	% FVC
HGS (kg)	0.72 (0.00)	0.59 (0.03)	0.59 (0.03)
KES (N)	0.57 (0.03)	0.12 (0.68)	0.08 (0.77)
KES/body weight (N/kg)	0.55 (0.03)	0.05 (0.87)	0.11 (0.70)

HGS, handgrip strength; kg, kilogram; KES, knee extension strength; N, Newton; m, meter; s, second; FVC, forced vital capacity; L, liter.
In parentheses, the p-value of the test for equality to zero of the correlation coefficient.

CORRELATION BETWEEN BODY COMPOSITION, MUSCLE STRENGTH, AND PHYSICAL FUNCTION

Knee extension strength measures and gait speed showed moderate correlation coefficient significantly different from zero (**Table 3**). On the other hand, the coefficient between HGS and the physical function variables were all significant, showing a moderate to strong correlation (**Table 3**). The linear correlation coefficients between couples of possible explicative variables of muscularity showed values oscillating between 0.01 and 0.58 in absolute value. The indices of adiposity, total fat % and FMI, had non-significant linear correlation coefficient with all the muscle strength and physical function variables (**Table 4**). On the contrary, the indices of muscularity showed moderate positive values (0.40–0.58) when associated with FFMI and ALMI (**Table 4**); moreover, the HGS, FVC, and % FVC are significantly different from zero. The goodness of fit of the relationship between the predictor variables (BMI and ALMI) and the dependent variables (HGS, KES, % FVC, gait

Table 4 | Linear correlation coefficients between potential dependent (lines) and explanatory (columns) variables.

	Total fat %	FMI	FFMI	ALMI
HGS (kg)	−0.21 (0.47)	0.03 (0.91)	0.58 (0.03)	0.51 (0.06)
KES (N)	0.20 (0.48)	0.36 (0.21)	0.43 (0.12)	0.48 (0.08)
Gait speed (m/s)	0.08 (0.79)	0.28 (0.34)	0.43 (0.13)	0.40 (0.15)
FVC (L)	−0.19 (0.51)	0.09 (0.75)	0.48 (0.08)	0.55 (0.04)
% FVC	−0.31 (0.28)	0.01 (0.96)	0.55 (0.04)	0.54 (0.05)

HGS, handgrip strength; kg, kilogram; KES, knee extension strength; N, Newton; m, meter; s, second; FVC, forced vital capacity; L, liter; FMI, fat mass index; FFMI, fat-free mass index; ALMI, appendicular lean mass index.

In parentheses, the p-value of the test for equality to zero of the correlation coefficient.

Table 5 | Linear models ($y_i = \beta x_i + e_i$) of separate relative contribution of body mass and muscularity to muscle strength and physical function and the *p*-value of the test for equality to zero of the adjusted coefficient of linear determination.

Dependent variables	Predictor variables	β	R^2	*p*-Value
HGS (Kg)	BMI	0.46	0.78	0.00
	ALMI	2.53	0.82	0.00
KES (N)	BMI	2.62	0.75	0.00
	ALMI	14.05	0.75	0.00
% FVC	BMI	2.74	0.85	0.00
	ALMI	14.97	0.89	0.00
Gait speed (m/s)	BMI	0.04	0.75	0.00
	ALMI	0.21	0.75	0.00

R^2, adjusted coefficient of linear determination; HGS, handgrip strength; kg, kilogram; KES, knee extension strength; N, Newton; FVC, forced vital capacity; m, meter; s, second; BMI, body mass index; ALMI, appendicular lean mass index.

speed) was measured by the adjusted R^2, which was always different from zero (**Table 5**). Its values are always highly significant and, therefore, suggest a good approximation of the suggested regression model.

DISCUSSION

This study shows that adult MD patients can be classified according to the definition criteria of sarcopenia (Cruz-Jentoft et al., 2010). Our patients in spite of varying degree of impairment of muscle function, from mild to severe, all had "severe sarcopenia" that is the combination of low muscle mass, low muscle strength, and low physical performance (Cruz-Jentoft et al., 2010). The studied patients were also defined "sarcopenic obese" having in addition to a severe decrease in lean body mass an increase in FM (Baumgartner et al., 2004; Stenholm et al., 2008). ALMI was markedly reduced in all patients and correlated with the residual muscle strength in the arms and legs, and with physical performances determined by gait speed and FVC. In addition, ALMI and muscle strength were significantly reduced in non-walkers as compared to walkers.

A similar alteration in body composition, that is, decrease in lean body mass and increase in FM, was reported in patients with different types of MD (Skalsky et al., 2008, 2009; Pruna et al., 2011). Patients with facioscapulohumeral MD had higher fat tissue mass and lower lean tissue mass, despite similar BMI than controls (Skalsky et al., 2008). Patients with myotonic dystrophy had lower regional FFM index and higher fat mass index than controls (Pruna et al., 2011). However, in these studies, body composition was compared with age-matched, able-bodies controls, and not with the older adults impeding the recognition of sarcopenia.

Body composition, assessed by DXA, has started to be included in clinical trials as a primary or secondary endpoint in addition to the evaluation of muscle strength and function (Kissel et al., 2001; Merlini et al., 2008a; Vuillerot et al., 2014). A randomized, double-blind, placebo-controlled trial of albuterol in facioscapulohumeral dystrophy showed that although albuterol did not improve global strength or function, it did increase muscle mass assessed by DXA and improve some measures of strength (Kissel et al., 2001). The influence of a 2-year steroid treatment on body composition measured by DXA was evaluated in 29 DMD boys (Vuillerot et al., 2014). The 21 boys of the steroid group treatment improved significantly in body composition through a significant increase in lean tissue mass. In the steroid-naive patients, there were no significant increases in the lean tissue mass but deterioration in body composition was confirmed by a significant increase in the percentage of body FM (Vuillerot et al., 2014).

Loss of muscle mass and increased intramuscular fibrosis characterize both aging and MD. Research has shown that skeletal muscle wasting in aging and in muscular dystrophic share some pathophysiological mechanisms, including mitochondrial dysfunction (Irwin et al., 2003; Marzetti et al., 2013), increased apoptosis (Marzetti and Leeuwenburgh, 2006; Merlini et al., 2008a; Calvani et al., 2013), abnormal modulation of autophagy (Wohlgemuth et al., 2010; Merlini et al., 2014), decline in satellite cells (Thornell, 2011; Jiang et al., 2014), increased generation of reactive oxygen species (Doria et al., 2012; Canton et al., 2014), and modification of signaling and stress response pathways (Deldicque, 2013; Marzetti et al., 2013; Canton et al., 2014). Therefore, a standard evaluation of sarcopenia may be of benefit for both conditions: aging and MD.

Altogether, this study shows that aging sarcopenia criteria can be used in the evaluation of patients with MD providing relevant information in terms of residual muscle mass, muscle strength, and physical function, which may justify its broader implementation in future research, clinical trials, and clinical practice.

ACKNOWLEDGMENTS

This study was funded by Telethon Foundation (grant no: GUP11007 to Luciano Merlini).

REFERENCES

Batsis, J. A., Barre, L. K., Mackenzie, T. A., Pratt, S. I., Lopez-Jimenez, F., and Bartels, S. J. (2013). Variation in the prevalence of sarcopenia and sarcopenic obesity in older adults associated with different research definitions: dual-energy X-ray absorptiometry data from the national health and nutrition examination survey 1999-2004. *J. Am. Geriatr. Soc.* 61, 974–980. doi:10.1111/jgs.12260

Baumgartner, R. N., Koehler, K. M., Gallagher, D., Romero, L., Heymsfield, S. B., Ross, R. R., et al. (1998). Epidemiology of sarcopenia among the elderly in New Mexico. *Am. J. Epidemiol.* 147, 755–763. doi:10.1093/oxfordjournals.aje.a009520

Baumgartner, R. N., Wayne, S. J., Waters, D. L., Janssen, I., Gallagher, D., and Morley, J. E. (2004). Sarcopenic obesity predicts instrumental activities of daily living disability in the elderly. *Obes. Res.* 12, 1995–2004. doi:10.1038/oby.2004.250

Beenakker, E. A., van der Hoeven, J. H., Fock, J. M., and Maurits, N. M. (2001). Reference values of maximum isometric muscle force obtained in 270 children aged 4-16 years by hand-held dynamometry. *Neuromuscul. Disord.* 11, 441–446. doi:10.1016/S0960-8966(01)00193-6

Bohannon, R. W., Peolsson, A., Massy-Westropp, N., Desrosiers, J., and Bear-Lehman, J. (2006). Reference values for adult grip strength measured with a Jamar dynamometer: a descriptive meta-analysis. *Physiotherapy* 92, 11–15. doi:10.1016/j.physio.2005.05.003

Calvani, R., Joseph, A. M., Adhihetty, P. J., Miccheli, A., Bossola, M., Leeuwenburgh, C., et al. (2013). Mitochondrial pathways in sarcopenia of aging and disuse muscle atrophy. *Biol. Chem.* 394, 393–414. doi:10.1515/hsz-2012-0247

Canton, M., Menazza, S., and Di Lisa, F. (2014). Oxidative stress in muscular dystrophy: from generic evidence to specific sources and targets. *J. Muscle Res. Cell. Motil.* 35, 23–36. doi:10.1007/s10974-014-9380-2

Coin, A., Sergi, G., Minicuci, N., Giannini, S., Barbiero, E., Manzato, E., et al. (2008). Fat-free mass and fat mass reference values by dual-energy X-ray absorptiometry (DEXA) in a 20-80 year-old Italian population. *Clin. Nutr.* 27, 87–94. doi:10.1016/j.clnu.2007.10.008

Cruz-Jentoft, A. J., Baeyens, J. P., Bauer, J. M., Boirie, Y., Cederholm, T., Landi, F., et al. (2010). Sarcopenia: European consensus on definition and diagnosis: report of the European Working Group on sarcopenia in older people. *Age Ageing* 39, 412–423. doi:10.1093/ageing/afq034

Deldicque, L. (2013). Endoplasmic reticulum stress in human skeletal muscle: any contribution to sarcopenia? *Front. Physiol.* 4, 236. doi:10.3389/fphys.2013.00236

Doria, E., Buonocore, D., Focarelli, A., and Marzatico, F. (2012). Relationship between human aging muscle and oxidative system pathway. *Oxid. Med. Cell. Longev.* 2012, 830257. doi:10.1155/2012/830257

Emery, A. E. (2002). The muscular dystrophies. *Lancet* 359, 687–695. doi:10.1016/S0140-6736(02)07815-7

Faulkner, J. A., Larkin, L. M., Claflin, D. R., and Brooks, S. V. (2007). Age-related changes in the structure and function of skeletal muscles. *Clin. Exp. Pharmacol. Physiol.* 34, 1091–1096. doi:10.1111/j.1440-1681.2007.04752.x

Fielding, R. A., Vellas, B., Evans, W. J., Bhasin, S., Morley, J. E., Newman, A. B., et al. (2011). Sarcopenia: an undiagnosed condition in older adults. Current consensus definition: prevalence, etiology, and consequences. International working group on sarcopenia. *J. Am. Med. Dir. Assoc.* 12, 249–256. doi:10.1016/j.jamda.2011.01.003

Fried, L. P., Tangen, C. M., Walston, J., Newman, A. B., Hirsch, C., Gottdiener, J., et al. (2001). Frailty in older adults: evidence for a phenotype. *J. Gerontol. A Biol. Sci. Med. Sci.* 56, M146–M156. doi:10.1093/gerona/56.3.M146

Gualandi, F., Curci, R., Sabatelli, P., Martoni, E., Bovolenta, M., Maraldi, N. M., et al. (2011). Macrophages: a minimally invasive tool for monitoring collagen VI myopathies. *Muscle Nerve* 44, 80–84. doi:10.1002/mus.21999

Gualandi, F., Urciuolo, A., Martoni, E., Sabatelli, P., Squarzoni, S., Bovolenta, M., et al. (2009). Autosomal recessive Bethlem myopathy. *Neurology* 73, 1883–1891. doi:10.1212/WNL.0b013e3181c3fd2a

Hasegawa, R., Islam, M. M., Lee, S. C., Koizumi, D., Rogers, M. E., and Takeshima, N. (2008). Threshold of lower body muscular strength necessary to perform ADL independently in community-dwelling older adults. *Clin. Rehabil.* 22, 902–910. doi:10.1177/0269215508094713

Irwin, W. A., Bergamin, N., Sabatelli, P., Reggiani, C., Megighian, A., Merlini, L., et al. (2003). Mitochondrial dysfunction and apoptosis in myopathic mice with collagen VI deficiency. *Nat. Genet.* 35, 367–371. doi:10.1038/ng1270

Jankowski, C. M., Gozansky, W. S., Van Pelt, R. E., Schenkman, M. L., Wolfe, P., Schwartz, R. S., et al. (2008). Relative contributions of adiposity and muscularity to physical function in community-dwelling older adults. *Obesity (Silver Spring)* 16, 1039–1044. doi:10.1038/oby.2007.84

Jiang, C., Wen, Y., Kuroda, K., Hannon, K., Rudnicki, M. A., and Kuang, S. (2014). Notch signaling deficiency underlies age-dependent depletion of satellite cells in muscular dystrophy. *Dis. Model Mech.* 7, 997–1004. doi:10.1242/dmm.015917

Kissel, J. T., McDermott, M. P., Mendell, J. R., King, W. M., Pandya, S., Griggs, R. C., et al. (2001). Randomized, double-blind, placebo-controlled trial of albuterol in facioscapulohumeral dystrophy. *Neurology* 57, 1434–1440. doi:10.1212/WNL.57.8.1434

Langlois, J. A., Keyl, P. M., Guralnik, J. M., Foley, D. J., Marottoli, R. A., and Wallace, R. B. (1997). Characteristics of older pedestrians who have difficulty crossing the street. *Am. J. Public Health* 87, 393–397. doi:10.2105/AJPH.87.3.393

Lauretani, F., Russo, C. R., Bandinelli, S., Bartali, B., Cavazzini, C., Di Iorio, A., et al. (2003). Age-associated changes in skeletal muscles and their effect on mobility: an operational diagnosis of sarcopenia. *J. Appl. Physiol.* 95, 1851–1860. doi:10.1152/japplphysiol.00246.2003

Lucioli, S., Giusti, B., Mercuri, E., Vanegas, O. C., Lucarini, L., Pietroni, V., et al. (2005). Detection of common and private mutations in the COL6A1 gene of patients with Bethlem myopathy. *Neurology* 64, 1931–1937. doi:10.1212/01.WNL.0000163990.00057.66

Martoni, E., Urciuolo, A., Sabatelli, P., Fabris, M., Bovolenta, M., Neri, M., et al. (2009). Identification and characterization of novel collagen VI non-canonical splicing mutations causing Ullrich congenital muscular dystrophy. *Hum. Mutat.* 30, E662–E672. doi:10.1002/humu.21022

Marzetti, E., Calvani, R., Cesari, M., Buford, T. W., Lorenzi, M., Behnke, B. J., et al. (2013). Mitochondrial dysfunction and sarcopenia of aging: from signaling pathways to clinical trials. *Int. J. Biochem. Cell Biol.* 45, 2288–2301. doi:10.1016/j.biocel.2013.06.024

Marzetti, E., and Leeuwenburgh, C. (2006). Skeletal muscle apoptosis, sarcopenia and frailty at old age. *Exp. Gerontol.* 41, 1234–1238. doi:10.1016/j.exger.2006.08.011

Merlini, L., Angelin, A., Tiepolo, T., Braghetta, P., Sabatelli, P., Zamparelli, A., et al. (2008a). Cyclosporin A corrects mitochondrial dysfunction and muscle apoptosis in patients with collagen VI myopathies. *Proc. Natl. Acad. Sci. U.S.A.* 105, 5225–5229. doi:10.1073/pnas.0800962105

Merlini, L., Martoni, E., Grumati, P., Sabatelli, P., Squarzoni, S., Urciuolo, A., et al. (2008b). Autosomal recessive myosclerosis myopathy is a collagen VI disorder. *Neurology* 71, 1245–1253. doi:10.1212/01.wnl.0000327611.01687.5e

Merlini, L., Bertini, E., Minetti, C., Mongini, T., Morandi, L., Angelini, C., et al. (2004). Motor function-muscle strength relationship in spinal muscular atrophy. *Muscle Nerve* 29, 548–552. doi:10.1002/mus.20018

Merlini, L., Mazzone, E. S., Solari, A., and Morandi, L. (2002). Reliability of hand-held dynamometry in spinal muscular atrophy. *Muscle Nerve* 26, 64–70. doi:10.1002/mus.10166

Merlini, L., Nishino, I., and Consortium for Autophagy in Muscular Dystrophies. (2014). 201st ENMC international workshop: autophagy in muscular dystrophies – translational approach, 1-3 November 2013, Bussum, The Netherlands. *Neuromuscul. Disord.* 24, 546–561. doi:10.1016/j.nmd.2014.03.009

Merlini, L., Solari, A., Vita, G., Bertini, E., Minetti, C., Mongini, T., et al. (2003). Role of gabapentin in spinal muscular atrophy: results of a multicenter, randomized Italian study. *J. Child Neurol.* 18, 537–541. doi:10.1177/08830738030180080501

Mijnarends, D. M., Meijers, J. M., Halfens, R. J., Ter Borg, S., Luiking, Y. C., Verlaan, S., et al. (2013). Validity and reliability of tools to measure muscle mass, strength, and physical performance in community-dwelling older people: a systematic review. *J. Am. Med. Dir. Assoc.* 14, 170–178. doi:10.1016/j.jamda.2012.10.009

Muscaritoli, M., Anker, S. D., Argiles, J., Aversa, Z., Bauer, J. M., Biolo, G., et al. (2010). Consensus definition of sarcopenia, cachexia and pre-cachexia: joint document elaborated by Special Interest Groups (SIG) "cachexia-anorexia in chronic wasting diseases" and "nutrition in geriatrics". *Clin. Nutr.* 29, 154–159. doi:10.1016/j.clnu.2009.12.004

Newman, A. B., Kupelian, V., Visser, M., Simonsick, E., Goodpaster, B., Nevitt, M., et al. (2003). Sarcopenia: alternative definitions and associations with lower extremity function. *J. Am. Geriatr. Soc.* 51, 1602–1609. doi:10.1046/j.1532-5415.2003.51534.x

Pepe, G., Giusti, B., Bertini, E., Brunelli, T., Saitta, B., Comeglio, P., et al. (1999). A heterozygous splice site mutation in COL6A1 leading to an in-frame deletion of the alpha1(VI) collagen chain in an Italian family affected by Bethlem myopathy. *Biochem. Biophys. Res. Commun.* 258, 802–807. doi:10.1006/bbrc.1999.0680

Ploutz-Snyder, L. L., Manini, T., Ploutz-Snyder, R. J., and Wolf, D. A. (2002). Functionally relevant thresholds of quadriceps femoris strength. *J. Gerontol. A Biol. Sci. Med. Sci.* 57, B144–B152. doi:10.1093/gerona/57.4.B144

Pruna, L., Chatelin, J., Pascal-Vigneron, V., and Kaminsky, P. (2011). Regional body composition and functional impairment in patients with myotonic dystrophy. *Muscle Nerve* 44, 503–508. doi:10.1002/mus.22099

Sabatelli, P., Gara, S. K., Grumati, P., Urciuolo, A., Gualandi, F., Curci, R., et al. (2011). Expression of the collagen VI alpha5 and alpha6 chains in normal human skin and in skin of patients with collagen VI-related myopathies. *J. Invest. Dermatol.* 131, 99–107. doi:10.1038/jid.2010.284

Sabatelli, P., Palma, E., Angelin, A., Squarzoni, S., Urciuolo, A., Pellegrini, C., et al. (2012). Critical evaluation of the use of cell cultures for inclusion in clinical trials of patients affected by collagen VI myopathies. *J. Cell. Physiol.* 227, 2927–2935. doi:10.1002/jcp.23039

Skalsky, A. J., Abresch, R. T., Han, J. J., Shin, C. S., and McDonald, C. M. (2008). The relationship between regional body composition and quantitative strength in facioscapulohumeral muscular dystrophy (FSHD). *Neuromuscul. Disord.* 18, 873–880. doi:10.1016/j.nmd.2008.07.005

Skalsky, A. J., Han, J. J., Abresch, R. T., Shin, C. S., and McDonald, C. M. (2009). Assessment of regional body composition with dual-energy X-ray absorptiometry in Duchenne muscular dystrophy: correlation of regional lean mass and quantitative strength. *Muscle Nerve* 39, 647–651. doi:10.1002/mus.21212

Stenholm, S., Harris, T. B., Rantanen, T., Visser, M., Kritchevsky, S. B., and Ferrucci, L. (2008). Sarcopenic obesity: definition, cause and consequences. *Curr. Opin. Clin. Nutr. Metab. Care* 11, 693–700. doi:10.1097/MCO.0b013e328312c37d

Tanko, L. B., Movsesyan, L., Mouritzen, U., Christiansen, C., and Svendsen, O. L. (2002). Appendicular lean tissue mass and the prevalence of sarcopenia among healthy women. *Metab. Clin. Exp.* 51, 69–74. doi:10.1053/meta.2002.28960

Thornell, L. E. (2011). Sarcopenic obesity: satellite cells in the aging muscle. *Curr. Opin. Clin. Nutr. Metab. Care* 14, 22–27. doi:10.1097/MCO.0b013e3283412260

van der Kooi, A. J., De Voogt, W. G., Bertini, E., Merlini, L., Talim, F. B., Ben Yaou, R., et al. (2006). Cardiac and pulmonary investigations in Bethlem myopathy. *Arch. Neurol.* 63, 1617–1621. doi:10.1001/archneur.63.11.1617

van der Ploeg, R. J., Fidler, V., and Oosterhuis, H. J. (1991). Hand-held myometry: reference values. *J. Neurol. Neurosurg. Psychiatr.* 54, 244–247. doi:10.1136/jnnp.54.3.244

Vuillerot, C., Braillon, P., Fontaine-Carbonnel, S., Rippert, P., Andre, E., Iwaz, J., et al. (2014). Influence of a two-year steroid treatment on body composition as measured by dual X-ray absorptiometry in boys with Duchenne muscular dystrophy. *Neuromuscul. Disord.* 24, 467–473. doi:10.1016/j.nmd.2014.03.002

WHO. (2000). Obesity: preventing and managing the global epidemic. Report of a WHO consultation. *World Health Organ. Tech. Rep. Ser.* 894, i–xii, 1–253.

Wohlgemuth, S. E., Seo, A. Y., Marzetti, E., Lees, H. A., and Leeuwenburgh, C. (2010). Skeletal muscle autophagy and apoptosis during aging: effects of calorie restriction and life-long exercise. *Exp. Gerontol.* 45, 138–148. doi:10.1016/j.exger.2009.11.002

7

Degeneration of neuromuscular junction in age and dystrophy

Rüdiger Rudolf [1,2,3]*, Muzamil Majid Khan [1,3], Siegfried Labeit [4] and Michael R. Deschenes [5]

[1] Institute of Molecular and Cell Biology, University of Applied Sciences Mannheim, Mannheim, Germany
[2] Institute of Medical Technology, University of Heidelberg and University of Applied Sciences Mannheim, Mannheim, Germany
[3] Institute of Toxicology and Genetics, Karlsruhe Institute of Technology, Eggenstein-Leopoldshafen, Germany
[4] Institute of Integrative Pathophysiology, University Medical Centre Mannheim, Mannheim, Germany
[5] Department of Kinesiology and Health Sciences, The College of William and Mary, Williamsburg, VA, USA

Correspondence:
Rüdiger Rudolf, Institute of Molecular and Cell Biology, University of Applied Sciences Mannheim, Paul-Wittsackstrasse 10, Mannheim 68163, Germany
e-mail: r.rudolf@hs-mannheim.de

Functional denervation is a hallmark of aging sarcopenia as well as of muscular dystrophy. It is thought to be a major factor reducing skeletal muscle mass, particularly in the case of sarcopenia. Neuromuscular junctions (NMJs) serve as the interface between the nervous and skeletal muscular systems, and thus they may receive pathophysiological input of both pre- and post-synaptic origin. Consequently, NMJs are good indicators of motor health on a systemic level. Indeed, upon sarcopenia and dystrophy, NMJs morphologically deteriorate and exhibit altered characteristics of primary signaling molecules, such as nicotinic acetylcholine receptor and agrin. Since a remarkable reversibility of these changes can be observed by exercise, there is significant interest in understanding the molecular mechanisms underlying synaptic deterioration upon aging and dystrophy and how synapses are reset by the aforementioned treatments. Here, we review the literature that describes the phenomena observed at the NMJ in sarcopenic and dystrophic muscle as well as to how these alterations can be reversed and to what extent. In a second part, the current information about molecular machineries underlying these processes is reported.

Keywords: neuromuscular junction, dystrophy, aging, sarcopenia, exercise therapy

INTRODUCTION

Sarcopenia, a term coined by Rosenberg, literally means "poverty of flesh" and originally referred to aging-related loss of muscle mass (Rosenberg, 1997). The etiology of this loss is most likely multi-factorial. Indeed, the functionality of skeletal muscle is subject to regulation by several different tissues. Primarily, these include muscle, tendons, skeleton, as well as central and peripheral nervous systems (and their supporting cells), but also hormonal glands, blood vessels, and others. Malfunctioning of any one of these components will ultimately affect the other constituents, although with different strength. This complexity of the motor system is certainly an important aspect that leads to the ambiguity in explaining the pathogenic mechanisms of many neuromuscular diseases. That is true even in disorders, in which simple genetic abnormalities are the sole initiating factor, as in the case of hereditary forms of muscular dystrophies. Indeed, although many muscular dystrophies are linked to mutations of different members of a single protein complex, i.e., the dystrophin-associated protein complex (DAPC), insight into the precise links between DAPC and the dystrophic symptoms remains limited. A similar uncertainty characterizes our understanding of the etiology of aging sarcopenia. While there is a general consensus that functional muscle denervation is one of the principal factors leading to sarcopenia, the origin and exact role of the partial silence between nerve and muscle are still debated as outlined below. Since many muscular dystrophies and sarcopenia share defects at the nerve–muscle synapse, i.e., the neuromuscular junction (NMJ), we analyze in this review whether this commonality could possibly reflect similar molecular origins and whether this would allow speculation about diagnostic or therapeutic interventions for these diseases.

COMMON FEATURES IN AGING AND DYSTROPHY WITH RESPECT TO THE NMJ

Before addressing features that are common or different in muscular dystrophy and sarcopenia, we need to briefly define both terms. *Muscular dystrophies*: these form a group of more than 30 different hereditary or acquired diseases, which are characterized by progressive degeneration of the musculoskeletal system leading in many cases to severe ambulation deficits and reduced lifespan. As excellently reviewed previously (Blake et al., 2002; Davies and Nowak, 2006; Mercuri and Muntoni, 2013), muscular dystrophies can be due to mutations in many different genes, including those encoding sarcomeric/sarcoplasmic proteins like titin or calpain 3, nuclear proteins such as lamin or emerin, and proteins of the sarcoplasmic reticulum like dystrophia myotonica protein kinase. Some forms of muscular dystrophy are also due to defective membrane repair (dysferlinopathy), but the largest part of dystrophies is connected to the DAPC and can be divided into two groups. Diseases originating from mutations in members of the DAPC are often called as dystrophinopathies, while conditions due to aberrant glycosylation of DAPC members (in particular, α-dystroglycan) are termed dystroglycanopathies. Duchenne muscular dystrophy is the most frequent form of dystrophinopathy, Fukuyama congenital muscular dystrophy, and

Walker–Warburg syndrome represent typical examples of dystroglycanopathies. Since the DAPC is highly abundant at the NMJ (Pilgram et al., 2009) and might play essential roles in maintaining it (see below), we will limit the discussion in the following text to dystrophinopathies and dystroglycanopathies. *Sarcopenia*: the European Working Group on Sarcopenia in Older People (Cruz-Jentoft et al., 2010), has defined sarcopenia as the loss of muscle mass (atrophy) and muscle strength (dynapenia) as a direct consequence of aging. Given that secondary conditions, like cancer, cirrhosis, or ovariectomy can also lead to (non-sarcopenic) atrophy upon aging, it is not always easy to determine if age or other reasons are the primary cause for muscle loss (Hepple, 2012). This has spurred interest in defining more specific characteristics for the clinical diagnosis of sarcopenia. In the following text, we will examine a few of these criteria (Hepple, 2012) and address to what extent these features are also present in muscular dystrophies.

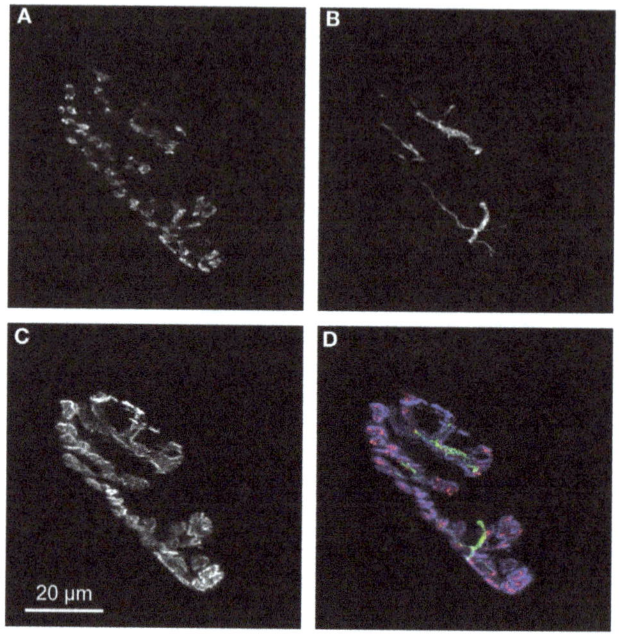

FIGURE 1 | Pre- and post-synapse exhibit perfect complementarity in young adult NMJs. **(A,B)** Pre-synaptic terminal as represented by motoneuronal markers for synaptic vesicles [synaptophysin **(A)**] and neuronal cytoskeleton [neurofilament **(B)**]. **(C)** Post-synaptic apparatus contains large amounts of AChRs directly juxtaposed to pre-synaptic ACh filled synaptic vesicles. **(D)** Overlay of synaptophysin (red), neurofilament (green), and AChR stainings (blue) nicely shows the perfect complementarity of pre- and post-synaptic portions of NMJ.

HISTOPATHOLOGICAL HALLMARKS OF SARCOPENIC MUSCLE

Apart from the eponymous loss in muscle mass, sarcopenic muscle is characterized by histopathological traits that can distinguish sarcopenia from other types of muscle atrophy. The first in a list of such parameters is the occurrence of fiber size heterogeneity in muscle from elderly people and analogous mouse/rat models (reviewed in Berger and Doherty, 2010; Hepple, 2012). Notably, while fiber size variability is not found in other types of atrophy like those related to cancer cachexia, it is a major feature of dystrophinopathies (Engel and Ozawa, 2004) and dystroglycanopathies (Taniguchi et al., 2006; Krag et al., 2011; Costa et al., 2013). Second, muscles from elderly exhibit extensive fiber type grouping. This means that a disproportionally large number of neighboring fibers exhibit the same fiber type. This has been found in both humans (Andersen, 2003) and murine models (Kanda and Hashizume, 1989; Rowan et al., 2011). Certainly, fiber type grouping is not very extensive in most muscular dystrophies, but the occurrence of smaller fiber groups was reported for samples from Becker muscular dystrophy (ten Houten and De Visser, 1984; Kaido et al., 1991) and also Duchenne muscular dystrophy (Engel and Ozawa, 2004). Another fiber type-related alteration is the co-expression of multiple myosin heavy chain isoforms, which is again indicative of sarcopenia (Andersen et al., 1999; Patterson et al., 2006; Rowan et al., 2012) and was also observed in Duchenne muscular dystrophy (Marini et al., 1991).

The above-mentioned alterations in fiber size, distribution of fiber type, and co-expression of multiple myosin heavy chain isoforms all suggest the occurrence of reiterating cycles of degeneration/regeneration as well as denervation followed by reinnervation of the affected fibers. Since paucity of neurotransmission is expected to modify the synapses of the involved fibers, it is intriguing that an additional common feature of aging sarcopenia (Valdez et al., 2010; Li et al., 2011) and muscular dystrophies (Lyons and Slater, 1991; Grady et al., 1997; Shiao et al., 2004) is fragmentation of NMJs. But what does fragmentation appear as? In normal mammalian muscle, AChRs densely cluster in winding, band-like arrays on the post-synaptic membrane. Mostly, these bands form a continuous structure also referred to as "pretzel"-like. To achieve maximally efficient neurotransmission, pre- and post-synaptic membranes exhibit the same band pattern (**Figure 1**). In aged and dystrophic muscle, however, the "pretzel" is fragmented into many individual gutters (Andonian and Fahim, 1987; Lyons and Slater, 1991) (see also **Figure 2**).

ORIGINS OF SYNAPTIC FRAGMENTATION MIGHT BE DIFFERENT

The cause of fragmentation of NMJs in aged and dystrophic muscle is rather unclear, but there are different possible explanations. First, it is conceivable that fragmentation of NMJs is due to degeneration of muscle fiber segments underlying the synapse. Subsequent regeneration would then create a patch-like appearance of the post-synaptic apparatus that could be mimicked by the pre-synaptic terminal through adaptive structural reorganization. This is a principal hypothesis for the occurrence of synaptic fragmentation in muscular dystrophy (Lyons and Slater, 1991) and was also suggested to play a role in the aging process in a longitudinal study in mice, where the same NMJs were followed over extended periods of time (Li et al., 2011). Results showed not a steady, progressive fragmentation, but rather complete fragmentation of individual synapses within short time ranges and mostly in conjunction with the appearance of central nuclei, a sign of regeneration. Feedback from the post- to pre-synaptic regions leading to adaptation of the pre-synaptic terminal to the scattered post-synaptic morphology could be mediated by Lrp4 (Yumoto et al., 2012), the co-receptor of MuSK in agrin-dependent signaling (Kim et al., 2008; Zhang et al., 2008).

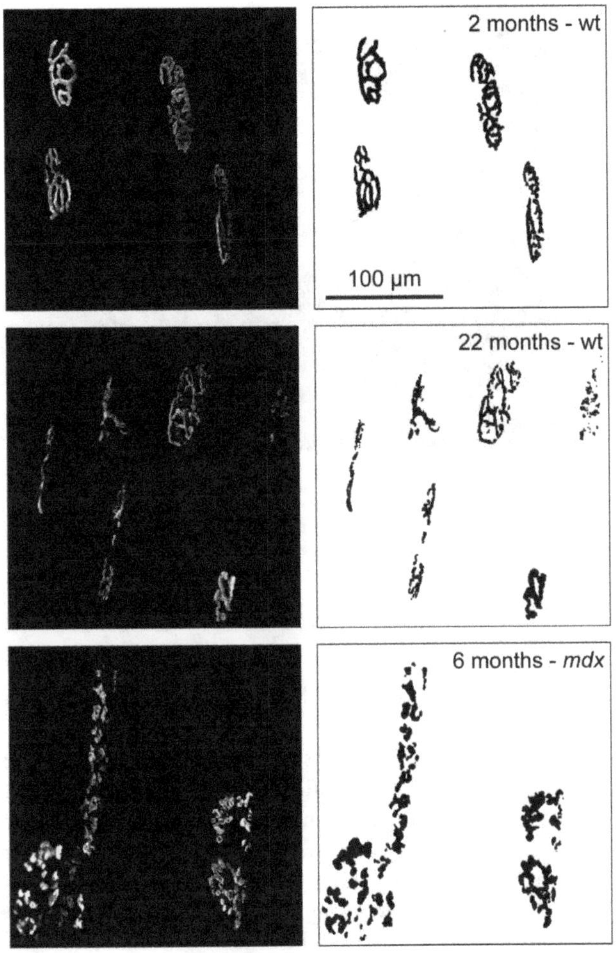

FIGURE 2 | The phenomenon of NMJ fragmentation during aging and dystrophy. Tibialis anterior muscles of wildtype (wt) or dystrophic *mdx* mice were injected with fluorescently labeled α-bungarotoxin to mark AChRs at the indicated ages and then imaged using *in vivo* confocal microscopy. Images show maximum intensity projections of several NMJs (left) and binarized pictures (right) to highlight the observation that in young wt AChRs form contiguous, "pretzel-like," bands while they align in fragmented clusters in aged wt and middle aged dystrophic muscles.

Another possible cause of NMJ fragmentation can be traced to the appearance of neuronal lesions or complete motor neuron death leading to muscle fiber denervation followed by reinnervation of the same post-synaptic apparatus by a new neuronal sprout from neighboring neurons. Indeed, in aging sarcopenia, there is wide spread consensus that denervation due to motor neuron apoptosis is a crucial feature. A fast decline in the number of alpha motor neuron cell bodies in the spinal cords of humans beyond the age of 60 was observed (Kawamura et al., 1977; Tomlinson and Irving, 1977; Berger and Doherty, 2010), and was accompanied by a decline in the number of motor units, i.e., the groups of muscle fibers innervated by individual motor neurons (Doherty et al., 1993). Since a massive reduction in the number of muscle fibers in aged muscle was also reported (Lexell, 1993), dying back of motor neurons due to loss of muscle fiber trophic signals could be a possible explanation of sarcopenia. Evidence that aging may induce peripheral nerve degeneration in muscle comes from a recent study in mice, which found signs of marked degeneration of pre- and post-synaptic portions of NMJs although counts of motor neuron somata at the level of the lumbar region did not reveal any difference between mice at 3 and 29 months of age (Chai et al., 2011). Peripheral degeneration of nerves in aged animals was also observed in other reports (Stanmore et al., 1978; Valdez et al., 2010) and investigations from other disease models imply that retrograde motor neuron death is possible (Wong and Martin, 2010). However, in Duchenne muscular dystrophy, motor neuron degeneration among patients has not been detected (Tomlinson et al., 1974) and intramuscular nerves appear normal (Engel and Ozawa, 2004). Given that massive muscle fiber death is occurring in Duchenne patients, it follows that retrograde motor neuron degeneration is not a logical consequence of muscle fiber loss. Finally, smaller rearrangements of molecular events could lead to a steady, slow decay of synaptic regions resulting in fragmented appearance of the synapse although findings in mice do not support this possibility (Li et al., 2011). However, it is unlikely that aging processes in rodents are fully comparable to those in humans, particularly with respect to slowly accumulating ones. In other words, it might well be that small rearrangements that are not visible within the 2–3-year lifespan of mice would in fact be detectable within the more than 80-year lifespan of humans. Before addressing the involvement of different molecular pathways in regulating NMJ morphology and function, we will first address how regular muscle activity affects NMJs. Due to the lack of studies on dystrophic muscle, the ensuing section focuses on the effects of training in healthy, young, and aged subjects and corresponding murine models.

ROLE OF EXERCISE ON MUSCLE PERFORMANCE IN AGED – FOCUS ON NMJ

There is growing epidemiological and experimental evidence suggesting that certain types of physical exercise are effective in offsetting age-related decline in muscle size and strength (reviewed e.g., in Berger and Doherty, 2010). Notably, life-long high-intensity physical activity significantly abates the loss of motor unit numbers (Power et al., 2010). Similar to the way in which chronic exercise training is capable of mitigating the loss of strength and muscle mass associated with aging, the same stimulus of regularly performed exercise appears to influence aging-related adaptations of the NMJ (Andonian and Fahim, 1987). This is evident with respect to both NMJ morphology and function. Moreover, our present understanding suggests that exercise training results in age-specific remodeling of the NMJ. That is, among young adults endurance training elicits an expansion of NMJ dimensions and this enlargement is evident in both the pre- and post-synaptic components of the NMJ. This is not surprising since there is convincing evidence that pre- and post-synaptic relationships of the NMJ are well maintained throughout aging and that this constancy is apparent even when examining the NMJs of muscles displaying different patterns of neuromuscular activity (Deschenes et al., 2013). It should be noted, however, that most of the exercise training studies conducted to date among aged animals have used only moderately aged rodents (i.e., 20–25 months). This is important as it has been reported that during advanced aging (>25 months) rodents display NMJ remodeling that is characterized by reduced dimensions rather than the expansion of synaptic size observed among animals with less advanced aging (Rosenheimer and Smith, 1985). Unclear at this point is how exercise training affects NMJ structure in these more senescent animals and if gender-specific differences occur.

Specific responses of NMJs to exercise training include an increase in total length of nerve terminal branching, a greater number of nerve terminal branches, and a more elaborate pattern of nerve terminal branching, i.e., branching complexity (Fahim, 1997; Deschenes et al., 2011). Accompanying this training-related amplification of nerve terminal branching is a greater total number of pre-synaptic vesicles containing the NMJ's neurotransmitter acetylcholine (ACh). The greater total nerve terminal branch length in the NMJs of trained muscles is necessary to secure increased numbers of ACh vesicles and total neurotransmitter in light of the fact that the number of vesicles supported by a given length of nerve terminal branching is consistent among young and aged, as well as in muscles with high or low recruitment patterns (Deschenes et al., 2013). It has also been established that the size of individual pre-synaptic vesicles is unaffected by training, again requiring the expression of greater numbers of vesicles if the total amount of stored ACh is to be increased (Fahim, 1997).

As expected in synapses exhibiting tight coupling of pre- and post-synaptic components, endurance training also promotes remodeling with respect to the number and distribution of AChRs at the muscle fiber's endplate region where post-synaptic depolarization occurs. Specific training-induced endplate modifications are characterized by a higher number of AChRs, which occupy a greater endplate area than in untrained muscle fibers (Deschenes et al., 1993, 2013; Cheng et al., 2013). The enhanced span of the AChR stained area is necessitated by the fact that the density of AChRs anchored within a given area within receptor clusters (i.e., stained area) does not change with training (Deschenes et al., 1993). Thus, to increase the total number of AChRs at the NMJ, the area anchoring these receptors must be expanded. This is precisely what is observed as a result of endurance training.

Other post-synaptic adaptations induced by training include a greater total perimeter length encompassing the entire endplate region, which includes clusters of receptors as well as interspersing sections of the endplate that do not express receptors. Training has also been found to increase the aggregate perimeter length encompassing only the stained clusters of AChRs without taking into account empty sections between those clusters (Deschenes et al., 2011). Finally, the dispersion of clusters of AChRs within the total endplate area – which includes stained AChR clusters and receptor void sections between those clusters – is sensitive to endurance training, with that stimulus responsible for a more compact, less dispersed distribution of stained receptor clusters (Deschenes et al., 2011). The quantitative technique used to assess the dispersion of AChR clusters within the total endplate area can be seen in **Figure 3**. As an aside, it is noteworthy that the expanded dimensions detected in run trained NMJs occur despite mild, e.g., 10–15%, atrophy in the size of the muscle fibers on which the NMJs reside (Deschenes et al., 1993, 2011). Clearly, the morphological modifications of NMJs brought about by endurance training cannot simply be attributed to similar remodeling of muscle fiber size.

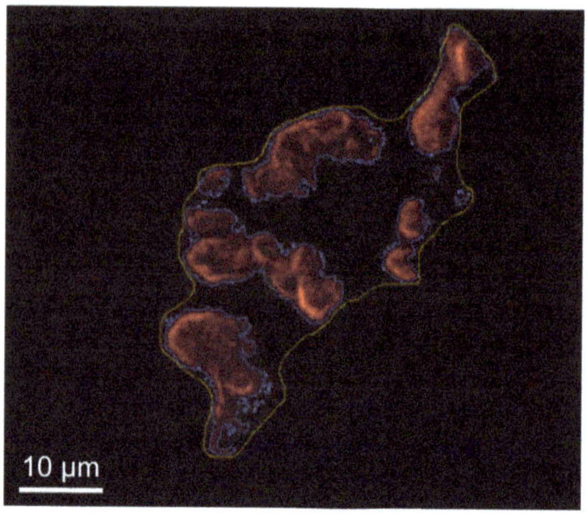

FIGURE 3 | Determination of post-synaptic ACh receptor cluster dispersion. Representative image of tracings made to determine total endplate area (yellow) and stained receptors clusters (blue) within that total area. To determine dispersion of AChRs within total endplate the stained area is divided by the total area and multiplied by 100.

A basic tenet of the biological sciences is that form and function are inextricably linked. The plasticity of the NMJ is another example of how form and function change hand-in-hand. That is, the endurance training-induced alterations of NMJ structure are associated with significant changes in synaptic transmission. Examples of such electrophysiological adaptations are training-induced elevations in quantal content, or the amount of neurotransmitter released from nerve terminals in response to a single electrical impulse. This is true despite the fact that unstimulated, or random release of ACh, is reduced among trained muscles (Fahim, 1997) suggesting a more secure anchoring of vesicles at pre-synaptic active zones. And during a continuous train of imposed electrical stimuli to the NMJ, there is a slighter degree of depression in post-synaptic response among trained compared to untrained neuromuscular systems (Fahim, 1997). This is viewed as evidence that trained NMJs are more adept not only at recycling the pre-synaptic ACh vesicles releasing neurotransmitter into the synaptic cleft, but also of maintaining sensitivity of the post-synaptic receptors to that ACh which is released.

In contrast to endurance training another form of exercise training, i.e., resistance training, or weight lifting, is known to promote significant muscle fiber hypertrophy (Kraemer et al., 1995). Mimicking the type, intensity, and volume of weight lifting that human athletes routinely perform has proven to be difficult with an animal model. Largely, because of this and because it is not practicable to visually examine the NMJs in human muscle as that synapse is located somewhere in the middle third of the length of the whole muscle and stains must be used to make it visible, much less is known about the effects of resistance training on the NMJ. But in one study using a model of rats climbing a ladder with resistance attached to their tails, it was shown that this mode of exercise brings about NMJ remodeling that is similar in nature to that observed with endurance training, albeit to a smaller extent. More specifically, a 7-week program of resistance training increased pre-synaptic area occupied by ACh containing vesicles, and post-synaptic endplate area stained for AChRs by ~15% – compared to ~30% with endurance training – with the coupling of ACh vesicles and receptors remaining constant (Deschenes et al., 1993, 2000). It appears then, that the stimulus of resistance training, while adequate to result in NMJ remodeling, is not capable of yielding the same degree of synaptic remodeling seen with endurance training.

Although a relatively new area of investigation, a number of studies have reported that aging does, indeed, modify the responsiveness of the NMJ to exercise training. For example, when young adult and aged rats participated in an identical 10-week program of treadmill running, training was shown to result in significant structural remodeling of NMJs (increased nerve terminal total branch length and number of branches, increased post-synaptic area occupied by ACh receptors, and perimeter length surrounding those receptors) in young animals, without such modifications occurring among aged rats (Deschenes et al., 2011). Upon close examination, however, it was apparent that aging alone had resulted in pre- and post-synaptic expansion, so that when aged rats performed endurance training, the effect was to reduce NMJ dimensions back to those observed in untrained young NMJs. **Figure 4** depicts the effects of exercise training on post-synaptic structure in young and aged NMJs. A similar age and exercise interaction on NMJ structure has recently been reported (Valdez et al., 2010). In that investigation, it was determined that aged mice displayed larger NMJs with more elaborate, and fragmented, architecture than those examined in young mice. But in aged mice given access to free running wheels, NMJs in exercised muscles were not morphologically distinct from those of young, untrained mice. These studies, along with a more recent report (Cheng et al., 2013), suggest that the morphological remodeling of NMJs associated with aging may be prevented or even reversed through regular participation in endurance type exercise. As aging modulates training-induced structural alterations of the NMJ, exercise-related adaptations in synaptic transmission across the NMJ are similarly affected by aging. Finally, although there is no information regarding the effect of controlled exercise on NMJs in dystrophic muscle, a recent trial documented beneficial impact of moderate bicycle training in a group of Duchenne patients (Jansen et al., 2013).

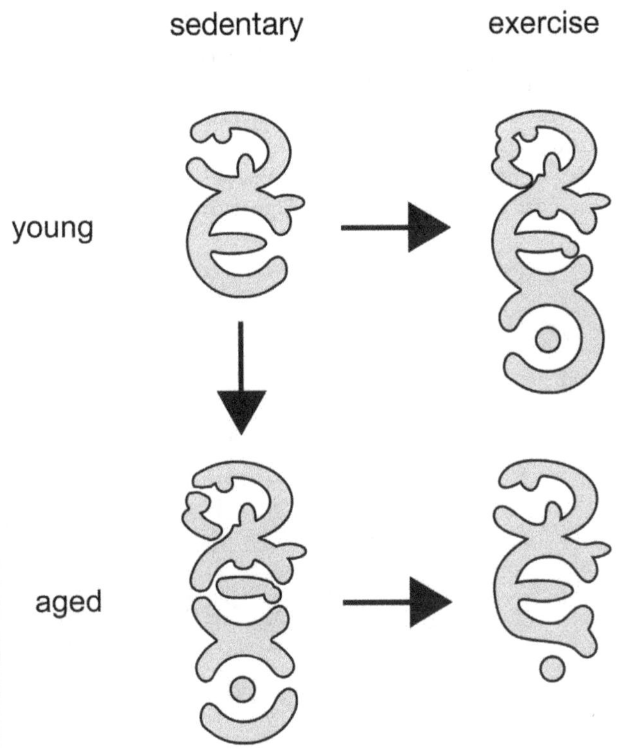

FIGURE 4 | Schematic representation of exercise-induced changes at post-synaptic membrane of NMJ of young adult and aged rodents. Both, exercise as well as the aging process come with augmented size of individual NMJs and increased branching complexity of AChR clusters within the NMJ organization. Aged NMJs are also often characterized by enhanced discontinuity of AChR cluster branches. Of note, exercise of aged animals partially reduces branching complexity, NMJ size, and fragmentation and, thus, leads to a morphology of synapses that resembles young adult sedentary NMJs. Relative density of AChR, indicated by gray scales, is always highest at the branch borders and does not significantly change under all conditions. Pre-synaptic branching and synaptic vesicle numbers (not shown) are largely modified in congruency with post-synaptic changes. However, upon aging partial loss of pre-to-post matching does frequently occur.

MOLECULAR CHARACTERISTICS AND BIOMARKERS AT NMJ

As outlined above, the sequence of events that results in fragmentation of NMJs has yet to be fully revealed. With respect to molecular pathways underlying pre- or post-synaptic processes leading to degeneration of the NMJ there have been recent advancements. Most studies that address the maintenance of the NMJ measure the coherence of the AChR clusters in "pretzel"-shaped arrays. This is mainly for two reasons: first, the AChR is the major ion channel of the post-synaptic apparatus and thus reflects gross morphological alterations of the NMJ with high fidelity. Second, visualization of its distribution, also *in vivo*, is greatly facilitated by the use of the snake venom, α-bungarotoxin, which does not permeate the cell membrane, but binds with extremely high specificity and affinity to AChRs and can be labeled with a variety of dyes, radioactive tracers, etc. To better understand possible scenarios that could affect NMJ morphology in general and AChRs in particular, it is useful to mention the principal steps of AChR lifecycle.

BIOGENESIS AND CLUSTERING OF AChRs

The AChR is a pentameric ligand-gated cation channel of the cys-loop family of ion channels with a wide expression in the central nervous system and skeletal muscle. In the latter, AChR subunit composition depends on the developmental state of the tissue. While embryonic and regenerating muscles express AChRs with a subunit composition of αγαδβ, adult intact muscle expresses receptors with αεαδβ composition (Witzemann et al., 1987, 1989; Gu and Hall, 1988). By substituting the ε subunit for the γ subunit, the gating properties of the channel change from displaying long open times with slow conductance, to brief open times with high ion conductance rates (Mishina et al., 1986; Schwarz et al., 2000).

The γ to ε switch was found to be essential, because mice lacking the adult-type AChRε subunit showed impaired neurotransmission, progressive muscle weakness, and died about 40–60 days after birth (Witzemann et al., 1996). The AChR life cycle starts with biogenesis and assembly of its subunits within the endoplasmic reticulum and then proceeds in the Golgi apparatus, where glycosylation occurs, before secretory vesicles transport the AChR to the post-synaptic membrane (**Figure 5**). Already during this transport, the 43 kDa receptor associated protein of the synapse (rapsyn) escorts the AChRs (Marchand et al., 2000, 2002) in a 1:1 fashion. At the membrane, AChRs are then clustered and maintained by the help of rapsyn that links AChRs to the underlying actin cytoskeleton via the DAPC (Gautam et al., 1995). This process is mainly mediated by the agrin/MuSK/Lrp4 signaling pathway (**Figure 5**) that is regulated by the presence of an active motor neuron pre-synaptic terminal. As recently reviewed

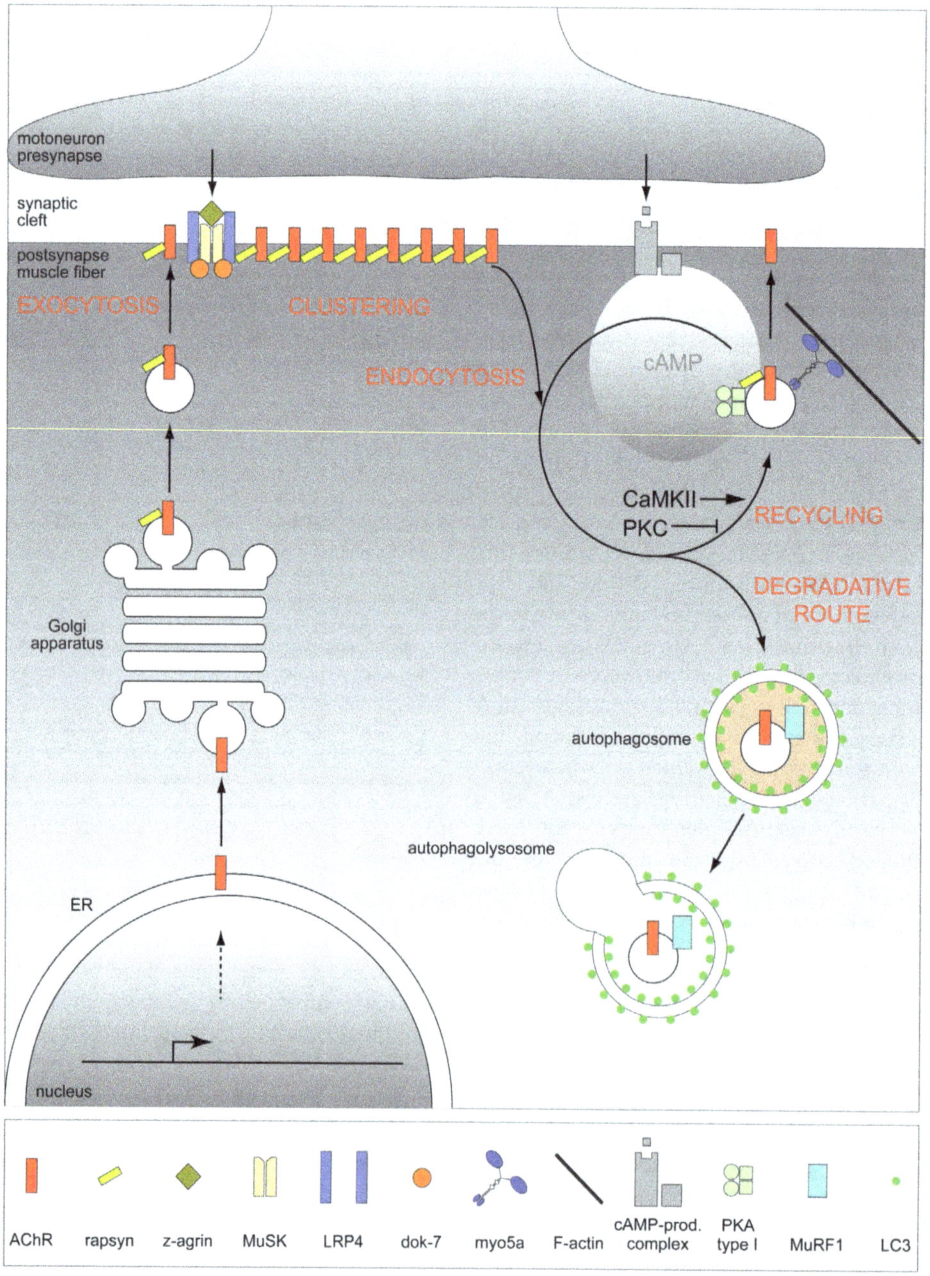

FIGURE 5 | Scheme depicting the putative life cycle of AChR at the vertebrate NMJ. Upon assembly in the ER and glycosylation in the Golgi apparatus, AChR is delivered by exocytosis to the post-synaptic membrane where it is clustered by means of agrin/MuSK/Lrp4/rapsyn complex, to fulfill its major function, i.e., mediating neuromuscular transmission. Subsequently, AChR is endocytosed and can then be recycled using a cooperative function of myosin Va, PKA type I, and rapsyn, or degraded, presumably via autophagic decay in a MuRF1-dependent manner. Decision-making between recycling or degradation appears to be subject to manifold signals including CaMKII and PKC.

(Punga and Ruegg, 2012), the large proteoglycan, neural agrin, activates the MuSK–Lrp4 complex to inhibit activity-dependent AChR cluster disassembly that occurs outside the reach of neuronal agrin. This involves the activation of effector molecules, primarily Dok-7 and rapsyn. Thus, the agrin/MuSK/Lrp4 pathway appears to perfectly explain the observed precise fit of pre- to post-synaptic portions of healthy NMJs by release of a neuronal signal and the subsequent response of muscle tissue. However, at least two factors complicate this concept. First, the agrin/MuSK/Lrp4 pathway is not the only regulator of AChR clustering. Indeed, a wealth of other signaling molecules also affects the presence of AChRs at the membrane, as reviewed previously (Wu et al., 2010). Second, it is increasingly appreciated that NMJ development and maintenance are not controlled in a simple unidirectional manner from nerve to muscle. For example, while agrin is dispensable for AChR cluster formation during development, cluster maintenance in the adult needs agrin to prohibit activity-induced cluster dispersal (see Kummer et al., 2006 for review). Furthermore, muscle-derived Lrp4 appears to also act in a retrograde manner, since it is necessary for early steps of pre-synaptic development *in vitro* and *in vivo* (Yumoto et al., 2012). In the context of aging research, it would be very interesting to know, whether Lrp4 also signals from muscle to nerve in adult tissue to maintain the nerve–muscle connectivity intact in a retrograde manner.

LIFE OR DEATH AFTER LEAVING THE CLUSTER

Although AChRs in intact and innervated muscle exhibit a high metabolic stability and are, thus, slowly turned over with a half-life of about 13 days, they are at some point removed from the post-synaptic region by endocytosis. Subsequent fates include storage in an intracellular compartment, recycling to the post-synaptic membrane in an activity-dependent manner, and degradation (**Figure 5**). Given that about 25% of all surface receptors are normally recycled within 4 days (Bruneau et al., 2005), positive or negative tuning of the decision between recycling and deterioration would also affect AChR density at the NMJ, and if recycling is lacking spatial precision, this could potentially lead to fragmentation of synapses due to receptor delivery at wrong sites. A couple of reports indicate that second messenger-triggered serine/threonine phosphorylation events are major determinants controlling the decision-making between recycling and degradation. Observations from different laboratories have revealed the positive and negative impacts of protein kinases A (PKA) and C (PKC), respectively, on AChR lifetime and recycling (Nelson et al., 2003; Röder et al., 2010; Martinez-Pena y Valenzuela et al., 2013). Furthermore, Ca^{2+}/calmodulin-dependent kinase II (CaMKII) also appears to trigger AChR recycling in an electrical stimulation and Ca^{2+}-dependent manner (Martinez-Pena y Valenzuela et al., 2010) (**Figure 5**).

The target molecules for these phosphorylation events are still unclear, but one obvious candidate is the AChR itself, which can be phosphorylated at different subunits by PKA and PKC (Miles et al., 1987; Huganir and Miles, 1989; Nimnual et al., 1998). A potential target for CaMKII at the NMJ could be myosin Va, which is crucial to recruit AChR-containing recycling carriers to the post-synaptic membrane (Röder et al., 2008; Yampolsky et al., 2010). Myosin V molecules are CaMKII-regulated motor proteins (Costa et al., 1999) and are also important for activity- and Ca^{2+}-dependent recycling of AMPA receptors at central synapses (Correia et al., 2008; Wang et al., 2008). Furthermore, myosin V is dependent on actin filaments to escort vesicles to their destination (Reck-Peterson et al., 2000; Walker et al., 2000). This might partially reflect the aberrant recycling of AChRs upon impairment of components of the DAPC (Martinez-Pena y Valenzuela et al., 2011; Schmidt et al., 2011), which is a major organizer of the actin cytoskeleton in skeletal muscle and the NMJ (Pilgram et al., 2009). Another general point that characterizes the organization of AChR recycling is the compartmentalization of signaling by virtue of anchoring molecules. While the cAMP necessary to recycle AChRs in a PKA-dependent manner appears to be located in certain microdomains (Röder et al., 2010), rapsyn was found to anchor PKA in close vicinity to the vesicles that harbor recycling AChRs and myosin Va (Röder et al., 2010; Choi et al., 2012). Similarly, absence of the CaMKII-anchoring protein αkap (which itself is a non-functional CaMKII), that is known to target CaMKII to different subcellular sites (Bayer et al., 1998; O'Leary et al., 2006; Singh et al., 2009), reduced AChR stability in myotubes (Mouslim et al., 2012). The presence and absence of αkap was claimed to be associated with decreased and increased ubiquitination, of AChRs (Mouslim et al., 2012), respectively, and regulation of this process might be directly linked to degradation of AChRs. While in this study, using myotubes and cell cultures, total AChR levels could be modulated using proteasome inhibitors (Mouslim et al., 2012), other reports show a role of lysosomal degradation of surface-exposed AChRs (Libby et al., 1980; Engel and Fumagalli, 1982; Clementi et al., 1983; Hyman and Froehner, 1983; Valkova et al., 2011). A likely explanation for the discrepancy regarding the degradation path of AChRs is the time-point at which they are to be eliminated. Whereas proteasome appears to be crucial for degradation of unassembled AChR subunits at the level of ER (Christianson and Green, 2004), lysosomal degradation should affect receptors after their endocytosis from the plasma membrane.

A recent study has looked at this latter degradation pathway in more detail and reported the involvement of autophagy that leads to loss of AChRs from the NMJ (Khan et al., 2014) (**Figure 5**) after ingestion of endosomal structures into autophagosomes that subsequently fuse with lysosomes to terminally digest the entire protein content as reviewed elsewhere (Shaid et al., 2013). AChR-containing endocytosed carriers were accompanied by the autophagy marker, LC3 and this was dependent on the presence of the LC3-activating enzyme, Atg7 (Khan et al., 2014). Notably, a strong increase in the amount of autophagic AChR-containing vesicles upon denervation was observed and this was completely blunted in the absence of the E3 ubiquitin ligase, MuRF1 (Khan et al., 2014). MuRF1 is also known as one of the central players in muscle atrophy (Bodine et al., 2001; Centner et al., 2001) and termed as atrogene (Lecker et al., 2004). This suggested a role of ubiquitination in sorting AChRs to autophagic decay, an assumption which was corroborated by the presence of the adaptor protein, p62/SQSTM1 in AChR-containing carriers (Khan et al., 2014). p62/SQSTM1 harbors both, ubiquitin binding site and LC3 interacting regions to bridge ubiquitinated target molecules to the autophagosomal membranes (Pankiv et al., 2007). So far, it is unclear, if ubiquitinated AChR serves as a direct target for selective autophagy or whether other molecules in complex with AChR do so.

PATHWAYS ALTERED IN AGING AND DYSTROPHY

The above discussion has mentioned a few molecular pathways that could potentially play a role in the deterioration of the NMJ. In the following text, actually observed alterations of these pathways in aging and dystrophy will be discussed. A recent genomic and proteomic profiling of aging rats revealed that a group of NMJ-related genes, including different subunits of AChR, MuSK, and Lrp4, are significantly up-regulated with age and weight loss (Ibebunjo et al., 2013). This has two implications. First, it corroborates an important involvement of functional denervation in the sarcopenia process, since synaptic genes are known targets upon denervation (Bodine et al., 2001; Furlow et al., 2013). Second, the MuSK pathway is apparently involved in the aging process of skeletal muscle. This is further substantiated by recent studies. First, tamoxifen-inducible conditional knock-out mice lacking agrin in a subset of motor neurons were recently created and analyzed (Samuel et al., 2012). Upon tamoxifen treatment of these mice, it took 2–3 months for agrin to detectably diminish in the affected neurons. Concurrently, NMJs displayed mild to severe morphological alterations. Notably, pre-synaptic decay seemed to follow deterioration of the post-synaptic apparatus, suggesting the involvement of retrograde signaling from muscle to nerve (Samuel et al., 2012). Five to six months after the administration of tamoxifen, there was marked withdrawal of motor axons and motor unit sizes were decreased (Samuel et al., 2012). Another important contribution was made by the finding that proteolytic cleavage of agrin induces early onset sarcopenia in young adult mice (Bütikofer et al., 2011). Agrin is cleaved at the NMJ by the protease, neuronal neurotrypsin, and this leads to the formation of 90 and 22 kDa N- and C-terminal fragments of agrin, respectively (Reif et al., 2007; Stephan et al., 2008). Notably, 4 months old transgenic mice overexpressing neurotrypsin in motor neurons displayed many facets of sarcopenia including reduced fiber number, fiber caliber heterogeneity, fiber type grouping, increased amount of type I fibers, and severely fragmented NMJs (Bütikofer et al., 2011). These findings suggest that destabilization of NMJ alone can be sufficient for leading to a pronounced sarcopenic phenotype and were substantiated by a recent study, where injection of a neurotrypsin-resistant agrin fragment stabilized NMJs and improved the phenotype of neurotrypsin-overexpressing mice (Hettwer et al., 2014). A recent clinical study identified significantly increased serum levels of the C-terminal agrin fragment in sarcopenic patients as compared to aged matched controls and a national blood donor cohort (Hettwer et al., 2013). Thus, agrin fragments appear to be not only promising candidates in the search for biomarkers in the field of sarcopenia diagnosis, but also carry hope for use as potential therapeutic agents. However, it needs to be mentioned that only about 38% of the sarcopenia patients displayed elevated levels of the agrin fragment in serum, indicating that sarcopenia is indeed likely a multi-factorial disease. This is also supported by the observation that aged transgenic mice lacking neurotrypsin, or overexpressing agrin develop sarcopenia (Bütikofer et al., 2011). Whether agrin signaling is modified or relevant in the context of NMJ maintenance in muscular dystrophies has yet to be explored.

Conversely, when considering second messenger handling as a major determinant of AChR turnover and NMJ continuity, this is definitely aberrant in dystrophic muscle while its role in sarcopenia is much less clear. With respect to dystrophies, alterations in Ca^{2+} and cAMP handling were previously reviewed (Carlson, 1998; Rudolf et al., 2013). Although to our knowledge there are no in-depth reports that have investigated modulation of second messenger signaling upon aging by means of *in vivo* approaches, genomic and proteomic profiling revealed a strong correlation between muscle loss and at least three members of the cAMP signaling system, i.e., adenylate cyclase 2, PKA type Iα, and phosphodiesterase 4a (Ibebunjo et al., 2013). Future work will be necessary to further tighten these links and to understand any possible relationship to age-related alterations of NMJ. Finally, NMJ remodeling and particularly, AChR turnover are affected by the autophagy process. So, what is the contribution of autophagy to sarcopenia and dystrophy? This question has recently been addressed in a nice review (Sandri et al., 2013). In brief, although to date genes that are involved in autophagy have not been found to be directly associated with dystrophinopathies and sarcopenia, autophagy is impaired in muscles of dystrophic mdx mice and Duchenne dystrophy patients (De Palma et al., 2012). Furthermore, treatment of mdx mice with the agonist, AICAR, for the autophagy-driving AMP kinase not only leads to increased autophagic flux but also improves the dystrophic phenotype significantly (Pauly et al., 2012). In general, a fine tuned balance of autophagy seems to be critical for keeping skeletal muscle intact (Neel et al., 2013). While too little autophagic activity might lead to accumulation of damaged organelles and proteins, such as mitochondria (Grumati et al., 2010) or sarcoplasmic reticulum (Russ et al., 2014), exacerbated autophagy would also entail muscle wasting.

CONCLUSION

In conclusion, the interplay between neurons and muscle is a principal component that appears to be altered in both sarcopenia and dystrophy. However, the origins of the degeneration in functional interaction between both tissues are likely to be different between those two conditions. Owing to anterograde and retrograde signaling cascades active at the NMJ, it can be envisaged that neuronal degradation may lead to muscle fiber atrophy as well as the reverse of this. Regardless, functional denervation might trigger several pathways leading to the morphological deterioration of NMJs and to altered turnover of AChRs. This could become important in the context of diagnosing and treating sarcopenia, given that with the appearance of agrin fragments, first biomarkers and therapeutic agents for a subset of sarcopenia are also apparent. Since the agrin/MuSK/Lrp4 pathway is a major but not exclusive regulator of NMJ maintenance, further research is needed to better understand these additional physiological signals that decide over NMJ morphology and AChR turnover.

ACKNOWLEDGMENTS

Siegfried Labeit and Rüdiger Rudolf are supported by Deutsche Forschungsgemeinschaft (LA668/15-1, RU923/7-1). Michael R. Deschenes is funded by NIH grant R15 AR060637-03. We acknowledge support by Deutsche Forschungsgemeinschaft and Open Access Publishing Fund of Karlsruhe Institute of Technology.

REFERENCES

Andersen, J. L. (2003). Muscle fibre type adaptation in the elderly human muscle. *Scand. J. Med. Sci. Sports* 13, 40–47. doi:10.1034/j.1600-0838.2003.00299.x

Andersen, J. L., Terzis, G., and Kryger, A. (1999). Increase in the degree of coexpression of myosin heavy chain isoforms in skeletal muscle fibers of the very old. *Muscle Nerve* 22, 449–454. doi:10.1002/(SICI)1097-4598(199904)22:4<449::AID-MUS4>3.0.CO;2-2

Andonian, M. H., and Fahim, M. A. (1987). Effects of endurance exercise on the morphology of mouse neuromuscular junctions during ageing. *J. Neurocytol.* 16, 589–599. doi:10.1007/BF01637652

Bayer, K. U., Harbers, K., and Schulman, H. (1998). alphaKAP is an anchoring protein for a novel CaM kinase II isoform in skeletal muscle. *EMBO J.* 17, 5598–5605. doi:10.1093/emboj/17.19.5598

Berger, M. J., and Doherty, T. J. (2010). Sarcopenia: prevalence, mechanisms, and functional consequences. *Interdiscip. Top. Gerontol.* 37, 94–114. doi:10.1159/000319997

Blake, D. J., Weir, A., Newey, S. E., and Davies, K. E. (2002). Function and genetics of dystrophin and dystrophin-related proteins in muscle. *Physiol. Rev.* 82, 291–329. doi:10.1152/physrev.00028.2001

Bodine, S. C., Latres, E., Baumhueter, S., Lai, V. K., Nunez, L., Clarke, B. A., et al. (2001). Identification of ubiquitin ligases required for skeletal muscle atrophy. *Science* 294, 1704–1708. doi:10.1126/science.1065874

Bruneau, E., Sutter, D., Hume, R. I., and Akaaboune, M. (2005). Identification of nicotinic acetylcholine receptor recycling and its role in maintaining receptor density at the neuromuscular junction in vivo. *J. Neurosci.* 25, 9949–9959. doi:10.1523/JNEUROSCI.3169-05.2005

Bütikofer, L., Zurlinden, A., Bolliger, M. F., Kunz, B., and Sonderegger, P. (2011). Destabilization of the neuromuscular junction by proteolytic cleavage of agrin results in precocious sarcopenia. *FASEB J.* 25, 4378–4393. doi:10.1096/fj.11-191262

Carlson, C. G. (1998). The dystrophinopathies: an alternative to the structural hypothesis. *Neurobiol. Dis.* 5, 3–15. doi:10.1006/nbdi.1998.0188

Centner, T., Yano, J., Kimura, E., McElhinny, A. S., Pelin, K., Witt, C. C., et al. (2001). Identification of muscle specific ring finger proteins as potential regulators of the titin kinase domain. *J. Mol. Biol.* 306, 717–726. doi:10.1006/jmbi.2001.4448

Chai, R. J., Vukovic, J., Dunlop, S., Grounds, M. D., and Shavlakadze, T. (2011). Striking denervation of neuromuscular junctions without lumbar motoneuron loss in geriatric mouse muscle. *PLoS ONE* 6:e28090. doi:10.1371/journal.pone.0028090

Cheng, A., Morsch, M., Murata, Y., Ghazanfari, N., Reddel, S. W., and Phillips, W. D. (2013). Sequence of age-associated changes to the mouse neuromuscular junction and the protective effects of voluntary exercise. *PLoS ONE* 8:e67970. doi:10.1371/journal.pone.0067970

Choi, K. R., Berrera, M., Reischl, M., Strack, S., Albrizio, M., Röder, I. V., et al. (2012). Rapsyn mediates subsynaptic anchoring of PKA type I and stabilisation of acetylcholine receptor in vivo. *J. Cell. Sci.* 125, 714–723. doi:10.1242/jcs.092361

Christianson, J. C., and Green, W. N. (2004). Regulation of nicotinic receptor expression by the ubiquitin-proteasome system. *EMBO J.* 23, 4156–4165. doi:10.1038/sj.emboj.7600436

Clementi, F., Sher, E., and Erroi, A. (1983). Acetylcholine receptor degradation: study of mechanism of action of inhibitory drugs. *Eur. J. Cell Biol.* 29, 274–280.

Correia, S. S., Bassani, S., Brown, T. C., Lise, M. F., Backos, D. S., El-Husseini, A., et al. (2008). Motor protein-dependent transport of AMPA receptors into spines during long-term potentiation. *Nat. Neurosci.* 11, 457–466. doi:10.1038/nn2063

Costa, C., Oliveira, J., Gonçalves, A., Santos, R., Bronze-da-Rocha, E., Rebelo, O., et al. (2013). A Portuguese case of Fukuyama congenital muscular dystrophy caused by a multi-exonic duplication in the fukutin gene. *Neuromuscul. Disord.* 23, 557–561. doi:10.1016/j.nmd.2013.03.005

Costa, M. C., Mani, F., Santoro, W. Jr, Espreafico, E. M., and Larson, R. E. (1999). Brain myosin-V, a calmodulin-carrying myosin, binds to calmodulin-dependent protein kinase II and activates its kinase activity. *J. Biol. Chem.* 274, 15811–15819. doi:10.1074/jbc.274.22.15811

Cruz-Jentoft, A. J., Baeyens, J. P., Bauer, J. M., Boirie, Y., Cederholm, T., Landi, F., et al. (2010). Sarcopenia: European consensus on definition and diagnosis: report of the European Working Group on sarcopenia in older people. *Age Ageing* 39, 412–423. doi:10.1093/ageing/afq034

Davies, K. E., and Nowak, K. J. (2006). Molecular mechanisms of muscular dystrophies: old and new players. *Nat. Rev. Mol. Cell Biol.* 7, 762–773. doi:10.1038/nrm2024

De Palma, C., Morisi, F., Cheli, S., Pambianco, S., Cappello, V., Vezzoli, M., et al. (2012). Autophagy as a new therapeutic target in Duchenne muscular dystrophy. *Cell Death Dis.* 3, e418. doi:10.1038/cddis.2012.159

Deschenes, M. R., Hurst, T. E., Ramser, A. E., and Sherman, E. G. (2013). Pre-to post-synaptic relationships of the neuromuscular junction are held constant across age and muscle fiber type. *Dev. Neurobiol.* 73, 744–753. doi:10.1002/dneu.22095

Deschenes, M. R., Judelson, D. A., Kraemer, W. J., Meskaitis, V. J., Volek, J. S., Nindl, B. C., et al. (2000). Effects of resistance training on neuromuscular junction morphology. *Muscle Nerve* 23, 1576–1581. doi:10.1002/1097-4598(200010)23:10<1576::AID-MUS15>3.0.CO;2-J

Deschenes, M. R., Maresh, C. M., Crivello, J. F., Armstrong, L. E., Kraemer, W. J., and Covault, J. (1993). The effects of exercise training of different intensities on neuromuscular junction morphology. *J. Neurocytol.* 22, 603–615. doi:10.1007/BF01181487

Deschenes, M. R., Roby, M. A., and Glass, E. K. (2011). Aging influences adaptations of the neuromuscular junction to endurance training. *Neuroscience* 190, 56–66. doi:10.1016/j.neuroscience.2011.05.070

Doherty, T. J., Vandervoort, A. A., and Brown, W. F. (1993). Effects of ageing on the motor unit: a brief review. *Can. J. Appl. Physiol.* 18, 331–358. doi:10.1139/h93-029

Engel, A. G., and Fumagalli, G. (1982). Mechanisms of acetylcholine receptor loss from the neuromuscular junction. *Ciba Found. Symp.* 90, 197–224.

Engel, A. G., and Ozawa, E. (2004). "Dystrophinopathies," in *Myology*, Vol. 2, eds A. G. Engel and C. Franzini-Armstrong (New-York, NY: McGraw-Hill), 961–1026.

Fahim, M. A. (1997). Endurance exercise modulates neuromuscular junction of C57BL/6NNia aging mice. *J. Appl. Physiol.* 83, 59–66.

Furlow, J. D., Watson, M. L., Waddell, D. S., Neff, E. S., Baehr, L. M., Ross, A. P., et al. (2013). Altered gene expression patterns in muscle ring finger 1 null mice during denervation- and dexamethasone-induced muscle atrophy. *Physiol. Genomics* 45, 1168–1185. doi:10.1152/physiolgenomics.00022.2013

Gautam, M., Noakes, P. G., Mudd, J., Nichol, M., Chu, G. C., Sanes, J. R., et al. (1995). Failure of postsynaptic specialization to develop at neuromuscular junctions of rapsyn-deficient mice. *Nature* 377, 232–236. doi:10.1038/377232a0

Grady, R. M., Teng, H., Nichol, M. C., Cunningham, J. C., Wilkinson, R. S., and Sanes, J. R. (1997). Skeletal and cardiac myopathies in mice lacking utrophin and dystrophin: a model for Duchenne muscular dystrophy. *Cell* 90, 729–738. doi:10.1016/S0092-8674(00)80533-4

Grumati, P., Coletto, L., Sabatelli, P., Cescon, M., Angelin, A., Bertaggia, E., et al. (2010). Autophagy is defective in collagen VI muscular dystrophies, and its reactivation rescues myofiber degeneration. *Nat. Med.* 16, 1313–1320. doi:10.1038/nm.2247

Gu, Y., and Hall, Z. W. (1988). Immunological evidence for a change in subunits of the acetylcholine receptor in developing and denervated rat muscle. *Neuron* 1, 117–125. doi:10.1016/0896-6273(88)90195-X

Hepple, R. T. (2012). Muscle atrophy is not always sarcopenia. *J. Appl. Physiol.* 113, 677–679. doi:10.1152/japplphysiol.00304.2012

Hettwer, S., Dahinden, P., Kucsera, S., Farina, C., Ahmed, S., Fariello, R., et al. (2013). Elevated levels of a C-terminal agrin fragment identifies a new subset of sarcopenia patients. *Exp. Gerontol.* 48, 69–75. doi:10.1016/j.exger.2012.03.002

Hettwer, S., Lin, S., Kucsera, S., Haubitz, M., Oliveri, F., Fariello, R. G., et al. (2014). Injection of a soluble fragment of neural agrin (NT-1654) considerably improves the muscle pathology caused by the disassembly of the neuromuscular junction. *PLoS ONE* 9:e88739. doi:10.1371/journal.pone.0088739

Huganir, R. L., and Miles, K. (1989). Protein phosphorylation of nicotinic acetylcholine receptors. *Crit. Rev. Biochem. Mol. Biol.* 24, 183–215. doi:10.3109/10409238909082553

Hyman, C., and Froehner, S. C. (1983). Degradation of acetylcholine receptors in muscle cells: effect of leupeptin on turnover rate, intracellular pool sizes, and receptor properties. *J. Cell Biol.* 96, 1316–1324. doi:10.1083/jcb.96.5.1316

Ibebunjo, C., Chick, J. M., Kendall, T., Eash, J. K., Li, C., Zhang, Y., et al. (2013). Genomic and proteomic profiling reveals reduced mitochondrial function and disruption of the neuromuscular junction driving rat sarcopenia. *Mol. Cell. Biol.* 33, 194–212. doi:10.1128/MCB.01036-12

Jansen, M., van Alfen, N., Geurts, A. C. H., and de Groot, I. J. M. (2013). Assisted bicycle training delays functional deterioration in boys with duchenne muscular dystrophy: the randomized controlled trial "no use is disuse". *Neurorehabil. Neural Repair* 27, 816–827. doi:10.1177/1545968313496326

Kaido, M., Arahata, K., Hoffman, E. P., Nonaka, I., and Sugita, H. (1991). Muscle histology in Becker muscular dystrophy. *Muscle Nerve* 14, 1067–1073. doi:10.1002/mus.880141105

Kanda, K., and Hashizume, K. (1989). Changes in properties of the medial gastrocnemius motor units in aging rats. *J. Neurophysiol.* 61, 737–746.

Kawamura, Y., O'Brien, P., Okazaki, H., and Dyck, P. J. (1977). Lumbar motoneurons of man II: the number and diameter distribution of large- and intermediate-diameter cytons in "motoneuron columns" of spinal cord of man. *J. Neuropathol. Exp. Neurol.* 36, 861–870. doi:10.1097/00005072-197709000-00010

Khan, M. M., Strack, S., Wild, F., Hanashima, A., Gasch, A., Brohm, K., et al. (2014). Role of autophagy, SQSTM1, SH3GLB1, and TRIM63 in the turnover of nicotinic acetylcholine receptors. *Autophagy* 10, 123–136. doi:10.4161/auto.26841

Kim, N., Stiegler, A. L., Cameron, T. O., Hallock, P. T., Gomez, A. M., Huang, J. H., et al. (2008). Lrp4 is a receptor for Agrin and forms a complex with MuSK. *Cell* 135, 334–342. doi:10.1016/j.cell.2008.10.002

Kraemer, W. J., Patton, J. F., Gordon, S. E., Harman, E. A., Deschenes, M. R., Reynolds, K., et al. (1995). Compatibility of high-intensity strength and endurance training on hormonal and skeletal muscle adaptations. *J. Appl. Physiol.* 78, 976–989.

Krag, T. O., Hauerslev, S., Sveen, M. L., Schwartz, M., and Vissing, J. (2011). Level of muscle regeneration in limb-girdle muscular dystrophy type 2I relates to genotype and clinical severity. *Skelet Muscle* 1, 31. doi:10.1186/2044-5040-1-31

Kummer, T. T., Misgeld, T., and Sanes, J. R. (2006). Assembly of the postsynaptic membrane at the neuromuscular junction: paradigm lost. *Curr. Opin. Neurobiol.* 16, 74–82. doi:10.1016/j.conb.2005.12.003

Lecker, S. H., Jagoe, R. T., Gilbert, A., Gomes, M., Baracos, V., Bailey, J., et al. (2004). Multiple types of skeletal muscle atrophy involve a common program of changes in gene expression. *FASEB J.* 18, 39–51. doi:10.1096/fj.03-0610com

Lexell, J. (1993). Ageing and human muscle: observations from Sweden. *Can. J. Appl. Physiol.* 18, 2–18. doi:10.1139/h93-002

Li, Y., Lee, Y. I., and Thompson, W. J. (2011). Changes in aging mouse neuromuscular junctions are explained by degeneration and regeneration of muscle fiber segments at the synapse. *J. Neurosci.* 31, 14910–14919. doi:10.1523/JNEUROSCI.3590-11.2011

Libby, P., Bursztajn, S., and Goldberg, A. L. (1980). Degradation of the acetylcholine receptor in cultured muscle cells: selective inhibitors and the fate of undegraded receptors. *Cell* 19, 481–491. doi:10.1016/0092-8674(80)90523-1

Lyons, P. R., and Slater, C. R. (1991). Structure and function of the neuromuscular junction in young adult mdx mice. *J. Neurocytol.* 20, 969–981. doi:10.1007/BF01187915

Marchand, S., Bignami, F., Stetzkowski-Marden, F., and Cartaud, J. (2000). The myristoylated protein rapsyn is cotargeted with the nicotinic acetylcholine receptor to the postsynaptic membrane via the exocytic pathway. *J. Neurosci.* 20, 521–528.

Marchand, S., Devillers-Thiery, A., Pons, S., Changeux, J. P., and Cartaud, J. (2002). Rapsyn escorts the nicotinic acetylcholine receptor along the exocytic pathway via association with lipid rafts. *J. Neurosci.* 22, 8891–8901.

Marini, J. F., Pons, F., Leger, J., Loffreda, N., Anoal, M., Chevallay, M., et al. (1991). Expression of myosin heavy chain isoforms in Duchenne muscular dystrophy patients and carriers. *Neuromuscul. Disord.* 1, 397–409. doi:10.1016/0960-8966(91)90003-B

Martinez-Pena y Valenzuela, I., Pires-Oliveira, M., and Akaaboune, M. (2013). PKC and PKA regulate AChR dynamics at the neuromuscular junction of living mice. *PLoS ONE* 8:e81311. doi:10.1371/journal.pone.0081311

Martinez-Pena y Valenzuela, I., Mouslim, C., and Akaaboune, M. (2010). Calcium/calmodulin kinase II-dependent acetylcholine receptor cycling at the mammalian neuromuscular junction in vivo. *J. Neurosci.* 30, 12455–12465. doi:10.1523/JNEUROSCI.3309-10.2010

Martinez-Pena y Valenzuela, I., Mouslim, C., Pires-Oliveira, M., Adams, M. E., Froehner, S. C., and Akaaboune, M. (2011). Nicotinic acetylcholine receptor stability at the NMJ deficient in alpha-syntrophin in vivo. *J. Neurosci.* 31, 15586–15596. doi:10.1523/JNEUROSCI.4038-11.2011

Mercuri, E., and Muntoni, F. (2013). Muscular dystrophies. *Lancet* 381, 845–860. doi:10.1016/S0140-6736(12)61897-2

Miles, K., Anthony, D. T., Rubin, L. L., Greengard, P., and Huganir, R. L. (1987). Regulation of nicotinic acetylcholine receptor phosphorylation in rat myotubes by forskolin and cAMP. *Proc. Natl. Acad. Sci. U.S.A.* 84, 6591–6595. doi:10.1073/pnas.84.18.6591

Mishina, M., Takai, T., Imoto, K., Noda, M., Takahashi, T., Numa, S., et al. (1986). Molecular distinction between fetal and adult forms of muscle acetylcholine receptor. *Nature* 321, 406–411. doi:10.1038/321406a0

Mouslim, C., Aittaleb, M., Hume, R. I., and Akaaboune, M. (2012). A role for the calmodulin kinase II-related anchoring protein (alphakap) in maintaining the stability of nicotinic acetylcholine receptors. *J. Neurosci.* 32, 5177–5185. doi:10.1523/JNEUROSCI.6477-11.2012

Neel, B. A., Lin, Y., and Pessin, J. E. (2013). Skeletal muscle autophagy: a new metabolic regulator. *Trends Endocrinol. Metab.* 24, 635–643. doi:10.1016/j.tem.2013.09.004

Nelson, P. G., Lanuza, M. A., Jia, M., Li, M. X., and Tomas, J. (2003). Phosphorylation reactions in activity-dependent synapse modification at the neuromuscular junction during development. *J. Neurocytol.* 32, 803–816. doi:10.1023/B:NEUR.0000020625.70284.a6

Nimnual, A. S., Chang, W., Chang, N. S., Ross, A. F., Gelman, M. S., and Prives, J. M. (1998). Identification of phosphorylation sites on AChR delta-subunit associated with dispersal of AChR clusters on the surface of muscle cells. *Biochemistry* 37, 14823–14832. doi:10.1021/bi9802824

O'Leary, H., Sui, X., Lin, P.-J., Volpe, P., and Bayer, K. U. (2006). Nuclear targeting of the CaMKII anchoring protein alphaKAP is regulated by alternative splicing and protein kinases. *Brain Res.* 1086, 17–26. doi:10.1016/j.brainres.2006.02.120

Pankiv, S., Clausen, T. H., Lamark, T., Brech, A., Bruun, J. A., Outzen, H., et al. (2007). p62/SQSTM1 binds directly to Atg8/LC3 to facilitate degradation of ubiquitinated protein aggregates by autophagy. *J. Biol. Chem.* 282, 24131–24145. doi:10.1074/jbc.M702824200

Patterson, M. F., Stephenson, G. M. M., and Stephenson, D. G. (2006). Denervation produces different single fiber phenotypes in fast- and slow-twitch hindlimb muscles of the rat. *Am. J. Physiol. Cell Physiol.* 291, C518–C528. doi:10.1152/ajpcell.00013.2006

Pauly, M., Daussin, F., Burelle, Y., Li, T., Godin, R., Fauconnier, J., et al. (2012). AMPK activation stimulates autophagy and ameliorates muscular dystrophy in the mdx mouse diaphragm. *Am. J. Pathol.* 181, 583–592. doi:10.1016/j.ajpath.2012.04.004

Pilgram, G. S., Potikanond, S., Baines, R. A., Fradkin, L. G., and Noordermeer, J. N. (2009). The roles of the dystrophin-associated glycoprotein complex at the synapse. *Mol. Neurobiol.* 41, 1–21. doi:10.1007/s12035-009-8089-5

Power, G. A., Dalton, B. H., Behm, D. G., Vandervoort, A. A., Doherty, T. J., and Rice, C. L. (2010). Motor unit number estimates in masters runners: use it or lose it? *Med. Sci. Sports Exerc.* 42, 1644–1650. doi:10.1249/MSS.0b013e3181d6f9e9

Punga, A. R., and Ruegg, M. A. (2012). Signaling and aging at the neuromuscular synapse: lessons learnt from neuromuscular diseases. *Curr. Opin. Pharmacol.* 12, 340–346. doi:10.1016/j.coph.2012.02.002

Reck-Peterson, S. L., Provance, D. W. Jr, Mooseker, M. S., and Mercer, J. A. (2000). Class V myosins. *Biochim. Biophys. Acta* 1496, 36–51. doi:10.1016/S0167-4889(00)00007-0

Reif, R., Sales, S., Hettwer, S., Dreier, B., Gisler, C., Wölfel, J., et al. (2007). Specific cleavage of agrin by neurotrypsin, a synaptic protease linked to mental retardation. *FASEB J.* 21, 3468–3478. doi:10.1096/fj.07-8800com

Röder, I. V., Choi, K. R., Reischl, M., Petersen, Y., Diefenbacher, M. E., Zaccolo, M., et al. (2010). Myosin Va cooperates with PKA RIalpha to mediate maintenance of the endplate in vivo. *Proc. Natl. Acad. Sci. U.S.A.* 107, 2031–2036. doi:10.1073/pnas.0914087107

Röder, V. I, Petersen, Y., Choi, K. R., Witzemann, V., Hammer, J. A. III, and Rudolf, R. (2008). Role of myosin Va in the plasticity of the vertebrate neuromuscular junction in vivo. *PLoS ONE* 3:e3871. doi:10.1371/journal.pone.0003871

Rosenberg, I. H. (1997). Sarcopenia: origins and clinical relevance. *J. Nutr.* 127, 990S–991S.

Rosenheimer, J. L., and Smith, D. O. (1985). Differential changes in the end-plate architecture of functionally diverse muscles during aging. *J. Neurophysiol.* 53, 1567–1581.

Rowan, S. L., Purves-Smith, F. M., Solbak, N. M., and Hepple, R. T. (2011). Accumulation of severely atrophic myofibers marks the acceleration of sarcopenia in slow and fast twitch muscles. *Exp. Gerontol.* 46, 660–669. doi:10.1016/j.exger.2011.03.005

Rowan, S. L., Rygiel, K., Purves-Smith, F. M., Solbak, N. M., Turnbull, D. M., and Hepple, R. T. (2012). Denervation causes fiber atrophy and myosin heavy chain co-expression in senescent skeletal muscle. *PLoS ONE* 7:e29082. doi:10.1371/journal.pone.0029082

Rudolf, R., Khan, M. M., Lustrino, D., Labeit, S., Kettelhut, ÍC., and Navegantes, L. C. C. (2013). Alterations of cAMP-dependent signaling in dystrophic skeletal muscle. *Front. Physiol.* 4:290. doi:10.3389/fphys.2013.00290

Russ, D. W., Wills, A. M., Boyd, I. M., and Krause, J. (2014). Weakness, SR function and stress in gastrocnemius muscles of aged male rats. *Exp. Gerontol.* 50, 40–44. doi:10.1016/j.exger.2013.11.018

Samuel, M. A., Valdez, G., Tapia, J. C., Lichtman, J. W., and Sanes, J. R. (2012). Agrin and synaptic laminin are required to maintain adult neuromuscular junctions. *PLoS ONE* 7:e46663. doi:10.1371/journal.pone.0046663

Sandri, M., Coletto, L., Grumati, P., and Bonaldo, P. (2013). Misregulation of autophagy and protein degradation systems in myopathies and muscular dystrophies. *J. Cell Sci.* 126, 5325–5333. doi:10.1242/jcs.114041

Schmidt, N., Akaaboune, M., Gajendran, N., Martinez-Pena, Y., Valenzuela, I., Wakefield, S., et al. (2011). Neuregulin/ErbB regulate neuromuscular junction development by phosphorylation of α-dystrobrevin. *J. Cell Biol.* 195, 1171–1184. doi:10.1083/jcb.201107083

Schwarz, H., Giese, G., Muller, H., Koenen, M., and Witzemann, V. (2000). Different functions of fetal and adult AChR subtypes for the formation and maintenance of neuromuscular synapses revealed in epsilon-subunit-deficient mice. *Eur. J. Neurosci.* 12, 3107–3116. doi:10.1046/j.1460-9568.2000.00195.x

Shaid, S., Brandts, C. H., Serve, H., and Dikic, I. (2013). Ubiquitination and selective autophagy. *Cell Death Differ.* 20, 21–30. doi:10.1038/cdd.2012.72

Shiao, T., Fond, A., Deng, B., Wehling-Henricks, M., Adams, M. E., Froehner, S. C., et al. (2004). Defects in neuromuscular junction structure in dystrophic muscle are corrected by expression of a NOS transgene in dystrophin-deficient muscles, but not in muscles lacking alpha- and beta1-syntrophins. *Hum. Mol. Genet.* 13, 1873–1884. doi:10.1093/hmg/ddh204

Singh, P., Salih, M., and Tuana, B. S. (2009). Alpha-kinase anchoring protein alphaKAP interacts with SERCA2A to spatially position Ca2+/calmodulin-dependent protein kinase II and modulate phospholamban phosphorylation. *J. Biol. Chem.* 284, 28212–28221. doi:10.1074/jbc.M109.044990

Stanmore, A., Bradbury, S., and Weddell, A. G. (1978). A quantitative study of peripheral nerve fibres in the mouse following the administration of drugs. 1. Age changes in untreated CBA mice from 3 to 21 months of age. *J. Anat.* 127, 101–115.

Stephan, A., Mateos, J. M., Kozlov, S. V., Cinelli, P., Kistler, A. D., Hettwer, S., et al. (2008). Neurotrypsin cleaves agrin locally at the synapse. *FASEB J.* 22, 1861–1873. doi:10.1096/fj.07-100008

Taniguchi, M., Kurahashi, H., Noguchi, S., Fukudome, T., Okinaga, T., Tsukahara, T., et al. (2006). Aberrant neuromuscular junctions and delayed terminal muscle fiber maturation in alpha-dystroglycanopathies. *Hum. Mol. Genet.* 15, 1279–1289. doi:10.1093/hmg/ddl045

ten Houten, R., and De Visser, M. (1984). Histopathological findings in Becker-type muscular dystrophy. *Arch. Neurol.* 41, 729–733. doi:10.1001/archneur.1984.04050180051017

Tomlinson, B. E., and Irving, D. (1977). The numbers of limb motor neurons in the human lumbosacral cord throughout life. *J. Neurol. Sci.* 34, 213–219. doi:10.1016/0022-510X(77)90069-7

Tomlinson, B. E., Walton, J. N., and Irving, D. (1974). Spinal cord limb motor neurones in muscular dystrophy. *J. Neurol. Sci.* 22, 305–327. doi:10.1016/0022-510X(74)90003-3

Valdez, G., Tapia, J. C., Kang, H., Clemenson, G. D. Jr, Gage, F. H., Lichtman, J. W., et al. (2010). Attenuation of age-related changes in mouse neuromuscular synapses by caloric restriction and exercise. *Proc. Natl. Acad. Sci. U.S.A.* 107, 14863–14868. doi:10.1073/pnas.1002220107

Valkova, C., Albrizio, M., Röder, I. V., Schwake, M., Betto, R., Rudolf, R., et al. (2011). Sorting receptor Rer1 controls surface expression of muscle acetylcholine receptors by ER retention of unassembled alpha-subunits. *Proc. Natl. Acad. Sci. U.S.A.* 108, 621–625. doi:10.1073/pnas.1001624108

Walker, M. L., Burgess, S. A., Sellers, J. R., Wang, F., Hammer, J. A. III, Trinick, J., et al. (2000). Two-headed binding of a processive myosin to F-actin. *Nature* 405, 804–807. doi:10.1038/35015592

Wang, Z., Edwards, J. G., Riley, N., Provance, D. W. Jr, Karcher, R., Li, X. D., et al. (2008). Myosin Vb mobilizes recycling endosomes and AMPA receptors for postsynaptic plasticity. *Cell* 135, 535–548. doi:10.1016/j.cell.2008.09.057

Witzemann, V., Barg, B., Criado, M., Stein, E., and Sakmann, B. (1989). Developmental regulation of five subunit specific mRNAs encoding acetylcholine receptor subtypes in rat muscle. *FEBS Lett.* 242, 419–424. doi:10.1016/0014-5793(89)80514-9

Witzemann, V., Barg, B., Nishikawa, Y., Sakmann, B., and Numa, S. (1987). Differential regulation of muscle acetylcholine receptor gamma- and epsilon-subunit mRNAs. *FEBS Lett.* 223, 104–112. doi:10.1016/0014-5793(87)80518-5

Witzemann, V., Schwarz, H., Koenen, M., Berberich, C., Villarroel, A., Wernig, A., et al. (1996). Acetylcholine receptor epsilon-subunit deletion causes muscle weakness and atrophy in juvenile and adult mice. *Proc. Natl. Acad. Sci. U.S.A.* 93, 13286–13291. doi:10.1073/pnas.93.23.13286

Wong, M., and Martin, L. J. (2010). Skeletal muscle-restricted expression of human SOD1 causes motor neuron degeneration in transgenic mice. *Hum. Mol. Genet.* 19, 2284–2302. doi:10.1093/hmg/ddq106

Wu, H., Xiong, W. C., and Mei, L. (2010). To build a synapse: signaling pathways in neuromuscular junction assembly. *Development* 137, 1017–1033. doi:10.1242/dev.038711

Yampolsky, P., Pacifici, P. G., Lomb, L., Giese, G., Rudolf, R., Röder, I. V., et al. (2010). Time lapse in vivo visualization of developmental stabilization of synaptic receptors at neuromuscular junctions. *J. Biol. Chem.* 285, 34589–34596. doi:10.1074/jbc.M110.168880

Yumoto, N., Kim, N., and Burden, S. J. (2012). Lrp4 is a retrograde signal for presynaptic differentiation at neuromuscular synapses. *Nature* 489, 438–442. doi:10.1038/nature11348

Zhang, B., Luo, S., Wang, Q., Suzuki, T., Xiong, W. C., and Mei, L. (2008). LRP4 serves as a coreceptor of agrin. *Neuron* 60, 285–297. doi:10.1016/j.neuron.2008.10.006

8

Borderlines between sarcopenia and mild late-onset muscle disease

Johanna Palmio[1]* and Bjarne Udd[1,2,3]

[1] Department of Neurology, Neuromuscular Research Center, Tampere University Hospital, University of Tampere, Tampere, Finland
[2] Department of Medical Genetics, Folkhälsan Institute of Genetics, University of Helsinki, Helsinki, Finland
[3] Department of Neurology, Vaasa Central Hospital, Vaasa, Finland

***Correspondence:**
Johanna Palmio, Department of Neurology, Neuromuscular Research Center, Tampere University Hospital, University of Tampere, P.O.Box 2000, Tampere FIN-33520, Finland
e-mail: johanna.palmio@uta.fi

Numerous natural or disease-related alterations occur in different tissues of the body with advancing age. Sarcopenia is defined as age-related decrease of muscle mass and strength beginning in mid-adulthood and accelerating in people older than 60 years. Pathophysiology of sarcopenia involves both neural and muscle dependent mechanisms and is enhanced by multiple factors. Aged muscles show loss in fiber number, fiber atrophy, and gradual increase in the number of ragged red fibers and cytochrome *c* oxidase-negative fibers. Generalized loss of muscle tissue and increased amount of intramuscular fat are seen on muscle imaging. However, the degree of these changes varies greatly between individuals, and the distinction between normal age-related weakening of muscle strength and clinically significant muscle disease is not always obvious. Because some of the genetic myopathies can present at a very old age and be mild in severity, the correct diagnosis is easily missed. We highlight this difficult borderline zone between sarcopenia and muscle disease by two examples: LGMD1D and myotonic dystrophy type 2. Muscle magnetic resonance imaging (MRI) is a useful tool to help differentiate myopathies from sarcopenia and to reach the correct diagnosis also in the elderly.

Keywords: sarcopenia, myopathy, late-onset, genetic, muscle imaging

INTRODUCTION

One of the most serious consequence of aging is its effects on skeletal muscle. The aging in muscle is a complex process to which various physiological and pathological mechanisms contribute (Cruz-Jentoft et al., 2010). Sarcopenia, featuring the normal age-related changes in muscle, is defined as the slow but progressing loss of skeletal muscle mass and strength occurring with advancing age (Morley et al., 2001). A term, skeletal muscle function deficit (SMFD), has also been introduced in an attempt to better define the muscle problems in advanced age (Correa-de-Araujo and Hadley, 2014). Although sarcopenia is part of the normal aging process, it has a great impact on health and functionality, because the mobility is impaired, the risk of falls and injuries is increased, ability to perform activities of daily living is decreased, and there is an increased risk of lost independence and death (Rolland et al., 2008). Sarcopenia is common in adults over the age of 65 years and its prevalence increases with age. The prevalence varies from 5 to 13% in 60- to 70-year olds and 11–50% for the population aged 80 years or older and depends on what diagnostic methods and definitions are used (Iannuzzi-Sucich et al., 2002; Wang and Bai, 2012; Patel et al., 2013).

Muscle mass is strongly age dependent. After the age of 50, approximately 1–2% of muscle mass is expected to be lost every year and between the ages of 20 and 80 years muscle mass is reduced up to 50% (Wang and Bai, 2012). Pathophysiology of sarcopenia involves both neural- and muscle-dependent mechanisms and is enhanced by multiple factors (Cruz-Jentoft et al., 2010). Continuous age-related decrease in the number of motor neurons leads to chronic denervation of muscle tissue. This is one of the most important factors leading to the loss of muscle fibers and total muscle mass, although multiple other factors contribute, such as decreased physical activity, altered hormonal status, especially anabolic hormones, decreased total caloric and protein intake, inflammatory mediators, and factors leading to altered protein synthesis (Doherty, 2003; Ryall et al., 2008). Muscle atrophy might be induced also by increased susceptibility to apoptosis caused by mitochondrial dysfunction (Edström et al., 2007). The degree of these changes varies greatly between individuals, and an accepted definition of sarcopenia for use in clinical practice is still lacking (Cruz-Jentoft et al., 2010).

Age-related generalized loss of muscle tissue and the decrease in muscle volume and thickness are seen in muscle imaging using different techniques, such as, magnetic resonance imaging (MRI), computed tomography (CT), or ultrasonography (**Figures 1A,B**). Also, increased amount of intramuscular and intermuscular fat is observed (Wattjes and Fischer, 2013).

PATHOLOGICAL CHANGES WITH AGING

Aged muscles show loss in fiber number and fiber size. Fiber size reduction is more prominent in type 2 fibers. The decrease in fiber number affects both fiber types but preferential loss is seen in type 2, resulting in increase in the proportion of type 1 fibers (Lexell et al., 1988). Some neurogenic changes due to motor neuron loss may be seen in muscle biopsies of very aged individuals: the "Checkerboard" appearance of the normal muscle fibers is less distinct and certain fiber grouping can be observed

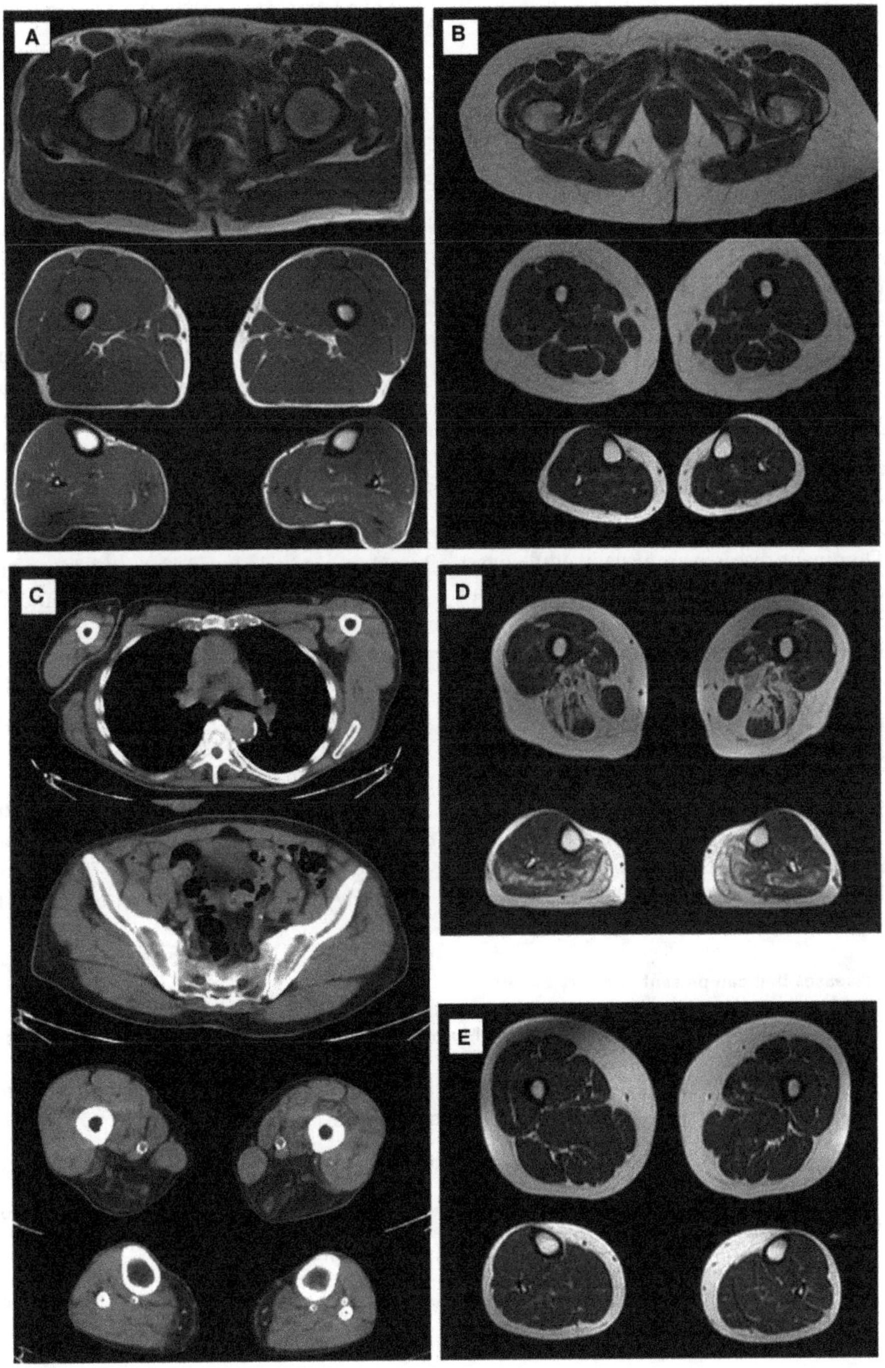

FIGURE 1 | Muscle imaging at different ages and diseases. Normal muscle imaging in a 40-year-old male **(A)**. Normal muscle imaging in a 73-year-old male with clear decrease in muscle volume **(B)**. Slight increase of diffuse fatty tissue is seen intramuscularly. Muscle CT in a 78-year-old male with LGMD2L shows dystrophic changes in the hamstrings and gastrocnemius medialis muscles **(C)**. Muscle MRI findings in a patient with LGMD1D at age 73 with typical fatty degenerative changes in the hamstring muscles and adductors at thigh level in the soleus and gastrocnemius muscles in the calves **(D)**. Muscle MRI in a patient with DM2 **(E)** shows that muscle volume is normal, and fatty degenerative changes are not seen at age 60.

in aging muscle tissue. The number of hybrid fibers, expressing more than a single myosin heavy chain isoform, is also increased (Doherty, 2003). Aging gradually increases the number of ragged red fibers (RRF) and cytochrome *c* oxidase (COX)-negative fibers (Müller-Höcker, 1992). There is no clear cut-point for the amount of these changes between normal aging and mitochondrial myopathies. Thus, in cases where there are more than occasional RRF or COX-negative fibers, late-onset mitochondrial or inflammatory myopathy (inclusion body myositis) should be considered.

MUSCULAR DYSTROPHIES

Usually genetic myopathies manifest at birth, in childhood, or early in adulthood, but many of them can also present at very old age (**Table 1**). Typically, muscular dystrophies present with slowly progressive weakness and muscle atrophy. Especially, if the symptoms are mild in severity and occur very late, the distinction between normal age-related weakening of muscle strength and clinically significant muscle disease is not always easy to make. Two entities with disease manifestations beginning at an old age are discussed in more detail.

LIMB-GIRDLE MUSCULAR DYSTROPHIES

Limb-girdle muscular dystrophies (LGMD) are a heterogeneous group of muscle diseases affecting hip and shoulder region first. There are eight autosomal dominant (LGMD1) and 23 autosomal recessive (LGMD2) genes or loci identified to date (Nigro and Savarese, 2014). Dominant diseases are usually adult-onset and milder than recessive forms, and comprise around 10% of all LGMD diseases. The age of onset of LGMD1 group of diseases is typically before the age of 50 (Nigro and Savarese, 2014) but occasional cases with later onset have been reported. LGMD1D is caused by heterozygous missense mutations in *DNAJB6* gene (Sarparanta et al., 2012). The muscle symptoms start in the proximal lower limbs at age 20–60 (Sandell et al., 2010). The weakness progresses very slowly and most of the patients remain ambulant even at very old age, although waddling gait is typical. In recessive LGMD diseases, the severity of the symptoms varies significantly. For example, LGMD2L disease caused by *ANO5* gene mutations can be very mild or even asymptomatic, especially in female patients (Penttilä et al., 2012). Of the patients examined in that study, one male patient's symptoms started at age 70, and at first, they were considered to be a consequence of statin use. He had, however, proximal weakness in the lower limb on examination and dystrophic changes on muscle MRI (Penttilä et al., 2012). Another male patient with a very mild LGMD2L disease is now 78 years old and still walking long distances without aid. His muscle CT showed relatively severe dystrophic changes (**Figure 1C**).

LGMD1D IN AN ELDERLY PATIENT

A 70-year-old sister, who at that time considered herself healthy, accompanied her brother to the hospital who was known to carry a *DNAJB6* mutation and who had more severe weakness and walking difficulties. She was found to carry the same mutation confirming the diagnosis of LGMD1D. At the first examination, she had mild weakness in the lower limbs, which progressed slowly during the follow-up of 10 years. Muscle MRI showed, nonetheless, dystrophic changes in her muscles compatible with the earlier findings of this disease (**Figure 1D**) (Sandell et al., 2013).

MYOTONIC DYSTROPHY TYPE 2

Myotonic dystrophies are the most common forms of muscular dystrophies in adults, but exact epidemiological data for myotonic dystrophy type 2 (DM2) are lacking. DM2 is, however, quite common at least in European populations. The mutation frequency is 1 in 1830 in the Finnish population, suggesting a clinical manifestation frequency of 1 in 5000 (Suominen et al., 2011). Dominantly inherited DM2 results from a (CCTG)n expansion in CNBP gene (formerly ZNF9 gene) (Liquori et al., 2001). The phenotype of

Table 1 | Genetic muscle diseases that can present at a very old age.

Muscle disease	Gene, locus	Mutation type	Age of onset
Tibial muscular dystrophy	*TTN* (titin), 2q31	Dominant, insertion–deletion, missense, truncating	35–40 distal weakness, rarely after 60 years; 60–80 proximal weakness
Welander distal myopathy	*TIA1*, 2p13	Dominant, missense	40–60 infrequently after 60 years
LGMD1A	*TTID* (myotilin), 5q31	Dominant, missense	50–60 up to 77 years
LGMD1D	*DNAJB6*, 7q36.3	Dominant, missense	20–50 up to 70 years
IBMPFD	*VCP*, 9p13.3	Dominant, missense	Mean age 42 can be over 60
Oculopharyngeal muscular dystrophy	*PAPBN1*, 14q11.2	Dominant/recessive, repeat expansion	50–60 or later in heterozygotes
DM1, late-onset oligosymptomatic	*DMPK*, 19q13.3	Dominant, repeat expansion	Over 50
DM2	*CNBP (ZNF9)*, 3q21	Dominant, repeat expansion	20–60, proximal weakness manifests later in typical cases
Acid maltase deficiency, adult-onset	*GAA* (acid α-glucosidase), 17q25.2-q25.3	Recessive, missense, nonsense, frameshift	Early adulthood up to 72 years
Mitochondrial myopathy	mtDNA defects	Dominant/recessive, maternal, sporadic, point mutations, deletions	Any age up to 70 years

LGMD, limb-girdle muscular dystrophies; IBMPFD, inclusion body myopathy with Paget disease and frontotemporal dementia; DM1, myotonic dystrophy type 1; DM2, myotonic dystrophy type 2; mtDNA, mitochondrial DNA.

DM2 is highly variable in severity, characterized by adult- or late-onset proximal muscle weakness, myalgia, and myotonia. Beyond the skeletal muscle symptoms, it is a multi-system disease and can cause cardiac conduction deficits, cataracts, and hormonal problems, such as insulin resistance, mild cerebral involvement, and liver enzyme elevation (Machuca-Tzili et al., 2005; Udd and Krahe, 2012).

DM2 IN ELDERLY PATIENTS

A 64-year-old female has had a slowly progressing myalgic syndrome for 15 years. The investigations begun when she experienced recurrent rhabdomyolysis at age 56 while on statin medication. Electromyogram showed spontaneous activity high frequency discharges and increased insertional activity but no myotonia. Between rhabdomyolysis periods, the levels of creatine kinase (CK) were normal. Myalgia reduced her physical performance; she was only able to walk 100 m at normal pace. Otherwise, the muscle strength was normal and muscle MRI was within normal limits (**Figure 1E**). Muscle biopsy showed minor changes suggestive of DM2: a subpopulation of highly atrophic type 2 fibers, nuclear clump fibers, and increased amount of internal nuclei. DNA analysis revealed (CCTG)n expansion in *CNBP* gene confirming the diagnosis of DM2. The mutation was transmitted by her mother, now at age 90. The mother was investigated after the diagnosis was made in the daughter and proved to have had some progressive walking difficulties and used a stick for walking since age 80. She had regular visits at the primary health care because of type 2 diabetes but her muscle weakness had not been noted as abnormal for age. At examination, she had moderate proximal lower limb weakness, even though she thought herself healthy for the age.

DISCUSSION

Muscle weakness, gradually worsening walking difficulties, muscle pain, and stiffness are common complaints in the elderly. Sarcopenia begins in mid-late adulthood, but the age of onset and the rate of muscle loss vary greatly between individuals. Normal age-related processes lead to certain findings in muscle histology and imaging studies. It is not always self-evident to consider the possibility of a late-onset myopathy as a cause of muscle symptoms in elderly people. However, old age should not limit investigations.

Comprehensive studies on myopathies in the elderly are scarce. Laguno et al. (2002) studied muscle biopsies from 239 patients over 65 years and diagnosed specific myopathies in 36% of them. Most of the causes of myopathies were other than genetic, i.e., inflammatory myopathies and vasculitis being the most frequent. They identified dystrophies or congenital myopathies in 9% and metabolic myopathies in 10% of the patients. Elderly patients showed more non-specific type 2 fiber atrophy and fewer normal muscle biopsies compared to younger patients (Laguno et al., 2002). This was also shown in a similar study by Lacomis et al. (1993). These studies proved that muscle biopsies are useful also in the elderly. The findings can be subtle or non-specific as in our patient with DM2, although together with the myalgic syndrome, they were suggestive of DM2.

DM2 is a heterogeneous disease, and in the mild end of the spectrum, not always obvious to suspect. This is particularly true for patients without myotonia even on EMG and with normal CK levels, as was the case in the DM2 patient and in the LGMD1D patient examples. Electromyogram is usually myopathic in muscular dystrophies but can be normal and without myotonia in DM2 (Udd and Krahe, 2012). Many DM2 patients experience myalgia, typically induced by exercise, as initial manifestation. The myalgic syndrome in DM2 cannot be distinguished from fibromyalgia (Udd and Krahe, 2012). Proximal muscle weakness manifests later, usually after 50–60 years of age, even though, patients can remain asymptomatic until old age. Rhabdomyolysis is not a known manifestation of DM2, and without rhabdomyolysis, our patient could still be undiagnosed. She has probably a second unknown cause for rhabdomyolysis. Otherwise, the muscle disease was quite mild and even milder in her mother showing the milder end of symptom severity of DM2.

Muscle MRI (or CT) is useful and currently a widely used tool to assess the distribution of affected muscles and to aid in obtaining targeted muscle biopsy. Dystrophic changes, i.e., fatty degenerative changes in muscle, are more reliably detected on MRI compared to clinical evaluation. The pattern of affected muscles can direct the diagnostic genetic investigations, which is explicit in the case of LGMD1D (Sandell et al., 2013). When evaluating a patient with a possibility of a neuromuscular disorder, a concomitant neurogenic disease is more prevalent in the elderly, such as neuropathy or degeneration of the lumbar vertebrae causing radiculopathy. Neurogenic and myogenic changes can, to some extent, be distinguished by muscle imaging and sometimes unnecessary investigations or even a surgical operation can be avoided by correct diagnosis.

The specific cause of the symptoms is the key to assess the right therapeutic and rehabilitation measures, and to estimate prognosis. A possibility of a genetic myopathy is important to bear in mind also in the patients with very late-onset symptoms. If a genetic muscle disease is diagnosed, it can have an impact for the wider family and genetic counseling can be applied. Muscle MRI is useful in the distinction and a recommended tool to help differentiate myopathies from sarcopenia and to reach the correct diagnosis also in the elderly.

AUTHOR CONTRIBUTIONS

Dr. Johanna Palmio: substantial contribution to the design of the work, drafting the work, final approval of the version to be published, and agreement to be accountable for all aspects of the work in ensuring that questions related to the accuracy or integrity of any part of the work are appropriately investigated and resolved. Dr. Bjarne Udd: substantial contribution to the design of the work, revising the work critically for important intellectual content, final approval of the version to be published, and agreement to be accountable for all aspects of the work in ensuring that questions related to the accuracy or integrity of any part of the work are appropriately investigated and resolved.

REFERENCES

Correa-de-Araujo, R., and Hadley, E. (2014). Skeletal muscle function deficit: a new terminology to embrace the evolving concepts of sarcopenia and age-related muscle dysfunction. *J. Gerontol. A Biol. Sci. Med. Sci.* 69, 591–594. doi:10.1093/gerona/glt208

Cruz-Jentoft, A. J., Baeyens, J. P., Bauer, J. M., Boirie, Y., Cederholm, T., and Landi, F. (2010). Sarcopenia: European consensus on definition and diagnosis: report of the European working group on sarcopenia in older people. *Age Ageing* 39, 412–423. doi:10.1093/ageing/afq034

Doherty, T. J. (2003). Physiology of aging. Invited review: aging and sarcopenia. *J. Appl. Physiol (1985).* 95, 1717–1727.

Edström, E., Altun, M., Bergman, E., Johnson, H., Kullberg, S., Ramírez-León, V., et al. (2007). Factors contributing to neuromuscular impairment and sarcopenia during aging. *Physiol. Behav.* 92, 129–135. doi:10.1016/j.physbeh.2007.05.040

Iannuzzi-Sucich, M., Prestwood, K. M., and Kenny, A. M. (2002). Prevalence of sarcopenia and predictors of skeletal muscle mass in healthy, older men and women. *J. Gerontol. A Biol. Sci. Med. Sci.* 57, M772–M777. doi:10.1093/gerona/57.12.M772

Lacomis, D., Chad, D. A., and Smith, T. W. (1993). Myopathy in the elderly: evaluation of the histopathologic spectrum and the accuracy of clinical diagnosis. *Neurology* 43, 825–828. doi:10.1212/WNL.43.4.825

Laguno, M., Miró, O., Perea, M., Picón, M., Urbano-Márquez, A., and Grau, J. M. (2002). Muscle diseases in elders: a 10-year retrospective study. *J. Gerontol. A Biol. Sci. Med. Sci.* 57, M378–M384. doi:10.1093/gerona/57.6.M378

Lexell, J., Taylor, C. C., and Sjostrom, M. (1988). What is the cause of the ageing atrophy? Total number, size and proportion of different fiber types studied in whole vastus lateralis muscle from 15- to 83-year-old men. *J. Neurol. Sci.* 84, 275–294. doi:10.1016/0022-510X(88)90132-3

Liquori, C. L., Ricker, K., Moseley, M. L., Jacobsen, J. F., Kress, W., Naylor, S. L., et al. (2001). Myotonic dystrophy type 2 caused by a CCTG expansion in intron 1 of ZNF9. *Science* 293, 864–867. doi:10.1126/science.1062125

Machuca-Tzili, L., Brook, D., and Hilton-Jones, D. (2005). Clinical and molecular aspects of the myotonic dystrophies: a review. *Muscle Nerve* 32, 1–18. doi:10.1002/mus.20301

Morley, J. E., Baumgartner, R. N., Roubenoff, R., Mayer, J., and Nair, K. S. (2001). Sarcopenia. *J. Lab. Clin. Med.* 137, 231–243. doi:10.1067/mlc.2001.113504

Müller-Höcker, J. (1992). Mitochondria and ageing. *Brain Pathol.* 2, 149–158. doi:10.1111/j.1750-3639.1992.tb00683.x

Nigro, V., and Savarese, M. (2014). Genetic basis of limb-girdle muscular dystrophies: the 2014 update. *Acta Myol.* 33, 1–12.

Patel, H. P., Syddall, H. E., Jameson, K., Robinson, S., Denison, H., Roberts, H. C., et al. (2013). Prevalence of sarcopenia in community-dwelling older people in the UK using the European working group on sarcopenia in older people (EWGSOP) definition: findings from the hertfordshire cohort study (HCS). *Age Ageing* 42, 378–384. doi:10.1093/ageing/afs197

Penttilä, S., Palmio, J., Suominen, T., Raheem, O., Evilä, A., Muelas Gomez, N., et al. (2012). Eight new mutations and the expanding phenotype variability in muscular dystrophy caused by ANO5. *Neurology* 78, 897–903. doi:10.1212/WNL.0b013e31824c4682

Rolland, Y., Czerwinski, S., Abellan Van Kan, G., Morley, J. E., Cesari, M., Onder, G., et al. (2008). Sarcopenia: its assessment, etiology, pathogenesis, consequences and future perspectives. *J. Nutr. Health Aging* 12, 433–450. doi:10.1007/BF02982704

Ryall, J. G., Schertzer, J. D., and Lynch, G. S. (2008). Cellular and molecular mechanisms underlying age-related skeletal muscle wasting and weakness. *Biogerontology* 9, 213–228. doi:10.1007/s10522-008-9131-0

Sandell, S., Huovinen, S., Sarparanta, J., Luque, H., Haapasalo, H., Hackman, P., et al. (2010). The enigma of 7q36 linked autosomal dominant limb girdle muscular dystrophy. *J. Neurol. Neurosurg. Psychiatr.* 81, 834–839. doi:10.1136/jnnp.2009.192351

Sandell, S., Mahjneh, I., Palmio, J., Tasca, G., Ricci, E., and Udd, B. (2013). "Pathognomonic" muscle imaging findings in DNAJB6 mutated LGMD1D. *Eur. J. Neurol.* 20, 1553–1559. doi:10.1111/ene.12239

Sarparanta, J., Jonson, P. H., Golzio, C., Sandell, S., Luque, H., Screen, M., et al. (2012). Mutations affecting the cytoplasmic functions of the co-chaperone DNAJB6 cause limb-girdle muscular dystrophy. *Nat. Genet.* 44, S1–S2. doi:10.1038/ng.1103

Suominen, T., Bachinski, L. L., Auvinen, S., Hackman, P., Baggerly, K. A., Angelini, C., et al. (2011). Population frequency of myotonic dystrophy: higher than expected frequency of myotonic dystrophy type 2 (DM2) mutation in Finland. *Eur. J. Hum. Genet.* 19, 776–782. doi:10.1038/ejhg.2011.23

Udd, B., and Krahe, R. (2012). The myotonic dystrophies: molecular, clinical, and therapeutic challenges. *Lancet Neurol.* 11, 891–905. doi:10.1016/S1474-4422(12)70204-1

Wang, C., and Bai, L. (2012). Sarcopenia in the elderly: basic and clinical issues. *Geriatr. Gerontol. Int.* 12, 388–396. doi:10.1111/j.1447-0594.2012.00851.x

Wattjes, M. P., and Fischer, D. (2013). "Normal aging muscle tissue," in *Neuromuscular Imaging*, eds M. P. Wattjes and D. Fischer (New York, NY: Springer), 101–107.

9

Pre-hospital dietary intake correlates with muscle mass at the time of fracture in older hip-fractured patients

Riccardo Calvani†, Anna Maria Martone†, Emanuele Marzetti, Graziano Onder, Giulia Savera, Maria Lorenzi, Elisabetta Serafini, Roberto Bernabei and Francesco Landi*

Department of Geriatrics, Neurosciences and Orthopedics, Teaching Hospital "Agostino Gemelli," Catholic University of the Sacred Heart School of Medicine, Rome, Italy

***Correspondence:**
Francesco Landi, Department of Geriatrics, Neurosciences and Orthopedics, Catholic University of the Sacred Heart School of Medicine, L.go A. Gemelli 8, Rome 00168, Italy e-mail: francesco.landi@rm.unicatt.it

† Riccardo Calvani and Anna Maria Martone have contributed equally to this work.

Background: Failure to meet an adequate dietary intake is involved in the pathogenesis of sarcopenia and osteoporosis, which in turn increase the risk for falls and fractures, respectively. Older people with hip fracture are often protein-malnourished at hospitalization. Whether low protein-energy intake is associated with muscle atrophy in hip-fractured patients is presently unknown. This information is necessary for the development of novel strategies to manage this especially vulnerable patient population. The aim of this study was, therefore, to explore the relationship between dietary intake and muscle mass in older hip-fractured patients.

Methods: Analyses were conducted in hip-fractured elderly admitted to an orthopedic and trauma surgery ward (University Hospital). Muscle mass was estimated by bioelectrical impedance analysis within 24 h from admission. Dietary information was collected via 24-h dietary recall and nutrient intake calculated by a nutrition software.

Results: Among 62 hip-fractured patients (mean age 84.6 ± 7.6 years, 84% women), the average energy intake was 929.2 ± 170.3 Kcal day^{-1}, with higher values reported by men (1.046.8 ± 231.4 Kcal day^{-1}) relative to women (906.5 ± 148.3 Kcal day^{-1}; $p = 0.01$). Absolute and normalized protein intake was 50.0 ± 13.5 g day^{-1} and 0.88 ± 0.27 g kg (body $weight)^{-1}$ day^{-1}, respectively, with no gender differences. A positive correlation was determined between total energy intake and muscle mass ($r = 0.384$; $p = 0.003$). Similarly, protein and leucine consumption was positively correlated with muscle mass ($r = 0.367$ and 0.311, respectively; $p = 0.005$ for both).

Conclusion: A low intake of calories, protein, and leucine is associated with reduced muscle mass in hip-fractured elderly. Given the relevance of sarcopenia as a risk factor for adverse outcomes in this patient population, our findings highlight the importance of a comprehensive dietary assessment for the detection of nutritional deficits predisposing to or aggravating muscle atrophy.

Keywords: sarcopenia, diet, recommended dietary allowance, leucine, disability, malnutrition, bioelectrical impedance analysis, muscle atrophy

INTRODUCTION

Hip fracture is a devastating event for elderly people, with over 25% per-year mortality and incomplete recovery of pre-fractural conditions in more than 50% of survivors (Maggi et al., 2010). Approximately 1.6 million older adults worldwide sustain a hip fracture annually (Hung et al., 2012). What is worse, due to the ongoing demographic transition, the incidence of hip fractures is projected to increase up to 2.6 million by 2025 and reach 4.5 million in 2050 (Cauley et al., 2014). This epidemiological figure has a dramatic impact from both healthcare and societal perspectives, given the enormous direct (e.g., acute in-hospital treatment, rehabilitation programs, and use of health services) and indirect costs (e.g., burden to families related to the patient's acquired or worsened disability) associated with hip fracture and its consequences (Pike et al., 2010). These considerations call for the development of novel strategies to improve the survival and functional recovery of this vulnerable patient population.

Among the factors that may impact the clinical outcome of hip-fractured elderly, the age-related loss of muscle mass and function (sarcopenia) emerges as serious candidate for interventions. Indeed, declines in muscle mass and strength are associated with poor functional recovery following hip fracture repair (Visser et al., 2000; D'Adamo et al., 2014). Given the role of protein–energy malnutrition as a risk factor for the development of sarcopenia (Calvani et al., 2013; Landi et al., 2013a; Martone et al., 2013), a suboptimal nutritional status may mediate, at least partly, the association between sarcopenia and poor clinical outcomes in older hip-fractured patients.

Malnutrition is commonly found in older adults admitted to hospital with hip fracture (Murphy et al., 2000). Moreover, older hip-fractured patients who enter the hospital undernourished do not usually meet the recommended dietary allowance (RDA) for protein [0.8 g kg (body weight)$^{-1}$ day^{-1}] (Miller et al., 2006). This in the face that a high protein intake reduces the risk of perioperative complications (Milne et al., 2009; Botella-Carretero et al., 2010), improves bone mineral density (Schürch et al., 1998; Tengstrand et al., 2007), and shortens the rehabilitation time in this patient population (Avenell and Handoll, 2005). Nevertheless, a debate is ongoing as to whether the current RDA for protein is sufficient to prevent major adverse events in older adults, especially in frail, critically ill patients (Bauer et al., 2013).

Although one may expect a relationship exists that links low protein and energy ingestion, muscle atrophy, and poor clinical outcomes, no studies have yet assessed the association between dietary intake and muscle wasting in hip-fractured older patients. If such an association does exist, it would imply that a potentially amenable causative factor of sarcopenia and related consequences may be proposed as a therapeutic target in standard clinical practice. The present study was, therefore, undertaken to verify the association between dietary intake and muscle atrophy in a sample of hip-fractured elderly, with the aim of providing the foundation for future intervention studies.

MATERIALS AND METHODS

STUDY SAMPLE

The study was performed between November 2012 and August 2013 among older adults admitted for hip fracture due to accidental fall to the Emergency Department (ED) of the Teaching Hospital "Agostino Gemelli," Catholic University of the Sacred Heart (Rome, Italy). Exclusion criteria were age < 65 years, presence of peripheral edema, bone metastasis, cognitive impairment (Cognitive Performance Scale < 3), presence of pacemaker or implantable cardioverter defibrillator, and unwillingness to take part to the study. The study was approved by the Institutional Review Board of the Catholic University of the Sacred Heart, and all participants signed a written consent before enrollment.

DATA COLLECTION

Information pertaining to demographic, clinical, functional, and lifestyle characteristics were collected by attending physicians upon admission to the Orthopedic and Trauma Surgery ward using the interRAI Acute Care instrument (Gray et al., 2008). Due to practical difficulties in obtaining accurate weight and height measurements in our patient population, body mass index (BMI) was calculated based on self-reported weight and height. However, an excellent agreement has been shown in older adults between self-reported and measured anthropometric parameters (Ng et al., 2011).

ASSESSMENT OF MUSCLE MASS

Whole-body fat-free mass was measured by bioelectrical impedance analysis (BIA) using a Quantum/S Bioelectrical Body Composition Analyzer (Akern Srl, Florence, Italy) with an operating frequency of 50 kHz at 800 μA, as previously described (Marzetti et al., 2014). Measurements were taken within 24 h from ED admission adopting standard conditions (NIH Expert Panel, 1996), with the subject in a supine position and surface electrodes placed on wrist and ankle contralateral to the side of the fracture. Muscle mass was estimated using the equation developed by Janssen et al. (2000). The skeletal muscle index (SMI) was obtained dividing absolute muscle mass by squared height (kg m^{-2}).

DIETARY ASSESSMENT

Pre-hospital dietary information was collected within 24 h from admission to the Orthopedic and Trauma Surgery ward via a dietary interview on nutritional habits. The nutrient intake was estimated by 24-h dietary recall of the day before fracture (Buzzard, 1998). Collected data were elaborated using a nutrition software (MètaDieta, ME.TE.DA. LLC, San Benedetto del Tronto, Italy) to estimate the daily intake of macro- and micronutrients.

STATISTICAL ANALYSES

All data are expressed as proportions (%) or mean ± standard deviation (SD). Differences between continuous variables were assessed by ANOVA comparisons or the Kruskal–Wallis test, as appropriate. Distributions of categorical variables were compared by the Fisher exact test. The Pearson's correlation test was used to assess the strength of association between variables. All tests were two sided, with significance set at $p < 0.05$. All analyses were run using the SPSS software (version 18, SPSS Inc., Chicago, IL, USA).

RESULTS

The main characteristics of the study sample are shown in **Table 1**. The mean age of participants was 84.6 ± 7.6 years, with no differences between genders. Women were predominant (84%), which is coherent with epidemiological data showing a higher incidence of hip fracture in the female gender (Cauley et al., 2014). Men showed a trend toward higher muscle mass values relative to women (SMI: 10.00 ± 2.70 kg m^{-2} and 8.83 ± 1.73 kg m^{-2}, respectively), but the difference did not reach the statistical significance ($p = 0.08$) (**Table 1**).

The mean pre-hospital energy intake was 929.2 ± 170.3 kcal day^{-1}, with a significantly higher energy consumption reported by men (1046.8 ± 231.4 vs. 906.5 ± 148.3 kcal day^{-1}; $p = 0.01$; **Table 1**). Pre-hospital protein intake was 50.0 ± 13.5 g day^{-1}, corresponding to 0.88 ± 0.27 g kg (body weight)$^{-1}$ day^{-1}, with no differences between genders (**Table 1**). Remarkably, more than 75% of participants reported protein consumption below 1.0 g kg^{-1} day^{-1}, which represents the minimum intake currently recommended for older people (Bauer et al., 2013; Deutz et al., 2014). Finally, the average leucine consumption was 3.97 ± 1.13 g day^{-1}, with similar values in men and women (**Table 1**). A positive correlation was determined between SMI and total daily energy intake ($r = 0.384$; $p = 0.003$; **Figure 1**). Positive, significant correlations were also found between SMI and both absolute ($r = 0.367$, $p = 0.005$; **Figure 2A**) and normalized daily protein intake ($r = 0.311$, $p = 0.01$; **Figure 2B**), as well as daily leucine consumption ($r = 0.360$, $p = 0.005$; **Figure 3**).

DISCUSSION

Hip fracture is a dramatic event for older adults due to its detrimental consequences on the individual health status and quality of life. Considerable efforts have, therefore, been directed toward the development of interventions aimed at reducing the incidence

Table 1 | Characteristics of study participants according to gender.

	Total ($n = 62$), n (%)	Men ($n = 10$), n (%)	Women ($n = 52$), n (%)	p value
Age (years) (mean ± SD)	84.6 ± 7.6	86.1 ± 4.7	84.4 ± 8.1	0.5
Pre-fracture ADL score (mean ± SD)[a]	1.4 ± 2.4	1.2 ± 2.2	0.8 ± 1.5	0.7
CPS score at admission (mean ± SD)[b]	0.8 ± 1.5	0.9 ± 1.6	0.8 ± 1.5	0.8
Number of diseases (mean ± SD)	4.8 ± 3.3	6.1 ± 2.9	4.6 ± 3.4	0.1
Number of medications (mean ± SD)	2.7 ± 1.7	4.1 ± 1.7	2.4 ± 1.6	0.03
BMI (mean ± SD)	22.0 ± 3.3	22.1 ± 2.8	23.2 ± 3.3	0.3
SMI ($kg\ m^{-2}$) (mean ± SD)	9.02 ± 1.9	10.00 ± 2.70	8.83 ± 1.73	0.08
Pre-fracture daily energy intake (kcal) (mean ± SD)	929.2 ± 170.3	1046.8 ± 231.4	906.5 ± 148.3	0.01
Pre-fracture daily protein intake (absolute) (g) (mean ± SD)	50.0 ± 13.5	55.3 ± 16.6	50.8 ± 14.0	0.2
Pre-fracture daily protein intake (normalized) ($g\ kg^{-1}$) (mean ± SD)	0.88 ± 0.27	0.86 ± 0.31	0.88 ± 0.26	0.9
Pre-fracture daily leucine intake (g) (mean ± SD)	3.97 ± 1.13	4.40 ± 1.39	3.89 ± 1.07	0.1

ADL: activities of daily living; BMI: body mass index; CPS: Cognitive Performance Scale; SMI: skeletal muscle index.

[a]ADL: 0 (no impairment), 7 (severe impairment).

[b]CPS: 0 (no impairment), 6 (severe impairment).

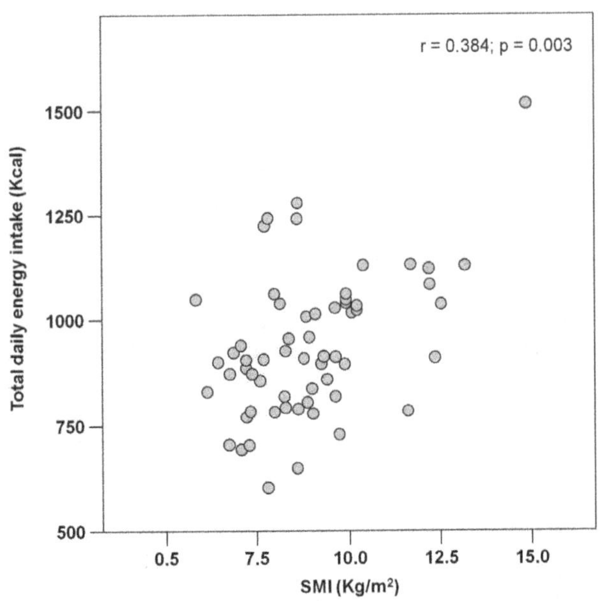

FIGURE 1 | Scatter plot of total daily energy intake and skeletal muscle index (SMI; $n = 62$).

of new fractures and improving health outcomes when the fracture has occurred (Hung et al., 2012; Pioli et al., 2014). Over the years, a shift of paradigm has emerged such that hip fracture is no longer considered as a condition limited to the bone. Rather, it represents a complex "geriatric syndrome" that affects the whole organism (Pioli et al., 2014). As such, it is becoming increasingly clear that the management of this condition requires a comprehensive, multidisciplinary approach that goes beyond fracture repair and osteoporosis treatment (Hung et al., 2012; Pioli et al., 2014). Our results should be considered against this complex clinical and pathophysiological backdrop.

Previous investigations have shown that older people with hip fracture are often energy and protein malnourished at the time of fracture (Lumbers et al., 2001) and that a high prevalence of sarcopenia is observed in this patient population (Di Monaco et al., 2011, 2012). The finding from the present study that these two phenomena are correlated with each other extends our knowledge on these frail patients and adds interesting cues on hip fracture management. Indeed, muscle wasting is a powerful risk factor for adverse outcomes among older adults hospitalized with acute conditions. For instance, recent data from members of our group have shown that among 770 older patients admitted to acute care units, participants with sarcopenia experienced a threefold higher in-hospital mortality as compared with non-sarcopenic patients (Vetrano et al., 2014). This association remained significant after adjustment for a number of potential confounders, including among others cancer, cardiovascular disease, chronic obstructive pulmonary disease, dementia, chronic kidney disease, and pre-hospital disability. Furthermore, reduced muscle mass and strength were found to predict poor mobility recovery following hip fracture repair (Visser et al., 2000; Di Monaco et al., 2007).

On the other hand, it is well established that an adequate intake of dietary protein is required for the preservation of lean body mass in late life (Calvani et al., 2013). For instance, in the Health, Aging, and Body Composition Study, older adults in the highest quintile of protein consumption lost nearly 40% less appendicular lean mass than did those in the lowest quintile over 3 years of follow-up, after adjustment for potential confounders (Houston et al., 2008). Notably, protein supplementation is *per se* sufficient at increasing muscle mass in older hospitalized patients (Bos et al., 2001). This effect may explain, at least partly, the improvement in clinical outcomes observed in hip-fractured elderly undergoing perioperative protein supplementation (Bauer et al., 2013).

A central aspect to consider is that a higher dietary protein ingestion is necessary for the promotion of muscle health in older persons relative to young adults (Bauer et al., 2013). In light of this evidence, the average protein intake recorded in our study sample

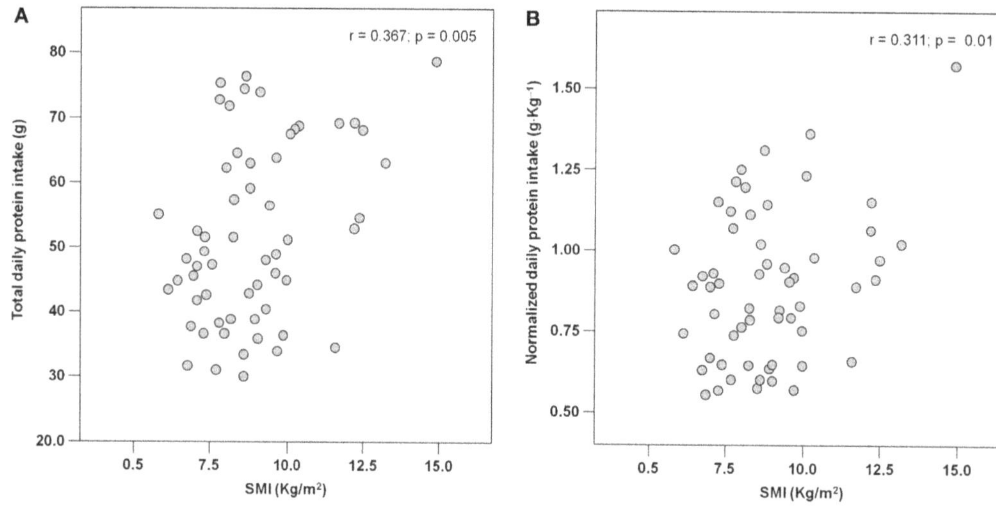

FIGURE 2 | Scatter plot of total (A) and normalized (B) protein intake and skeletal muscle index (SMI; $n = 62$).

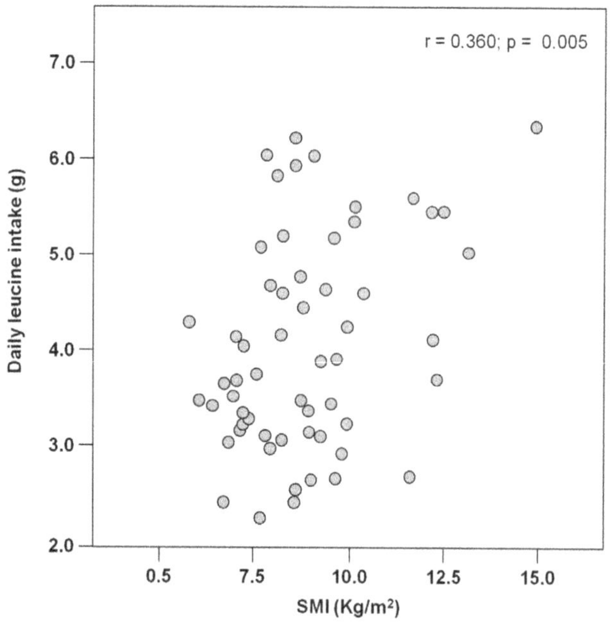

FIGURE 3 | Scatter plot of daily leucine intake and skeletal muscle index (SMI; $n = 62$).

(0.88 g kg^{-1} day^{-1}), albeit slightly above the RDA for protein, may not still be sufficient to sustain optimal muscle protein synthesis. Notably, over 75% of participants did not reach the protein intake currently recommended for older adults (1.0 g kg^{-1} day^{-1}), and only 8% reported a protein consumption between 1.2 and 1.5 g kg^{-1} day^{-1}, which is the amount recommended by the Society for Sarcopenia, Cachexia, and Wasting Disease to maximize muscle health in advanced age (Morley et al., 2010).

Besides quantity, the quality of ingested protein plays an important role in the context of muscle health (Calvani et al., 2013; Landi et al., 2013b). In particular, given the role of leucine as the master dietary regulator of muscle protein turnover, supplementation with protein sources enriched with this essential amino acid is thought to offer the greatest advantage in terms of preservation of muscle mass and function (Paddon-Jones and Rasmussen, 2009; Landi et al., 2013b). This evidence is in line with our finding in that both total protein ingestion and leucine consumption are positively correlated with muscle mass in hip-fractured elderly patients (**Figures 2** and **3**).

Albeit dealing with a highly relevant issue, our study presents several limitations that need to be discussed. First of all, the study is exploratory in nature, evident by the relatively small sample size. In addition, the cross-sectional design does not allow determining the impact of low protein-energy intake and reduced muscle mass on out-of-hospital survival and functional recovery. Along the same line, the specific impact of individual nutrients on muscle mass could not be established. Although BIA is an established technique for the estimation of lean body mass (Kyle et al., 2003), it does not represent the gold standard for the quantification of muscle mass (Cesari et al., 2012). However, BIA measurements were taken directly at the patient bed, which allowed minimizing discomfort in the pre-operative phase. The lack of a control group of non-hip-fractured older subjects does not allow establishing whether their nutritional habits differ substantially from those of hip-fractured elderly. For the same reason, no information can be provided on eventual differences in the relationship between dietary intake and muscle mass among fractured and non-fractured older adults. Finally, dietary assessment in older adults poses special challenges due to possible memory and cognitive impairment, hearing problems, or biases in diet reporting (Thompson and Subar, 2012). Indeed, because of the high prevalence of chronic illnesses in this age group, it is likely that prescription diets (e.g., low sodium, low fat, and high fiber) are recommended. However, individuals may report what they should eat rather than what they actually eat. Alternatively, subjects on special diets may be more accurate in reporting their actual food consumption. The dietary assessment tool chosen for the present investigation allowed collecting reliable information about food consumption, while avoiding drops in concentration due to excessively long interviews (Adamson et al., 2009). In addition, the exclusion of cognitively impaired patients increased the accuracy and reliability of dietary testing.

CONCLUSION

The worldwide epidemic of hip fractures and the dramatic impact on the individual's health and functionality urge the development of effective strategies for the management of this condition. The recognition of sarcopenia as a major risk factor for adverse outcomes in this patient population indicates that the skeletal muscle may represent a critical target for interventions. The association between low intake of calories, protein and leucine, and reduced muscle mass in hip-fractured older patients revealed by the present study highlights the importance of a comprehensive dietary assessment for the early detection of nutritional deficits, which may aggravate muscle wasting. The evidence provided by this investigation could eventually serve as the foundation for the design of studies testing whether the implementation of nutritional interventions targeting the skeletal muscle (e.g., protein and leucine supplementation) improves the clinical outcomes of older hip-fractured patients.

ACKNOWLEDGMENTS

This study was partly supported by the "Centro studi Achille e Linda Lorenzon" and by grants of the Italian Ministry for Education, Universities and Research (MIUR – linea D1 2012 and MIUR – linea D3 2014), and the Innovative Medicines Initiative Joint Undertaking (IMI – JU 115621). The authors wish to thank Dr. Ornella Bianchi (Catholic University of Rome) for her invaluable help with data collection.

REFERENCES

Adamson, A. J., Collerton, J., Davies, K., Foster, E., Jagger, C., Stamp, E., et al. (2009). Nutrition in advanced age: dietary assessment in the Newcastle 85+ study. *Eur. J. Clin. Nutr.* 63(Suppl. 1), S6–S18. doi:10.1038/ejcn.2008.60

Avenell, A., and Handoll, H. H. (2005). Nutritional supplementation for hip fracture aftercare in older people. *Cochrane Database Syst. Rev* 2, CD001880. doi:10.1002/14651858.CD001880.pub3

Bauer, J., Biolo, G., Cederholm, T., Cesari, M., Cruz-Jentoft, A. J., Morley, J. E., et al. (2013). Evidence-based recommendations for optimal dietary protein intake in older people: a position paper from the PROT-AGE study group. *J. Am. Med. Dir. Assoc.* 14, 542–559. doi:10.1016/j.jamda.2013.05.021

Bos, C., Benamouzig, R., Bruhat, A., Roux, C., Valensi, P., Ferrière, F., et al. (2001). Nutritional status after short-term dietary supplementation in hospitalized malnourished geriatric patients. *Clin. Nutr.* 20, 225–233. doi:10.1054/clnu.2000.0387

Botella-Carretero, J. I., Iglesias, B., Balsa, J. A., Arrieta, F., Zamarrón, I., and Vázquez, C. (2010). Perioperative oral nutritional supplements in normally or mildly undernourished geriatric patients submitted to surgery for hip fracture: a randomized clinical trial. *Clin. Nutr.* 29, 574–579. doi:10.1016/j.clnu.2010.01.012

Buzzard, M. (1998). "24-Hour dietary recall and food record methods," in *Nutritional Epidemiology*, ed. W. Willet (Oxford: Oxford University Press), 50–73.

Calvani, R., Miccheli, A., Landi, F., Bossola, M., Cesari, M., Leeuwenburgh, C., et al. (2013). Current nutritional recommendations and novel dietary strategies to manage sarcopenia. *J. Frailty Aging* 2, 38–53.

Cauley, J. A., Chalhoub, D., Kassem, A. M., and Fuleihan, G. E. H. (2014). Geographic and ethnic disparities in osteoporotic fractures. *Nat. Rev. Endocrinol.* 10, 338–351. doi:10.1038/nrendo.2014.51

Cesari, M., Fielding, R. A., Pahor, M., Goodpaster, B., Hellerstein, M., Abellan van Kan, A., et al. (2012). Biomarkers of sarcopenia in clinical trials-recommendations from the international working group on sarcopenia. *J. Cachexia Sarcopenia Muscle* 3, 181–190. doi:10.1007/s13539-012-0078-2

D'Adamo, C. R., Hawkes, W. G., Miller, R. R., Jones, M., Hochberg, M., Yu-Yahiro, J., et al. (2014). Short-term changes in body composition after surgical repair of hip fracture. *Age Ageing* 43, 275–280. doi:10.1093/ageing/aft198

Deutz, N. E., Bauer, J. M., Barazzoni, R., Biolo, G., Boirie, Y., Bosy-Westphal, A., et al. (2014). Protein intake and exercise for optimal muscle function with aging: recommendations from the ESPEN expert group. *Clin. Nutr.* doi:10.1016/j.clnu.2014.04.007

Di Monaco, M., Castiglioni, C., Vallero, F., Di Monaco, R., and Tappero, R. (2012). Sarcopenia is more prevalent in men than in women after hip fracture: a cross-sectional study of 591 inpatients. *Arch. Gerontol. Geriatr.* 55, e48–e52. doi:10.1016/j.archger.2012.05.002

Di Monaco, M., Vallero, F., Di Monaco, R., and Tappero, R. (2011). Prevalence of sarcopenia and its association with osteoporosis in 313 older women following a hip fracture. *Arch. Gerontol. Geriatr.* 52, 71–74. doi:10.1016/j.archger.2010.02.002

Di Monaco, M., Vallero, F., Di Monaco, R., Tappero, R., and Cavanna, A. (2007). Muscle mass and functional recovery in men with hip fracture. *Am. J. Phys. Med. Rehabil.* 86, 818–825. doi:10.1097/PHM.0b013e318151fec7

Gray, L. C., Bernabei, R., Berg, K., Finne-Soveri, H., Fries, B. E., Hirdes, J. P., et al. (2008). Standardizing assessment of elderly people in acute care: the interRAI acute care instrument. *J. Am. Geriatr. Soc.* 56, 536–541. doi:10.1111/j.1532-5415.2007.01590.x

Houston, D. K., Nicklas, B. J., Ding, J., Harris, T. B., Tylavsky, F. A., Newman, A. B., et al. (2008). Dietary protein intake is associated with lean mass change in older, community-dwelling adults: the Health, Aging, and Body Composition (Health ABC) Study. *Am. J. Clin. Nutr.* 87, 150–155.

Hung, W. W., Egol, K. A., Zuckerman, J. D., and Siu, A. L. (2012). Hip fracture management: tailoring care for the older patient. *JAMA* 307, 2185–2194. doi:10.1001/jama.2012.4842

Janssen, I., Heymsfield, S. B., Baumgartner, R. N., and Ross, R. (2000). Estimation of skeletal muscle mass by bioelectrical impedance analysis. *J. Appl. Physiol. (1985)* 89, 465–471.

Kyle, U. G., Genton, L., Hans, D., and Pichard, C. (2003). Validation of a bioelectrical impedance analysis equation to predict appendicular skeletal muscle mass (ASMM). *Clin. Nutr.* 22, 537–543. doi:10.1016/S0261-5614(03)00048-7

Landi, F., Liperoti, R., Russo, A., Giovannini, S., Tosato, M., Barillaro, C., et al. (2013a). Association of anorexia with sarcopenia in a community-dwelling elderly population: results from the ilSIRENTE study. *Eur. J. Nutr.* 52, 1261–1268. doi:10.1007/s00394-012-0437-y

Landi, F., Marzetti, E., and Bernabei, R. (2013b). Perspective: protein: what kind, how much, when? *J. Am. Med. Dir. Assoc.* 14, 66–67. doi:10.1016/j.jamda.2012.09.020

Lumbers, M., New, S. A., Gibson, S., and Murphy, M. C. (2001). Nutritional status in elderly female hip fracture patients: comparison with an age-matched home living group attending day centres. *Br. J. Nutr.* 85, 733–740.

Maggi, S., Siviero, P., Wetle, T., Besdine, R. W., Saugo, M., Crepaldi, G., et al. (2010). A multicenter survey on profile of care for hip fracture: predictors of mortality and disability. *Osteoporos. Int.* 21, 223–231. doi:10.1007/s00198-009-0936-8

Martone, A. M., Onder, G., Vetrano, D. L., Ortolani, E., Tosato, M., Marzetti, E., et al. (2013). Anorexia of aging: a modifiable risk factor for frailty. *Nutrients* 5, 4126–4133. doi:10.3390/nu5104126

Marzetti, E., Lorenzi, M., Antocicco, M., Bonassi, S., Celi, M., Mastropaolo, S., et al. (2014). Shorter telomeres in peripheral blood mononuclear cells from older persons with sarcopenia: results from an exploratory study. *Front. Aging Neurosci.* 6:233. doi:10.3389/fnagi.2014.00233

Miller, M. D., Bannerman, E., Daniels, L. A., and Crotty, M. (2006). Lower limb fracture, cognitive impairment and risk of subsequent malnutrition: a prospective evaluation of dietary energy and protein intake on an orthopaedic ward. *Eur. J. Clin. Nutr.* 60, 853–861. doi:10.1038/sj.ejcn.1602390

Milne, A. C., Potter, J., Vivanti, A., and Avenell, A. (2009). Protein and energy supplementation in elderly people at risk from malnutrition. *Cochrane Database Syst. Rev.* 2, CD003288. doi:10.1002/14651858.CD003288.pub3

Morley, J. E., Argiles, J. M., Evans, W. J., Bhasin, S., Cella, D., Deutz, N. E., et al. (2010). Nutritional recommendations for the management of sarcopenia. *J. Am. Med. Dir. Assoc.* 11, 391–396. doi:10.1016/j.jamda.2010.04.014

Murphy, M. C., Brooks, C. N., New, S. A., and Lumbers, M. L. (2000). The use of the mini-nutritional assessment (MNA) tool in elderly orthopaedic patients. *Eur. J. Clin. Nutr.* 54, 555–562. doi:10.1038/sj.ejcn.1601055

Ng, S. P., Korda, R., Clements, M., Latz, I., Bauman, A., Bambrick, H., et al. (2011). Validity of self-reported height and weight and derived body mass index in middle-aged and elderly individuals in Australia. *Aust. N. Z. J. Public Health* 35, 557–563. doi:10.1111/j.1753-6405.2011.00742.x

NIH Expert Panel. (1996). Bioelectrical impedance analysis in body composition measurement: National Institutes of Health Technology Assessment Conference Statement. *Am. J. Clin. Nutr.* 64, 524S–532S.

Paddon-Jones, D., and Rasmussen, B. B. (2009). Dietary protein recommendations and the prevention of sarcopenia. *Curr. Opin. Clin. Nutr. Metab. Care* 12, 86–90. doi:10.1097/MCO.0b013e32831cef8b

Pike, C., Birnbaum, H. G., Schiller, M., Sharma, H., Burge, R., and Edgell, E. T. (2010). Direct and indirect costs of non-vertebral fracture patients with osteoporosis in the US. *Pharmacoeconomics* 28, 395–409. doi:10.2165/11531040-000000000-00000

Pioli, G., Barone, A., Mussi, C., Tafaro, L., Bellelli, G., Falaschi, P., et al. (2014). The management of hip fracture in the older population. Joint position statement by Gruppo Italiano Ortogeriatria (GIOG). *Aging Clin. Exp. Res.* 26, 547–553. doi:10.1007/s40520-014-0198-y

Schürch, M. A., Rizzoli, R., Slosman, D., Vadas, L., Vergnaud, P., and Bonjour, J. P. (1998). Protein supplements increase serum insulin-like growth factor-I levels and attenuate proximal femur bone loss in patients with recent hip fracture. A randomized, double-blind, placebo-controlled trial. *Ann. Intern. Med.* 128, 801–809. doi:10.7326/0003-4819-128-10-199805150-00002

Tengstrand, B., Cederholm, T., Söderqvist, A., and Tidermark, J. (2007). Effects of protein-rich supplementation and nandrolone on bone tissue after a hip fracture. *Clin. Nutr.* 26, 460–465. doi:10.1016/j.clnu.2007.03.007

Thompson, F. E., and Subar, A. F. (2012). " Dietary assessment methodology," in *Nutrition in the Prevention and Treatment of Disease*, 3d Edn, eds A. M. Coulston, C. J. Boushey, and M. Ferruzzi (London: Academic Press), 5–46. doi:10.1016/B978-0-12-391884-0.00001-9

Vetrano, D. L., Landi, F., Volpato, S., Corsonello, A., Meloni, E., Bernabei, R., et al. (2014). Association of sarcopenia with short- and long-term mortality in older adults admitted to acute care wards: results from the CRIME study. *J. Gerontol. A Biol. Sci. Med. Sci.* 69, 1154–1161. doi:10.1093/gerona/glu034

Visser, M., Harris, T. B., Fox, K. M., Hawkes, W., Hebel, J. R., Yahiro, J. Y., et al. (2000). Change in muscle mass and muscle strength after a hip fracture: relationship to mobility recovery. *J. Gerontol. A Biol. Sci. Med. Sci.* 55, M434–M440. doi:10.1093/gerona/55.8.M434

10

Aggresome–autophagy involvement in a sarcopenic patient with rigid spine syndrome and a p.C150R mutation in *FHL1* gene

Patrizia Sabatelli[1,2], Silvia Castagnaro[3], Francesca Tagliavini[1,2], Martina Chrisam[3], Francesca Sardone[1,2], Laurence Demay[4], Pascale Richard[5], Spartaco Santi[1,2], Nadir M. Maraldi[1], Luciano Merlini[2], Marco Sandri[6,7] and Paolo Bonaldo[3]*

[1] Institute of Molecular Genetics, CNR-National Research Council of Italy, Bologna, Italy
[2] SC Laboratory of Musculoskeletal Cell Biology, Rizzoli Orthopedic Institute, Bologna, Italy
[3] Department of Molecular Medicine, University of Padova, Padova, Italy
[4] UF Cardiogénétique et Myogénétique, Service de Biochimie Métabolique, Groupe Hospitalier Pitié-Salpêtrière, Paris, France
[5] UF Cardiogénétique et Myogénétique, Centre de Génétique, Hôpitaux Universitaires de la Pitié Salpêtrière, Paris, France
[6] Dulbecco Telethon Institute, Venetian Institute of Molecular Medicine, Padova, Italy
[7] Department of Biomedical Science, University of Padova, Padova, Italy

***Correspondence:**
Paolo Bonaldo, Department of Molecular Medicine, University of Padova, Via U. Bassi 58/B, Padova I-35131, Italy
e-mail: bonaldo@bio.unipd.it

The four-and-half LIM domain protein 1 (FHL1) is highly expressed in skeletal and cardiac muscle. Mutations of the *FHL1* gene have been associated with diverse chronic myopathies including reducing body myopathy, rigid spine syndrome (RSS), and Emery–Dreifuss muscular dystrophy. We investigated a family with a mutation (p.C150R) in the second LIM domain of *FHL1*. In this family, a brother and a sister were affected by RSS, and their mother had mild lower limbs weakness. The 34-year-old female had an early and progressive rigidity of the cervical spine and severe respiratory insufficiency. Muscle mass evaluated by DXA was markedly reduced, while fat mass was increased to 40%. CT scan showed an almost complete substitution of muscle by fibro-adipose tissue. Muscle biopsy showed accumulation of FHL1 throughout the cytoplasm and around myonuclei into multiprotein aggregates with aggresome/autophagy features as indicated by ubiquitin, p62, and LC3 labeling. DNA deposits, not associated with nuclear lamina components and histones, were also detected in the aggregates, suggesting nuclear degradation. Ultrastructural analysis showed the presence of dysmorphic nuclei, accumulation of tubulofilamentous and granular material, and perinuclear accumulation of autophagic vacuoles. These data point to involvement of the aggresome–autophagy pathway in the pathophysiological mechanism underlying the muscle pathology of *FHL1* C150R mutation.

Keywords: myopathy, sarcopenia, FHL1, autophagy, protein aggregates

INTRODUCTION

Four-and-half LIM domain protein 1 (FHL1) is a cysteine-rich double zinc-finger protein encoded by the *FHL1* gene, localized on chromosome X (Dawid et al., 1995; Kadrmas and Beckerle, 2004). To date, three distinct FHL1 splicing isoforms have been identified (Brown et al., 1999; Morgan and Madgwick, 1999; Ng et al., 2001; Purcell et al., 2004; Johannessen et al., 2006; McGrath et al., 2006). FHL1A, also known as skeletal muscle LIM protein 1, is the full-length protein. FHL1B, or SLIMMER, is composed of the first three LIM domains and contains nuclear localization and export sequences and a RBP-J binding region. FHL1C, or KyoT2, is the shortest isoform, which contains only the first two LIM domains and a RBP-J binding region and interacts with PIAS1 (Taniguchi et al., 1998; Wang et al., 2007).

Four-and-half LIM domain protein 1 is highly expressed in skeletal and cardiac muscles (Lee et al., 1998; Brown et al., 1999; Greene et al., 1999; Morgan and Madgwick, 1999), where it localizes in the myofibrillar sarcomeres and in the sarcolemma (Bertrand et al., 2014). This protein has been demonstrated to be involved in several processes, including cellular architecture (McGrath et al., 2003, 2006), myoblast differentiation (Lee et al., 2012), mechanotransduction (Sheikh et al., 2008), and myofiber size (Cowling et al., 2008). FHL1 binds signaling and cytoskeletal proteins as well as transcription factors, acting as a transcriptional regulator of nuclear factor of activated T cells (NFATc1) to enhance the expression of genes that increase myofiber size (Cowling et al., 2008).

Mutations in the *FHL1* gene are responsible for a number of muscular disorders, which exhibit a broad spectrum of clinical features and disease severity ranging from severe childhood onset to milder adult-onset disorders. The diseases described so far include X-linked myopathy with postural muscle atrophy (XMPMA) (Windpassinger et al., 2008), reducing body myopathy (RBM) (Schessl et al., 2009; Shalaby et al., 2009; Selcen et al., 2011; Schreckenbach et al., 2013), X-linked dominant scapuloperoneal myopathy (Quinzii et al., 2008; Chen et al., 2010), rigid spine syndrome (RSS) (Shalaby et al., 2008), hypertrophic cardiomyopathy (Friedrich et al., 2012), and Emery–Dreifuss muscular dystrophy

(Gueneau et al., 2009; Knoblauch et al., 2010). RBM is characterized by the presence of intracellular protein aggregates called "reducing bodies (RBs)" mainly containing mutated FHL1 protein, cytoskeletal and intermediate filament proteins, and components of the unfolded protein response pathway (Liewluck et al., 2007). Although scapuloperoneal myopathy, XMPMA, RSS, hypertrophic cardiomyopathy, and Emery–Dreifuss muscular dystrophy share some overlapping clinical features and muscle pathology with RBM, the involvement of protein aggregation in these disorders remains unclear (Wilding et al., 2014).

Reducing bodies morphologically resemble aggresomes, structures proposed to facilitate the sequestration, and degradation of toxic misfolded proteins. Non-functional, damaged, and/or misfolded proteins are removed from the cell by the ubiquitin proteasome system. However, when the capacity of the proteasome is impaired or overwhelmed, polyubiquitinated misfolded proteins cannot be properly cleared and accumulate into the aggresome (Goldberg, 2003; Kawaguchi et al., 2003). Accumulating evidence suggests that aggresomes are substrates for autophagy. Autophagy is a degradation pathway that mediates bulk clearance of cytosolic proteins and organelles by the lysosome in a highly regulated process involving the coordinated actions of a large number of autophagy-related (Atg) genes. In response to particular stimuli, such as proteasomal dysfunction, an isolation membrane forms and expands to sequester portions of cytoplasm into double membrane structures called autophagosomes. The autophagosomes eventually fuse with lysosomes and their contents are degraded by lysosomal hydrolases. One hypothesis is that aggresomes may concentrate aggregated proteins for more efficient autophagic degradation (Bjorkoy et al., 2005, 2006; Iwata et al., 2005). Recent evidence indicates that aggresome formation is mediated by dynein/dynactin-mediated transport of misfolded proteins to the centrosome and involves several regulators, including the E3 ubiquitin-protein ligase parkin (Olzmann et al., 2008). Aggresome clearance is mediated by ubiquitin-binding proteins such as p62/SQSTM1 (Kirkin et al., 2009), an adaptor protein that decides the fate of protein degradation either through the ubiquitin proteasome system or the autophagy–lysosome pathway (Komatsu et al., 2007; Kirkin et al., 2009; Komatsu and Ichimura, 2010). Here, we report evidence of aggresome and autophagy involvement in the muscle of a sarcopenic patient with RSS and p.C150R mutation in the *FHL1* gene.

MATERIALS AND METHODS

GENOTYPING

The six coding exons and introns boundaries of FHL1 (NM_001159702) were screened for mutations by PCR on DNA from peripheral lymphocytes using primer pairs with a universal sequence (Table on demand). Exon 5 was sequenced with primers:

5PUF: 5′–ACCGTTAGTATGCGAGTTGGATTCAGGCAC
TGGATCCTA – 3′

5PUR: 5′–TCGGATAGTCAGTCGTTTGCTGTCGTGAGG
ATGGAATG – 3′.

Analysis of sequences was done with SeqScape software (Applied Biosystem).

MUSCLE BIOPSY

Peroneal muscle biopsy of the 34-year-old female was performed after written informed consent, and approval was obtained from the Ethics Committee of the Rizzoli Orthopedic Institute. The muscle sample was frozen in melting isopentane and stored in liquid nitrogen.

HISTOCHEMISTRY AND IMMUNOHISTOCHEMICAL ANALYSIS

Standard histochemical study was performed, and congophilic deposits were identified by Congo red staining (Bioptica) following the manufacturer's instructions. Cytochrome oxidase activity was assessed by conventional method. Acridine-orange staining was performed as previously reported (Darzynkiewicz, 1994). For double staining with menadione–nitro blue tetrazolium and anti-FHL1 antibodies, 10 μm-thick frozen sections were incubated with menadione-NBT solution in Gomori-Tris-HCl buffer at pH 7.4, without the addition of α-glycerophosphate substrate (Brooke and Neville, 1972), followed by incubation with anti-FHL1 antibody (Aviva System) and TRITC conjugated anti-rabbit secondary antibody (DAKO). Seven micrometer-thick non-fixed frozen sections were incubated with antibodies against laminin α2 chain, collagen VI, parkin (Millipore), desmin, developmental myosin heavy chain (d-MHC), fast myosin heavy chain, dystrophin (DYS1, DYS2, and DYS3 antibodies), emerin, lamin A/C (Novocastra), LC3 (Novus Biologicals), p62 (Progen Biotechnik), pericentrin, α-B-crystallin (Abcam), ubiquitin (Santa Cruz Biotechnologies), and histones (Chemicon), and revealed with FITC or TRITC conjugated anti-rabbit, anti-mouse, or anti-guinea pig secondary antibodies. Samples were stained with DAPI, mounted with anti-fading reagent (Molecular Probes), and observed with a Nikon epifluorescent/light microscope.

CONFOCAL IMAGING

The confocal imaging was performed with a A1-R confocal laser scanning microscope (Nikon), equipped with a Nikon 60×, 1.4 NA objective, and with a 488 and 561 nm laser lines to excite FITC (green) and TRITC (red) fluorescence signals. The 3D images were processed by stacking up 20–25 consecutive confocal images with surface shaded reconstruction. No deconvolution was applied to the images.

TRANSMISSION ELECTRON MICROSCOPY

Muscle biopsy was fixed with 2.5% glutaraldehyde in 0.1 M cacodylate buffer pH 7.4 for 3 h at 4°C, post-fixed with 1% osmium tetroxide in cacodylate buffer for 2 h, dehydrated in an ethanol series, infiltrated with propylene oxide and embedded in Epon 812 resin. Ultrathin sections were stained with uranyl acetate and lead citrate (Reynolds) and examined under a Philips EM400 operating at 100 kV.

WESTERN BLOTTING

Twenty micrometer-thick frozen sections were cut from the muscle biopsy of a healthy individual and of the proband patient. Sections were taken from two different portions of the patient muscle biopsy (referred as P_a and P_b). Muscle sections were lysed in 150 μl lysis buffer (50 mM Tris, pH 7.5, 150 mM NaCl, 10 mM $MgCl_2$, 1 mM EDTA, 10% glycerol, 0.5 mM DTT, 2%

sodium dodecyl sulfate, 1% Triton X-100) supplemented with phosphatase inhibitors (Sigma-Aldrich) and protease inhibitors (Roche), heated at 70°C for 10 min and centrifuged at 16,100 g for 10 min at 4°C. The protein content of each lysate was determined by the BCA Protein Assay kit (Pierce) and 30 μg of total proteins were separated by SDS-PAGE (Invitrogen) and immunoblotted as previously described (Chen et al., 2014). Membranes were probed with primary antibodies against FHL1 (ab23937 Abcam), LC3 (Thermo Scientific), p62 (Progen Biotechnik), ubiquitin (Cell Signaling Technologies), beclin 1 (Cell Signaling), BNIP3 (Sigma), vinculin (Sigma), or GAPDH (Millipore). Proteins were revealed with anti-rabbit, -mouse (Bethyl), -goat (Santa Cruz Biotechnologies), or -guinea pig (Sigma) HRP-conjugated secondary antibodies using the ECL reagent (Pierce-Thermo Scientific). Densitometric quantification of protein bands was performed by the ImageJ software (US National Institute of Health). Western blotting and quantifications are representative of at least three independent experiments.

RESULTS

The proband is a 34-year-old woman who noticed the inability to extend the right thumb at age 20. Soon after, she manifested neck weakness and limitation of flexion. Progression of weakness was rapid and she started to have difficulty in climbing stairs and getting up from the floor. At age 24, she started falling several times while walking. At age 26, the patient lost ambulation and was wheelchair bound. Examination at age 34 showed an atrophic phenotype with marked diffuse muscle wasting and weakness and prominent contractures. She had normal facial muscle strength, a minimal residual motor function in the elbow extensors and in the right biceps, but was profoundly weak in all the other muscles. She revealed marked contractures involving proximal and distal joints. The most striking contractures were in the neck muscles causing a fixed hyperextended neck that was also impossible to move in any direction. She showed a progressive decline in the respiratory function with a forced vital capacity 59% of predicted at age 25, 45% at age 27, and 13% at age 34. She refused to undergo mechanical ventilation. Cardiac investigation, including echocardiography and Holter, revealed no cardiac involvement. Muscle CT showed that all muscles were atrophic and substituted by fat and connective tissue, including the axial muscles, with a minimal sparing of the rectus femoris and vastus lateralis on the left, and of the peroneus on the right (**Figure 1A**). She was underweight (BMI = 17.1). However, according to her body composition, as revealed by DXA, she was sarcopenic/obese (appendicular lean body mass index of 3.27 kg/m^2 and total body fat of 44.4%) (Baumgartner et al., 2004). Her brother had a similar atrophic phenotype with marked rigidity of the spine and diffuse contractures but with more rapid progression, as he lost ambulation at age 18 and underwent tracheostomy at age 28. Their mother at age 58 had a mild lower limbs weakness and no contractures.

Sequencing of the *FHL1* gene in the index case identified a single missense mutation c.448T > C in exon 5 resulting in the replacement at codon 150 of a cysteine residue with an arginine residue (p.Cys150Arg). Nucleotide c.448 and residue p.150 of the *FHL1* gene are highly conserved among species and evolution, and all prediction softwares conclude for a pathogenic mutation. Analysis of the family showed that her brother and mother also have the same *FHL1* mutation.

Muscle biopsy showed fiber size variability, numerous internal nuclei, and increased endomysial and perimysial tissue. Several muscle fibers showed menadione-NBT positive aggregates, consistent with the presence of RBs (**Figure 1B**). RBs were devoid of oxidative enzyme activity and displayed an intense congophilia, indicative of the presence of amyloid deposits. Immunohistochemistry with FHL1 antibody revealed the presence of protein aggregates in about 20% of muscle fibers. Consistent with previous reports (Selcen et al., 2011; Feldkirchner et al., 2013; Bertrand et al., 2014), FHL1 deposits were detected throughout the cytoplasm and around myonuclei. Double staining with menadione-NBT revealed that FHL1 deposits strongly correlated with RBs, although with a more diffuse pattern. Desmin and α-B-crystallin (not shown) were strongly up-regulated in affected muscle fibers but they did not co-localize with FHL1 deposits (**Figure 1** and data not shown). Sarcolemmal components, such as dystrophin and laminin α2, were not detected in RBs; collagen VI was increased in the endomysium and perimysium, possibly as a consequence of active fibrosis (data not shown).

Reducing bodies displayed aggresome features as indicated by association with ubiquitin and with the luminal endoplasmic reticulum chaperone Grp78, in agreement with a previous work (Wilding et al., 2014). Consistent with aggresome formation, parkin, an E3 ubiquitin ligase involved in retrograde transport of misfolded proteins to centrosome (Garcia-Mata et al., 1999), and pericentrin, a marker of centrosome, were increased in affected myofibers (**Figure 2A**). Western blot analysis showed a patient-specific increase of ubiquitin (**Figure 2B**), confirming the massive presence of aberrant ubiquitinated proteins. Western blotting for FHL1 in the soluble fraction of patient muscle biopsy showed no significant change of FHL1 protein levels with respect to the control (**Figure 2C**).

Confocal imaging revealed a clear co-localization of FHL1 with p62 labeling (**Figure 2D**). FHL1/p62-positive aggregates also stained with DAPI, indicating the presence of nuclear material. Interestingly, DAPI-positive structures were not surrounded by nuclear lamina, as indicated by the absence of lamin A/C (**Figure 3A**) and emerin (not shown). In addition, DAPI-positive structures did not associate with histones (**Figure 3B**) and displayed an intense red fluorescence when stained with acridine orange (**Figure 3C**), a metachromatic dye that differentially stains double-stranded DNA and single-stranded DNA or RNA. Notably, DNase treatment strongly reduced the acridine-orange staining (**Figure 3D**). Altogether, these data suggest that FHL1/p62 aggregates also include single-stranded DNA, possibly due to nuclear degradation.

Recent studies have suggested that aggresomes are substrates for autophagy (Yao, 2010). LC3 immunolabeling on the patient muscle biopsy revealed the presence of autophagosomes in proximity of p62 aggregates (**Figure 4A**), suggesting the involvement of the autophagic pathway in aggresome clearance. Moreover, analysis of the protein levels of several autophagic markers showed a strong accumulation of p62, confirming the presence of an elevated number of aggresomes (**Figures 4B,C**). Notably, Beclin 1 and BNIP3, two well-known positive regulators of autophagy, were

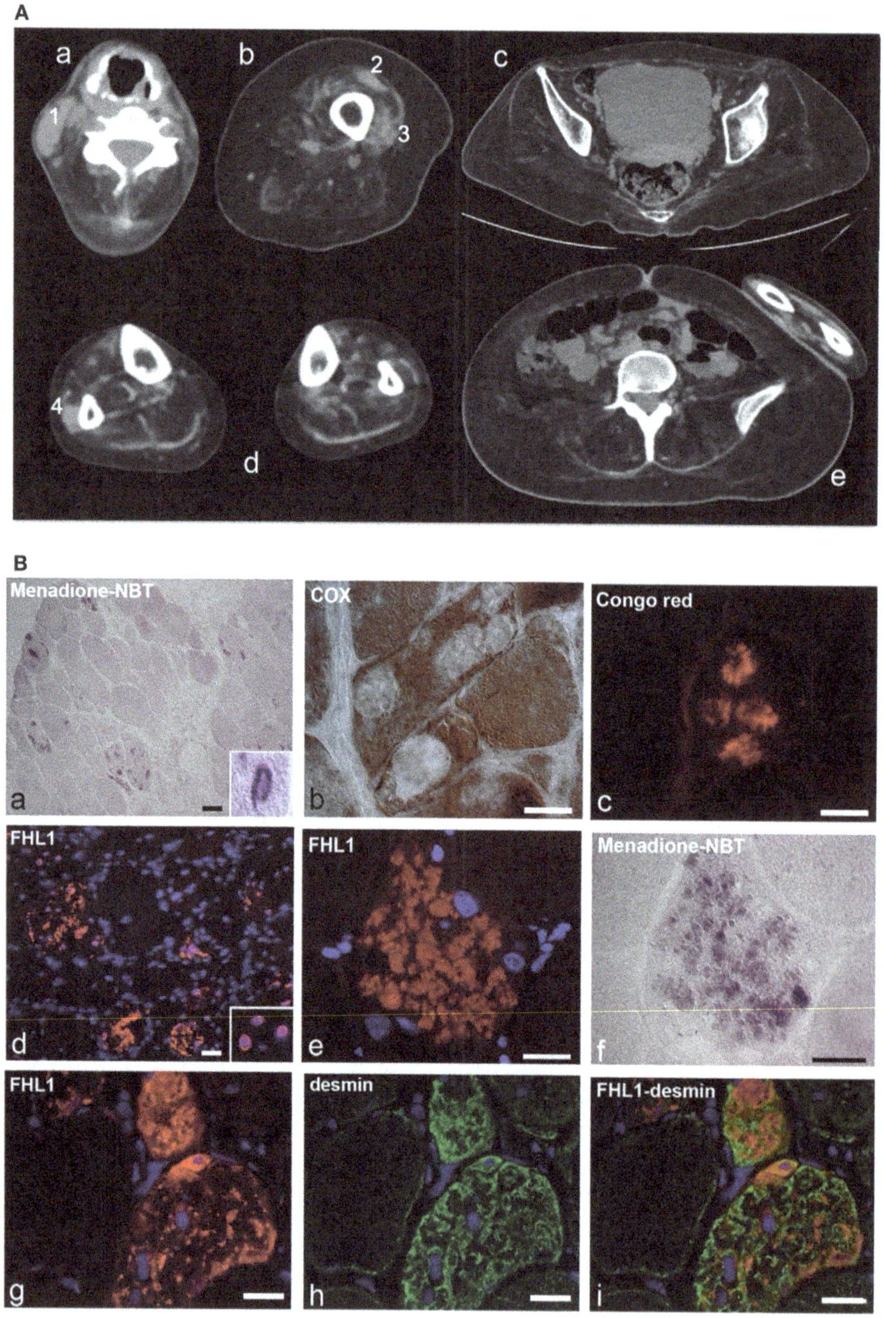

FIGURE 1 | (A) Patient with FHL1 mutation: index case. Muscle CT imaging of the neck (a), left thigh (b), pelvis (c), lower legs (d), and abdominal (e) muscles. In the neck, there is a relative preservation of the left sternocleidomastoideus (1) and almost complete involvement of all the other muscles (a). In the left thigh, only the rectus femoris (2) and vastus lateralis (3) are relatively spared (b). In the pelvis (c) and in the abdomen (e), there is a marked degeneration of all muscles. In the lower legs, only the peroneus (4) of the right leg is relatively spared (d). **(B)** Histochemistry and immunohistochemical analysis of patient muscle biopsy. Cross-sections show the presence of RBs in several muscle fibers, as revealed by menadione-NBT staining (a). Granular deposits are detectable at the nuclear rim of some myonuclei (a, inset). RBs appear devoid of oxidative activity (cytochrome oxidase, COX in b) and display affinity to Congo red staining (c). Immunofluorescence analysis of FHL1 shows protein accumulation throughout the cytoplasm of several muscle fibers (d) and around myonuclei (d, inset). FHL1 immunolabeling (e), followed by menadione-NBT staining (f), demonstrates that FHL1 accumulates in RBs (f). Double labeling for FHL1 and desmin (g–i) shows a marked increase of desmin in FHL1-accumulating myofibers. Scale bar, 20 μm.

strongly increased in the patient biopsy, indicating that autophagy induction is taking place, likely in response to the need of clearing the accumulating aggregates. This was further confirmed by the slight increase of LC3 lipidation observed in the patient biopsy (**Figures 4B,C**). All together, these data indicate that autophagy is strongly induced in the muscle biopsy from the patient.

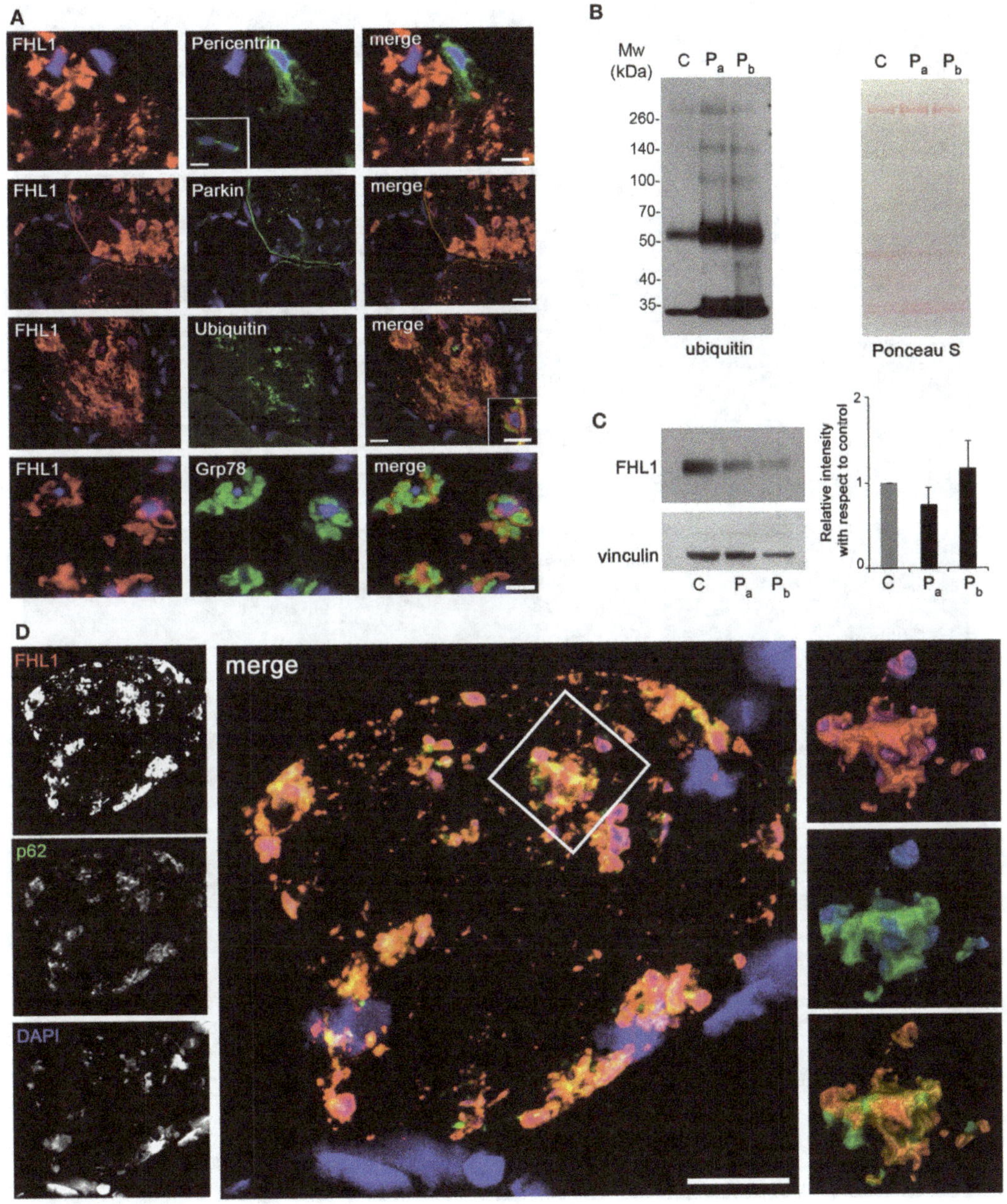

FIGURE 2 | (A) Double labeling of FHL1 with pericentrin, parkin, ubiquitin, and Grp78 in cross-sections of patient muscle biopsy. Scale bar, 20 μm. **(B)** Western blot analysis for ubiquitin in total protein extracts from muscle biopsies derived from a healthy donor **(C)** and from the patient (two different fragments of the index case biopsy, P_a and P_b). Increased reactivity for ubiquitin is clearly detectable in patient extracts. Ponceau S staining is shown as loading control. **(C)** Western blot analysis for FHL1 and vinculin in total protein extracts from muscle biopsies derived from a healthy donor **(C)** and from the index case (P_a and P_b). Quantification of the FHL1 protein level showing the relative western blot intensity with respect to control. Densitometric quantification was performed by three independent western blot experiments ($P > 0.05$, P_a and P_b vs C). **(D)** Confocal immunofluorescence imaging of the patient muscle biopsy labeled with FHL1 antibody (red), p62 antibody (green), and DAPI (blue). The maximum intensity projections of the single channels (white) are shown on the left, the merged image of confocal projections are shown in the middle, and the 3D surface shaded reconstruction of an enlargement of the area defined by the white box is shown on the right. Scale bar, 10 μm.

Ultrastructural analysis showed cytoplasmic bodies and tubulofilamentous material associated with nuclear alterations and autophagic vacuoles (**Figure 5**). Tubulofilamentous aggregates ranged from 14 to 1.2 nm. Dysmorphic nuclei showed condensed heterochromatin, ribonucleoprotein aggregates, enlarged nucleoli, and condensed granular material at the outer face of the nuclear cisterna. In addition, a reduced number of nuclear pores were also detected in nuclei with hypercondensed heterochromatin. Autophagic vacuoles, and in particular autophagolysosomes as indicated by the presence of a single membrane, were frequently

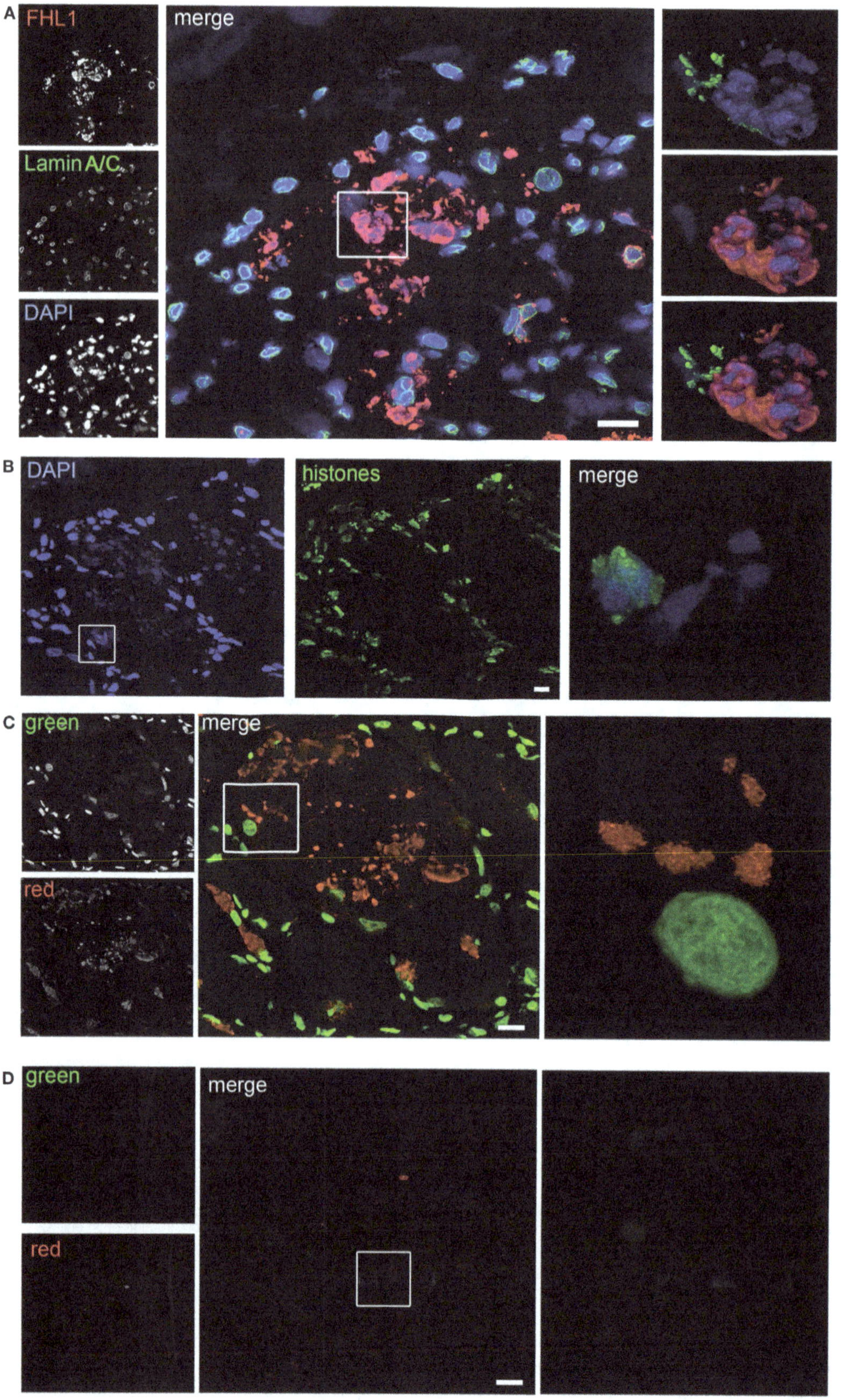

FIGURE 3 | Continued

FIGURE 3 | Continued
(A) Confocal immunofluorescence imaging of the patient muscle biopsy labeled with FHL1 antibody (red), lamin A/C antibody (green), and DAPI (blue). The maximum intensity projections of red and green channels (white) are shown on the left, the merged image of confocal projections are shown in the middle, and the 3D surface shaded reconstruction of an enlargement of the area defined by the white box is shown on the right. **(B)** Confocal immunofluorescence imaging of the patient muscle biopsy labeled with an anti-histones antibody (green) and DAPI (blue), together with 3D surface shaded reconstruction (merge). **(C)** Acridine-orange staining. The maximum intensity projections of the single channels (white) are shown on the left, the merged image of confocal projections are shown in the middle, and the 3D surface shaded reconstruction of an enlargement of the area defined by the white box is shown on the right. **(D)** Acridine-orange staining after DNase digestion on frozen sections of the patient's muscle biopsy showing that the treatment completely removed nuclear and RBs associated DNA. The maximum intensity projections of the red and green channels (white) are shown on the left, the merged image of confocal projections are shown in the middle, and the 3D surface shaded reconstruction of the area defined by box is shown on the right. Scale bar, 10 μm.

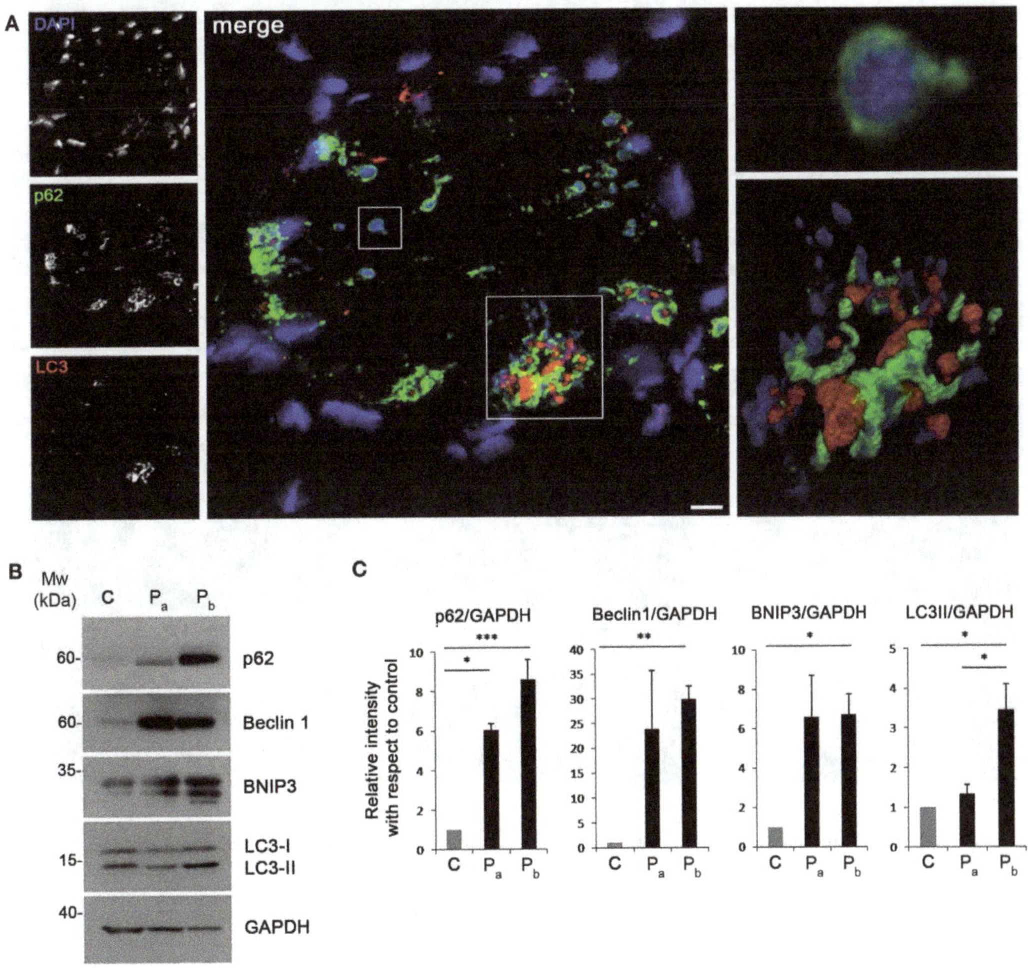

FIGURE 4 | (A) Confocal immunofluorescence imaging of the patient muscle biopsy labeled with LC3 antibody (red), p62 antibody (green), and DAPI (blue). The maximum intensity projections of the single channels (white) are shown on the left, the merged image of confocal projections are shown in the middle, and the 3D surface shaded reconstruction of an enlargement of the areas defined by the white boxes are shown on the right. Scale bar, 10 μm. **(B)** Western blot analysis for the autophagic markers LC3, Beclin 1, BNIP3, and p62 in muscle biopsies derived from a healthy donor **(C)** and from the index case (P_a and P_b). GAPDH was used as a loading control. **(C)** Quantification of the protein levels showing the relative western blot intensity with respect to control. Densitometric quantification was performed by three independent western blot experiments (***$P < 0.001$; **$P < 0.01$; *$P < 0.05$).

found in proximity of altered nuclei. Other inclusions consisted of myelinic bodies and aggregates of sarcoplasmic reticulum.

DISCUSSION

In this work, we provided data showing that aggresome and autophagy are involved in the pathophysiological defects underlying the muscle pathology of a sarcopenic patient with RSS and carrying a *FHL1* p.C150R mutation.

In our family, the female index case and her brother had a typical RSS (Moghadaszadeh et al., 2001). The p.C150R mutation has already been reported in patients with RSS (Schessl et al., 2010; Selcen et al., 2011). Interestingly, another female patient

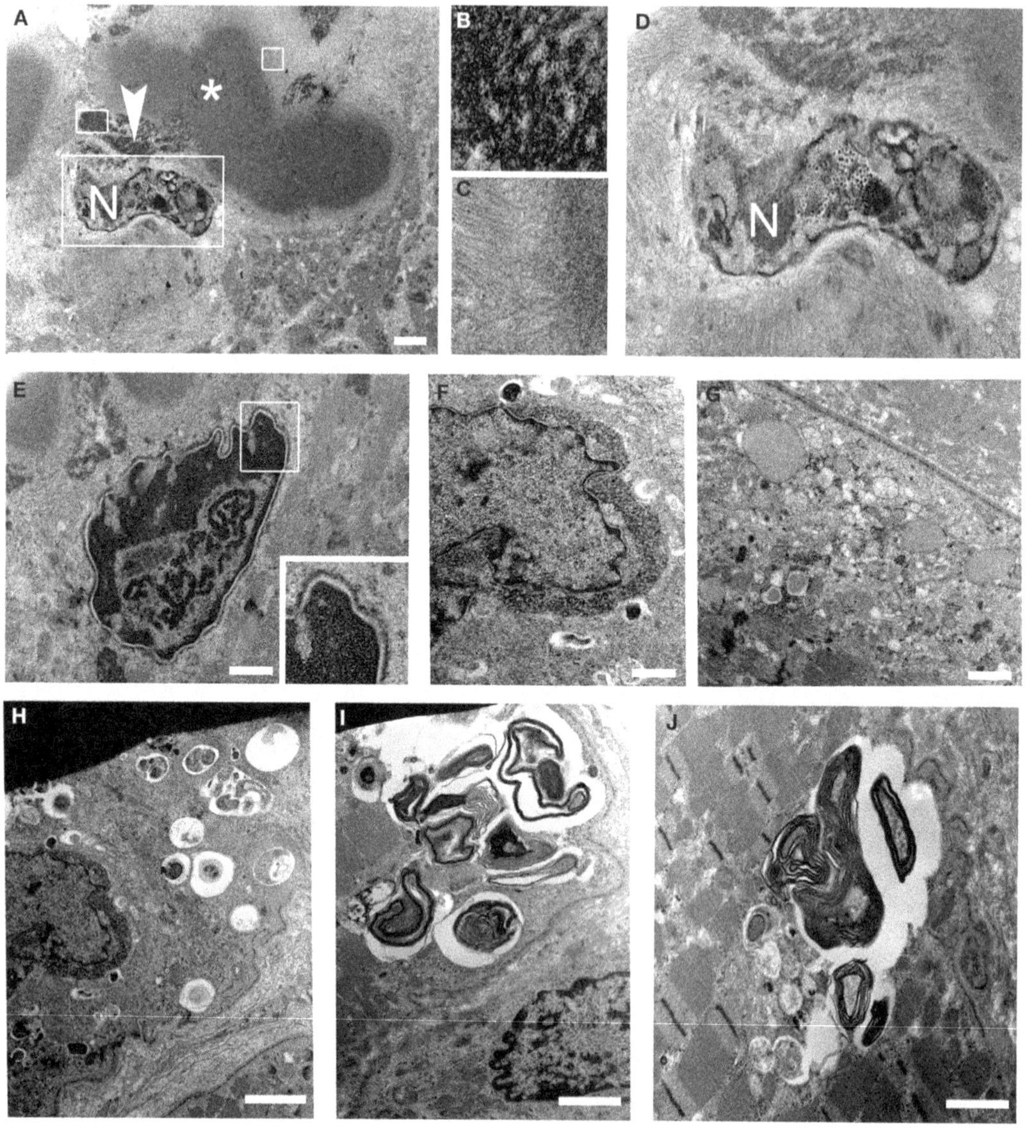

FIGURE 5 | Transmission electron microscopy of patient muscle biopsy. **(A–D)** Images showing cytoplasmic body (asterisk) and tubulofilamentous aggregates (arrowhead) close to degenerated nuclei (N). Higher magnification of the areas defined by boxes in **(A)** is shown in **(B–D)**. **(E,F)** Images showing altered nuclei with granular material accumulated at the nuclear rim. **(G)** Images showing dilated sarcoplasmic reticulum filled with amorphous material in a myofiber. **(H–J)** Images showing autophagic vacuoles and myelin figures close to nuclei and throughout some sarcomeres of muscle fibers. Scale bar, 500 nm.

(Selcen et al., 2011) presented extensor pollicis weakness, which was the first symptom noticed by our index case. Our patient had an atrophic phenotype. Underweight by body mass index, she was recognized to be sarcopenic-obese as determined by DXA given the marked reduction of lean body mass with relative increase of fat mass (Baumgartner et al., 2004). The sarcopenic condition was also reflected in the muscle CT that showed diffuse end stage degeneration. The brother of the index case had a severe progressive course; he lost ambulation at age 18, and underwent tracheostomy at age 28. In previously reported families, male patients were the most affected, while female carriers showed varying manifestations usually mild and some were asymptomatic (Schessl et al., 2010; Selcen et al., 2011). In our family, the two female patients had a very different course: severe and progressive in the index case and mild in her mother who was ambulant and without spine rigidity at age 58. Because of X chromosome inactivation, heterozygous women are mosaic for X-linked gene expression. This may explain the much milder phenotype in the mother compared with that of her daughter (Schessl et al., 2010; Selcen et al., 2011). The less affected mother was also much less atrophic, pointing to a possible differential activation of muscle atrophy pathways. However, no muscle biopsy of the mother was available, and X-inactivation studies were not performed in this family.

Muscle findings included menadione-NBT-positive aggregates, consistent with RBs, which also contained FHL1. The same *FHL1* mutation was previously reported in a family with RBM phenotype (Schessl et al., 2010) and in two patients with RBs and myofibrillar myopathy (Selcen et al., 2011). Also in those patients, the mutated FHL1 protein accumulated in RBs, pointing to a causative effect of this mutation in RB formation. The mutated cysteine residue localizes in the second LIM domain of the protein and it is expected to affect all FHL1 isoforms, i.e., full-length FHL1A and the shorter FHL1B and FHL1C polypeptides. Cys150 is a crucial coordinating residue in the second LIM domain (Michelsen et al., 1994) and mutations occurring at this site are predicted to induce protein misfolding. It has been proposed that the accumulation of misfolded FHL1 polypeptides results in the characteristic RB aggregates observed in muscle of RBM patients as well as in C2C12 myoblasts transfected with the mutant FHL1 protein (Schessl et al., 2008).

Aggresomes are structures proposed to facilitate the sequestration and degradation of toxic misfolded proteins. In agreement with previous reports (Bertrand et al., 2014), the RBs of the proband displayed characteristics of aggresomes, as indicated by the increase of proteins involved in aggresome formation and by the accumulation of ubiquitin, Grp78, p62, and cytoskeletal components, such as desmin and α-B-crystallin. Moreover, the FHL1-containing aggresomes were mainly accumulated around nuclei. It is well known that aggresome formation is mediated by the dynein/dynactin-mediated transport of misfolded proteins to the centrosome, as confirmed by the presence of aggresomes in the perinuclear region and matching with centrosome markers (Olzmann et al., 2008). In muscle cells, the centrosome undergoes redistribution at the nuclear rim during differentiation (Bugnard et al., 2005). This pattern persists in adult muscle (Srsen et al., 2009), as indicated by the localization of centrosome markers on the outer membrane of the nuclear cisterna. This peculiar positioning of the centrosome at the nuclear rim of muscle cells accounts for the recruitment of granular material with aggresome-like features we observed in nuclei of the *FHL1* mutated muscle fibers. In addition, we found that nuclei with perinuclear granular material appeared dysmorphic, with dramatic changes of the nuclear envelope and hypercondensed heterochromatin. These data, in addition to the finding of single-stranded DNA in aggresomes, suggest that the aggresome accumulation at the nuclear rim may induce nuclear degradation. This hypothesis is consistent with the alterations of the nuclear envelope in cells containing inclusion bodies that were described in patients affected by Huntington disease and in transgenic mice expressing mutant huntingtin (Waelter et al., 2001).

We also found that Grp78, an endoplasmic reticulum chaperone up-regulated during the unfolded protein response, was strongly increased and associated to the FHL1 deposits in the proband muscle biopsy. This finding is in agreement with previous work showing increased expression of Grp78 and unfolded protein response in patients with RBM (Liewluck et al., 2007). However, the association of Grp78 with aggresomes may be also due to retrograde transport from the endoplasmic reticulum, as hypothesized by the formation of aggresome-like inclusion bodies induced by mutant huntingtin (Garcia-Mata et al., 2002).

The association of FHL1 with p62 we detected in the proband muscle biopsy indicates that the mutant FHL1 protein is targeted to degradative pathways. p62 is a multifunctional protein containing a number of protein–protein interaction motifs that are involved in protein aggregation and degradation (Moscat and Diaz-Meco, 2009a,b). It has been hypothesized that p62 may act as a critical ubiquitin chain-targeting factor that shuttles substrates for proteasomal degradation (Seibenhener et al., 2004). On the other hand, a role for p62 in aggregate formation for autophagic degradation was also hypothesized (Komatsu et al., 2007; Kirkin et al., 2009; Komatsu and Ichimura, 2010). The strong increase of Beclin 1 and BNIP3 levels we detected in the patient biopsy indicates that autophagy induction is taking place, likely to help the clearance of accumulating aggregates. This is further confirmed by the slight increase of LC3 lipidation and by the accumulation of LC3 deposits in proximity to aggresomes in the proband muscle. The presence of autophagic vacuoles and myelin figures further confirms the involvement of the autophagic pathway in the pathophysiological alterations of this patient. Interestingly, the presence of autophagosomes and autophagic vacuoles was also reported in muscle biopsies of RBM patients (Bertrand et al., 2014). It is also interesting to consider that FHL1 null mice, lacking global FHL1 expression and without aggregates accumulation, display susceptibility to autophagy, as indicated by increased LC3 lipidation in skeletal muscle (Domenighetti et al., 2014). These findings point to a causative role of FHL1 deficiency in autophagy activation, and indicate that activation of the autophagic pathway in FHL1-related myopathies may be a common pathophysiological mechanism, independent from the accumulation of protein aggregates. Although future studies of the autophagic flux in muscle cells from patients and animal models for FHL1 deficiency are needed in order to understand in detail how and to which extent deregulation of autophagy contributes to the pathogenesis of FHL1-related myopathies, our data demonstrate for the first time the coexistence of aggresomes and autophagy in the muscle biopsy of a patient with severe sarcopenia caused by p.C150R mutation in *FHL1*. These findings add new insights in delineating the altered mechanisms involved in the pathogenesis of *FHL1*-associated diseases.

ACKNOWLEDGMENTS

This work was supported by the Italian Ministry of Education, University and Research (FIRB RBAP10KCNS to Patrizia Sabatelli, and FIRB RBAP11Z3YA_003 to Paolo Bonaldo), and by "5 per mille" 2010 Rizzoli Orthopaedic Institute.

REFERENCES

Baumgartner, R. N., Wayne, S. J., Waters, D. L., Janssen, I., Gallagher, D., and Morley, J. E. (2004). Sarcopenic obesity predicts instrumental activities of daily living disability in the elderly. *Obes. Res.* 12, 1995–2004. doi:10.1038/oby.2004.250

Bertrand, A. T., Bonnemann, C. G., and Bonne, G. (2014). 199th ENMC international workshop: FHL1 related myopathies, June 7-9, 2013, Naarden, the Netherlands. *Neuromuscul. Disord.* 24, 453–462. doi:10.1016/j.nmd.2014.02.002

Bjorkoy, G., Lamark, T., Brech, A., Outzen, H., Perander, M., Overvatn, A., et al. (2005). p62/SQSTM1 forms protein aggregates degraded by autophagy and has a protective effect on huntingtin-induced cell death. *J. Cell Biol.* 171, 603–614. doi:10.1083/jcb.200507002

Bjorkoy, G., Lamark, T., and Johansen, T. (2006). p62/SQSTM1: a missing link between protein aggregates and the autophagy machinery. *Autophagy* 2, 138–139. doi:10.4161/auto.2.2.2405

Brooke, M. H., and Neville, H. E. (1972). Reducing body myopathy. *Neurology* 22, 829–840. doi:10.1212/WNL.22.8.829

Brown, S., Mcgrath, M. J., Ooms, L. M., Gurung, R., Maimone, M. M., and Mitchell, C. A. (1999). Characterization of two isoforms of the skeletal muscle LIM protein 1, SLIM1. Localization of SLIM1 at focal adhesions and the isoform slimmer in the nucleus of myoblasts and cytoplasm of myotubes suggests distinct roles in the cytoskeleton and in nuclear-cytoplasmic communication. *J. Biol. Chem.* 274, 27083–27091.

Bugnard, E., Zaal, K. J., and Ralston, E. (2005). Reorganization of microtubule nucleation during muscle differentiation. *Cell Motil. Cytoskeleton* 60, 1–13. doi:10.1002/cm.20042

Chen, D. H., Raskind, W. H., Parson, W. W., Sonnen, J. A., Vu, T., Zheng, Y., et al. (2010). A novel mutation in FHL1 in a family with X-linked scapuloperoneal myopathy: phenotypic spectrum and structural study of FHL1 mutations. *J. Neurol. Sci.* 296, 22–29. doi:10.1016/j.jns.2010.06.017

Chen, P., Cescon, M., Megighian, A., and Bonaldo, P. (2014). Collagen VI regulates peripheral nerve myelination and function. *FASEB J.* 28, 1145–1156. doi:10.1096/fj.13-239533

Cowling, B. S., Mcgrath, M. J., Nguyen, M. A., Cottle, D. L., Kee, A. J., Brown, S., et al. (2008). Identification of FHL1 as a regulator of skeletal muscle mass: implications for human myopathy. *J. Cell Biol.* 183, 1033–1048. doi:10.1083/jcb.200804077

Darzynkiewicz, Z. (1994). Simultaneous analysis of cellular RNA and DNA content. *Methods Cell Biol.* 41, 401–420. doi:10.1016/S0091-679X(08)61731-8

Dawid, I. B., Toyama, R., and Taira, M. (1995). LIM domain proteins. *C. R. Acad. Sci. III, Sci. Vie* 318, 295–306.

Domenighetti, A. A., Chu, P. H., Wu, T., Sheikh, F., Gokhin, D. S., Guo, L. T., et al. (2014). Loss of FHL1 induces an age-dependent skeletal muscle myopathy associated with myofibrillar and intermyofibrillar disorganization in mice. *Hum. Mol. Genet.* 23, 209–225. doi:10.1093/hmg/ddt412

Feldkirchner, S., Walter, M. C., Muller, S., Kubny, C., Krause, S., Kress, W., et al. (2013). Proteomic characterization of aggregate components in an intrafamilial variable FHL1-associated myopathy. *Neuromuscul. Disord.* 23, 418–426. doi:10.1016/j.nmd.2013.02.006

Friedrich, F. W., Wilding, B. R., Reischmann, S., Crocini, C., Lang, P., Charron, P., et al. (2012). Evidence for FHL1 as a novel disease gene for isolated hypertrophic cardiomyopathy. *Hum. Mol. Genet.* 21, 3237–3254. doi:10.1093/hmg/dds157

Garcia-Mata, R., Bebok, Z., Sorscher, E. J., and Sztul, E. S. (1999). Characterization and dynamics of aggresome formation by a cytosolic GFP-chimera. *J. Cell Biol.* 146, 1239–1254. doi:10.1083/jcb.146.6.1239

Garcia-Mata, R., Gao, Y. S., and Sztul, E. (2002). Hassles with taking out the garbage: aggravating aggresomes. *Traffic* 3, 388–396. doi:10.1034/j.1600-0854.2002.30602.x

Goldberg, A. L. (2003). Protein degradation and protection against misfolded or damaged proteins. *Nature* 426, 895–899. doi:10.1038/nature02263

Greene, W. K., Baker, E., Rabbitts, T. H., and Kees, U. R. (1999). Genomic structure, tissue expression and chromosomal location of the LIM-only gene, SLIM1. *Gene* 232, 203–207. doi:10.1016/S0378-1119(99)00125-0

Gueneau, L., Bertrand, A. T., Jais, J. P., Salih, M. A., Stojkovic, T., Wehnert, M., et al. (2009). Mutations of the FHL1 gene cause Emery-Dreifuss muscular dystrophy. *Am. J. Hum. Genet.* 85, 338–353. doi:10.1016/j.ajhg.2009.07.015

Iwata, A., Riley, B. E., Johnston, J. A., and Kopito, R. R. (2005). HDAC6 and microtubules are required for autophagic degradation of aggregated huntingtin. *J. Biol. Chem.* 280, 40282–40292. doi:10.1074/jbc.M508786200

Johannessen, M., Moller, S., Hansen, T., Moens, U., and Van Ghelue, M. (2006). The multifunctional roles of the four-and-a-half-LIM only protein FHL2. *Cell. Mol. Life Sci.* 63, 268–284. doi:10.1007/s00018-005-5438-z

Kadrmas, J. L., and Beckerle, M. C. (2004). The LIM domain: from the cytoskeleton to the nucleus. *Nat. Rev. Mol. Cell Biol.* 5, 920–931. doi:10.1038/nrm1499

Kawaguchi, Y., Kovacs, J. J., Mclaurin, A., Vance, J. M., Ito, A., and Yao, T. P. (2003). The deacetylase HDAC6 regulates aggresome formation and cell viability in response to misfolded protein stress. *Cell* 115, 727–738. doi:10.1016/S0092-8674(03)00939-5

Kirkin, V., Lamark, T., Sou, Y. S., Bjorkoy, G., Nunn, J. L., Bruun, J. A., et al. (2009). A role for NBR1 in autophagosomal degradation of ubiquitinated substrates. *Mol. Cell* 33, 505–516. doi:10.1016/j.molcel.2009.01.020

Knoblauch, H., Geier, C., Adams, S., Budde, B., Rudolph, A., Zacharias, U., et al. (2010). Contractures and hypertrophic cardiomyopathy in a novel FHL1 mutation. *Ann. Neurol.* 67, 136–140. doi:10.1002/ana.21839

Komatsu, M., and Ichimura, Y. (2010). Physiological significance of selective degradation of p62 by autophagy. *FEBS Lett.* 584, 1374–1378. doi:10.1016/j.febslet.2010.02.017

Komatsu, M., Waguri, S., Koike, M., Sou, Y. S., Ueno, T., Hara, T., et al. (2007). Homeostatic levels of p62 control cytoplasmic inclusion body formation in autophagy-deficient mice. *Cell* 131, 1149–1163. doi:10.1016/j.cell.2007.10.035

Lee, J. Y., Chien, I. C., Lin, W. Y., Wu, S. M., Wei, B. H., Lee, Y. E., et al. (2012). Fhl1 as a downstream target of Wnt signaling to promote myogenesis of C2C12 cells. *Mol. Cell. Biochem.* 365, 251–262. doi:10.1007/s11010-012-1266-2

Lee, S. M., Tsui, S. K., Chan, K. K., Garcia-Barcelo, M., Waye, M. M., Fung, K. P., et al. (1998). Chromosomal mapping, tissue distribution and cDNA sequence of four-and-a-half LIM domain protein 1 (FHL1). *Gene* 216, 163–170. doi:10.1016/S0378-1119(98)00302-3

Liewluck, T., Hayashi, Y. K., Ohsawa, M., Kurokawa, R., Fujita, M., Noguchi, S., et al. (2007). Unfolded protein response and aggresome formation in hereditary reducing-body myopathy. *Muscle Nerve* 35, 322–326. doi:10.1002/mus.20691

McGrath, M. J., Cottle, D. L., Nguyen, M. A., Dyson, J. M., Coghill, I. D., Robinson, P. A., et al. (2006). Four and a half LIM protein 1 binds myosin-binding protein C and regulates myosin filament formation and sarcomere assembly. *J. Biol. Chem.* 281, 7666–7683. doi:10.1074/jbc.M512552200

McGrath, M. J., Mitchell, C. A., Coghill, I. D., Robinson, P. A., and Brown, S. (2003). Skeletal muscle LIM protein 1 (SLIM1/FHL1) induces alpha 5 beta 1-integrin-dependent myocyte elongation. *Am. J. Physiol. Cell Physiol.* 285, C1513–C1526. doi:10.1152/ajpcell.00207.2003

Michelsen, J. W., Sewell, A. K., Louis, H. A., Olsen, J. I., Davis, D. R., Winge, D. R., et al. (1994). Mutational analysis of the metal sites in an LIM domain. *J. Biol. Chem.* 269, 11108–11113.

Moghadaszadeh, B., Petit, N., Jaillard, C., Brockington, M., Roy, S. Q., Merlini, L., et al. (2001). Mutations in SEPN1 cause congenital muscular dystrophy with spinal rigidity and restrictive respiratory syndrome. *Nat. Genet.* 29, 17–18. doi:10.1038/ng713

Morgan, M. J., and Madgwick, A. J. (1999). The LIM proteins FHL1 and FHL3 are expressed differently in skeletal muscle. *Biochem. Biophys. Res. Commun.* 255, 245–250. doi:10.1006/bbrc.1999.0179

Moscat, J., and Diaz-Meco, M. T. (2009a). p62 at the crossroads of autophagy, apoptosis, and cancer. *Cell* 137, 1001–1004. doi:10.1016/j.cell.2009.05.023

Moscat, J., and Diaz-Meco, M. T. (2009b). To aggregate or not to aggregate? A new role for p62. *EMBO Rep.* 10, 804. doi:10.1038/embor.2009.172

Ng, E. K., Lee, S. M., Li, H. Y., Ngai, S. M., Tsui, S. K., Waye, M. M., et al. (2001). Characterization of tissue-specific LIM domain protein (FHL1C) which is an alternatively spliced isoform of a human LIM-only protein (FHL1). *J. Cell. Biochem.* 82, 1–10. doi:10.1002/jcb.1110

Olzmann, J. A., Li, L., and Chin, L. S. (2008). Aggresome formation and neurodegenerative diseases: therapeutic implications. *Curr. Med. Chem.* 15, 47–60. doi:10.2174/092986708783330692

Purcell, N. H., Darwis, D., Bueno, O. F., Muller, J. M., Schule, R., and Molkentin, J. D. (2004). Extracellular signal-regulated kinase 2 interacts with and is negatively regulated by the LIM-only protein FHL2 in cardiomyocytes. *Mol. Cell. Biol.* 24, 1081–1095. doi:10.1128/MCB.24.3.1081-1095.2004

Quinzii, C. M., Vu, T. H., Min, K. C., Tanji, K., Barral, S., Grewal, R. P., et al. (2008). X-linked dominant scapuloperoneal myopathy is due to a mutation in the gene encoding four-and-a-half-LIM protein 1. *Am. J. Hum. Genet.* 82, 208–213. doi:10.1016/j.ajhg.2007.09.013

Schessl, J., Columbus, A., Hu, Y., Zou, Y., Voit, T., Goebel, H. H., et al. (2010). Familial reducing body myopathy with cytoplasmic bodies and rigid spine revisited: identification of a second LIM domain mutation in FHL1. *Neuropediatrics* 41, 43–46. doi:10.1055/s-0030-1254101

Schessl, J., Taratuto, A. L., Sewry, C., Battini, R., Chin, S. S., Maiti, B., et al. (2009). Clinical, histological and genetic characterization of reducing body myopathy caused by mutations in FHL1. *Brain* 132, 452–464. doi:10.1093/brain/awn325

Schessl, J., Zou, Y., Mcgrath, M. J., Cowling, B. S., Maiti, B., Chin, S. S., et al. (2008). Proteomic identification of FHL1 as the protein mutated in human reducing body myopathy. *J. Clin. Invest.* 118, 904–912. doi:10.1172/JCI34450

Schreckenbach, T., Henn, W., Kress, W., Roos, A., Maschke, M., Feiden, W., et al. (2013). Novel FHL1 mutation in a family with reducing body myopathy. *Muscle Nerve* 47, 127–134. doi:10.1002/mus.23500

Seibenhener, M. L., Babu, J. R., Geetha, T., Wong, H. C., Krishna, N. R., and Wooten, M. W. (2004). Sequestosome 1/p62 is a polyubiquitin chain binding protein involved in ubiquitin proteasome degradation. *Mol. Cell. Biol.* 24, 8055–8068. doi:10.1128/MCB.24.18.8055-8068.2004

Selcen, D., Bromberg, M. B., Chin, S. S., and Engel, A. G. (2011). Reducing bodies and myofibrillar myopathy features in FHL1 muscular dystrophy. *Neurology* 77, 1951–1959. doi:10.1212/WNL.0b013e31823a0ebe

Shalaby, S., Hayashi, Y. K., Goto, K., Ogawa, M., Nonaka, I., Noguchi, S., et al. (2008). Rigid spine syndrome caused by a novel mutation in four-and-a-half LIM domain 1 gene (FHL1). *Neuromuscul. Disord.* 18, 959–961. doi:10.1016/j.nmd.2008.09.012

Shalaby, S., Hayashi, Y. K., Nonaka, I., Noguchi, S., and Nishino, I. (2009). Novel FHL1 mutations in fatal and benign reducing body myopathy. *Neurology* 72, 375–376. doi:10.1212/01.wnl.0000341311.84347.a0

Sheikh, F., Raskin, A., Chu, P. H., Lange, S., Domenighetti, A. A., Zheng, M., et al. (2008). An FHL1-containing complex within the cardiomyocyte sarcomere mediates hypertrophic biomechanical stress responses in mice. *J. Clin. Invest.* 118, 3870–3880. doi:10.1172/JCI34472

Srsen, V., Fant, X., Heald, R., Rabouille, C., and Merdes, A. (2009). Centrosome proteins form an insoluble perinuclear matrix during muscle cell differentiation. *BMC Cell Biol.* 10:28. doi:10.1186/1471-2121-10-28

Taniguchi, Y., Furukawa, T., Tun, T., Han, H., and Honjo, T. (1998). LIM protein KyoT2 negatively regulates transcription by association with the RBP-J DNA-binding protein. *Mol. Cell. Biol.* 18, 644–654.

Waelter, S., Boeddrich, A., Lurz, R., Scherzinger, E., Lueder, G., Lehrach, H., et al. (2001). Accumulation of mutant huntingtin fragments in aggresome-like inclusion bodies as a result of insufficient protein degradation. *Mol. Biol. Cell* 12, 1393–1407. doi:10.1091/mbc.12.5.1393

Wang, J., Qin, H., Liang, J., Zhu, Y., Liang, L., Zheng, M., et al. (2007). The transcriptional repression activity of KyoT2 on the Notch/RBP-J pathway is regulated by PIAS1-catalyzed SUMOylation. *J. Mol. Biol.* 370, 27–38. doi:10.1016/j.jmb.2007.04.010

Wilding, B. R., Mcgrath, M. J., Bonne, G., and Mitchell, C. A. (2014). FHL1 mutants that cause clinically distinct human myopathies form protein aggregates and impair myoblast differentiation. *J. Cell. Sci.* 127, 2269–2281. doi:10.1242/jcs.140905

Windpassinger, C., Schoser, B., Straub, V., Hochmeister, S., Noor, A., Lohberger, B., et al. (2008). An X-linked myopathy with postural muscle atrophy and generalized hypertrophy, termed XMPMA, is caused by mutations in FHL1. *Am. J. Hum. Genet.* 82, 88–99. doi:10.1016/j.ajhg.2007.09.004

Yao, T. P. (2010). The role of ubiquitin in autophagy-dependent protein aggregate processing. *Genes Cancer* 1, 779–786. doi:10.1177/1947601910383277

11

Melanocytes from patients affected by Ullrich congenital muscular dystrophy and Bethlem myopathy have dysfunctional mitochondria that can be rescued with cyclophilin inhibitors

Alessandra Zulian[1,2], Francesca Tagliavini[3,4], Erika Rizzo[1,2], Camilla Pellegrini[4], Francesca Sardone[3,4], Nicoletta Zini[3,4], Nadir Mario Maraldi[3], Spartaco Santi[3,4], Cesare Faldini[5], Luciano Merlini[4], Valeria Petronilli[1,2], Paolo Bernardi[1,2]* and Patrizia Sabatelli[3,4]*

[1] *Department of Biomedical Sciences, University of Padova, Padova, Italy*
[2] *CNR Neuroscience Institute, Padova, Italy*
[3] *CNR National Research Council of Italy, Institute of Molecular Genetics, Bologna, Italy*
[4] *SC Laboratory of Musculoskeletal Cell Biology, IOR, Bologna, Italy*
[5] *Rizzoli Orthopaedic Institute, University of Bologna, Bologna, Italy*

***Correspondence:**
Paolo Bernardi, Department of Biomedical Sciences, University of Padova, Via Ugo Bassi 58/B, Padova I-35131, Italy
e-mail: bernardi@bio.unipd.it;
Patrizia Sabatelli, Institute of Molecular Genetics-CNR, Bologna I-40136, Italy
e-mail: sabatelli@area.bo.cnr.it

Ullrich congenital muscular dystrophy and Bethlem myopathy are caused by mutations in collagen VI (ColVI) genes, which encode an extracellular matrix protein; yet, mitochondria play a major role in disease pathogenesis through a short circuit caused by inappropriate opening of the permeability transition pore, a high-conductance channel, which causes a shortage in ATP production. We find that melanocytes do not produce ColVI yet they bind it at the cell surface, suggesting that this protein may play a trophic role and that its absence may cause lesions similar to those seen in skeletal muscle. We show that mitochondria in melanocytes of Ullrich congenital muscular dystrophy and Bethlem myopathy patients display increased size, reduced matrix density, and disrupted cristae, findings that suggest a functional impairment. In keeping with this hypothesis, mitochondria (i) underwent anomalous depolarization after inhibition of the F-ATP synthase with oligomycin, and (ii) displayed decreased respiratory reserve capacity. The non-immunosuppressive cyclophilin inhibitor NIM811 prevented mitochondrial depolarization in response to oligomycin in melanocytes from both Ullrich congenital muscular dystrophy and Bethlem myopathy patients, and partially restored the respiratory reserve of melanocytes from one Bethlem myopathy patient. These results match our recent findings on melanocytes from patients affected by Duchenne muscular dystrophy (Pellegrini et al., 2013), and suggest that skin biopsies may represent a minimally invasive tool to investigate mitochondrial dysfunction and to evaluate drug efficacy in ColVI-related myopathies and possibly in other muscle wasting conditions like aging sarcopenia.

Keywords: collagen VI, muscular dystrophy, mitochondria, melanocytes, permeability transition, cyclophilin inhibitors

INTRODUCTION

Collagen VI (ColVI) is an extracellular matrix (ECM) protein that forms a complex microfibrillar network; it is present in several organs including skeletal muscle, where it is localized just outside the basement membrane (Kuo et al., 1997). ColVI is constituted by three chains (α1, α2, and α3) encoded by different genes (*COL6A1*, *COL6A2*, and *COL6A3*, respectively). Three additional ColVI chains have recently been identified (α4, α5, α6), which are similar to α3 but display a more restricted tissue distribution (Gara et al., 2008). Deficiency of ColVI due to mutations in *COL6A1*, *COL6A2*, or *COL6A3* gives rise to three main muscle disorders, Ullrich congenital muscular dystrophy (UCMD, MIM #254090) (Ullrich, 1930; Camacho Vanegas et al., 2001), Bethlem myopathy (BM, MIM #158810) (Bethlem and Wijngaarden, 1976), and myosclerosis myopathy (MIM #255600) (Merlini et al., 2008b). UCMD is a severe disorder characterized by congenital muscle weakness with axial and proximal joint contractures and coexisting distal joint hypermobility (Bertini and Pepe, 2002). BM is characterized by slowly progressive axial and proximal muscle weakness with finger flexion contractures (Merlini et al., 1994). Myosclerosis myopathy is a recessive disorder characterized by progressive contractures affecting all joints (Merlini et al., 2008b). However, it should be noted that the clinical features of ColVI muscular dystrophy can be extremely heterogenous, ranging from

Abbreviations: BM, Bethlem myopathy; ColVI, collagen VI; Cs, cyclosporin; DEJ, dermal–epidermal junction; ECM, extracellular matrix; FCCP, carbonylcyanide-*p*-trifluoromethoxyphenyl hydrazone; OCR, oxygen consumption rate; PTP, mitochondrial permeability transition pore; TMRM, tetramethylrhodamine methyl ester; UCMD, Ullrich congenital muscular dystrophy.

mild to severe myopathy with progressive muscular dystrophy (Jöbsis et al., 1999). Consistent with the idea that these disorders represent a clinical continuum, about 70 different mutations of the *COL6* genes have so far been described in ColVI myopathies (Pepe et al., 2002; Lampe and Bushby, 2005). Patients affected by ColVI muscular dystrophies frequently display skin alterations. Patients with the UCMD phenotype usually present follicular hyperkeratosis over the extensor surfaces of upper and lower limbs, soft velvety skin on the palms and soles, and tendency to develop keloids or "cigarette paper" scars, skin features that may be present also in BM patients (Lampe and Bushby, 2005). Although the mechanism linking ColVI deficiency to skin lesions has not been established, it has recently been shown that melanocytes affect fibroblast proliferation and collagen production, contributing to the generation of hypertrophic scars and keloids (Gao et al., 2013).

Collagen VI myopathies share a common pathogenesis linked to deregulation of the mitochondrial permeability transition pore (PTP), an inner membrane high-conductance channel that forms from dimers of the mitochondrial F-ATP synthase under conditions of Ca^{2+} overload and oxidative stress (Bernardi, 2013; Giorgio et al., 2013) and is desensitized by cyclosporin (Cs) A. Oxidative stress is specifically involved in the pathogenesis of myopathy in the *Col6a1*$^{-/-}$ mouse model (Menazza et al., 2010; Sorato et al., 2014); and the resulting myofiber damage is amplified by impaired clearance of defective mitochondria (Grumati et al., 2010). PTP-dependent mitochondrial dysfunction appears to be involved also in other forms of muscular dystrophy, including those caused by lack of δ-sarcoglycan and laminin-2 (Millay et al., 2008), as well as of dystrophin (Millay et al., 2008; Reutenauer et al., 2008; Wissing et al., 2010; Pellegrini et al., 2013). These studies generated pharmacological strategies aimed at rescuing the mitochondrial defect through desensitization of the PTP, and encouraging results have been obtained with the use of CsA and its non-immunosuppressive analogs Debio025 and NIM811 in animal models and in a pilot trial in patients (Irwin et al., 2003; Angelin et al., 2007; Merlini et al., 2008a; Tiepolo et al., 2009; Telfer et al., 2010; Zulian et al., 2014).

Translation of the pharmacological strategies tested in animal models to muscular dystrophy patients is particularly complex, and often requires invasive procedures. Cell cultures derived from muscle biopsies can be used for genetic and mechanistic studies, but in the case of ColVI myopathies the disease phenotype is lost after a few passages, a likely result of *in vitro* selection of apoptosis-resistant cells (Sabatelli et al., 2012b). Melanocytes are the pigment-producing cells of the skin, localized to the basal layer of human epidermis. They are polarized cells performing specific functions at the basolateral and apical membranes, which explains the differential composition of the membrane at these sites (Pinon and Wehrle-Haller, 2011). At the basal layer, melanocytes attach to the dermal–epidermal junction (DEJ), a specialized structure with a fundamental role in maintaining attachment of the epidermis to the dermis and providing skin resistance against shearing forces (Santiago-Walker et al., 2009). Melanocytes do express muscle-specific proteins including the mDP427 dystrophin isoform at the interface with the DEJ (Pellegrini et al., 2013). We have recently demonstrated that melanocytes possess properties similar to those of myoblasts from Duchenne muscular dystrophy patients, and represent a promising cellular model to monitor the response of dystrophinopathies to pharmacological treatments (Pellegrini et al., 2013). Here, we have explored whether mitochondrial dysfunction can be detected in melanocytes from UCMD and BM patients, and whether these cells are a potential alternative to the use of muscle-derived cells in the study and therapy of ColVI myopathies.

MATERIALS AND METHODS

PATIENTS

Skin biopsies from two healthy subjects and four ColVI muscular dystrophy patients (two UCMD and two BM) were collected. All patients were previously diagnosed by genetic, and/or histochemical and biochemical analysis. UCMD patient 1 (UCMD1) carried a *COL6A2* homozygous mutation in exon 28 [UCMD-5 patient in Tagliavini et al. (2014)]; UCMD patient 2 (UCMD2) displayed typical UCMD features, severe deficiency of ColVI in muscle biopsies and defective ColVI secretion in cultured skin fibroblasts; BM patients 1 (BM1) and 2 (BM2) carried heterozygous mutations in *COL6A1* and *COL6A3*, respectively [patients BM-5 and BM-6, respectively, in Tagliavini et al. (2014)]. All participants provided written informed consent, and approval was obtained from the Ethics Committee of the Rizzoli Orthopaedic Institute (Bologna, Italy).

CELL CULTURES

Skin fragments were cut into small pieces and the epidermis was separated from the dermis after overnight incubation in 0.5% dispase II (Roche) at 4°C. Melanocytes were maintained in M254 culture medium (GIBCO) supplemented with phorbol-12-myristate 13-acetate, transferrin, hydrocortisone, insulin, bovine pituitary extract, basic fibroblast growth factor, and fetal calf serum (HMGS supplement, GIBCO). Melanocyte-fibroblast co-cultures were obtained by plating fibroblasts onto coverslips in DMEM growth medium until they reached 70% confluence; after 1 day melanocytes were seeded onto the fibroblast cultures and grown in M254 medium supplemented with 0.25 mM L-ascorbic acid (Sigma). ColVI-enriched, conditioned medium was obtained by treating confluent skin fibroblast cultures from healthy donors with DMEM medium supplemented with 0.25 mM L-ascorbic acid. After 24 h, the medium was collected, centrifuged at low speed to remove cell debris and diluted 1:1 with M254 medium. Normal melanocytes plated onto coverslips were grown with ColVI-enriched medium for 24 h before immunohistochemical analysis with anti-ColVI antibody (Millipore). To assess the effect of cyclophilin inhibitors on mitochondrial morphology, melanocytes from patients and healthy subjects were treated with 0.8 μM NIM811 diluted in M254 medium for 2 h at 37°C before processing for immunofluorescence and transmission electron microscopy.

IMMUNOFLUORESCENCE ANALYSIS

Cultured melanocytes were fixed with methanol at −20°C for 7 min, washed with phosphate-buffered saline, and incubated with antibodies against NG2 (Millipore), integrin β1 (Millipore), pMEL-17 (Monosan), ColVI (Millipore), or Tom20 (Santa Cruz). All antibodies were revealed with secondary anti-rabbit or anti-mouse TRITC or FITC-conjugated antibodies (DAKO). Samples were mounted with an anti-fading reagent (Molecular Probes) and analyzed with a A1-R confocal laser microscope (Nikon) equipped with a Nikon Plan Apo TIRF 100×, 1.45 NA objective, and with 405 and 561 nm laser lines to elicit DAPI (blue) and TRITC (red) fluorescence signals. Z-stacks were collected at optical resolution of 120 nm/pixel with pinhole diameter set to 1 Airy unit and z-step size to 150 nm. All image analyses were performed using NIS-Elements software (Nikon). For mitochondrial morphometric analysis, maximum intensity projections were generated. Analysis was limited to regions of interest at the periphery of cells, where individual mitochondria are readily resolved. Images were thresholded and converted to binary images. Image segmentation was performed on the binary mask, and number and length of discrete features was measured. The statistical significance of the differences between the experimental points was evaluated by Student's t-test.

TRANSMISSION ELECTRON MICROSCOPY

Skin biopsy fragments and melanocytes grown onto uncoated well plates were fixed with 2.5% glutaraldehyde in 0.1 M cacodylate buffer for 2 h and post-fixed with 1% osmium tetroxide. After dehydration, samples were detached with propylene oxide, embedded in Epon812 epoxy resin, and observed with a Philips EM400 electron microscope operated at 100 kV after cutting ultrathin sections. For rotary shadowing electron microscopy analysis, melanocyte-fibroblast co-cultures were incubated with anti-ColVI antibody diluted 1:25 in culture medium at 37°C for 2 h. After several washes with culture medium, samples were incubated with anti-mouse IgG 5 nm gold-conjugated antibody diluted 1:20 in culture medium for 1 h at 37°C. Negative controls were performed in the absence of primary antibody. After immunolabeling cells were fixed with 2.5% glutaraldehyde in 0.1 M cacodylate buffer and 1% osmium tetroxide, dehydrated in ethanol and critical point-dried. Thereafter, the slides were rotary-shadowed with platinum at 45°C and coated with carbon at 90°C in a Balzers BAF 400D Freeze Fracture as previously described (Zhang et al., 2002).

MITOCHONDRIAL MEMBRANE POTENTIAL

Mitochondrial membrane potential was measured based on the accumulation of tetramethylrhodamine methyl ester (TMRM, Molecular Probes) (Angelin et al., 2007). Primary cultures of melanocytes obtained as described above from healthy donors, UCMD, and BM patients were seeded onto 24-mm-diameter round glass coverslips and grown for 2 days in M254 culture medium with HMGS supplement (GIBCO). The medium was then replaced with serum-free M254 medium supplemented with 10 nM TMRM for 30 min, and cellular fluorescence images were acquired with an Olympus IX71/IX51 inverted microscope, equipped with a xenon light source (75 W) for epifluorescence illumination and with a 12-bit digital cooled CCD camera (Micromax, Princeton Instruments). Data were acquired and analyzed using Cell R Software (Olympus). For detection of fluorescence, 568 ± 25 nm band-pass excitation and 585 nm long-pass emission filter settings were used. Images were collected with exposure time of 100 ms using a 40×, 1.3 NA oil immersion objective (Nikon). The extent of cell and hence mitochondrial loading with potentiometric probes is affected by the activity of the plasma membrane multidrug resistance pump. In order to normalize the loading conditions, in all experiments with TMRM the medium was supplemented with 1.6 μM CsH, which inhibits the multidrug resistance pump but not the PTP (Bernardi et al., 1999). At the end of each experiment, mitochondria were fully depolarized by the addition of 4 μM of the protonophore carbonyl cyanide-p-trifluoromethoxyphenyl hydrazone (FCCP). Clusters of several mitochondria were identified as regions of interest, and fields not containing cells were taken as background. Sequential digital images were acquired every 5 min and the average fluorescence intensity of all relevant regions was recorded and stored for subsequent analysis.

OXYGEN CONSUMPTION RATE

Oxygen consumption rate (OCR) was measured with the XF24 Extracellular Flux Analyzer (Seahorse Bioscience, Billerica, MA, USA). Melanocytes were seeded in XF24 cell culture microplates at 6×10^4 cells/well for patient UCMD1 and 13×10^4 cells/well for patients UCMD2 and BM1 (the same cell densities were used for the matched cultures from healthy donors) in 0.2 ml of M254 culture medium with HMGS supplement and incubated at 37°C in 5% CO_2 for 24 h. Experiments were carried out on confluent monolayers. Assay were initiated by replacing the growth medium in each well with 0.67 ml of serum-free M254 prewarmed at 37°C. Cells were incubated at 37°C for 30 min to allow temperature and pH equilibration. A titration with FCCP was performed for each cell type in order to determine the optimal FCCP concentration (i.e., the concentration that stimulates respiration maximally), which was found to be 1 μM for cells from healthy donors, 0.8 μM for patient UCMD1, 0.4–0.6 μM for patient UCMD2, and 0.4 μM for patient BM1. After an OCR baseline was established, 70 μl of a solution containing oligomycin, FCCP, rotenone, or antimycin A were sequentially added to each well to reach final concentrations of 1 μg/ml oligomycin, FCCP as stated above, and 1 μM for rotenone and antimycin A. Data are expressed as pmol of O_2 per minute per 6×10^4 (UCMD1) or 13×10^4 (UCMD2, BM1) cells. At the end of each experiment, the medium was removed from each well and the total protein content per well was quantified. Cells were lysed at 4°C in a buffer composed of 140 mM NaCl, 20 mM Tris-HCl pH 7.4, 5 mM EDTA, 10% glycerol, 1% Triton X-100 (0.1 ml/well) in the presence of phosphatase and protease inhibitors (Sigma). Lysates were then cleared by centrifugation at $13{,}000 \times g$ for 30 min at 4°C, and proteins were quantified using a BCA Protein Assay Kit (Thermo Scientific-Pierce).

RESULTS

MELANOCYTES BIND COLLAGEN VI MICROFILAMENTS

To define their interactions with ColVI, we studied pure cultures of melanocytes from healthy donors in the presence of ascorbic acid, which allows hydroxylation of proline and lysine residues and secretion of ColVI *in vitro* (Colombatti and Bonaldo, 1987). ColVI could not be detected in the ECM or inside the cells (**Figure 1A**, left panel), indicating that melanocytes do not synthesize and secrete this protein. However, when melanocytes were treated with a ColVI-enriched medium obtained from skin fibroblasts (**Figure 1A**, middle panel) or co-cultured with ColVI-producing skin fibroblasts (**Figure 1A**, right panel) a clear association of ColVI with the cell surface was detected. Rotary shadowing immunoelectron microscopic analysis with anti-ColVI antibody

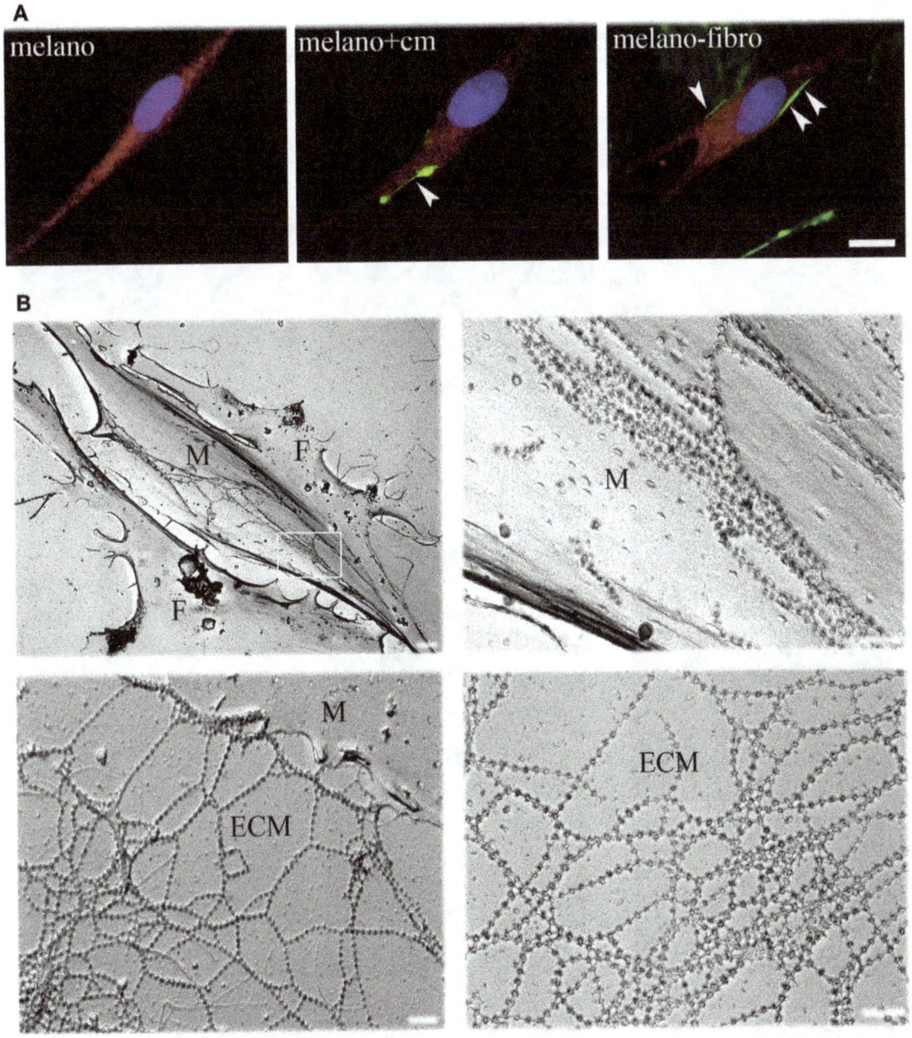

FIGURE 1 | Immunofluorescence analysis and EM rotary shadowing of melanocyte cultures. (A) Double labeling for ColVI (green) and *p*-MEL17 (red) on melanocyte cultures under basal conditions (melano), after treatment with ColVI-enriched medium conditioned by skin fibroblasts (melano + cm), and of melanocytes co-cultured with skin fibroblasts (melano + fibro); scale bar, 10 μm. **(B)** Rotary shadowing electron microscopy analysis of melanocytes co-cultured with fibroblasts. Melanocytes (M, upper left panel) display the typical bipolar shape compared to the flat morphology of fibroblasts (F). Typical ColVI "beaded" microfilaments, identified by 5 nm colloidal gold particles, are visible both at the melanocytes cell surface (top right panel) and in the ECM (bottom panels). Microfilaments formed parallel rows when attached to the cell surface (upper right panel, which is a magnification of the boxed area in the upper left panel), and web-like structures when deposited in the ECM (lower panels). Scale bar, 400 nm.

confirmed the presence of ColVI microfilaments onto the cell membrane of melanocytes (M), which can easily be distinguished from fibroblasts (F) because of their elongated, bipolar shape (**Figure 1B**, upper left panel). Microfilaments displayed the typical "beaded" pattern with a periodicity of 100 nm, and formed parallel rows when attached to the melanocyte cell surface (**Figure 1B**, upper right panel), while they formed web-like structures when deposited in the ECM (**Figure 1B**, lower panels).

MELANOCYTES FROM UCMD AND BM DISPLAY ALTERATIONS OF THE MITOCHONDRIAL NETWORK

Skin biopsies of healthy donors and of UCMD patients were studied by ultrastructural analysis. Mitochondrial changes, including increased size, reduced matrix density, and disrupted cristae consistent with swelling, were frequently found in patients (**Figure 2A**, arrows in middle and right panels), while mitochondria in melanocytes of healthy controls had the expected features (**Figure 2A**, left panel). Occurrence of mitochondrial alterations was also detected in melanocyte cultures obtained from both UCMD and BM patients. The mitochondrial reticulum, as monitored by immunofluorescence analysis of the outer membrane protein Tom20, appeared fragmented along the cytoplasmic extensions as indicated by the presence of a punctate labeling pattern (**Figure 2B**). Ultrastructural analysis showed changes similar to those detected in skin, with mitochondria of irregular size and focal swelling (**Figure 2C**, arrows).

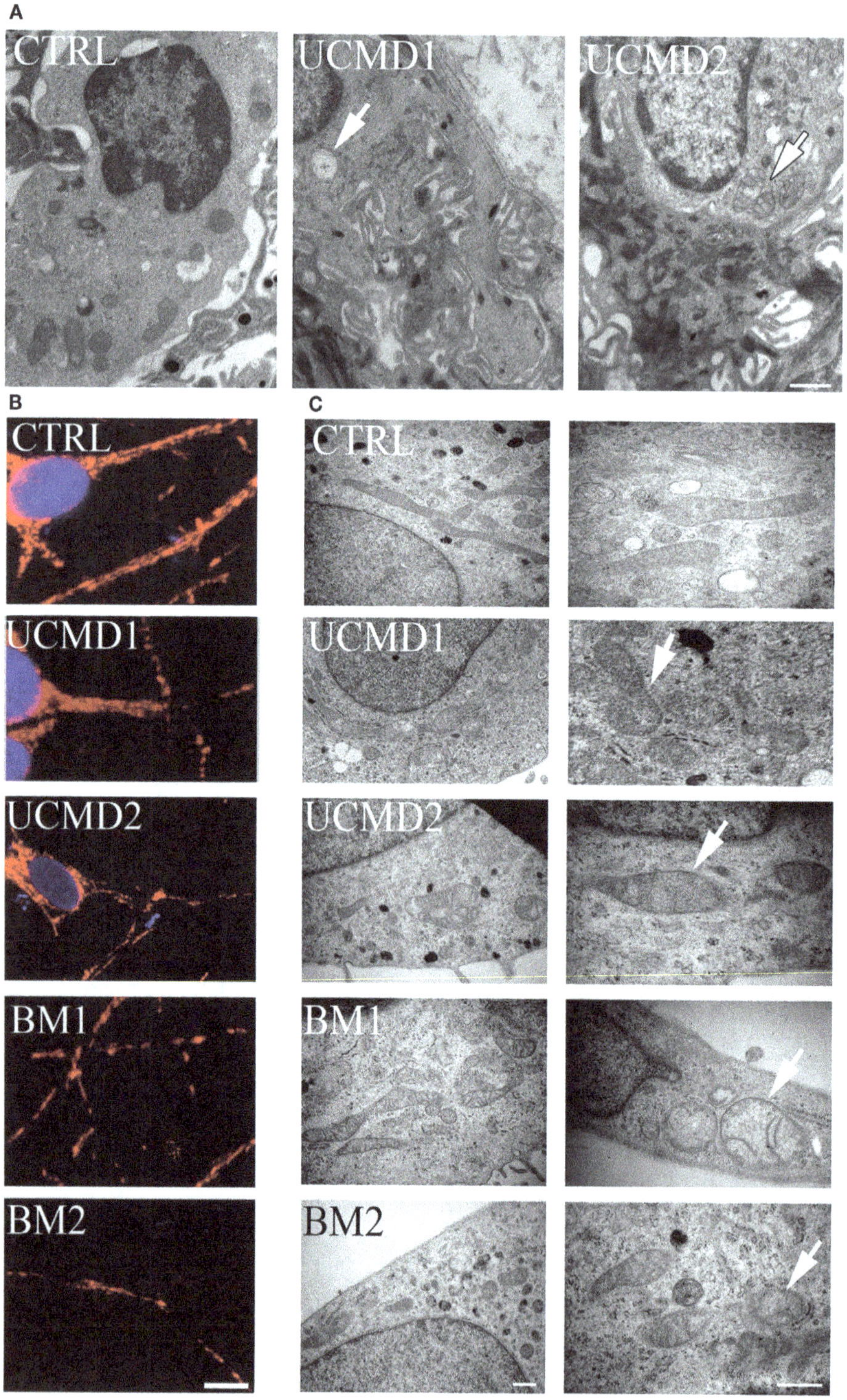

FIGURE 2 | Morphological analysis of skin biopsies and melanocyte cultures. **(A)** Ultrastructural analysis of melanocytes in epon-embedded skin biopsies from healthy donor (CTRL) and patients UCMD1 and UCMD2 showing altered mitochondria (arrows) in patient melanocytes; scale bar, 1 μm. **(B)** Confocal imaging of melanocyte cultures from patients UCMD1, UCMD2, BM1, and BM2 and from healthy donor (CTRL) labeled with an anti-Tom20 antibody. Patient melanocytes display a fragmented and discontinuous mitochondrial network compared to the long and branched pattern of the cells from healthy donor; scale bar, 20 μm. **(C)** Ultrastructural analysis of melanocyte cultures from a healthy donor and patients, showing the presence of enlarged mitochondria with a few cristae (arrows) in all patients; scale bar, 500 nm.

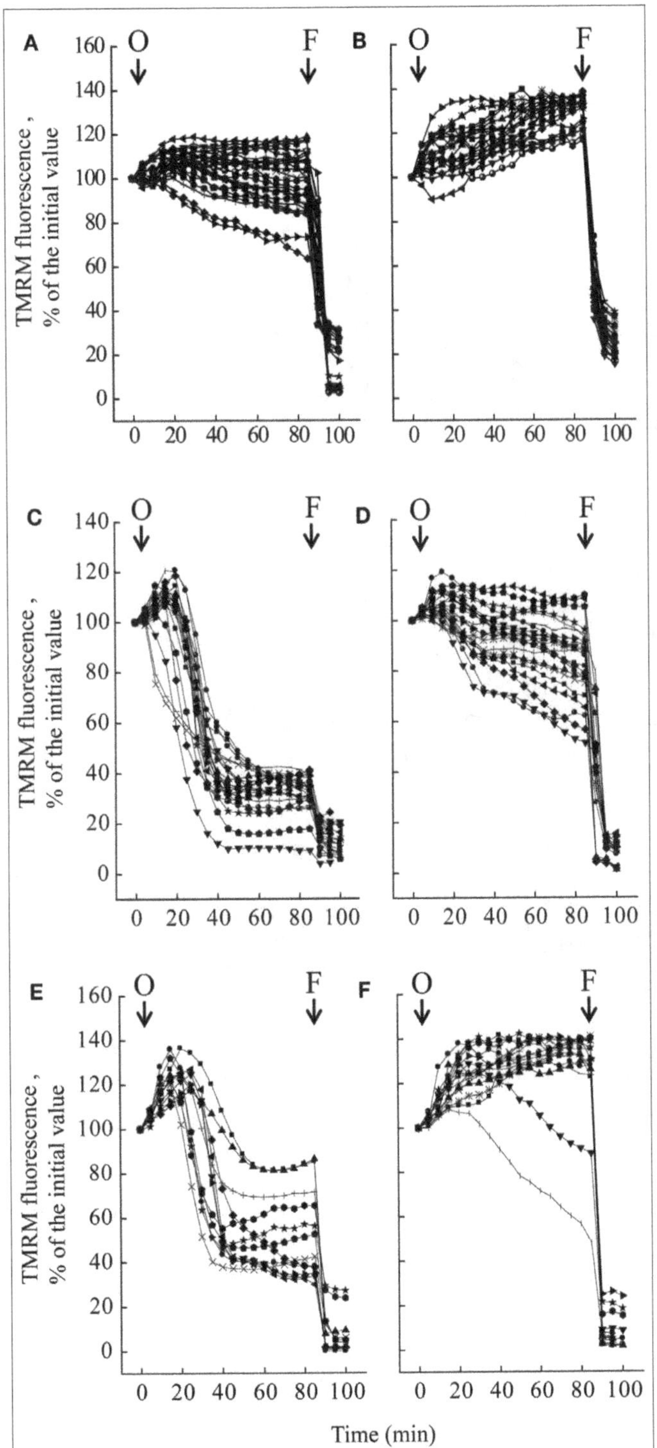

FIGURE 3 | Effect of oligomycin on mitochondrial membrane potential in melanocytes. Melanocytes from one healthy donor **(A,B)**, from patient UCMD2 **(C,D)** and from patient BM1 **(E,F)** were loaded with TMRM and studied by epifluorescence microscopy as described (Pellegrini et al., 2013). Where indicated (arrows), 6 μM oligomycin (O) and 4 μM FCCP (F) were added. In the experiments of **(B,D,F)**, cells had been treated with 0.8 μM NIM811 for 30 min before beginning the recordings. Each line reports mitochondrial fluorescence of one individual cell.

MITOCHONDRIA OF UCMD AND BM MELANOCYTES DISPLAY A LATENT DYSFUNCTION

We studied mitochondrial function in primary cultures of melanocytes obtained from one healthy donor and from patients UCMD2 and BM1. Irrespective of the presence of NIM811, addition of oligomycin to melanocytes from healthy donor was followed by an initial fluorescence increase (i.e., the expected hyperpolarization), which was readily followed by depolarization (i.e., probe release with decreased mitochondrial fluorescence) upon addition of the protonophore FCCP (**Figures 3A,B**). At variance from melanocytes from healthy donor, upon addition of oligomycin melanocytes from patients UCMD2 (**Figure 3C**) and BM1 (**Figure 3E**) underwent rapid mitochondrial depolarization after the initial hyperpolarization. Consistent with a key role of the PTP in onset of depolarization, the response to oligomycin was normalized by the cyclophilin inhibitor NIM811, a CsA analog devoid of immunosuppressive activity that desensitizes the PTP without inhibiting calcineurin (Zulian et al., 2014) (**Figures 3D,F**). Treatment with NIM811 normalized mitochondrial morphology of UCMD1, UCMD2, and BM1, improving the mitochondrial reticulum extension as indicated by increased mitochondrial length (**Figures 4A,B**). Ultrastructural analysis confirmed that treatment with NIM811 restored mitochondrial matrix density and cristae organization in patient melanocytes (**Figure 4C**), without affecting mitochondria of melanocytes from the healthy patient (**Figures 4B,C**). It should be noted that NIM811 inhibits all CyP isoforms, and that an isoform-selective inhibitor is only available for CyPA (Daum et al., 2009); yet, since mitochondria lack other Cs-binding proteins (Nicolli et al., 1996), we conclude that the mitochondrial effects of NIM811 are mediated by inhibition of CyPD. Taken together, these results demonstrate that UCMD and BM melanocytes display the same PTP-dependent latent mitochondrial dysfunction previously identified in primary muscle-derived cell cultures from *Col6a1*$^{-/-}$ mice (Irwin et al., 2003), UCMD and BM patients (Angelin et al., 2007), and zebrafish with ColVI myopathy (Telfer et al., 2010; Zulian et al., 2014).

MITOCHONDRIAL RESPIRATORY RESERVE CAPACITY IS DECREASED IN MELANOCYTE CULTURES FROM UCMD AND BM PATIENTS

We measured the OCR of primary cultures of melanocytes from UCMD and BM patients with the sensitive Seahorse technology (Wu et al., 2007). Basal respiration largely reflects mitochondrial oxygen consumption, which in aerobic, non-transformed cells fulfills the needs for ATP synthesis; addition of oligomycin inhibits the F-ATP synthase, and therefore, "removes" the fraction of respiration linked to ATP synthesis. Inspection of the response of melanocytes from healthy donors (**Figures 5A–C**, closed circles) reveals that a large fraction of the basal OCR is linked to ATP synthesis, as shown by the inhibitory effect of oligomycin (residual oxygen consumption is non-mitochondrial, see below). Melanocytes could be stimulated well above the basal respiratory level by addition of the protonophore FCCP, which stimulates respiration maximally, demonstrating that they have a large respiratory reserve (the difference between OCR after the addition of FCCP and basal OCR). Addition of rotenone (selective inhibitor of respiratory complex I) almost completely inhibited the OCR,

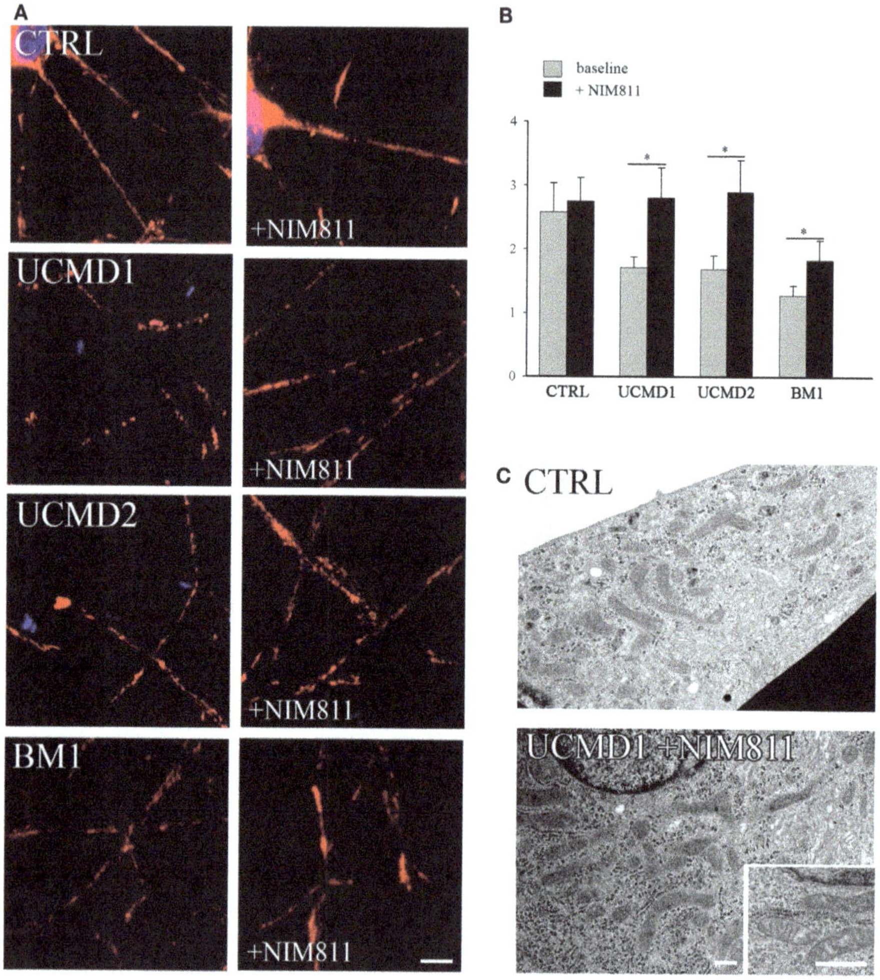

FIGURE 4 | Effect of NIM811 on mitochondrial morphology. **(A)** Melanocytes from a healthy donor, and from UCMD1, UCMD2, and BM1 patients were treated with 0.8 μM NIM811 for 2 h and labeled with anti-Tom20 antibody. Scale bar, 5 μm. **(B)** Mitochondrial length (μm) was quantified and is reported as mean ± SEM; *t*-test; $^{*}P < 0.05$; **(C)** Ultrastructural analysis of melanocytes from a healthy donor (CTRL) and patient UCMD1 (representative of all patients), after treatment with NIM811 (UCMD1 + NIM811). Scale bar, 300 nm.

no further decrease being seen with the addition of antimycin A (selective inhibitor of complex III). Finally, NIM811 had no effect in the response of melanocytes from healthy donors to oligomycin, FCCP, rotenone, and antimycin A (**Figures 5B,C** closed triangles). Melanocytes from patients UCMD1, UCMD2, and BM1 displayed a marked decrease of the respiratory reserve, which became apparent after the addition of FCCP (open circles in **Figures 5A–C**, respectively). In patient BM1, maximal respiration was partially restored by NIM811 but the effect was not statistically significant (**Figure 5C**). Thus, assessing whether the lower respiratory activity of melanocytes from patients depends on PTP opening will require further work. We also tested the effect of FCCP on basal respiration (i.e., in the absence of oligomycin) with identical results (data not shown). The statistical analysis of these experiments is presented in **Figures 5A'–C'**. Resting ATP levels were not altered in melanocytes from ColVI patients (results not shown), as also observed in myoblast cultures (Angelin et al., 2008). These findings, which match the maintenance of a normal mitochondrial membrane potential under resting conditions, are consistent with a latent rather than overt mitochondrial dysfunction in cultured melanocytes from the patients.

DISCUSSION

Epidermal melanocytes interact with the underlying ECM of derma via the DEJ, a specialized adhesion structure consisting of ECM components that include ColVI (Sabatelli et al., 2011). Adhesion of melanocytes to the DEJ involves components common to the muscle cell sarcolemma. Like muscle cells, melanocytes express mDp427 dystrophin (Pellegrini et al., 2013), which bridges the cytoskeleton and the ECM through α, β dystroglycan (Herzog et al., 2004) and the α2 chain of laminin (Sewry et al., 1996). In addition, the DEJ basement membrane is enriched in ColVI, which includes the α5 and α6 chains (Sabatelli et al., 2011) as also recently shown for the endomysium of human muscle (Sabatelli et al., 2012a). ColVI microfilament organization is influenced by the interactions of ColVI with its binding partners (Wiberg et al.,

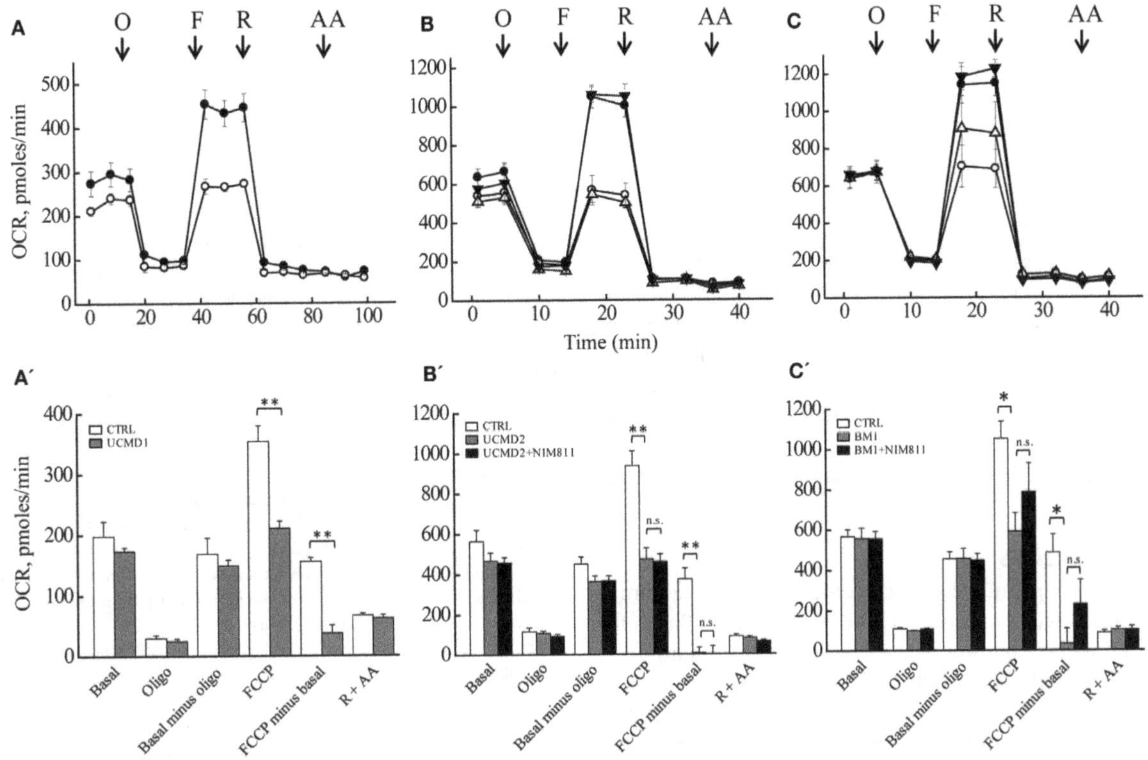

FIGURE 5 | Oxygen consumption rate of melanocytes. OCR of melanocytes from a healthy donor (closed circles in all panels), of patients (open circles in all panels) UCMD1 **(A)**, UCMD2 **(B)**, and BM1 **(C)** was measured in 24-well Seahorse plates [60,000 cells/well for **(A)** and 130,000 cells/well for **(B,C)**]. Where indicated (arrows) 1 μg/ml oligomycin (O), FCCP as detailed in Section "Materials and Methods" (F), 1 μM rotenone (R), and 1 μM antimycin A (AA) were added. In **(B,C)**, triangles report respiration of melanocytes from healthy donor (closed symbols) or UCMD2 and BM1 patients (open symbols) treated with 0.8 μM NIM811 1 h before beginning the recording. Data in each panel are mean of at least four independent determinations in triplicate ± SEM. **(A′–C′)** OCR before (Basal) and after the sequential addition of oligomycin (Oligo), FCCP, rotenone, and antimycin A. Data were analyzed with ANOVA. $*P < 0.05$; $**P < 0.005$; n.s., not significant.

2002). Our findings demonstrate that, like myoblasts (Zou et al., 2008; Sabatelli et al., 2012b), melanocytes do not produce ColVI, yet they bind the protein at the cell surface (Kawahara et al., 2008). Melanocytes do express NG2 proteoglycan (results not shown), which acts as a ColVI receptor (Campoli et al., 2010) together with integrins (Pfaff et al., 1993; Zambruno et al., 1993). The pattern of melanocyte surface labeling with ColVI microfibrils is consistent with receptor-mediated interactions. Interestingly, lack of ColVI affects melanocyte mitochondria in the same way as it affects mitochondria in skeletal muscle, suggesting that this ECM protein exerts a trophic role in the skin as well, consistent with the lesions detected in UCMD and BM patients (Lampe and Bushby, 2005). Indeed, UCMD and BM melanocytes display the same PTP-dependent latent mitochondrial dysfunction previously identified in primary muscle-derived cell cultures from *Col6a1*$^{-/-}$ mice (Irwin et al., 2003), UCMD and BM patients (Angelin et al., 2007), and zebrafish with ColVI myopathy (Zulian et al., 2014) that manifests itself as an oligomycin-induced depolarization. We have interpreted oligomycin-induced depolarization as a secondary event following mitochondrial Ca^{2+} overload; this would be a consequence of decreased activity of ATP-dependent Ca^{2+} pumps, resulting in cytosolic Ca^{2+} overload because of decreased Ca^{2+} extrusion at the plasma membrane and decreased Ca^{2+} uptake from the endo-sarcoplasmic reticulum (Angelin et al., 2008).

The reason why maximal respiration is decreased in melanocytes from ColVI muscular dystrophy patients is not easy to dissect in intact cells, but prominent possibilities are increased cytochrome *c* release through both PTP-dependent and -independent mechanisms (Clerc et al., 2012), and PTP-dependent pyridine nucleotide depletion (Vinogradov et al., 1972; Di Lisa et al., 2001). Short openings of the PTP that cannot be detected by TMRM redistribution do take place in isolated mitochondria (Hüser et al., 1998; Hüser and Blatter, 1999) and have also been documented *in situ* (Petronilli et al., 1999). The PTP open time can be increased by Ca^{2+} overload synergistically with arachidonic acid produced by activation of $cPLA_2$ (Petronilli et al., 2001; Scorrano et al., 2001; Penzo et al., 2004) leading to cytochrome *c* release (Petronilli et al., 2001), depletion of matrix pyridine nucleotides (Di Lisa et al., 2001), and respiratory inhibition (Vinogradov et al., 1972). Since we found ultrastructural and functional alterations of mitochondria compatible with increased PTP opening in melanocytes from UCMD and BM patients, we suspect that PTP opening is responsible for decreased maximal respiratory capacity as well. Some support for this interpretation comes from the partial restoration of respiration in patient BM1 after treatment with the cyclophilin inhibitor NIM811, which desensitizes the PTP.

The present results show that skin melanocytes from UCMD and BM patients faithfully reproduce the mitochondrial dysfunction and ultrastructural alterations that characterize myoblasts and myofibers from the same patients (Merlini and Bernardi, 2008). These findings may also help to understand the pathogenesis of the skin lesions in patients affected by ColVI muscular dystrophies, and closely match recent results on melanocytes derived from a patient affected by Duchenne muscular dystrophy (Pellegrini et al., 2013). Taken together, our results suggest that melanocytes can become a useful tool to study and monitor other muscle diseases as well, and that skin biopsies may represent a convenient and minimally invasive alternative procedure to monitor muscle genetic diseases and to assess potential therapies *ex vivo*.

ACKNOWLEDGMENTS

We thank Dr. Stefano Squarzoni for the rotary shadowing immunoelectron microscope experiment, and Novartis AG (Basel) for providing NIM811. Funding sources: This work was supported by TELETHON Italy (GUP11007 to Luciano Merlini, Patrizia Sabatelli, and Nadir Mario Maraldi and GGP11082 to Nadir Mario Maraldi and Paolo Bernardi), FIRB 2010 RBAP10KCNS and "5 per mille" 2011 Rizzoli Orthopaedic Institute.

REFERENCES

Angelin, A., Bonaldo, P., and Bernardi, P. (2008). Altered threshold of the mitochondrial permeability transition pore in Ullrich congenital muscular dystrophy. *Biochim. Biophys. Acta* 1777, 893–896. doi:10.1016/j.bbabio.2008.03.026

Angelin, A., Tiepolo, T., Sabatelli, P., Grumati, P., Bergamin, N., Golfieri, C., et al. (2007). Mitochondrial dysfunction in the pathogenesis of Ullrich congenital muscular dystrophy and prospective therapy with cyclosporins. *Proc. Natl. Acad. Sci. U.S.A.* 104, 991–996. doi:10.1073/pnas.0610270104

Bernardi, P. (2013). The mitochondrial permeability transition pore: a mystery solved? *Front. Physiol.* 4:95. doi:10.3389/fphys.2013.00095

Bernardi, P., Scorrano, L., Colonna, R., Petronilli, V., and Di Lisa, F. (1999). Mitochondria and cell death. Mechanistic aspects and methodological issues. *Eur. J. Biochem.* 264, 687–701. doi:10.1046/j.1432-1327.1999.00725.x

Bertini, E., and Pepe, G. (2002). Collagen type VI and related disorders: Bethlem myopathy and Ullrich scleroatonic muscular dystrophy. *Eur. J. Paediatr. Neurol.* 6, 193–198. doi:10.1053/ejpn.2002.0593

Bethlem, J., and Wijngaarden, G. K. (1976). Benign myopathy, with autosomal dominant inheritance. A report on three pedigrees. *Brain* 99, 91–100. doi:10.1093/brain/99.1.91

Camacho Vanegas, O., Bertini, E., Zhang, R. Z., Petrini, S., Minosse, C., Sabatelli, P., et al. (2001). Ullrich scleroatonic muscular dystrophy is caused by recessive mutations in collagen type VI. *Proc. Natl. Acad. Sci. U.S.A.* 98, 7516–7521. doi:10.1073/pnas.121027598

Campoli, M., Ferrone, S., and Wang, X. (2010). Functional and clinical relevance of chondroitin sulfate proteoglycan 4. *Adv. Cancer Res.* 109, 73–121. doi:10.1016/B978-0-12-380890-5.00003-X

Clerc, P., Carey, G. B., Mehrabian, Z., Wei, M., Hwang, H., Girnun, G. D., et al. (2012). Rapid detection of an ABT-737-sensitive primed for death state in cells using microplate-based respirometry. *PLoS ONE* 7:e42487. doi:10.1371/journal.pone.0042487

Colombatti, A., and Bonaldo, P. (1987). Biosynthesis of chick type VI collagen. II. Processing and secretion in fibroblasts and smooth muscle cells. *J. Biol. Chem.* 262, 14461–14466.

Daum, S., Schumann, M., Mathea, S., Aumuller, T., Balsley, M. A., Constant, S. L., et al. (2009). Isoform-specific inhibition of cyclophilins. *Biochemistry* 48, 6268–6277. doi:10.1021/bi9007287

Di Lisa, F., Menabò, R., Canton, M., Barile, M., and Bernardi, P. (2001). Opening of the mitochondrial permeability transition pore causes depletion of mitochondrial and cytosolic NAD^+ and is a causative event in the death of myocytes in postischemic reperfusion of the heart. *J. Biol. Chem.* 276, 2571–2575. doi:10.1074/jbc.M006825200

Gao, F. L., Jin, R., Zhang, L., and Zhang, Y. G. (2013). The contribution of melanocytes to pathological scar formation during wound healing. *Int. J. Clin. Exp. Med.* 6, 609–613.

Gara, S. K., Grumati, P., Urciuolo, A., Bonaldo, P., Kobbe, B., Koch, M., et al. (2008). Three novel collagen VI chains with high homology to the alpha3 chain. *J. Biol. Chem.* 283, 10658–10670. doi:10.1074/jbc.M709540200

Giorgio, V., von Stockum, S., Antoniel, M., Fabbro, A., Fogolari, F., Forte, M., et al. (2013). Dimers of mitochondrial ATP synthase form the permeability transition pore. *Proc. Natl. Acad. Sci. U.S.A.* 110, 5887–5892. doi:10.1073/pnas.1217823110

Grumati, P., Coletto, L., Sabatelli, P., Cescon, M., Angelin, A., Bertaggia, E., et al. (2010). Autophagy is defective in collagen VI muscular dystrophies, and its reactivation rescues myofiber degeneration. *Nat. Med.* 16, 1313–1320. doi:10.1038/nm.2247

Herzog, C., Has, C., Franzke, C. W., Echtermeyer, F. G., Schlötzer-Schrehardt, U., Kröger, S., et al. (2004). Dystroglycan in skin and cutaneous cells: beta-subunit is shed from the cell surface. *J. Invest. Dermatol.* 122, 1372–1380. doi:10.1111/j.0022-202X.2004.22605.x

Hüser, J., and Blatter, L. A. (1999). Fluctuations in mitochondrial membrane potential caused by repetitive gating of the permeability transition pore. *Biochem. J.* 343(Pt 2), 311–317. doi:10.1042/0264-6021:3430311

Hüser, J., Rechenmacher, C. E., and Blatter, L. A. (1998). Imaging the permeability pore transition in single mitochondria. *Biophys. J.* 74, 2129–2137. doi:10.1016/S0006-3495(98)77920-2

Irwin, W. A., Bergamin, N., Sabatelli, P., Reggiani, C., Megighian, A., Merlini, L., et al. (2003). Mitochondrial dysfunction and apoptosis in myopathic mice with collagen VI deficiency. *Nat. Genet.* 35, 267–271. doi:10.1038/ng1270

Jöbsis, G. J., Boers, J. M., Barth, P. G., and de Visser, M. (1999). Bethlem myopathy: a slowly progressive congenital muscular dystrophy with contractures. *Brain* 122(Pt 4), 649–655. doi:10.1093/brain/122.4.649

Kawahara, G., Ogawa, M., Okada, M., Malicdan, M. C., Goto, Y., Hayashi, Y. K., et al. (2008). Diminished binding of mutated collagen VI to the extracellular matrix surrounding myocytes. *Muscle Nerve* 38, 1192–1195. doi:10.1002/mus.21030

Kuo, H. J., Maslen, C. L., Keene, D. R., and Glanville, R. W. (1997). Type VI collagen anchors endothelial basement membranes by interacting with type IV collagen. *J. Biol. Chem.* 272, 26522–26529. doi:10.1074/jbc.272.42.26522

Lampe, A. K., and Bushby, K. M. (2005). Collagen VI related muscle disorders. *J. Med. Genet.* 42, 673–685. doi:10.1136/jmg.2002.002311

Menazza, S., Blaauw, B., Tiepolo, T., Toniolo, L., Braghetta, P., Spolaore, B., et al. (2010). Oxidative stress by monoamine oxidases is causally involved in myofiber damage in muscular dystrophy. *Hum. Mol. Genet.* 19, 4207–4215. doi:10.1093/hmg/ddq339

Merlini, L., Angelin, A., Tiepolo, T., Braghetta, P., Sabatelli, P., Zamparelli, A., et al. (2008a). Cyclosporin A corrects mitochondrial dysfunction and muscle apoptosis in patients with collagen VI myopathies. *Proc. Natl. Acad. Sci. U.S.A.* 105, 5225–5229. doi:10.1073/pnas.0800962105

Merlini, L., Martoni, E., Grumati, P., Sabatelli, P., Squarzoni, S., Urciuolo, A., et al. (2008b). Autosomal recessive myosclerosis myopathy is a collagen VI disorder. *Neurology* 71, 1245–1253. doi:10.1212/01.wnl.0000327611.01687.5e

Merlini, L., and Bernardi, P. (2008). Therapy of collagen VI-related myopathies (Bethlem and Ullrich). *Neurotherapeutics* 5, 613–618. doi:10.1016/j.nurt.2008.08.004

Merlini, L., Morandi, L., Granata, C., and Ballestrazzi, A. (1994). Bethlem myopathy: early-onset benign autosomal dominant myopathy with contractures. Description of two new families. *Neuromuscul. Disord.* 4, 503–511. doi:10.1016/0960-8966(94)90091-4

Millay, D. P., Sargent, M. A., Osinska, H., Baines, C. P., Barton, E. R., Vuagniaux, G., et al. (2008). Genetic and pharmacologic inhibition of mitochondrial-dependent necrosis attenuates muscular dystrophy. *Nat. Med.* 14, 442–447. doi:10.1038/nm1736

Nicolli, A., Basso, E., Petronilli, V., Wenger, R. M., and Bernardi, P. (1996). Interactions of cyclophilin with the mitochondrial inner membrane and regulation of the permeability transition pore, a cyclosporin A-sensitive channel. *J. Biol. Chem.* 271, 2185–2192. doi:10.1074/jbc.271.4.2185

Pellegrini, C., Zulian, A., Gualandi, F., Manzati, E., Merlini, L., Michelini, M. E., et al. (2013). Melanocytes-A novel tool to study mitochondrial dysfunction in Duchenne muscular dystrophy. *J. Cell Physiol.* 228, 1323–1331. doi:10.1002/jcp.24290

Penzo, D., Petronilli, V., Angelin, A., Cusan, C., Colonna, R., Scorrano, L., et al. (2004). Arachidonic acid released by phospholipase A2 activation triggers Ca^{2+}-dependent apoptosis through the mitochondrial pathway. *J. Biol. Chem.* 279, 25219–25225. doi:10.1074/jbc.M310381200

Pepe, G., Bertini, E., Bonaldo, P., Bushby, K., Giusti, B., de Visser, M., et al. (2002). Bethlem myopathy (BETHLEM) and Ullrich scleroatonic muscular dystrophy: 100th ENMC international workshop, 23-24 November 2001, Naarden, The Netherlands. *Neuromuscul. Disord.* 12, 984–993. doi:10.1016/S0960-8966(02)00139-6

Petronilli, V., Miotto, G., Canton, M., Brini, M., Colonna, R., Bernardi, P., et al. (1999). Transient and long-lasting openings of the mitochondrial permeability transition pore can be monitored directly in intact cells by changes in mitochondrial calcein fluorescence. *Biophys. J.* 76, 725–734. doi:10.1016/S0006-3495(99)77239-5

Petronilli, V., Penzo, D., Scorrano, L., Bernardi, P., and Di Lisa, F. (2001). The mitochondrial permeability transition, release of cytochrome c and cell death. Correlation with the duration of pore openings in situ. *J. Biol. Chem.* 276, 12030–12034. doi:10.1074/jbc.M010604200

Pfaff, M., Aumailley, M., Specks, U., Knolle, J., Zerwes, H. G., and Timpl, R. (1993). Integrin and Arg-Gly-Asp dependence of cell adhesion to the native and unfolded triple helix of collagen type VI. *Exp. Cell Res.* 206, 167–176. doi:10.1006/excr.1993.1134

Pinon, P., and Wehrle-Haller, B. (2011). Integrins: versatile receptors controlling melanocyte adhesion, migration and proliferation. *Pigment Cell Melanoma Res.* 24, 282–294. doi:10.1111/j.1755-148X.2010.00806.x

Reutenauer, J., Dorchies, O. M., Patthey-Vuadens, O., Vuagniaux, G., and Ruegg, U. T. (2008). Investigation of Debio 025, a cyclophilin inhibitor, in the dystrophic mdx mouse, a model for Duchenne muscular dystrophy. *Br. J. Pharmacol* 155, 574–584. doi:10.1038/bjp.2008.285

Sabatelli, P., Gara, S. K., Grumati, P., Urciuolo, A., Gualandi, F., Curci, R., et al. (2011). Expression of the collagen VI alpha5 and alpha6 chains in normal human skin and in skin of patients with collagen VI-related myopathies. *J. Invest. Dermatol.* 131, 99–107. doi:10.1038/jid.2010.284

Sabatelli, P., Gualandi, F., Gara, S. K., Grumati, P., Zamparelli, A., Martoni, E., et al. (2012a). Expression of collagen VI alpha5 and alpha6 chains in human muscle and in Duchenne muscular dystrophy-related muscle fibrosis. *Matrix Biol.* 31, 187–196. doi:10.1016/j.matbio.2011.12.003

Sabatelli, P., Palma, E., Angelin, A., Squarzoni, S., Urciuolo, A., Pellegrini, C., et al. (2012b). Critical evaluation of the use of cell cultures for inclusion in clinical trials of patients affected by collagen VI myopathies. *J. Cell. Physiol.* 227, 2927–2935. doi:10.1002/jcp.23039

Santiago-Walker, A., Li, L., Haass, N. K., and Herlyn, M. (2009). Melanocytes: from morphology to application. *Skin Pharmacol. Physiol.* 22, 114–121. doi:10.1159/000178870

Scorrano, L., Penzo, D., Petronilli, V., Pagano, F., and Bernardi, P. (2001). Arachidonic acid causes cell death through the mitochondrial permeability transition. Implications for tumor necrosis factor-α apoptotic signaling. *J. Biol. Chem.* 276, 12035–12040. doi:10.1074/jbc.M010603200

Sewry, C. A., Philpot, J., Sorokin, L. M., Wilson, L. A., Naom, I., Goodwin, F., et al. (1996). Diagnosis of merosin (laminin-2) deficient congenital muscular dystrophy by skin biopsy. *Lancet* 347, 582–584. doi:10.1016/S0140-6736(96)91274-X

Sorato, E., Menazza, S., Zulian, A., Sabatelli, P., Gualandi, F., Merlini, L., et al. (2014). Monoamine oxidase inhibition prevents mitochondrial dysfunction and apoptosis in myoblasts from patients with collagen VI myopathies. *Free Radic. Biol. Med.* 75C, 40–47. doi:10.1016/j.freeradbiomed.2014.07.006

Tagliavini, F., Pellegrini, C., Sardone, F., Squarzoni, S., Paulsson, M., Wagener, R., et al. (2014). Defective collagen VI alpha6 chain expression in the skeletal muscle of patients with collagen VI-related myopathies. *Biochim. Biophys. Acta* 1842, 1604–1612. doi:10.1016/j.bbadis.2014.05.033

Telfer, W. R., Busta, A. S., Bonnemann, C. G., Feldman, E. L., and Dowling, J. J. (2010). Zebrafish models of collagen VI-related myopathies. *Hum. Mol. Genet.* 19, 2433–2444. doi:10.1093/hmg/ddq126

Tiepolo, T., Angelin, A., Palma, E., Sabatelli, P., Merlini, L., Nicolosi, L., et al. (2009). The cyclophilin inhibitor Debio 025 normalizes mitochondrial function, muscle apoptosis and ultrastructural defects in *Col6a1*$^{-/-}$ myopathic mice. *Br. J. Pharmacol.* 157, 1045–1052. doi:10.1111/j.1476-5381.2009.00316.x

Ullrich, O. (1930). Kongenitale, atonisch-sklerotische Muskeldystrophie, ein weiterer Typus der heredodegenerativen Erkrankungen des neuromuskulaeren Systems. *Z. Ges. Neurol. Psychiatr.* 126, 171–201. doi:10.1007/BF02864097

Vinogradov, A., Scarpa, A., and Chance, B. (1972). Calcium and pyridine nucleotide interaction in mitochondrial membranes. *Arch. Biochem. Biophys.* 152, 646–654. doi:10.1016/0003-9861(72)90261-5

Wiberg, C., Heinegård, D., Wenglén, C., Timpl, R., and Mörgelin, M. (2002). Biglycan organizes collagen VI into hexagonal-like networks resembling tissue structures. *J. Biol. Chem.* 277, 49120–49126. doi:10.1074/jbc.M206891200

Wissing, E. R., Millay, D. P., Vuagniaux, G., and Molkentin, J. D. (2010). Debio-025 is more effective than prednisone in reducing muscular pathology in mdx mice. *Neuromuscul. Disord.* 20, 753–760. doi:10.1016/j.nmd.2010.06.016

Wu, M., Neilson, A., Swift, A. L., Moran, R., Tamagnine, J., Parslow, D., et al. (2007). Multiparameter metabolic analysis reveals a close link between attenuated mitochondrial bioenergetic function and enhanced glycolysis dependency in human tumor cells. *Am. J. Physiol. Cell Physiol.* 292, C125–C136. doi:10.1152/ajpcell.00247.2006

Zambruno, G., Marchisio, P. C., Melchiori, A., Bondanza, S., Cancedda, R., and De Luca, M. (1993). Expression of integrin receptors and their role in adhesion, spreading and migration of normal human melanocytes. *J. Cell Sci.* 105(Pt 1), 179–190.

Zhang, R. Z., Sabatelli, P., Pan, T. C., Squarzoni, S., Mattioli, E., Bertini, E., et al. (2002). Effects on collagen VI mRNA stability and microfibrillar assembly of three COL6A2 mutations in two families with Ullrich congenital muscular dystrophy. *J. Biol. Chem.* 277, 43557–43564. doi:10.1074/jbc.M207696200

Zou, Y., Zhang, R. Z., Sabatelli, P., Chu, M. L., and Bonnemann, C. G. (2008). Muscle interstitial fibroblasts are the main source of collagen VI synthesis in skeletal muscle: implications for congenital muscular dystrophy types Ullrich and Bethlem. *J. Neuropathol. Exp. Neurol.* 67, 144–154. doi:10.1097/nen.0b013e3181634ef7

Zulian, A., Rizzo, E., Schiavone, M., Palma, E., Tagliavini, F., Blaauw, B., et al. (2014). NIM811, a cyclophilin inhibitor without immunosuppressive activity, is beneficial in collagen VI congenital muscular dystrophy models. *Hum. Mol. Genet.* 23, 5353–5363. doi:10.1093/hmg/ddu254

12

Electrical stimulation counteracts muscle decline in seniors

Helmut Kern[1,2†], Laura Barberi[3†], Stefan Löfler[2], Simona Sbardella[3], Samantha Burggraf[2], Hannah Fruhmann[2], Ugo Carraro[2,4], Simone Mosole[2,4], Nejc Sarabon[5], Michael Vogelauer[1], Winfried Mayr[6], Matthias Krenn[6], Jan Cvecka[7], Vanina Romanello[8], Laura Pietrangelo[9], Feliciano Protasi[9], Marco Sandri[8], Sandra Zampieri[2,10] and Antonio Musaro[3,10]*

[1] *Institute of Physical Medicine and Rehabilitation, Wilhelminenspital, Vienna, Austria*
[2] *Ludwig Boltzmann Institute of Electrical Stimulation and Physical Rehabilitation, Vienna, Austria*
[3] *DAHFMO-Unit of Histology and Medical Embryology, Institute Pasteur Cenci-Bolognetti, IIM, Sapienza University of Rome, Rome, Italy*
[4] *Laboratory of Translation Myology, Department of Biomedical Sciences, University of Padova, Padova, Italy*
[5] *Science and Research Centre, Institute for Kinesiology Research, University of Primorska, Koper, Slovenia*
[6] *Center of Medical Physics and Biomedical Engineering, Medical University of Vienna, Vienna, Austria*
[7] *Faculty of Physical Education and Sport, Comenius University, Bratislava, Slovakia*
[8] *Dulbecco Telethon Institute at Venetian Institute of Molecular Medicine, Padova, Italy*
[9] *CeSI-Center for Research on Aging & DNICS – Department of Neuroscience, Imaging and Clinical Sciences, University G. d'Annunzio of Chieti, Chieti, Italy*
[10] *Center for Life Nano Science@Sapienza, Istituto Italiano di Tecnologia, Rome, Italy*

Correspondence:
Antonio Musaro, Unit of Histology and Medical Embryology, Via A. Scarpa 14, Rome 00161, Italy
e-mail: antonio.musaro@uniroma1.it

† Helmut Kern and Laura Barberi have contributed equally to this work.

The loss in muscle mass coupled with a decrease in specific force and shift in fiber composition are hallmarks of aging. Training and regular exercise attenuate the signs of sarcopenia. However, pathologic conditions limit the ability to perform physical exercise. We addressed whether electrical stimulation (ES) is an alternative intervention to improve muscle recovery and defined the molecular mechanism associated with improvement in muscle structure and function. We analyzed, at functional, structural, and molecular level, the effects of ES training on healthy seniors with normal life style, without routine sport activity. ES was able to improve muscle torque and functional performances of seniors and increased the size of fast muscle fibers. At molecular level, ES induced up-regulation of IGF-1 and modulation of MuRF-1, a muscle-specific atrophy-related gene. ES also induced up-regulation of relevant markers of differentiating satellite cells and of extracellular matrix remodeling, which might guarantee shape and mechanical forces of trained skeletal muscle as well as maintenance of satellite cell function, reducing fibrosis. Our data provide evidence that ES is a safe method to counteract muscle decline associated with aging.

Keywords: electrical stimulation, aging, muscle performance, muscle atrophy, IGF-1, extracellular matrix, satellite cells, microRNA

INTRODUCTION

There is considerable clinical interest in therapeutic strategies to counteract muscle wasting associated with aging.

Skeletal muscle is particularly susceptible to the effects of aging, undergoing a steady reduction in function and losing up to a third of its mass and strength. This decline in functional performance is due to an overall decrease in muscle integrity, as fibrosis and fat accumulation replace functional contractile tissue, and to loss of the fastest most powerful fibers (Scicchitano et al., 2009; Vinciguerra et al., 2010).

At present, it is clear that the most efficient method that has been used to counteract age-related muscle weakness is long term physical exercise (Paffenbarger et al., 1994). Physical exercise increases protein synthesis, turnover and satellite cell number, stimulates appetite, increases IGF-1 expression levels, and capillary bed density. We recently reported that physical exercise in seniors preserves muscle morphology and ultrastructure, guarantees a greater maximal isometric force and function, and modulates the expression of genes related to autophagy and reactive oxygen species detoxification (Mosole et al., 2014; Zampieri et al., 2014). Nevertheless, certain pathologic conditions and aging limit the effectiveness of exercise and, therefore, the benefits from it.

An alternative effective intervention to improve muscle recovery is electrical stimulation (ES) (Quittan et al., 2001; Nuhr et al., 2004; Bax et al., 2005; Strasser et al., 2009). ES has been used in clinical settings for rehabilitation purposes, as an alternative therapeutic approach to counteract neuromuscular disability, as well as for muscle strengthening and maintenance of muscle mass in seniors (Maddocks et al., 2013). In addition, there are studies showing that patients with knee osteoarthritis can benefit from the use of ES alone or as an adjunct therapy (Rosemffet et al., 2004; Levine et al., 2013). ES directly stimulates skeletal muscle protein synthesis rates (Wall et al., 2012). Although controversial results have been published as consequence of varying protocols (e.g., training 3–7 times a week, training period from 3–12 weeks) and stimulation parameters (e.g., stimulation duration 2–30 s, stimulation frequency 8–80 Hz) (Giggins et al., 2012; de Oliveira Melo et al., 2013), ES represents a promising adjuvant treatment to attenuate muscle disability. Nevertheless, the molecular mechanisms by which ES exerts its specific anabolic effects on skeletal muscle remain to be elucidated.

Based on our documented clinical experience on the use of ES to rescue permanently denervated skeletal muscles in paraplegics (Kern et al., 2004, 2008, 2010; Ashley et al., 2007; Boncompagni et al., 2007), we verified whether ES can be proposed as a therapeutic tool to rehabilitate skeletal muscle of sedentary seniors.

We demonstrated that ES mimics the beneficial effects of physical exercise in muscle of aging individuals and we defined the molecular signature underlying these effects.

MATERIALS AND METHODS

SUBJECTS ENROLLED IN THE STUDY

Sixteen subjects (eight male and eight female) (73.1 ± 6.9 years, 81.7 ± 14.7 kg, 170.3 ± 11.2 cm) were recruited for the study. All of the subjects were volunteers who signed an informed consent and received detailed information about the functional test protocols, the trainings, and muscle biopsies. Approval from the national committee for medical ethics was obtained at the beginning of the study (EK08-102-0608). All subjects included were healthy and declared not to have any specific physical/disease issue and were instructed to maintain their normal daily activities during the training period. Various functional tests, force measurement, and muscle biopsy were performed twice, namely 1 week before and 1 week after 9 weeks of ES training.

ELECTRICAL STIMULATION TRAINING

Subjects were exposed to regular neuromuscular ES training (swelling current) for a period of 9 weeks, starting two times a week for the first 3 weeks and then switched to three times a week for the next 6 weeks, amounting to a total of 24 training sessions (3×10 min each session). ES training was performed with a two channel custom-built battery-powered stimulator (Krenn et al., 2011) at home by the subjects themselves after detailed instructions. The subjects applied two conductive rubber electrodes ($9\,cm \times 14\,cm$; $126\,cm^2$), which were attached to the skin by wet sponge on the anterior thigh on both sides (left/right). The electrode pairs for left and right thigh were connected to the two channels of the stimulator. This allowed independent activation of the left and right thigh muscles, which were stimulated in an alternative manner. Each repetition (i.e., ES evoked muscle contraction) was evoked by a 3.5 s train (60 Hz) of electrical pulses (rectangular, biphasic, width 0.6 ms). Consecutive contractions of the same thigh were separated by 4.5 s intervals. In this study, constant voltage stimulation devices were applied. The subjects were instructed to increase the stimulation intensity until their maximum sensory tolerance level was reached. With this intensity all of the subjects achieved full knee extension. Nevertheless, the applied current and voltage was recorded by the stimulation device for each training session. The mean stimulation current was 128 ± 16 mA and voltage of 39 ± 14 V.

FORCE MEASUREMENT

An isometric measurement on a dynamometer (S2P Ltd., Lubljana, Slovenia) as described (Šarabon et al., 2013a,b) with 90° hip flexion and 60° knee flexion (full knee extension = 0°) was performed three times at each leg to assess the maximal isometric torque of the left and right knee extensors. The mean of the best values of each leg were taken for further analyses.

FUNCTIONAL TESTS

A complete set of functional tests to access mobility and function in activities of daily living (ADL) was designed and applied to each of the subjects. These tests included: time up and go test (TUGT) (Podsiadlo and Richardson, 1991) where the subjects were asked to stand up from a standard chair, walk a distance of 3 m, turn around, walk back to the chair, and sit down again all as fast as possible; short physical performance battery (SPPB) (Guralnik et al., 1994) to evaluate the lower extremities function by using tests of gait speed (2.4 m), standing balance (side-by-side, semi-tandem, and tandem stance for 10 s) and the time which the subject needed to rise from a chair for five times as quickly as possible with the arms folded across their chest; 12 flight Stair Test (Suzuki et al., 2001) where the participant was instructed to ascend and descend the stairs after reaching the top (12th) step as quick and safe as possible; and 10 m-walking test with habitual and fastest walking speed (but not running) (Šarabon et al., 2010a,b) where each speed was performed three times, the time was measured and average velocity calculated.

MUSCLE BIOPSIES

Muscle biopsies were harvested as described (Kern et al., 2004) from the vastus lateralis muscle 15–20 cm proximal of the joint space of the knee, with the Bergström needle inserted perpendicular to the fiber direction. The biopsies before training were taken 10 days after the initial assessment at inclusion to the study, ES training started 14 days later. Post-training biopsies were taken 7 days after the last training session. The final functional assessment was done 4 days after the last training session. About 50–70 mg of tissue was harvested from both legs of the subjects.

Histological analysis

For light microscopy analyses, serial cryosections (8 μ thick) from frozen muscle biopsies were mounted on polysine™ glass slides, air-dried, and stained either with Hematoxylin–Eosin (HE) or for myofibrillar ATPases to evaluate muscle fiber type using conventional techniques as described (Rossini et al., 2002). Slow-type muscle fibers are dark-stained, while the fast-type fibers are light-stained following pre-incubation at pH 4.35.

Morphometric analysis

The mean myofiber diameter and the percentage of slow and fast-type muscle fibers were evaluated from stained cross sections in accordance with our previous published methods (Rossini et al., 2002; Carraro et al., 2005; Ashley et al., 2007; Biral et al., 2008; Kern et al., 2008, 2010). Images were acquired using a Zeiss microscope connected to a Leica DC300F camera. Morphometry analysis was performed using Scion Image software (2000 Scion Corporation, Inc.).

IMMUNOFLUORESCENCE ANALYSIS

Muscle sections were incubated either for 1 h at room temperature (RT) or overnight at 4°C, with anti-neural adhesion molecule (N-CAM) rabbit polyclonal antibody (Chemicon, Italy), anti-Pax7 mouse monoclonal antibody (DSHB, Iowa), or anti-laminin rabbit polyclonal antibody (Sigma, Italy) 1:100 diluted in PBS, respectively, as described (Zampieri et al., 2010; Mosole et al., 2014).

Sections were then incubated for 1 h at RT with Cy3 or Alexa Fluor® 488 dye conjugated antibodies against rabbit (Chemicon, Italy) or mouse IgG (Life technologies, Italy). Sections were then mounted on glass slides using ProLong Gold antifade reagent with DAPI (Life Technologies). Quantitation of Pax7 positive cells were performed on captured images from random fields counting a minimum of 300 fibers per biopsy.

GENE EXPRESSION ANALYSES AND miRNA

Total RNA extraction from human muscle biopsies before and after ES was performed with tissue lyser (Qiagen) in TriRiagentTM (Sigma) and small RNAs were purified using PureLink miRNA Isolation Kit (Invitrogen). This RNA fraction, containing microRNA (miRNA), was reverse-transcribed using the TaqMan® MicroRNA Reverse Transcription Kit (Life Technologies); the other RNA fraction, containing mRNA, was reverse-transcribed using a QuantiTect Reverse Transcription kit (Qiagen). The reverse-transcription reactions were performed according to the manufacturers' instructions. Quantitative PCR was performed on an ABI PRISM 7500 SDS (Applied Biosystems, USA), using pre-made 6-carboxyfluorescein (FAM)-labeled TaqMan assays for GAPDH, IGF-1 Ea, IGF-1 Eb, IGF-1 Ec, IGF-1 pan, Myostatin, Collagen I, III, VI (Applied Biosystems, USA). FAM-labeled TaqMan MicroRNA Assays for miR-1, miR-133a, miR-206, miR-29, and U6 snRNA (Applied Biosystems, USA) were performed as described. Quantitative RT-PCR sample values were normalized to the expression of GAPDH mRNA or U6 snRNA. The relative level for each gene and miRNA was calculated using the 2-DDCt method (Livak and Schmittgen, 2001) and reported as mean fold change in gene expression.

STATISTICAL ANALYSES

SPSS Statistics software package, version 17.0 was used to evaluate differences between the measurements in parameters of torque, functional tests, muscle morphometry, and molecular data. Normal distribution was obtained with Shapiro–Wilk-Test, the two-tailed paired and unpaired Student's t-test and Wilcoxon-Test were used for normal and not normal distributed variables, respectively. For differences presented in percentage the 95% confidence interval (CI) was calculated. The level of significance was set to $p < 0.05$.

RESULTS

ELECTRICAL STIMULATION IMPROVES FUNCTIONAL PERFORMANCES AFTER 9 WEEKS OF TRAINING

To assess mobility, frailty, and risk of falling, behavior analyses in challenging conditions as TUGT and SPPB is recommended (Freiberger et al., 2013; Viana et al., 2013).

With ES training, we improved (i.e., shortened) the *TUGT* time ($-16.4\% \pm 6.1$ CI, $p < 0.0005$) and increased the *SPPB Score* ($+11.2\% \pm 6.8$ CI, $p < 0.005$) (**Table 1**), resulting in a greater mobility in seniors recruited for this study.

For older adults, the ability to rise from a chair and sit down five times consecutively is a parameter to measure the degree of independence (Corrigan and Bohannon, 2001; Freiberger et al., 2013) and is considered as an index of muscle strength (Bohannon, 1997). Since the test is specific to lower body strength and power, the significant pre-post-test improvement ($-23.9\% \pm 8.6$ CI, $p < 0.005$) of the 5× Chair Rise Test indicates a sufficient training effect of ES (**Table 1**).

The maximum isometric torque, an important factor for gait and physical function and a key factor against sarcopenia (Cruz-Jentoft, 2013) developed by the Quadriceps ($+6.0\% \pm 4.9$ CI, $p < 0.05$), was significantly improved by ES training (**Table 1**).

The ability to climb stairs in a secure and fast manner is an essential eccentric and concentric strength performance of the lower extremities in daily life (Rejeski et al., 1995). The significant decrease of stair test time ($-21.1\% \pm 10.8$ CI, $p < 0.05$) in our ES-treated subjects indicates a greater performance and safety for the ADL (**Table 1**).

Gait speed is relevant to the functioning of seniors in the community and an important predictor for the onset of disability, commonly used by physical therapists and other clinicians (Guralnik et al., 2000; Bohannon and Williams Andrews, 2011) and known as good predictor for frailty (Cruz-Jentoft, 2013; Viana et al., 2013). The significant increase of the 10 m test habitual as well as fastest walking speed ($+5.3\% \pm 4.6$ CI, $p < 0.05$ and $+4.9\% \pm 3.7$ CI, $p < 0.05$, respectively) supports the functional changes and are good indicators of prevention of frailty and falls (**Table 1**).

ELECTRICAL STIMULATION MAINTAINS MUSCLE MASS AND ENHANCES SATELLITE CELLS ACTIVATION, PROMOTING MUSCLE ADAPTATION

We also monitored whether the aforementioned functional benefit, exerted by ES, was associated with a morphological gain. ES training maintained the overall mean myofiber diameter (**Figures 1A,B; Table 2**), while significantly increased the diameter of fast-type myofibers and decreased that of slow fibers type (**Figures 1C,D; Table 2**). Changes in fiber-type distribution were also observed, even though not significantly (**Table 2**).

Of note, no sign of fibrosis and/or inflammatory cell infiltration was detected in treated muscles (**Figure 1**). Moreover, ultrastructural analysis did not reveal alterations in muscle structure between pre- and post-trained muscles, nor differences in the frequency and position of calcium release units (CRUs) and mitochondria between the two groups of samples (data not shown).

A critical role in muscle homeostasis and regeneration is exerted by satellite cells (Carosio et al., 2011), which can be also activated by different stimuli, including physical exercise (Kadi et al., 1999; Snijders et al., 2009; Walker et al., 2012).

To verify whether ES promotes a similar response of exercise, we analyzed the expression of relevant molecular markers of activated and committed satellite cells such as N-CAM, Pax7, and myogenin (Carosio et al., 2011). Immunofluorescence analysis revealed that ES induced a significant increase in the percentage of N-CAM (**Figure 2A**) and Pax7 (**Figure 2B** left and right panels) expressing cells, along with a significant increase in myogenin expression, analyzed by RT-PCR analysis (**Figure 2C**). Recent studies have shown that muscle cell proliferation and differentiation are mediated by a collection of muscle-specific miRNAs (van Rooij et al., 2008). miR-206 is expressed in early phases of differentiation,

Table 1 | Force measurements and functional tests of seniors with muscle weakness before and after ES training.

	Pre	Post	Improvement	*t*-test
ALL (*N* = 16)				
Torque (Nm/kg)	1.42 ± 0.34	1.51 ± 0.38	6.0 ± 4.9	***p* < 0.05**
TUGT (s)	8.42 ± 1.95	7.04 ± 1.09	−16.4 ± 6.1	***p* < 0.0005**
5× chair rise (s)	13.85 ± 3.33	10.53 ± 3.63	−23.9 ± 8.6	***p* < 0.005[a]**
SPPB score	10.06 ± 1.39	11.19 ± 1.22	11.2 ± 6.8	***p* < 0.005[a]**
Stair test (s)	15.09 ± 3.48	11.90 ± 2.32	−21.1 ± 10.8	***p* < 0.05**
10 m test habitual (m/s)	1.20 ± 0.19	1.26 ± 0.18	5.3 ± 4.6	***p* < 0.05**
10 m test fast (m/s)	1.58 ± 0.28	1.66 ± 0.24	4.9 ± 3.7	***p* < 0.05**
FEMALE (*N* = 8)				
Torque (Nm/kg)	1.35 ± 0.32	1.45 ± 0.37	7.5 ± 7.4	**0.058**
TUGT (s)	9.13 ± 1.82	7.58 ± 0.96	−16.9 ± 9.0	***p* < 0.05**
5× chair rise (s)	13.52 ± 3.30	9.01 ± 1.19	−33.3 ± 12.5	***p* < 0.005**
SPPB score	10.13 ± 1.55	11.75 ± 0.46	16.0 ± 12.1	***p* < 0.05[a]**
Stair test (s)	15.26 ± 2.83	11.12 ± 1.70	−27.2 ± 16.6	**0.054**
10 m test habitual (m/s)	1.09 ± 0.16	1.17 ± 0.14	7.4 ± 8.3	**0.117**
10 m test fast (m/s)	1.41 ± 0.15	1.51 ± 0.14	6.5 ± 6.3	**0.075**
MALE (*N* = 8)				
Torque (Nm/kg)	1.50 ± 0.36	1.57 ± 0.41	4.5 ± 6.7	**0.208[a]**
TUGT (s)	7.71 ± 1.92	6.49 ± 0.97	−15.8 ± 8.8	***p* < 0.05**
5× chair rise (s)	14.22 ± 3.60	12.28 ± 4.74	−13.7 ± 9.4	***p* < 0.05**
SPPB score	10.0 ± 1.31	10.63 ± 1.51	6.3 ± 3.6	***p* < 0.05**
Stair test (s)	14.92 ± 4.37	12.69 ± 2.77	−15.0 ± 13.1	**0.161**
10 m test habitual (m/s)	1.31 ± 0.16	1.35 ± 0.17	3.5 ± 3.9	**0.125**
10 m test fast (m/s)	1.74 ± 0.29	1.81 ± 0.22	3.5 ± 4.0	**0.173**

Values are given as mean ± SD; BMI, body mass index; TUGT, timed up and go test; SPPB, short physical performance battery. Improvement values are presented as difference in percentage ±95% confidence interval.

[a]Wilcoxon-Test.

whereas the expression of miR-1 is a marker of terminal differentiation and controls the expression of relevant enzymes in the response to oxidative stress (Chen et al., 2006; Rao et al., 2006; Cacchiarelli et al., 2010). Real time PCR analysis (**Figure 2C**) revealed a significant up-regulation of miR-206 and an increase of miR-1 expression in ES stimulated muscle compared to control muscle.

CHARACTERIZATION OF MOLECULAR PATHWAYS INVOLVED IN ES-MEDIATED MUSCLE ADAPTATION

To determine the adaptation changes of gene expression due to ES, we performed RT-PCR to quantify shifts in mRNA levels of a selected panel of genes involved in muscle growth and plasticity, in pre-trained (used as control) and electrical stimulated (treated) aged muscles. One of the key factors involved in skeletal muscle adaptations and growth is insulin-like growth factor-1 (IGF-1) (Musarò et al., 2001; Berg and Bang, 2004; Adamo and Farrar, 2006; Scicchitano et al., 2009; Kern et al., 2011).

We analyzed the expression of the different isoforms of IGF-1. In humans, three mRNA variants (known as IGF-1Ea, IGF-1Eb, and IGF-1Ec) with alternatively spliced ends have been identified (Scicchitano et al., 2009; Vinciguerra et al., 2010). **Figure 3A** shows that ES promoted a significant increase in the mRNA expression of total (pan) IGF-1 and of IGF-1Ea, IGF-1Eb, and IGF-1Ec isoforms.

To verify whether ES stimulates not only anabolic pathways, but negatively modulates muscle catabolism, we analyzed the expression of factors associated with relevant proteolytic systems such as the ubiquitin-proteasome and the autophagy-lysosome systems (Vinciguerra et al., 2010). Atrogin-1 and MuRF-1 are muscle-specific atrophy-related ubiquitin ligases and are responsible for the increased protein degradation through the ubiquitin-proteasome system (Vinciguerra et al., 2010). We found a significant down-regulation of MuRF-1 and a reduced trend in atrogin-1 expression in the post-training group (**Figure 3B**). The autophagy-related genes Beclin1, Bnip3, and p62 did not change in trained muscles indicating that ES do not modulate the autophagy pathway (**Figure 3B**).

Another key modulator of muscle mass is myostatin (Elliott et al., 2012). Myostatin has been described as a negative regulator of skeletal muscle mass and regeneration and a target of miR-206 (Clop et al., 2006). Surprisingly, real time PCR revealed an up-regulation of myostatin mRNA in ES-treated muscle compared to control pre-trained muscle (**Figure 3C**).

The age-related decrease in muscle mass involves a selective loss of fast glycolytic fibers (Type II) over slow oxidative fibers (Type I) (Alnaqeeb and Goldspink, 1987). Although the Type I fibers are energetically more efficient than Type II fibers, so that senescent muscle should become progressively more resistant to fatigue, they are also greatly decreased in their force-generating capacity, exhibiting restricted contractile options in terms of speed and power output. Since ES involved an improvement in

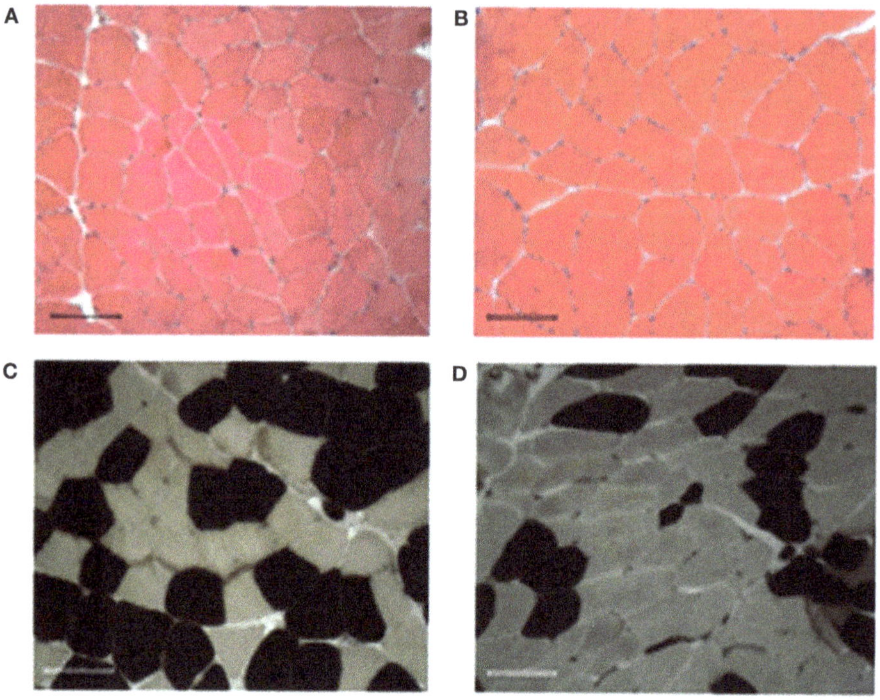

FIGURE 1 | Muscle morphology and fiber-type distribution. All muscle biopsies present well-packed myofibers, without signs of fibrosis, and inflammatory cell infiltration before **(A)** or after 9 weeks of training **(B)**. The training induced an increase of either diameter and percentage of the fast-type fibers [brown stained **(C,D)**]. Bar 100 μm.

muscle strength and power, we analyzed one of the key factors involved in oxidative metabolism and fiber-type switching, namely PGC1α (Lin et al., 2002). Of note, PGC1α was down-regulated in ES-treated muscles (**Figure 3D**), indicating a maintenance of the fastest more powerful phenotype. Since down-regulation of PGC1α could point to altered mitochondrial function and therefore to potential increase in ROS production, we monitored the expression of Nrf2, a transcription factor that has a central role in oxidative stress response in worms, flies, and mice. Importantly, expression of the gene Nrf2 did not change with ES (**Figure 3E**).

Interestingly, muscle extracellular matrix (ECM) constitutes a vital adaptation in providing protection against contraction-induced injury in human skeletal muscle (Mackey et al., 2011).

To support this hypothesis, we analyzed, by real time PCR, the expression of adhesion-promoting matrix components, demonstrating a significant up-regulation of collagen types I and III in ES muscle compared to control pre-trained muscle (**Figure 4**). Of note, ECM represents also a niche component of satellite cells. One of the matrix components that might play a role in maintaining satellite cell function is collagen VI (Urciuolo et al., 2013). Real time PCR analysis revealed a significant increase in Collagen VI expression in ES-trained muscle compared to pre-trained muscle (**Figure 4**).

Interestingly, the up-regulation of ECM regulators was not associated with accumulation of fibrotic tissue, as revealed by histological analysis (**Figure 1**), suggesting that ECM remodeling is indeed an important homeostatic event promoted by ES.

Table 2 | Mean myofiber diameter and fiber-type distribution in skeletal muscle biopsies pre- and post-training.

	Pre	Post	Difference	*t*-test
All fibers				
Size (μm)	49.6 ± 15.6	49.5 ± 15.8	−0.3%	N.S
Fast-type fibers				
Size (μm)	46.8 ± 14.4	47.8 ± 15.8	+2.2%	**$p < 0.0001$**
Percentage	45%	49%	+8.9%	N.S
Slow-type fibers				
Size (μm)	50.4 ± 14.8	48.4 ± 16.7	−3.6%	**$p < 0.0001$**
Percentage	55%	51%	−7.2%	N.S

The overall mean myofiber diameter did not significantly change after 9 weeks of training, while a significant increase of fast-type mean myofiber diameter was observed. Values are given in mean ± SD. Bold font indicates statistically significant values. N.S, No statistically significant.

To support this evidence, we analyzed the expression of miR-29, which controls the extracellular proteins and the fibrotic process (van Rooij et al., 2008; Cacchiarelli et al., 2010; He et al., 2013). qRT-PCR revealed that ES promotes a significant increase in miR-29 expression (**Figure 4**), suggesting that mir-29 controls fibrosis in ES stimulated muscle.

DISCUSSION

Electrical stimulation has been proved to be very effective in restoring muscle mass and function in denervated muscles (Kern et al.,

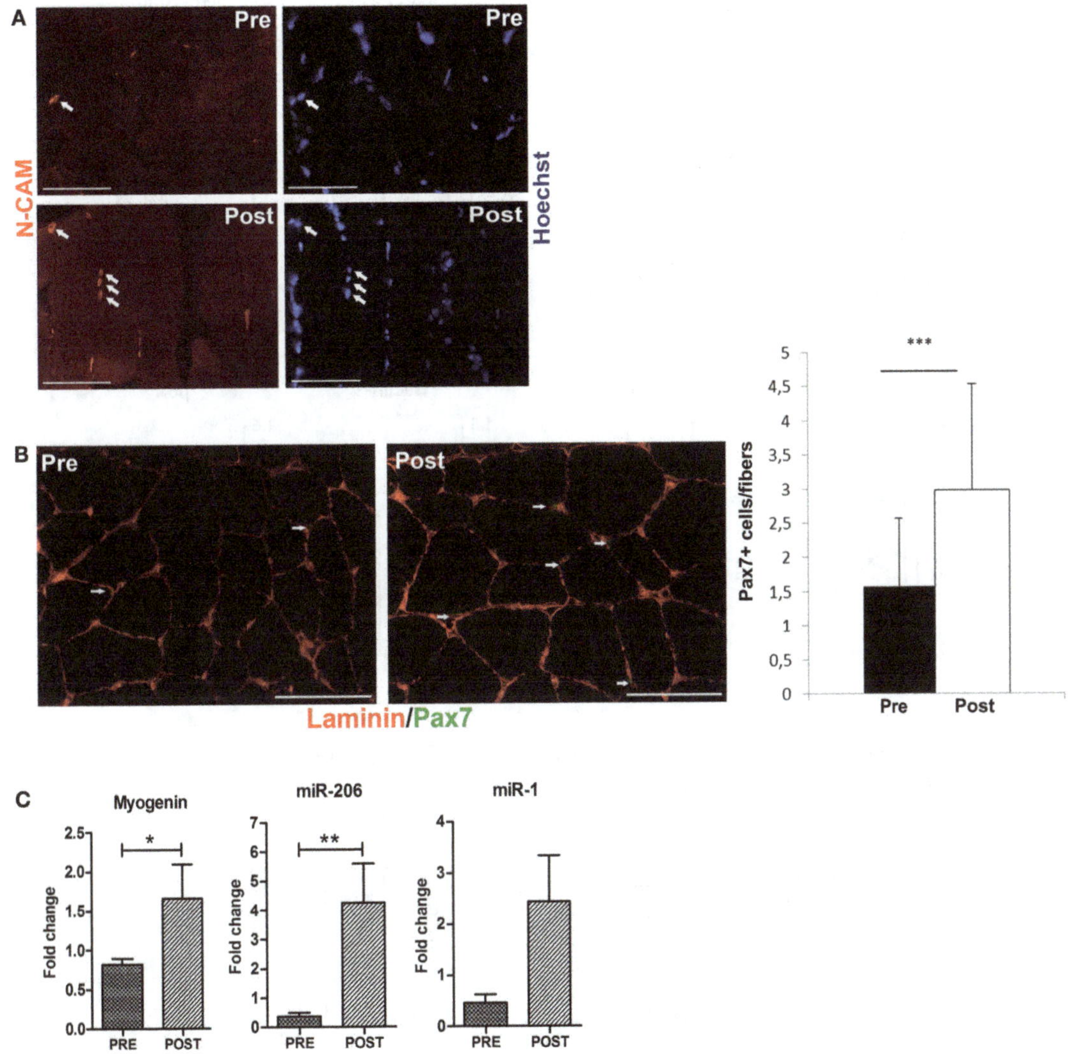

FIGURE 2 | Electrical stimulation induces an increase of satellite cells. **(A)** Representative immunofluorescence analysis for N-CAM expression (red stained, arrowed). N-CAM expressing cells are increased in post-trained muscle compared with the pre-training condition. Nuclei are counterstained in blue with Hoechst. Bar 100 μm. **(B)** Representative co-immunofluorescence analyses of laminin (red staining) and Pax7 (green staining) expression in skeletal muscle biopsies comparing pre- to post-training conditions. The number of Pax7 positive cells (arrowed) is increased in biopsies of post-trained subjects, compared to the pre-training ones. Bar 100 μm. Right panel: percentage of Pax7+ cells in pre-trained and post-ES-trained muscles. Data are represented as average ± SD. $^{***}p < 0.0001$. **(C)** Real time PCR analysis for myogenin, miR-206, and miR-1 expression in pre-trained (PRE) and post-ES-trained (POST) muscles. Data are represented as average ± SEM. $n = 16$. $^{*}p < 0.05$; $^{**}p < 0.005$.

2004, 2008, 2010; Carraro et al., 2005; Ashley et al., 2007; Maddocks et al., 2013).

The aim of the present study was to verify whether ES can be used to improve muscle function in elderly individuals. It is well documented that training and regular exercise can attenuate the pathological signs of sarcopenia, increasing muscle strength while decreasing fall risk. Nevertheless, certain pathologic conditions (e.g., sarcopenia, osteoarthritis, disuse associated atrophy, muscular dystrophies, trauma, and injuries) limit the ability to perform physical exercise. An alternative effective intervention to improve muscle recovery is ES.

We evaluated the functional performance of ES-trained subject and analyzed the molecular signature of ES-mediated effects on skeletal muscle. In our study, we did not include untreated controls but we compared the functional performance of same subjects before and after ES training.

The results collected here suggest that ES, similarly to physical exercise, attenuate the functional decline associated with aging, improving muscle strength and mass, maintaining the overall size of muscle fibers (decreasing during aging), activating satellite cell, and guaranteeing muscle adaptation. Thus, ES should be protective for sarcopenia.

All functional tests and maximal isometric torque showed significant improvements after 9 weeks of ES training, counteracting age-depended mobility ability, frailty, risk of falling, while improving functional performance and ADL. Of note, the ES-treated

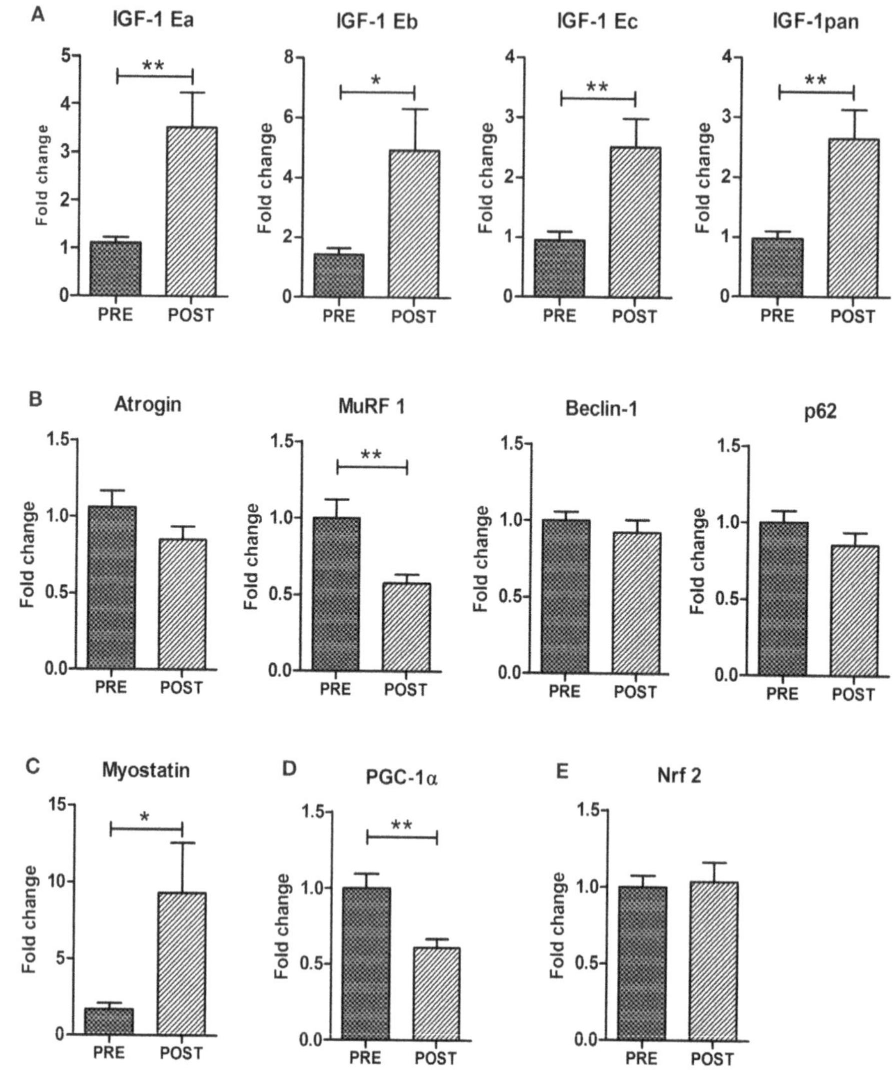

FIGURE 3 | Expression analyses of genes controlling muscle mass and metabolism. Real time PCR analysis for the expression of IGF-1 isoforms (total IGF-1pan, IGF-1Ea, IGF-1Eb, IGF-1Ec) **(A)** Atrogin-1, MurF-1, Beclin1, p62 **(B)**, Myostatin **(C)**, PGC1α **(D)**, and Nrf2 **(E)**. Data are represented as average ± SEM. $n = 16$. $^{**}p < 0.005$; $^{***}p < 0.0005$.

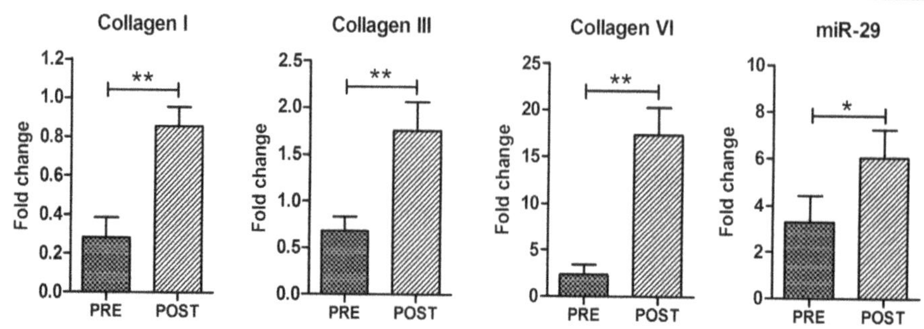

FIGURE 4 | Electrical stimulation promotes ECM remodeling. Real time PCR analysis for Collagen I, Collagen III, Collagen VI, and miR-29. Data are represented as average ± SEM. $n = 16$. $^{*}p < 0.05$; $^{***}p < 0.0005$.

subjected performed similarly to a 6-week resistance trained older adults (70.6 ± 6.1 years) (Fragala et al., 2014), assessed with TUGT, 5× Chair Rise and gait time.

It has been reported that female subjects displayed higher sensory and supramotor excitability to surface ES (Maffiuletti et al., 2008). In our study, the intensity (current) was very similar in all (male and female) subjects, which were instructed to increase the stimulation intensity until their maximum sensory tolerance level was reached. None of them declared problematic events during training sessions, and both males and females reported slight pain clinically not relevant at rest before ES, without changes through ES training. In the functional tests, the males were generally stronger and faster than females except chair rise (females faster) and stair test (equal). Both males and females improved in all tests but females gained in percentage nearly twice as males. This could be explained taking into consideration that the electrodes we used in our study covered a relative larger area of the thigh in female than male and therefore activated more motor-points by stimulation. This results in training of a larger volume of the quadriceps muscles similar to the observation reported by Maffiuletti et al. (2008). We suggest, for all therapeutic applications of ES that aim to improve force and quality of muscle structure, to use electrode sizes greater than 100 cm^2 to cover larger portions of the muscle and at the same time to create less discomfort due to low current density at the electrode-skin interface (Kern, 2014).

At molecular level, we demonstrated that ES promotes the modulation of factors associated with muscle growth and induces a remodeling of ECM. Our findings demonstrated that ES of 73.1 years old healthy sedentary seniors, increases expression of IGF-1 and of relevant biomarkers of activated satellite cells and myoblasts, reduces expression of muscle-specific atrophy-related ubiquitin ligase genes, and promotes the remodeling of myofibers and of ECM.

IGF-1 plays an important anabolic role in skeletal muscle and it is an important modulator of muscle growth and regeneration. Different evidences indicate that, during muscle regeneration, IGF-IEb levels is responsible for activating and for proliferating satellite cells; IGF-1Ea is responsible for myoblast differentiation and IGF-1Ec expression is normally up-regulated in response to mechanical signals (Matheny et al., 2010). Thus, our data suggests that ES stimulates the expression of different isoforms of IGF-1 in muscle, guaranteeing muscle homeostasis and protection against age-related sarcopenia. In fact, increased levels of IGF-1 were associated with a reduced level of expression of MuRF-1, a gene involved in muscle atrophy.

Among potential molecular mechanisms activated by exercise, autophagy might play a critical role for metabolic adaptation (Lira et al., 2013; Ferraro et al., 2014; Vainshtein et al., 2014). In particular, it has been reported that autophagy is an essential process for skeletal muscle adaptation and physical performance after endurance training (Lira et al., 2013). Conversely, we did not observe significant activation of autophagic pathway in ES-treated subjects. This can be justified considering that the up-regulation of autophagic-relevant markers is an early event and then they returned to basal levels shortly after the stimulus. We analyzed the muscle biopsies 7 days after the last ES treatments, a time point that might not sustain the activation of autophagic pathways. Further analysis will clarify and address this point.

Of note, myostatin was up-regulated in ES-treated muscles. We can interpret this result considering that myostatin may be produced locally by skeletal muscle cells to limit the muscle growth stimulated by IGF-1, guaranteeing an appropriate organ size (Shyu et al., 2005).

The up-regulation of myostatin can be also explained considering that ES guarantees a balance between satellite cells activation and differentiation. In fact, skeletal muscle differentiation is a complex and highly regulated process characterized by morphological changes, which include myoblast proliferation, alignment, elongation, and fusion into multinucleated myotubes. This is a balanced process dynamically coordinated by positive and negative signals. Recent studies revealed that IGF-1 also stimulates the expression of myostatin and it has been suggested that myostatin and IGF-1 positively coordinate myogenesis (Kurokawa et al., 2009; Valdés et al., 2013). Interestingly, it has been recently reported that myostatin stimulates C2C12 proliferation, and this effect occurred in the presence of IGF-1 (Rodgers et al., 2014). Thus, it is possible that in our experimental model the modulation of myostatin is independent by miR-206 expression/activity; however, myostatin and the relevant markers of activated and differentiating satellite cells are part of the mechanism for muscle adaptation induced by ES.

Interestingly, the up-regulation of collagen VI and ECM remodeling suggests that ES strengths key component of the satellite cell niche (Urciuolo et al., 2013). It has been recently suggested that ES stimulates satellite cells and a strengthened ECM, factors that are likely to be involved in protecting the muscle from damage on exposure to subsequent injuring stimuli (Mackey et al., 2011).

These results are also in agreement with morphometric analyses, which showed an increase of the percentage and diameter of the fast-type fibers.

Of clinical interest was the up-regulation of miR-29, which control fibrosis in different tissues, including skeletal muscle (Cacchiarelli et al., 2010). Considering that sarcopenia involves a decrease in muscle integrity as fibrotic invasions replace functional contractile tissue, and a progressive loss of the most powerful fast fibers, our data clearly indicate that ES improves muscle function and mass and protects against accumulation of fibrosis, regulating key factors, and signaling of muscle homeostasis and growth.

Altogether, the molecular data support our clinical findings that neuromuscular ES positively influences excitability and recruitment of stimulated muscle fibers resulting in greater force and better coordination guaranteeing, ADL, exercise programs, and rehabilitation strategies.

In conclusion, a three times a week ES is an effective therapy to improve molecular adaptations of muscle, counteracting muscle atrophy, and improving functional outcomes with positive influence on quality of life of seniors.

AUTHOR CONTRIBUTIONS

Helmut Kern, Samantha Burggraf, Nejc Sarabon, Matthias Krenn, Jan Cvecka: designed the clinical work, recruited senior subjects and made clinical evaluation, drafted the work, reviewed the work. Helmut Kern, Stefan Löfler, Michael Vogelauer, Winfried Mayr, Hannah Fruhmann: collected human biopsies and samples; designed the ES protocol, performed functional evaluation on senior subjects, acquisition, statistical analysis, and interpretation of clinical data, drafted the work, reviewed the work. Laura Barberi, Simona Sbardella, Vanina Romanello, Marco Sandri, Antonio Musaro: perform molecular analysis, acquisition, statistic analysis, and interpretation of gene expression data, reviewed the work. Laura Pietrangelo, Feliciano Protasi: performed electron microscopy analysis, measured frequency, and position of CRUs and mitochondria, acquisition, statistical analysis, and interpretation of data, drafted the work, reviewed the work. Sandra Zampieri, Ugo Carraro: performed histological analysis, acquisition, statistic analysis, and interpretation of data; drafted the work, reviewed the work. Antonio Musaro, Marco Sandri, Helmut Kern, Ugo Carraro, Feliciano Protasi, Sandra Zampieri: designed and organized the experiments, interpreted the results, critically revised the work. Antonio Musaro: wrote the paper. All authors approved the final version of the manuscript.

ACKNOWLEDGMENTS

This study was supported by PRIN; European Regional Development Fund-Cross Border Cooperation Programme SLOVAKIA–AUSTRIA (Interreg-Iva) project "Mobilität im Alter" MOBIL N_00033; Austrian Federal Ministry of Science and Research; Ludwig Boltzmann Society (Vienna); Telethon (GGP13013 to Antonio Musaro and 13213 to Feliciano Protasi); AFM; ASI.

REFERENCES

Adamo, M. L., and Farrar, R. P. (2006). Resistance training, and IGF involvement in the maintenance of muscle mass during the aging process. *Ageing Res. Rev.* 5, 310–331. doi:10.1016/j.arr.2006.05.001

Alnaqeeb, M. A., and Goldspink, G. (1987). Changes in fibre type, number and diameter in developing and ageing skeletal muscle. *J. Anat.* 153, 31–45.

Ashley, Z., Salmons, S., Boncompagni, S., Protasi, F., Russold, M., Lanmuller, H., et al. (2007). Effects of chronic electrical stimulation on long-term denervated muscles of the rabbit hind limb. *J. Muscle Res. Cell. Motil.* 28, 203–217. doi:10.1007/s10974-007-9119-4

Bax, L., Staes, F., and Verhagen, A. (2005). Does neuromuscular electrical stimulation strengthen the quadriceps femoris? A systematic review of randomised controlled trials. *Sports Med.* 35, 191–212. doi:10.2165/00007256-200535030-00002

Berg, U., and Bang, P. (2004). Exercise and circulating insulin-like growth factor I. *Horm. Res.* 62, 50–58. doi:10.1159/000080759

Biral, D., Kern, H., Adami, N., Boncompagni, S., Protasi, F., and Carraro, U. (2008). Atrophy-resistant fibers in permanent peripheral denervation of human skeletal muscle. *Neurol. Res.* 30, 137–144. doi:10.1179/174313208X281145

Bohannon, R. W. (1997). Isometric strength data. *Arch. Phys. Med. Rehabil.* 78, 566–567. doi:10.1016/S0003-9993(97)90181-7

Bohannon, R. W., and Williams Andrews, A. (2011). Normal walking speed: a descriptive meta-analysis. *Physiotherapy* 97, 182–189. doi:10.1016/j.physio.2010

Boncompagni, S., Kern, H., Rossini, K., Hofer, C., Mayr, W., Carraro, U., et al. (2007). Structural differentiation of skeletal muscle fibers in the absence of innervation in humans. *Proc. Natl. Acad. Sci. U.S.A.* 104, 19339–19344. doi:10.1073/pnas.0709061104

Cacchiarelli, D., Martone, J., Girardi, E., Cesana, M., Incitti, T., Morlando, M., et al. (2010). MicroRNAs involved in molecular circuitries relevant for the Duchenne muscular dystrophy pathogenesis are controlled by the dystrophin/nNOS pathway. *Cell Metab.* 12, 341–351. doi:10.1016/j.cmet.2010.07.008

Carosio, S., Berardinelli, M. G., Aucello, M., and Musarò, A. (2011). Impact of ageing on muscle cell regeneration. *Ageing Res. Rev.* 10, 35–42. doi:10.1016/j.arr.2009.08.001

Carraro, U., Rossini, K., Mayr, W., and Kern, H. (2005). Muscle fiber regeneration in human permanent lower motoneuron denervation: relevance to safety and effectiveness of ES-training, which induces muscle recovery in SCI subjects. *Artif. Organs* 29, 187–191. doi:10.1111/j.1525-1594.2005.29032.x

Chen, J. F., Mandel, E. M., Thomson, J. M., Wu, Q., Callis, T. E., Hammond, S. M., et al. (2006). The role of microRNA-1 and microRNA-133 in skeletal muscle proliferation and differentiation. *Nat. Genet.* 38, 228–233. doi:10.1038/ng1725

Clop, A., Marcq, F., Takeda, H., Pirottin, D., Tordoir, X., Bibé, B., et al. (2006). A mutation creating a potential illegitimate microRNA target site in the myostatin gene affects muscularity in sheep. *Nat. Genet.* 38, 813–818. doi:10.1038/ng1810

Corrigan, D., and Bohannon, R. W. (2001). Relationship between knee extension force and stand-up performance in community-dwelling elderly women. *Arch. Phys. Med. Rehabil.* 82, 1666–1672. doi:10.1053/apmr.2001.26811

Cruz-Jentoft, A. J. (2013). Perspective: protein and exercise for frailty and sarcopenia: still learning. *J. Am. Med. Dir. Assoc.* 14, 69–71. doi:10.1016/j.jamda.2012.09.024

de Oliveira Melo, M., Aragão, F. A., and Vaz, M. A. (2013). Neuromuscular electrical stimulation for muscle strengthening in elderly with knee osteoarthritis – a systematic review. *Complement. Ther. Clin. Pract.* 19, 27–31. doi:10.1016/j.ctcp.2012.09.002

Elliott, B., Renshaw, D., Getting, S., and Mackenzie, R. (2012). The central role of myostatin in skeletal muscle and whole body homeostasis. *Acta Physiol. (Oxf.)* 205, 324–340. doi:10.1111/j.1748-1716.2012.02423.x

Ferraro, E., Giammarioli, A. M., Chiandotto, S., Spoletini, I., and Rosano, G. (2014). Exercise-induced skeletal muscle remodeling and metabolic adaptation: redox signaling and role of autophagy. *Antioxid. Redox Signal.* 21, 154–176. doi:10.1089/ars.2013.5773

Fragala, M. S., Fukuda, D. H., Stout, J. R., Townsend, J. R., Emerson, N. S., Boone, C. H., et al. (2014). Muscle quality index improves with resistance exercise training in older adults. *Exp. Gerontol.* 53, 1–6. doi:10.1016/j.exger.2014.01.027

Freiberger, E., Blank, W. A., Salb, J., Geilhof, B., Hentschke, C., Landendoerfer, P., et al. (2013). Effects of a complex intervention on fall risk in the general practitioner setting: a cluster randomized controlled trial. *Clin. Interv. Aging* 8, 1079–1088. doi:10.2147/CIA.S46218

Giggins, O., Fullen, B., and Coughlan, G. (2012). Neuromuscular electrical stimulation in the treatment of knee osteoarthritis: a systematic review and meta-analysis. *Clin. Rehabil.* 26, 867–881. doi:10.1177/0269215511431902

Guralnik, J. M., Ferrucci, L., Pieper, C. F., Leveille, S. G., Markides, K. S., Ostir, G. V., et al. (2000). Lower extremity function and subsequent disability: consistency across studies, predictive models, and value of gait speed alone compared with the short physical performance battery. *J. Gerontol. A Biol. Sci. Med. Sci.* 55, M221–M231. doi:10.1093/gerona/55.4.M221

Guralnik, J. M., Simonsick, E. M., Ferrucci, L., Glynn, R. J., Berkman, L. F., Blazer, D. G., et al. (1994). A short physical performance battery assessing lower extremity function: association with self-reported disability and prediction of mortality and nursing home admission. *J. Gerontol.* 49, M85–M94. doi:10.1093/geronj/49.2.M85

He, Y., Huang, C., Lin, X., and Li, J. (2013). MicroRNA-29 family, a crucial therapeutic target for fibrosis diseases. *Biochimie* 95, 1355–1359. doi:10.1016/j.biochi.2013.03.010

Kadi, F., Eriksson, A., Holmner, S., Butler-Browne, G. S., and Thornell, L. E. (1999). Cellular adaptation of the trapezius muscle in strength-trained athletes. *Histochem. Cell Biol.* 111, 189–195. doi:10.1007/s004180050348

Kern, H. (2014). Functional electrical stimulation on paraplegic patients. *Eur. J. Transl. Myol.* 24, 75–157. doi:10.4081/bam.2014.2.75

Kern, H., Boncompagni, S., Rossini, K., Mayr, W., Fanò, G., Zanin, M. E., et al. (2004). Long-term denervation in humans causes degeneration of both contractile and excitation-contraction coupling apparatus that can be reversed by functional electrical stimulation (ES). A role for myofiber regeneration? *J. Neuropathol. Exp. Neurol.* 63, 919–931.

Kern, H., Carraro, U., Adami, N., Biral, D., Hofer, C., Forstner, C., et al. (2010). Home-based functional electrical stimulation rescues permanently denervated muscles in paraplegic patients with complete lower motor neuron lesion. *Neurorehabil. Neural Repair* 24, 709–721. doi:10.1177/1545968310366129

Kern, H., Hofer, C., Mödlin, M., Mayr, W., Vindigni, V., Zampieri, S., et al. (2008). Stable muscle atrophy in long-term paraplegics with complete upper motor neuron lesion from 3- to 20-year SCI. *Spinal Cord* 46, 293–304. doi:10.1038/sj.sc.3102131

Kern, H., Pelosi, L., Coletto, L., Musarò, A., Sandri, M., Vogelauer, M., et al. (2011). Atrophy/hypertrophy cell signaling in muscles of young athletes trained with vibrational-proprioceptive stimulation. *Neurol. Res.* 33, 998–1009. doi:10.1179/016164110X12767786356633

Krenn, M., Haller, M., Bijak, M., Unger, E., Hofer, C., Kern, H., et al. (2011). Safe neuromuscular electrical stimulator designed for the elderly. *Artif. Organs* 35, 253–256. doi:10.1111/j.1525-1594.2011.01217.x

Kurokawa, M., Sato, F., Aramaki, S., Soh, T., Yamauchi, N., and Hattori, M. A. (2009). Monitor of the myostatin autocrine action during differentiation of embryonic chicken myoblasts into myotubes: effect of IGF-I. *Mol. Cell. Biochem.* 331, 193–199. doi:10.1007/s11010-009-0158-6

Levine, M., McElroy, K., Stakich, V., and Cicco, J. (2013). Comparing conventional physical therapy rehabilitation with neuromuscular electrical stimulation after TKA. *Orthopedics* 36, e319–e324. doi:10.3928/01477447-20130222-20

Lin, J., Wu, H., Tarr, P. T., Zhang, C. Y., Wu, Z., Boss, O., et al. (2002). Transcriptional co-activator PGC-1 alpha drives the formation of slow-twitch muscle fibres. *Nature* 418, 797–801. doi:10.1038/nature00904

Lira, V. A., Okutsu, M., Zhang, M., Greene, N. P., Laker, R. C., Breen, D. S., et al. (2013). Autophagy is required for exercise training-induced skeletal muscle adaptation and improvement of physical performance. *FASEB J.* 27, 4184–4193. doi:10.1096/fj.13-228486

Livak, K. J., and Schmittgen, T. D. (2001). Analysis of relative gene expression data using real-time quantitative PCR and the 2(-Delta Delta C(T)). *Methods* 25, 402–408. doi:10.1006/meth.2001.1262

Mackey, A. L., Brandstetter, S., Schjerling, P., Bojsen-Moller, J., Qvortrup, K., Pedersen, M. M., et al. (2011). Sequenced response of extracellular matrix deadhesion and fibrotic regulators after muscle damage is involved in protection against future injury in human skeletal muscle. *FASEB J.* 25, 1943–1959. doi:10.1096/fj.10-176487

Maddocks, M., Gao, W., Higginson, I. J., and Wilcock, A. (2013). Neuromuscular electrical stimulation for muscle weakness in adults with advanced disease. *Cochrane Database Syst. Rev.* 1, 1–30. doi:10.1002/14651858.CD009419.pub2

Maffiuletti, N. A., Herrero, A. J., Jubeau, M., Impellizzeri, F. M., and Bizzini, M. (2008). Differences in electrical stimulation thresholds between men and women. *Ann. Neurol.* 63, 507–512. doi:10.1002/ana.21346

Matheny, R. W. Jr, Nindl, B. C., and Adamo, M. L. (2010). Minireview: mechano-growth factor: a putative product of IGF-I gene expression involved in tissue repair and regeneration. *Endocrinology* 151, 865–875. doi:10.1210/en.2009-1217

Mosole, S., Carraro, U., Kern, H., Loefler, S., Fruhmann, H., Vogelauer, M., et al. (2014). Long-term high-level exercise promotes muscle reinnervation with age. *J. Neuropathol. Exp. Neurol.* 73, 284–294. doi:10.1097/NEN.0000000000000032

Musarò, A., McCullagh, K., Paul, A., Houghton, L., Dobrowolny, G., Molinaro, M., et al. (2001). Localized Igf-1 transgene expression sustains hypertrophy and regeneration in senescent skeletal muscle. *Nat. Genet.* 27, 195–200. doi:10.1038/84839

Nuhr, M. J., Pette, D., Berger, R., Quittan, M., Crevenna, R., Huelsman, M., et al. (2004). Beneficial effects of chronic low-frequency stimulation of thigh muscles in patients with advanced chronic heart failure. *Eur. Heart J.* 25, 136–143. doi:10.1016/j.ehj.2003.09.027

Paffenbarger, R. S. Jr, Kampert, J. B., Lee, I. M., Hyde, R. T., Leung, R. W., and Wing, A. L. (1994). Changes in physical activity and other lifeway patterns influencing longevity. *Med. Sci. Sports Exerc.* 26, 857–865. doi:10.1249/00005768-199407000-00008

Podsiadlo, D., and Richardson, S. (1991). The timed "Up & Go": a test of basic functional mobility for frail elderly persons. *J. Am. Geriatr. Soc.* 39, 142–148.

Quittan, M., Wiesinger, G. F., Sturm, B., Puig, S., Mayr, W., Sochor, A., et al. (2001). Improvement of thigh muscles by neuromuscular electrical stimulation in patients with refractory heart failure: a single-blind, randomized, controlled trial. *Am. J. Phys. Med. Rehabil.* 80, 206–214. doi:10.1097/00002060-200103000-00011

Rao, P. K., Kumar, R. M., Farkhondeh, M., Baskerville, S., and Lodish, H. F. (2006). Myogenic factors that regulate expression of muscle-specific microRNAs. *Proc. Natl. Acad. Sci. U.S.A.* 103, 8721–8726. doi:10.1073/pnas.0602831103

Rejeski, W. J., Ettinger, W. H. Jr, Schumaker, S., James, P., Burns, R., and Elam, J. T. (1995). Assessing performance-related disability in patients with knee osteoarthritis. *Osteoarthr. Cartil.* 3, 157–167. doi:10.1016/S1063-4584(05)80050-0

Rodgers, B. D., Wiedeback, B. D., Hoversten, K. E., Jackson, M. F., Walker, R. G., and Thompson, T. B. (2014). Myostatin stimulates, not inhibits, C2C12 myoblast proliferation. *Endocrinology* 155, 670–675. doi:10.1210/en.2013-2107

Rosemffet, M. G., Schneeberger, E. E., Citera, G., Sgobba, M. E., Laiz, C., Schmulevich, H., et al. (2004). Effects of functional electrostimulation on pain, muscular strength, and functional capacity in patients with osteoarthritis of the knee. *J. Clin. Rheumatol.* 10, 246–249. doi:10.1097/01.rhu.0000141831.40350.91

Rossini, K., Zanin, M. E., Podhorska-Okolow, M., and Carraro, U. (2002). To stage and quantify regenerative myogenesis in human long-term permanent denervated muscle. *Basic Appl. Myol.* 12, 277–286.

Šarabon, N., Loefler, S., Cvecka, J., Sedliak, M., and Kern, H. (2013a). Strength training in elderly people improves static balance: a randomized controlled trial. *Eur. J. Transl. Myol.* 23, 85–89. doi:10.4081/bam.2013.3.85

Šarabon, N., Rošker, J., Fruhmann, H., Burggraf, S., Loefler, S., and Kern, H. (2013b). Reliability of maximal voluntary contraction related parameters measured by a portable isometric knee dynamometer. *Phys. Med. Rehabil. Kuror.* 23, 22–27. doi:10.1055/s-0032-1331190

Šarabon, N., Loefler, S., Fruhmann, H., Burggraf, S., and Kern, H. (2010a). Reduction and technical simplification of testing protocol for walking based on repeatability analyses: an Interreg IVa pilot study. *Eur. J. Transl. Myol.* 1, 181–186. doi:10.4081/bam.2010.4.181

Šarabon, N., Rošker, J., Loefler, S., and Kern, H. (2010b). Sensitivity of body sway parameters during quiet standing to manipulation of support surface size. *J. Sport Sci. Med.* 9, 431–438.

Scicchitano, B. M., Rizzuto, E., and Musarò, A. (2009). Counteracting muscle wasting in aging and neuromuscular diseases: the critical role of IGF-1. *Aging* (Albany NY) 1, 451–457.

Shyu, K. G., Ko, W. H., Yang, W. S., Wang, B. W., and Kuan, P. (2005). Insulin-like growth factor-1 mediates stretch-induced upregulation of myostatin expression in neonatal rat cardiomyocytes. *Cardiovasc. Res.* 68, 405–414. doi:10.1016/j.cardiores.2005.06.028

Snijders, T., Verdijk, L. B., and van Loon, L. J. (2009). The impact of sarcopenia and exercise training on skeletal muscle satellite cells. *Ageing Res. Rev.* 8, 328–338. doi:10.1016/j.arr.2009.05.003

Strasser, E. M., Stättner, S., Karner, J., Klimpfinger, M., Freynhofer, M., Zaller, V., et al. (2009). Neuromuscular electrical stimulation reduces skeletal muscle protein degradation and stimulates insulin-like growth factors in an age- and current-dependent manner: a randomized, controlled clinical trial in major abdominal surgical patients. *Ann. Surg.* 249, 738–743. doi:10.1097/SLA.0b013e3181a38e71

Suzuki, T., Bean, J. F., and Fielding, R. A. (2001). Muscle power of the ankle flexors predicts functional performance in community-dwelling older women. *J. Am. Geriatr. Soc.* 49, 1161–1167. doi:10.1046/j.1532-5415.2001.49232.x

Urciuolo, A., Quarta, M., Morbidoni, V., Gattazzo, F., Molon, S., Grumati, P., et al. (2013). Collagen VI regulates satellite cell self-renewal and muscle regeneration. *Nat. Commun.* 4, 1964–1989. doi:10.1038/ncomms2964

Vainshtein, A., Grumati, P., Sandri, M., and Bonaldo, P. (2014). Skeletal muscle, autophagy, and physical activity: the ménage à trois of metabolic regulation in health and disease. *J. Mol. Med.* 92, 127–137. doi:10.1007/s00109-013-1096-z

Valdés, J. A., Flores, S., Fuentes, E. N., Osorio-Fuentealba, C., Jaimovich, E., and Molina, A. (2013). IGF-1 induces IP3-dependent calcium signal involved in the regulation of myostatin gene expression mediated by NFAT during myoblast differentiation. *J. Cell. Physiol.* 228, 1452–1463. doi:10.1002/jcp.24298

van Rooij, E., Liu, N., and Olson, E. N. (2008). MicroRNAs flex their muscles. *Trends Genet.* 24, 159–166. doi:10.1016/j.tig.2008.01.007

Viana, J. U., Silva, S. L., Torres, J. L., Dias, J. M., Pereira, L. S., and Dias, R. C. (2013). Influence of sarcopenia and functionality indicators on the frailty profile of community-dwelling elderly subjects: a cross-sectional study. *Braz. J. Phys. Ther.* 17, 373–381. doi:10.1590/S1413-35552012005000102

Vinciguerra, M., Musaro, A., and Rosenthal, N. (2010). Regulation of muscle atrophy in aging and disease. *Adv. Exp. Med. Biol.* 694, 211–233. doi:10.1007/978-1-4419-7002-2_15

Walker, D. K., Fry, C. S., Drummond, M. J., Dickinson, J. M., Timmerman, K. L., Gundermann, D. M., et al. (2012). PAX7+ satellite cells in young and older adults following resistance exercise. *Muscle Nerve* 46, 51–59. doi:10.1002/mus.23266

Wall, B. T., Dirks, M. L., Verdijk, L. B., Snijders, T., Hansen, D., Vranckx, P., et al. (2012). Neuromuscular electrical stimulation increases muscle protein synthesis in elderly type 2 diabetic men. *Am. J. Physiol. Endocrinol. Metab.* 303, 614–623. doi:10.1152/ajpendo.00138.2012

Zampieri, S., Doria, A., Adami, N., Biral, D., Vecchiato, M., Savastano, S., et al. (2010). Subclinical myopathy in patients affected with newly diagnosed colorectal cancer at clinical onset of disease: evidence from skeletal muscle biopsies. *Neurol. Res.* 32, 20–25. doi:10.1179/016164110X12556180205997

Zampieri, S., Pietrangelo, L., Loefler, S., Fruhmann, H., Vogelauer, M., Burggraf, S., et al. (2014). Lifelong physical exercise delays age-associated skeletal muscle decline. *J. Gerontol. A Biol. Sci. Med. Sci.* doi:10.1093/gerona/glu006

13

Skeletal muscle homeostasis in Duchenne muscular dystrophy: modulating autophagy as a promising therapeutic strategy

Clara De Palma[1], Cristiana Perrotta[1], Paolo Pellegrino[1], Emilio Clementi[1,2]* and Davide Cervia[1,3]*

[1] Unit of Clinical Pharmacology, Department of Biomedical and Clinical Sciences "L. Sacco", National Research Council-Institute of Neuroscience, University Hospital "L. Sacco", University of Milan, Milan, Italy

[2] Scientific Institute IRCCS Eugenio Medea, Bosisio Parini, Italy

[3] Department for Innovation in Biological, Agro-Food and Forest Systems, University of Tuscia, Viterbo, Italy

***Correspondence:**
Emilio Clementi, Department of Biomedical and Clinical Sciences "L. Sacco", Università di Milano, Via G.B. Grassi 74, Milano 20157, Italy
e-mail: emilio.clementi@unimi.it;
Davide Cervia, Department for Innovation in Biological, Agro-Food and Forest Systems, Università della Tuscia, Largo dell'Università snc, Blocco D, Viterbo 01100, Italy
e-mail: d.cervia@unitus.it

Muscular dystrophies are a group of genetic and heterogeneous neuromuscular disorders characterized by the primary wasting of skeletal muscle. In Duchenne muscular dystrophy (DMD), the most severe form of these diseases, the mutations in the dystrophin gene lead to muscle weakness and wasting, exhaustion of muscular regenerative capacity, and chronic local inflammation leading to substitution of myofibers by connective and adipose tissue. DMD patients suffer from continuous and progressive skeletal muscle damage followed by complete paralysis and death, usually by respiratory and/or cardiac failure. No cure is yet available, but several therapeutic approaches aiming at reversing the ongoing degeneration have been investigated in preclinical and clinical settings. Autophagy is an important proteolytic system of the cell and has a crucial role in the removal of proteins, aggregates, and organelles. Autophagy is constantly active in skeletal muscle and its role in tissue homeostasis is complex: at high levels, it can be detrimental and contribute to muscle wasting; at low levels, it can cause weakness and muscle degeneration, due to the unchecked accumulation of damaged proteins and organelles. The causal relationship between DMD pathogenesis and dysfunctional autophagy has been recently investigated. At molecular level, the Akt axis is one of the key dysregulated pathways, although the molecular events are not completely understood. The aim of this review is to describe and discuss the clinical relevance of the recent advances dissecting autophagy and its signaling pathway in DMD. The picture might pave the way for the development of interventions that are able to boost muscle growth and/or prevent muscle wasting.

Keywords: skeletal muscle, Duchenne muscular dystrophy, muscle wasting, autophagy, Akt–mTOR axis, *mdx* mice, therapeutic target

PATHOLOGICAL FEATURES OF DYSTROPHIN DEFICIENCY

Duchenne muscular dystrophy (DMD) is the most frequent and lethal form of muscular dystrophy, affecting 1 out of 3,500 newborns (Govoni et al., 2013). DMD is an X-linked disorder caused by mutations of the largest gene of the human genome, the dystrophin gene. So far, more than 4,700 mutations have been identified and classified as deletions (65.8%), duplications (13.6%), and point mutations (micro-insertions, microdeletions, and nonsense, missense, and splicing mutations; 20.6%) (Magri et al., 2011). Mutations that change the reading frame of the gene generally result in premature stop codons with complete loss of dystrophin in DMD muscles. Other mutations can result in the generation of a smaller size-dystrophin or in a lesser amount of the protein being produced leading to the allelic dystrophinopathy disorder known as Becker muscular dystrophy, a disease milder than DMD, affecting 1 of 18,518 male births (Emery, 1991).

The diagnosis of DMD and Becker muscular dystrophy is based on careful analysis of the clinical features and confirmed by additional investigations including muscle biopsy and/or genetic testing. In particular, DMD is characterized by an early onset before 3 years of age, then ambulation loss occurs between 10 and 14 years of age, and finally death takes place between 20 and 30 years of age (Davies et al., 1988).

The most impaired muscle in DMD patients is the diaphragm, and its wasting is responsible for the respiratory failure (reduced wall and lung compliance, hypoventilation, hypercapnia, and hypoxemia) and thus death (Fayssoil et al., 2010; Mosqueira et al., 2013). DMD also affects cardiac muscle, and to a lesser extent, smooth muscle (Fayssoil et al., 2010; Mosqueira et al., 2013). More than 90% of DMD patients are affected by some degree of cardiomyopathy (Fayssoil et al., 2010; Mosqueira et al., 2013), which causes a progressive reduction in the ejection fraction, which may hesitate in heart failure with or without concomitant arrhythmias (Jefferies et al., 2005). The onset of cardiomyopathy is variable, starting from 18 years of age in DMD patients (Spurney, 2011; Politano and Nigro, 2012). Cardiac decline is observed also in Becker muscular dystrophy patients, which progresses faster than skeletal muscle decline (Bushby et al., 2010).

Functionally, dystrophic skeletal muscles are more susceptible to eccentric contraction than the healthy ones (Lynch et al., 2000). In response to this type of injury, altered muscle fibers undergo repeated cycles of necrosis and regeneration, during which satellite cells, the primary myogenic precursor cells of the muscle, activate muscle regeneration process (Le Grand and Rudnicki, 2007; Biressi and Rando, 2010). However, the regenerative process is rather inefficient and the repeated cycles of necrosis and regeneration lead to satellite cell depletion and gradual replacement of muscle by fat and connective tissue; this process is responsible for progressive muscle wasting and weakness. This may be attributed to a great extent to the loss of dystrophin.

Dystrophin is essential for maintenance of muscle membrane integrity; it is a scaffolding protein that recruits other structural and signaling proteins to the sarcolemma, forming a well-organized multimeric dystrophin-associated glycoprotein complex. The dystrophin-associated glycoprotein complex is composed of several transmembrane and peripheral proteins, depending on the tissue, in particular it encloses different sarcoplasmic proteins [α- and β-dystrobrevins, α1-, β1-, β2-, γ1-, and γ2-syntrophins, and neuronal nitric oxide synthase (nNOS)], transmembrane proteins (β-dystroglycan, α-, β-, γ-, δ-, ε-, and ζ-sarcoglycans, sarcospan, and caveolin-3), and extracellular proteins (α-dystroglycan and laminin). Dystrophin-associated glycoprotein complex plays a key role in the mechanical stabilization of the sarcolemma during muscle contractions (Straub and Campbell, 1997), and acts as a scaffold for different proteins implicated in intracellular signaling. The proteins inside dystrophin-associated glycoprotein complex are tightly connected to each other and abnormalities affecting one of these proteins lead to changes in the others impairing muscle function. Of importance, the disruption of the dystrophin-associated glycoprotein complex in DMD also causes the delocalization of the nNOS from sarcolemma, leading to a reduced generation of NO. NO is important in skeletal muscle physiology as it controls excitation–contraction coupling and energy balance (De Palma and Clementi, 2012). The loss of NO-dependent signaling pathways contributes significantly to impair muscle bulk and force generation with increased fatigability (De Palma and Clementi, 2012). Moreover, the loss of sarcolemmal nNOS contributes to increase the muscle fibers susceptibility to ischemia during exercise, and to mechanical damage resulting in a focal muscle injury, dependent on muscle use (Thomas, 2013).

MOUSE MODELS

In DMD, different mouse models with mutations in dystrophin gene have been generated. The *mdx* mouse on C57BL/10ScSn genetic background (C57BL/10ScSn-Dmd^{mdx}, here referred as "*mdx* mouse") (Coulton et al., 1988) shows a point mutation in exon 23, generating an early stop codon and leading to the absence of full-length dystrophin (Willmann et al., 2009). Other models bearing different mutations have been also generated, as for instance *mdx*2cv, *mdx*3cv, *mdx*4cv, or *mdx*5cv mouse (Im et al., 1996), *mdx*52 (with mutation on exon 52; Araki et al., 1997), and *mdx*/utr$^{-/-}$ (*mdx* mouse with additional knockout of utrophin) (Deconinck et al., 1997).

Among these models, the *mdx* mouse is the most commonly used (Nakamura and Takeda, 2011). The mutation on exon 23 is wide spread and affects one-third of DMD patients (Willmann et al., 2009). *mdx* mice have a shorter life compared to controls and display a decreased relative muscle force, whereas absolute muscle force is unaffected. Isolated muscles show a reduced force contraction, even if lacking standard condition of analysis is difficult to compare results from different groups.

Degeneration, regeneration, and necrosis are processes observed in young *mdx* mice (2–4 weeks) that result in increased number of regenerating-centronucleated fibers and in the heterogeneity of myofibers area (McGeachie et al., 1993). Necrotic fibers can be found at any age with very high frequency after 18 months (Nakamura and Takeda, 2011). Muscles undergo frequent cycles of necrosis/regeneration, associated with weakness and muscle loss. These cycles of regeneration lead to a muscle phenotype milder than the one observed in human patients. Fibrosis appears to be much less than in DMD patients, except for diaphragm muscle (Nakamura and Takeda, 2011). Although the *mdx* mouse diaphragm reproduces the degenerative changes of DMD, respiratory complications are visible only in 16-month-old mice (Stedman et al., 1991; Nakamura and Takeda, 2011). Muscle pathology can be worsened by forced exercise; this is a viable strategy to worsen the disease phenotype and better reveal the efficacy of new therapies.

Of importance, *mdx* mouse also displays cardiomyopathy, characterized by fibrosis and presence of necrosis and inflammation, thus sharing some aspects of DMD-patients cardiomyopathy and constitute a good model to investigate cardio-protective candidate molecules (Quinlan et al., 2004).

AUTOPHAGY AND ITS ROLE IN SKELETAL MUSCLE HOMEOSTASIS

Autophagy is a crucial mechanism involved in the turnover of cell components both in constitutive and catabolic (stress, nutrient deprivation, cytokines, amino acids deprivation) conditions. Autophagy classically functions as a physiological process to degrade cytoplasmic components, protein aggregates, and/or organelles, and as a regulator of cellular architecture. Autophagy in mammals generally protects the cells from death and defective autophagy can be associated with several diseases including cancer, neurodegenerative diseases, infectious diseases, and metabolic diseases (Cervia et al., 2013; Jiang and Mizushima, 2014; Schneider and Cuervo, 2014).

So far, three different mechanisms of autophagy have been described: macroautophagy, microautophagy, and chaperone-mediated autophagy. The most part of the information on autophagy in skeletal muscle is about macroautophagy, a process characterized by membranes that grow in size to generate double membrane-structures termed autophagosome, that enclose organelles, portion of cytoplasm, or protein aggregates. In this process, small ubiquitin-like proteins are required for the formation of autophagosomes and they are covalently bound to phosphatidylethanolamine.

Autophagy was considered initially as a non-specific degradation mechanism, but over the years selective forms of autophagy have been identified. For instance, selective removal of organelles, such as mitochondria or peroxisomes occurs *via* specific types of autophagy, termed mitophagy or peroxophagy, respectively.

AUTOPHAGIC SIGNALING

The molecular signaling pathway leading to autophagy is very complex and regulated by autophagy-related genes (Atgs), which are connected with the formation of autophagosomes (Hurley and Schulman, 2014). The protein products of Atgs are organized in five functional groups, namely: (i) the Unc-51-like kinase (Ulk):Atg13:FIP200 initiation complex (Ganley et al., 2009; Hosokawa et al., 2009); (ii) the beclin1:hVps34[phosphatidylinositol 3 (PI3) kinase]:Atg14L nucleation complex (Itakura et al., 2008); (iii) the PI3–phosphate-binding WIPI-1/2 complex (Proikas-Cezanne et al., 2004; Vergne et al., 2009); (iv) the Atg5–Atg12 conjugation complex activated by Atg7 (Mizushima et al., 1998); and (v) the Atg8 (LC3) conjugation system (Kabeya et al., 2000). These protein complexes participate at specific stages in the autophagic process: initiation, formation, elongation, and fusion (Mehrpour et al., 2010; Awan and Deng, 2014); they are also controlled by several other signaling pathways that fine tune autophagy to regulate the pace of autophagosome formation.

A key player in the control of autophagy is the mammalian target of rapamycin (mTOR), which together with raptor (regulatory associated protein of mTOR), G protein β-subunit-like protein (GβL) and proline-rich Akt substrate of 40 kDa (PRAS40) forms the multiprotein complex, mTORC1. The activity of mTOR, a negative regulator of autophagy, depends on several positive signals including normoxia, amino acid supply, high energy levels, or growth factors. Upon stimulation by growth factors or nutrients (glucose, amino acids), mTORC1 negatively regulates the macromolecular initiation complex Ulk:Atg13:FIP200 leading to autophagy suppression (Ganley et al., 2009; Hosokawa et al., 2009; Wong et al., 2013). Conversely, starvation and energy depletion, which stimulate autophagy, inhibit mTORC1, leading to the activation of Ulk (Jung et al., 2010; Kim et al., 2011; Mihaylova and Shaw, 2011).

The main signaling pathway controlling mTORC1 is the PI3 kinase/Akt pathway activated by the binding of growth factors or insulin to their cell surface receptors. Activated Akt in turn phosphorylates and inhibits the tuberous sclerosis complex 2 (TSC2), thus preventing the formation of the inhibitory TSC1/TSC2 heterodimer. This inhibition allows the small GTPase Rheb to activate directly mTORC1 (Long et al., 2005a,b; Huang and Manning, 2009) and to inhibit autophagy. Another signaling pathway controlling mTOR is the adenosine monophosphate-activated protein kinase (AMPK) pathway activated under energy-low conditions (Alers et al., 2012). Activated AMPK is known to regulate mTORC1 activity mainly through the phosphorylation and consequent activation of the negative regulator TSC2 (Inoki et al., 2003). However, the discovery that TSC2-deficient cells can respond to a decrease in energy levels has led to the investigation of additional mechanisms. Recently, it has been demonstrated that both mTORC1 and AMPK can act on the same substrate, Ulk1, with opposite effects: mTORC1 inhibits Ulk1 activation by phosphorylating Ser757; conversely, AMPK activates Ulk1 through its phosphorylation on Ser317 and Ser777 (Kim et al., 2011).

Additional proteins have been found to be associated with mTOR, i.e., rictor (rapamycin-insensitive companion of mTOR), GβL, SAPK-interacting protein 1 (SIN1), and protein observed with rictor (PROTOR), to form the multiprotein complex mTORC2 (Sarbassov et al., 2006). mTORC2 is involved in the phosphorylation and activation of Akt, thereby promoting its prosurvival action. Through this activation, mTOR determines the downregulation of the transcription factor Forkhead Box O3 (FoxO3), particularly important in muscle where it stimulates autophagy by enhancing the expression of genes including Atg12, Ulk1, Atg4b, and Gabarapl1 (Mammucari et al., 2007).

AUTOPHAGY LEVELS AND SKELETAL MUSCLE IMPAIRMENT

The role of autophagy in skeletal muscle has been investigated extensively (Sandri, 2010; Neel et al., 2013). Muscle mass represents 40–50% of the human body and is one of the most important sites for the regulation of metabolism. Excessive protein degradation in the skeletal muscle is detrimental for the economy of the body and can lead to death. Studies in mice with muscle-specific inactivation of autophagic genes have been used to identify the role of autophagy in muscles (Sandri, 2010; Neel et al., 2013). Briefly, ablation of Atg7 gene led to an altered muscle structure, with sarcomere disorganization and myofibers degeneration due to activation of an unfolded protein response, accumulation of abnormal mitochondria, enhanced oxidative stress, and increased concentration of polyubiquitinated proteins (Masiero et al., 2009). Altogether, these effects accounted for muscle weakness, atrophy, and other signs of myopathy such as an irregular distribution of fibers' shape as well as fibers with a vacuolated cytosol. In general, the blocking of basal autophagy in muscle enhanced the accumulation of damaged and dysfunctional mitochondria, suggesting that mitophagy was impaired and critical to maintain muscle homeostasis (Masiero et al., 2009). Further, muscle-specific $Atg5^{-/-}$ mice displayed an atrophic phenotype in the fibers of the fast type, associated to accumulation of autophagic substrates, for instance, ubiquitinated proteins (Raben et al., 2008). In particular, in fast muscles of $Atg5^{-/-}$ mice, the size and density of lysosomes were increased and their distribution on the microtubules altered. Microtubules displayed a more linear organization compared to that of wild-type mice, demonstrating that autophagy is crucial also for the correct arrangement of microtubules (Raben et al., 2008).

Finally, in studies in which the transcription of FoxO3 was upregulated an enhanced autophagy–lysosome system was observed, especially during muscle wasting and the factor itself was enough to enhance autophagy process and to trigger atrophy (Mammucari et al., 2007). Noteworthy, a recent study showed that mice lacking the nutrient-deprivation autophagy factor-1, displayed muscle weakness, associated with an increased autophagy, dysregulation of calcium and accumulation of enlarged mitochondria (Chang et al., 2012).

The lesson from these results is complex and indicates a dual role for autophagy in skeletal muscle homeostasis: at high levels, it can be detrimental and contribute to muscle atrophy; at low levels, it can cause weakness and muscle degeneration, due to the unchecked accumulation of damaged proteins and organelles (Sandri, 2010; Sandri et al., 2013). Thus, a proper autophagic process is vital for both functional skeletal muscle, which controls the support and movement of the skeleton, and muscle metabolism (Neel et al., 2013).

DEREGULATION OF AUTOPHAGY IN DUCHENNE MUSCULAR DYSTROPHY

The fact that manipulation of animal models to dysregulate autophagy also leads to muscle pathology has prompted studies to investigate whether this process is altered in muscle diseases (Neel et al., 2013; Sandri et al., 2013). Of interest, our understanding on the role of detective autophagy in different forms of inherited muscular dystrophies, including Bethlem myopathy, Ullrich congenital muscular dystrophy, merosin-deficient congenital muscular dystrophy, and Emery–Dreifuss muscular dystrophy has emerged in the past 5 years (Sandri et al., 2013).

As initially postulated from indirect evidence, deficient autophagy was suggested to contribute to DMD pathogenesis. The presence of swollen and damaged mitochondria, protein aggregation, and distension of sarcoplasmic reticulum, which are cyto-pathological hallmarks of DMD, are often observed when autophagy is impaired (Culligan et al., 2002; Zhao et al., 2007). In addition, activation of Akt was significantly higher in muscles from *mdx* mice and dystrophin-deficient primary myotubes, thereby suggesting a defective autophagic process (Dogra et al., 2006; Peter and Crosbie, 2006). In line with these observations, DMD patients were found to exhibit a similar pattern of Akt activation (Peter and Crosbie, 2006).

The causal relationship between DMD pathogenesis and dysfunctional autophagy has been investigated more recently in studies addressing this issue specifically. A severe impairment of autophagy was indeed demonstrated by biochemical and ultrastructural analyses in muscles from patients affected by DMD and *mdx* mice. In particular, these muscles display a significant reduction in the lipidated form of the protein LC3, which is a common marker of autophagy induction (De Palma et al., 2012; Bibee et al., 2014). The reduction in lipidated LC3 has been found to be accompanied by clear signs of impaired autophagy at the ultrastructural level, i.e., by the presence of damaged organelles, the increase in the signaling adaptor p62 protein (a marker inversely correlated with autophagic flux), and the decrease of Bnip3, a mitochondrial protein, which recruits LC3 to mitochondria (De Palma et al., 2012; Bibee et al., 2014). Recent studies have also shown a role for the TNF receptor-associated factor 6 (TRAF6) as an important regulator of autophagy. In skeletal muscle of *mdx* mice, the activity of TRAF6 is increased and its absence correlates with a reduced autophagy (Hindi et al., 2014). Strikingly, this study also reported that the inhibition of TRAF6 signaling deteriorates muscle pathology at later stages of disease progression. It has been thus hypothesized that the initial inhibition of autophagy in young *mdx* mice in the absence of TRAF6 gene may be a protective mechanism to preserve skeletal muscle mass. Autophagy emerges then as an essential process for the clearance of defunct cellular organelles and a continued inhibition of autophagy exaggerates dystrophic phenotype (Hindi et al., 2014). The beneficial effects of activating autophagy in *mdx* mice have been also confirmed by overexpressing peroxisome proliferator-activated receptor γ coactivator 1α (PGC-1a), a transcriptional coactivator, which is a powerful mediator of muscle plasticity (Hollinger et al., 2013) and by pharmacological treatment with an agonist drug against the energy sensor AMPK, i.e., 5-aminoimidazole-4-carboxamide-1-β-D-ribofuranoside (AICAR) (Pauly et al., 2012). In particular, AICAR treatment led to a significant activation of the autophagy, as indicated by the characteristic biochemical changes of increased lipidated LC3 content, an upregulation of other prototypical autophagy-associated proteins, and to significant improvements in both muscle structure and maximum force-generating capacity (Pauly et al., 2012).

From a functional point of view, it has been recently shown that voluntary exercise in *mdx* mice enhances markers of autophagy to or above the levels observed in healthy mice, thus suggesting that beneficial autophagy can be induced by exercise (Hulmi et al., 2013). In agreement with these data, fasting induced autophagy in wild-type and *mdx* mice diaphragm (Spitali et al., 2013). Interestingly in *mdx* mice, the ability of upregulating autophagy appears restricted to certain muscles: *tibialis anterior* muscle of *mdx* mice are unable to enhance autophagy in response to fasting, which induces autophagy in *tibialis anterior* muscle of wild-type mice.

MOLECULAR CHARACTERISTICS

The defect in autophagy of *mdx* mouse muscles is accompanied by persistent activation of the Akt–mTOR axis (**Figure 1**) and its related autophagy-inhibiting pathways, and the concomitant downregulation of several autophagy-inducing genes (Dogra et al., 2006; Peter and Crosbie, 2006; De Palma et al., 2012). In particular, Akt activation has been established to occur at very early, pre-necrotic stages of disease pathogenesis, with a progressive increase with disease worsening (Peter and Crosbie, 2006). This high activation of Akt stimulates in turn the mTOR-dependent pathways whereas the mTOR-independent axis is not significantly altered (Dogra et al., 2006; Peter and Crosbie, 2006). The involvement of the mTOR axis in the pathogenesis of *mdx* mice is demonstrated also by the effects of the mTOR-targeting, immunosuppressant drug rapamycin. Oral or injected rapamycin treatment has been shown to improve histopathological features of dystrophy (Eghtesad et al., 2011) and the treatment with rapamycin-loaded nanoparticles (RNPs) has been shown to increase skeletal muscle strength in both young and adult mice concomitantly to an increased mTOR-dependent autophagy (Bibee et al., 2014). Consistently, *mdx* mice treatment with a long-term low-protein diet reactivates autophagy in muscle fibers, with increased lipidation of LC3, reduced levels of p62, normalization of Akt and mTOR signaling, a reduced accumulation of damaged organelles, and a significant recovery of muscle inflammation, fibrosis, myofiber damage and muscle function (De Palma et al., 2012). Since the long-term low-protein diet was shown to preserve the regenerating ability of *mdx* mouse muscle, it is tempting to speculate that physiological levels of autophagy maintain the number and function of myogenic precursor cells.

The picture is not completely clear and some controversies still exist and issues remain to be solved. Spitali et al. (2013) reported that autophagy levels and Akt axis activation in *mdx* mice is similar to wild-type control mice. Likewise, a study on Akt–mTOR axis activation in very old *mdx* mice correlated the advancing of age with a reduction in mTOR signaling in dystrophic muscles (Mouisel et al., 2010). In another study, however, it was also reported that mTOR activation is increased by age in diaphragm muscle of wild-type mice, but not in *mdx* mice, while similar levels of mTOR activation were found in *tibialis anterior* muscles

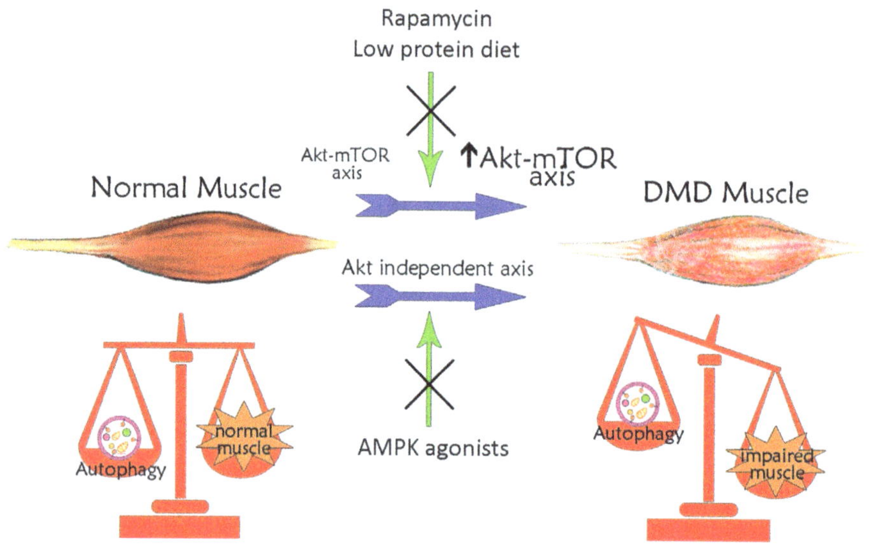

FIGURE 1 | Schematic illustration of the correlation between autophagy and Duchenne muscular dystrophy. Basal autophagy levels are required for muscle homeostasis and for the maintenance of healthy myofibers. In DMD, muscle autophagy is impaired contributing to muscle degeneration. This autophagy inhibition is dependent on the iper-activation of Akt–mTOR axis. Treatments with rapamycin or low-protein diet, acting on Akt pathway, restore autophagy ameliorating DMD muscle phenotype and function. The impaired autophagy may also occur independently of Akt. Treatments with AMPK agonists, which increase AMPK activation, counteract the Akt-independent axes enhancing autophagy and inducing a positive effect in DMD muscle.

(Eghtesad et al., 2011). Although these data are apparently difficult to reconcile, different confounding factors may explain them, as for instance the fact that *mdx* mice undergo extensive muscle regeneration between 6 and 12 weeks. Furthermore, the fact that the regulation of autophagy in *mdx* mice was indicated to differ depending on the muscle type (Spitali et al., 2013) should be taken into consideration, with the glycolytic muscles showing a process of vesicles formation significantly greater than oxidative muscles (Mizushima et al., 2004).

Autophagy can be modulated in *mdx* mice also through mTOR-independent mechanisms (**Figure 1**). Chronic AICAR administration induced autophagy in *mdx* muscles, with a significant upregulation of Ulk1 and an increased expression of Bnip3 in the absence of mTOR inhibition (Pauly et al., 2012). In addition, it has been suggested that TRAF6 regulation of Akt signaling is independent of TRAF6 regulation of autophagy (Hindi et al., 2014). The evidence for potentially augmented autophagic signaling may thus be suggestive of an adaptive response to attempt to rid dystrophic myofibers of defective and/or detrimental constituents, such as dysfunctional mitochondria (Ljubicic and Jasmin, 2013). The complex and apparently contrasting evidence on the role of authophagy in *mdx* mice suggests that the autophagic machinery in these mice is more complex than in wild-type mice and that a systematic analysis taking into account the variable of time has to be undertaken to clarify each single aspect in distinct muscles and during disease progression.

THERAPEUTIC IMPLICATIONS OF CORRECTIVE AUTOPHAGY IN DUCHENNE MUSCULAR DYSTROPHY

At present, there is no satisfactory therapy for DMD. The treatment with corticosteroids is the actual gold standard. Treatment with glucocorticoids significantly delays the impairment of muscle force and function, extends ambulation period, and retards the onset of pulmonary failure, cardiomyopathy, and scoliosis (Bushby et al., 2010). These effects, however, are often only temporary and associated with severe side effects. More than 25% of patients are not treated with glucocorticoids due to adverse effects, such as obesity, immune suppression, bone demineralization, associated with negative behavioral changes, or lack of response (Bushby et al., 2010). This strongly indicates an urgent requirement of new clinical intervention for DMD patients.

The genetic approaches [exon skipping, viral vector-mediated gene delivery, and cell therapy (Pichavant et al., 2011; Mendell et al., 2012)], currently being investigated, show some degree of success and some of them have been recently granted orphan status by either the European Medicines Agency or the Food and Drug Administration (http://orphandruganaut.wordpress.com/2013/12/14/duchenne-muscular-dystrophy-2013-fda-orphan-drug-designations-2/). They, however, are directed to specific subsets of population and cannot restore fully the damage already caused by the disease to the muscle. Alternative strategies are therefore needed and to this end identification of suitable therapeutic targets is necessary.

In this context, pharmacological modulation of autophagy can be considered a possible strategy aimed at delaying muscle degeneration (**Figure 1**). As mentioned above, the AICAR activating AMPK, ameliorated phenotypic and functional features of dystrophic muscle (Pauly et al., 2012). AMPK pharmacological agonists exist; they are clinically approved and AICAR has been tested for ischemic damage in the heart and used in clinical trial for metabolic disorders (Ljubicic and Jasmin, 2013). The beneficial effects of AICAR in dystrophic muscle could be due to a well-known effect in stimulating the slow, oxidative phenotype (Ljubicic et al., 2011). It could also be due to induction of autophagic pathways, since AICAR stimulates the removal of damaged mitochondria via mitophagy (Pauly et al., 2012).

A second pharmacological approach that targets autophagy has been proposed by Bibee et al. (2014) in which RNPs were used to successfully enhance grip strength and the left-ventricular ejection fraction in *mdx* mice, ameliorating both physical and cardiac performances. These effects with RNPs have been achieved after administration of only eight doses of RNPs, with the final dose within the range of recommended oral doses for immune-suppressive therapy in patients. Interestingly, oral administration of rapamycin at pharmacological doses was of no efficacy on muscle strength. It appears that the way RNPs worked was via autophagy induction, dependent on nanoparticles delivery of the drug: rapamycin was locally delivered at high concentration thus becoming able to trigger autophagy (Bibee et al., 2014). Interestingly, at least in the *mdx* mice also corticosteroids induce autophagy and this may contribute to explain their beneficial effects.

Autophagy cannot certainly be envisaged as a stand-alone therapeutic option. Low-protein diet regimen has been recently hypothesized to be safely usable in the treatment of DMD patients in combination with pharmacological treatment and cell and gene therapies (De Palma et al., 2012). RPNs and low-protein diet might also be used in combination with corticosteroids to act as steroids sparing drugs, reducing their toxic effects. Low-protein diet has been demonstrated safe and useful also in Col6a1-deficient mouse, considered an animal model of Bethlem myopathy (Grumati et al., 2010). Of interest, a very recent clinical study showed a clear induction of autophagy with a low-protein diet regimen in muscles from Becker and Ulrich patients (Merlini and Nishino, 2014), further suggesting that also in humans a strategy of autophagy reactivation is applicable.

CONCLUSION

Autophagy has emerged as a key process whose dysregulation contributes to the pathogenesis of several muscular dystrophies. The relevance of this process is that its normalization by pharmacological approaches leads to an amelioration of the dystrophic phenotype. While drugs targeting autophagy have good perspective in terms of therapy, we still need to refine them, by identifying appropriate targets in the autophagic pathway against which to design selected modulating drugs.

ACKNOWLEDGMENTS

This work was supported by: "Ministero della Salute" "Giovani Ricercatori 2011–2012" grant to Clara De Palma and "Ricerca corrente 2014" grant to Emilio Clementi; "Ministero dell'Istruzione, Università e Ricerca," PRIN 2010–2011 grants to Emilio Clementi and Davide Cervia; European Community's framework program FP7/2007–2013 under the agreement no. 223098 (OPTISTEM) and no. 241440 (ENDOSTEM) to Emilio Clementi.

REFERENCES

Alers, S., Loffler, A. S., Wesselborg, S., and Stork, B. (2012). Role of AMPK-mTOR-Ulk1/2 in the regulation of autophagy: cross talk, shortcuts, and feedbacks. *Mol. Cell. Biol.* 32, 2–11. doi:10.1128/MCB.06159-11

Araki, E., Nakamura, K., Nakao, K., Kameya, S., Kobayashi, O., Nonaka, I., et al. (1997). Targeted disruption of exon 52 in the mouse dystrophin gene induced muscle degeneration similar to that observed in Duchenne muscular dystrophy. *Biochem. Biophys. Res. Commun.* 238, 492–497. doi:10.1006/bbrc.1997.7328

Awan, M. U., and Deng, Y. (2014). Role of autophagy and its significance in cellular homeostasis. *Appl. Microbiol. Biotechnol.* 98, 5319–5328. doi:10.1007/s00253-014-5721-8

Bibee, K. P., Cheng, Y. J., Ching, J. K., Marsh, J. N., Li, A. J., Keeling, R. M., et al. (2014). Rapamycin nanoparticles target defective autophagy in muscular dystrophy to enhance both strength and cardiac function. *FASEB J.* 28, 2047–2061. doi:10.1096/fj.13-237388

Biressi, S., and Rando, T. A. (2010). Heterogeneity in the muscle satellite cell population. *Semin. Cell Dev. Biol.* 21, 845–854. doi:10.1016/j.semcdb.2010.09.003

Bushby, K., Finkel, R., Birnkrant, D. J., Case, L. E., Clemens, P. R., Cripe, L., et al. (2010). Diagnosis and management of Duchenne muscular dystrophy, part 1: diagnosis, and pharmacological and psychosocial management. *Lancet Neurol.* 9, 77–93. doi:10.1016/S1474-4422(09)70271-6

Cervia, D., Perrotta, C., Moscheni, C., De Palma, C., and Clementi, E. (2013). Nitric oxide and sphingolipids control apoptosis and autophagy with a significant impact on Alzheimer's disease. *J. Biol. Regul. Homeost. Agents* 27, 11–22.

Chang, N. C., Nguyen, M., Bourdon, J., Risse, P. A., Martin, J., Danialou, G., et al. (2012). Bcl-2-associated autophagy regulator Naf-1 required for maintenance of skeletal muscle. *Hum. Mol. Genet.* 21, 2277–2287. doi:10.1093/hmg/dds048

Coulton, G. R., Curtin, N. A., Morgan, J. E., and Partridge, T. A. (1988). The mdx mouse skeletal muscle myopathy: II. Contractile properties. *Neuropathol. Appl. Neurobiol.* 14, 299–314. doi:10.1111/j.1365-2990.1988.tb00890.x

Culligan, K., Banville, N., Dowling, P., and Ohlendieck, K. (2002). Drastic reduction of calsequestrin-like proteins and impaired calcium binding in dystrophic mdx muscle. *J. Appl. Physiol.* 92, 435–445. doi:10.1152/japplphysiol.00903.2001

Davies, K. E., Smith, T. J., Bundey, S., Read, A. P., Flint, T., Bell, M., et al. (1988). Mild and severe muscular dystrophy associated with deletions in Xp21 of the human X chromosome. *J. Med. Genet.* 25, 9–13. doi:10.1136/jmg.25.1.9

De Palma, C., and Clementi, E. (2012). Nitric oxide in myogenesis and therapeutic muscle repair. *Mol. Neurobiol.* 46, 682–692. doi:10.1007/s12035-012-8311-8

De Palma, C., Morisi, F., Cheli, S., Pambianco, S., Cappello, V., Vezzoli, M., et al. (2012). Autophagy as a new therapeutic target in Duchenne muscular dystrophy. *Cell Death Dis.* 3, e418. doi:10.1038/cddis.2012.159

Deconinck, A. E., Rafael, J. A., Skinner, J. A., Brown, S. C., Potter, A. C., Metzinger, L., et al. (1997). Utrophin-dystrophin-deficient mice as a model for Duchenne muscular dystrophy. *Cell* 90, 717–727. doi:10.1016/S0092-8674(00)80532-2

Dogra, C., Changotra, H., Wergedal, J. E., and Kumar, A. (2006). Regulation of phosphatidylinositol 3-kinase (PI3K)/Akt and nuclear factor-kappa B signaling pathways in dystrophin-deficient skeletal muscle in response to mechanical stretch. *J. Cell. Physiol.* 208, 575–585. doi:10.1002/jcp.20696

Eghtesad, S., Jhunjhunwala, S., Little, S. R., and Clemens, P. R. (2011). Rapamycin ameliorates dystrophic phenotype in mdx mouse skeletal muscle. *Mol. Med.* 17, 917–924. doi:10.2119/molmed.2010.00256

Emery, A. E. (1991). Population frequencies of inherited neuromuscular diseases – a world survey. *Neuromuscul. Disord.* 1, 19–29. doi:10.1016/0960-8966(91)90039-U

Fayssoil, A., Nardi, O., Orlikowski, D., and Annane, D. (2010). Cardiomyopathy in Duchenne muscular dystrophy: pathogenesis and therapeutics. *Heart Fail. Rev.* 15, 103–107. doi:10.1007/s10741-009-9156-8

Ganley, I. G., Lam du, H., Wang, J., Ding, X., Chen, S., and Jiang, X. (2009). ULK1.ATG13.FIP200 complex mediates mTOR signaling and is essential for autophagy. *J. Biol. Chem.* 284, 12297–12305. doi:10.1074/jbc.M900573200

Govoni, A., Magri, F., Brajkovic, S., Zanetta, C., Faravelli, I., Corti, S., et al. (2013). Ongoing therapeutic trials and outcome measures for Duchenne muscular dystrophy. *Cell. Mol. Life Sci.* 70, 4585–4602. doi:10.1007/s00018-013-1396-z

Grumati, P., Coletto, L., Sabatelli, P., Cescon, M., Angelin, A., Bertaggia, E., et al. (2010). Autophagy is defective in collagen VI muscular dystrophies, and its reactivation rescues myofiber degeneration. *Nat. Med.* 16, 1313–1320. doi:10.1038/nm.2247

Hindi, S. M., Sato, S., Choi, Y., and Kumar, A. (2014). Distinct roles of TRAF6 at early and late stages of muscle pathology in the mdx model of Duchenne muscular dystrophy. *Hum. Mol. Genet.* 23, 1492–1505. doi:10.1093/hmg/ddt536

Hollinger, K., Gardan-Salmon, D., Santana, C., Rice, D., Snella, E., and Selsby, J. T. (2013). Rescue of dystrophic skeletal muscle by PGC-1alpha involves restored expression of dystrophin-associated protein complex components and satellite cell signaling. *Am. J. Physiol. Regul. Integr. Comp. Physiol.* 305, R13–R23. doi:10.1152/ajpregu.00221.2012

Hosokawa, N., Hara, T., Kaizuka, T., Kishi, C., Takamura, A., Miura, Y., et al. (2009). Nutrient-dependent mTORC1 association with the ULK1-Atg13-FIP200 complex required for autophagy. *Mol. Biol. Cell* 20, 1981–1991. doi:10.1091/mbc.E08-12-1248

Huang, J., and Manning, B. D. (2009). A complex interplay between Akt, TSC2 and the two mTOR complexes. *Biochem. Soc. Trans.* 37, 217–222. doi:10.1042/BST0370217

Hulmi, J. J., Oliveira, B. M., Silvennoinen, M., Hoogaars, W. M., Pasternack, A., Kainulainen, H., et al. (2013). Exercise restores decreased physical activity levels and increases markers of autophagy and oxidative capacity in myostatin/activin-blocked mdx mice. *Am. J. Physiol. Endocrinol. Metab.* 305, E171–E182. doi:10.1152/ajpendo.00065.2013

Hurley, J. H., and Schulman, B. A. (2014). Atomistic autophagy: the structures of cellular self-digestion. *Cell* 157, 300–311. doi:10.1016/j.cell.2014.01.070

Im, W. B., Phelps, S. F., Copen, E. H., Adams, E. G., Slightom, J. L., and Chamberlain, J. S. (1996). Differential expression of dystrophin isoforms in strains of mdx mice with different mutations. *Hum. Mol. Genet.* 5, 1149–1153. doi:10.1093/hmg/5.8.1149

Inoki, K., Zhu, T., and Guan, K. L. (2003). TSC2 mediates cellular energy response to control cell growth and survival. *Cell* 115, 577–590. doi:10.1016/S0092-8674(03)00929-2

Itakura, E., Kishi, C., Inoue, K., and Mizushima, N. (2008). Beclin 1 forms two distinct phosphatidylinositol 3-kinase complexes with mammalian Atg14 and UVRAG. *Mol. Biol. Cell* 19, 5360–5372. doi:10.1091/mbc.E08-01-0080

Jefferies, J. L., Eidem, B. W., Belmont, J. W., Craigen, W. J., Ware, S. M., Fernbach, S. D., et al. (2005). Genetic predictors and remodeling of dilated cardiomyopathy in muscular dystrophy. *Circulation* 112, 2799–2804. doi:10.1161/CIRCULATIONAHA.104.528281

Jiang, P., and Mizushima, N. (2014). Autophagy and human diseases. *Cell Res.* 24, 69–79. doi:10.1038/cr.2013.161

Jung, C. H., Ro, S. H., Cao, J., Otto, N. M., and Kim, D. H. (2010). mTOR regulation of autophagy. *FEBS Lett.* 584, 1287–1295. doi:10.1016/j.febslet.2010.01.017

Kabeya, Y., Mizushima, N., Ueno, T., Yamamoto, A., Kirisako, T., Noda, T., et al. (2000). LC3, a mammalian homologue of yeast Apg8p, is localized in autophagosome membranes after processing. *EMBO J.* 19, 5720–5728. doi:10.1093/emboj/19.21.5720

Kim, J., Kundu, M., Viollet, B., and Guan, K. L. (2011). AMPK and mTOR regulate autophagy through direct phosphorylation of Ulk1. *Nat. Cell Biol.* 13, 132–141. doi:10.1038/ncb2152

Le Grand, F., and Rudnicki, M. A. (2007). Skeletal muscle satellite cells and adult myogenesis. *Curr. Opin. Cell Biol.* 19, 628–633. doi:10.1016/j.ceb.2007.09.012

Ljubicic, V., and Jasmin, B. J. (2013). AMP-activated protein kinase at the nexus of therapeutic skeletal muscle plasticity in Duchenne muscular dystrophy. *Trends Mol. Med.* 19, 614–624. doi:10.1016/j.molmed.2013.07.002

Ljubicic, V., Miura, P., Burt, M., Boudreault, L., Khogali, S., Lunde, J. A., et al. (2011). Chronic AMPK activation evokes the slow, oxidative myogenic program and triggers beneficial adaptations in mdx mouse skeletal muscle. *Hum. Mol. Genet.* 20, 3478–3493. doi:10.1093/hmg/ddr265

Long, X., Lin, Y., Ortiz-Vega, S., Yonezawa, K., and Avruch, J. (2005a). Rheb binds and regulates the mTOR kinase. *Curr. Biol.* 15, 702–713. doi:10.1016/j.cub.2005.02.053

Long, X., Ortiz-Vega, S., Lin, Y., and Avruch, J. (2005b). Rheb binding to mammalian target of rapamycin (mTOR) is regulated by amino acid sufficiency. *J. Biol. Chem.* 280, 23433–23436. doi:10.1074/jbc.C500169200

Lynch, G. S., Rafael, J. A., Chamberlain, J. S., and Faulkner, J. A. (2000). Contraction-induced injury to single permeabilized muscle fibers from mdx, transgenic mdx, and control mice. *Am. J. Physiol. Cell Physiol.* 279, C1290–C1294.

Magri, F., Govoni, A., D'Angelo, M. G., Del Bo, R., Ghezzi, S., Sandra, G., et al. (2011). Genotype and phenotype characterization in a large dystrophinopathic cohort with extended follow-up. *J. Neurol.* 258, 1610–1623. doi:10.1007/s00415-011-5979-z

Mammucari, C., Milan, G., Romanello, V., Masiero, E., Rudolf, R., Del Piccolo, P., et al. (2007). FoxO3 controls autophagy in skeletal muscle in vivo. *Cell Metab.* 6, 458–471. doi:10.1016/j.cmet.2007.11.001

Masiero, E., Agatea, L., Mammucari, C., Blaauw, B., Loro, E., Komatsu, M., et al. (2009). Autophagy is required to maintain muscle mass. *Cell Metab.* 10, 507–515. doi:10.1016/j.cmet.2009.10.008

McGeachie, J. K., Grounds, M. D., Partridge, T. A., and Morgan, J. E. (1993). Age-related changes in replication of myogenic cells in mdx mice: quantitative autoradiographic studies. *J. Neurol. Sci.* 119, 169–179. doi:10.1016/0022-510X(93)90130-Q

Mehrpour, M., Esclatine, A., Beau, I., and Codogno, P. (2010). Overview of macroautophagy regulation in mammalian cells. *Cell Res.* 20, 748–762. doi:10.1038/cr.2010.82

Mendell, J. R., Rodino-Klapac, L., Sahenk, Z., Malik, V., Kaspar, B. K., Walker, C. M., et al. (2012). Gene therapy for muscular dystrophy: lessons learned and path forward. *Neurosci. Lett.* 527, 90–99. doi:10.1016/j.neulet.2012.04.078

Merlini, L., and Nishino, I. (2014). 201St ENMC international workshop: autophagy in muscular dystrophies – translational approach, 1-3 November 2013, Bussum, The Netherlands. *Neuromuscul. Disord.* 24, 546–561. doi:10.1016/j.nmd.2014.03.009

Mihaylova, M. M., and Shaw, R. J. (2011). The AMPK signalling pathway coordinates cell growth, autophagy and metabolism. *Nat. Cell Biol.* 13, 1016–1023. doi:10.1038/ncb2329

Mizushima, N., Sugita, H., Yoshimori, T., and Ohsumi, Y. (1998). A new protein conjugation system in human. The counterpart of the yeast Apg12p conjugation system essential for autophagy. *J. Biol. Chem.* 273, 33889–33892. doi:10.1074/jbc.273.51.33889

Mizushima, N., Yamamoto, A., Matsui, M., Yoshimori, T., and Ohsumi, Y. (2004). In vivo analysis of autophagy in response to nutrient starvation using transgenic mice expressing a fluorescent autophagosome marker. *Mol. Biol. Cell* 15, 1101–1111. doi:10.1091/mbc.E03-09-0704

Mosqueira, M., Zeiger, U., Forderer, M., Brinkmeier, H., and Fink, R. H. (2013). Cardiac and respiratory dysfunction in Duchenne muscular dystrophy and the role of second messengers. *Med. Res. Rev.* 33, 1174–1213. doi:10.1002/med.21279

Mouisel, E., Vignaud, A., Hourde, C., Butler-Browne, G., and Ferry, A. (2010). Muscle weakness and atrophy are associated with decreased regenerative capacity and changes in mTOR signaling in skeletal muscles of venerable (18-24-month-old) dystrophic mdx mice. *Muscle Nerve* 41, 809–818. doi:10.1002/mus.21624

Nakamura, A., and Takeda, S. (2011). Mammalian models of Duchenne Muscular Dystrophy: pathological characteristics and therapeutic applications. *J. Biomed. Biotechnol.* 2011, 184393. doi:10.1155/2011/184393

Neel, B. A., Lin, Y., and Pessin, J. E. (2013). Skeletal muscle autophagy: a new metabolic regulator. *Trends Endocrinol. Metab.* 24, 635–643. doi:10.1016/j.tem.2013.09.004

Pauly, M., Daussin, F., Burelle, Y., Li, T., Godin, R., Fauconnier, J., et al. (2012). AMPK activation stimulates autophagy and ameliorates muscular dystrophy in the mdx mouse diaphragm. *Am. J. Pathol.* 181, 583–592. doi:10.1016/j.ajpath.2012.04.004

Peter, A. K., and Crosbie, R. H. (2006). Hypertrophic response of Duchenne and limb-girdle muscular dystrophies is associated with activation of Akt pathway. *Exp. Cell Res.* 312, 2580–2591. doi:10.1016/j.yexcr.2006.04.024

Pichavant, C., Aartsma-Rus, A., Clemens, P. R., Davies, K. E., Dickson, G., Takeda, S., et al. (2011). Current status of pharmaceutical and genetic therapeutic approaches to treat DMD. *Mol. Ther.* 19, 830–840. doi:10.1038/mt.2011.59

Politano, L., and Nigro, G. (2012). Treatment of dystrophinopathic cardiomyopathy: review of the literature and personal results. *Acta Myol.* 31, 24–30.

Proikas-Cezanne, T., Waddell, S., Gaugel, A., Frickey, T., Lupas, A., and Nordheim, A. (2004). WIPI-1alpha (WIPI49), a member of the novel 7-bladed WIPI protein family, is aberrantly expressed in human cancer and is linked to starvation-induced autophagy. *Oncogene* 23, 9314–9325. doi:10.1038/sj.onc.1208331

Quinlan, J. G., Hahn, H. S., Wong, B. L., Lorenz, J. N., Wenisch, A. S., and Levin, L. S. (2004). Evolution of the mdx mouse cardiomyopathy: physiological and morphological findings. *Neuromuscul. Disord.* 14, 491–496. doi:10.1016/j.nmd.2004.04.007

Raben, N., Hill, V., Shea, L., Takikita, S., Baum, R., Mizushima, N., et al. (2008). Suppression of autophagy in skeletal muscle uncovers the accumulation of ubiquitinated proteins and their potential role in muscle damage in Pompe disease. *Hum. Mol. Genet.* 17, 3897–3908. doi:10.1093/hmg/ddn292

Sandri, M. (2010). Autophagy in skeletal muscle. *FEBS Lett.* 584, 1411–1416. doi:10.1016/j.febslet.2010.01.056

Sandri, M., Coletto, L., Grumati, P., and Bonaldo, P. (2013). Misregulation of autophagy and protein degradation systems in myopathies and muscular dystrophies. *J. Cell. Sci.* 126, 5325–5333. doi:10.1242/jcs.114041

Sarbassov, D. D., Ali, S. M., Sengupta, S., Sheen, J. H., Hsu, P. P., Bagley, A. F., et al. (2006). Prolonged rapamycin treatment inhibits mTORC2 assembly and Akt/PKB. *Mol. Cell* 22, 159–168. doi:10.1016/j.molcel.2006.03.029

Schneider, J. L., and Cuervo, A. M. (2014). Autophagy and human disease: emerging themes. *Curr. Opin. Genet. Dev.* 26C, 16–23. doi:10.1016/j.gde.2014.04.003

Spitali, P., Grumati, P., Hiller, M., Chrisam, M., Aartsma-Rus, A., and Bonaldo, P. (2013). Autophagy is impaired in the tibialis anterior of dystrophin null mice. *PLoS Curr.* 5. doi:10.1371/currents.md.e1226cefa851a2f079bbc406c0a21e80

Spurney, C. F. (2011). Cardiomyopathy of Duchenne muscular dystrophy: current understanding and future directions. *Muscle Nerve* 44, 8–19. doi:10.1002/mus.22097

Stedman, H. H., Sweeney, H. L., Shrager, J. B., Maguire, H. C., Panettieri, R. A., Petrof, B., et al. (1991). The mdx mouse diaphragm reproduces the degenerative changes of Duchenne muscular dystrophy. *Nature* 352, 536–539. doi:10.1038/352536a0

Straub, V., and Campbell, K. P. (1997). Muscular dystrophies and the dystrophin-glycoprotein complex. *Curr. Opin. Neurol.* 10, 168–175. doi:10.1097/00019052-199704000-00016

Thomas, G. D. (2013). Functional muscle ischemia in Duchenne and Becker muscular dystrophy. *Front. Physiol.* 4:381. doi:10.3389/fphys.2013.00381

Vergne, I., Roberts, E., Elmaoued, R. A., Tosch, V., Delgado, M. A., Proikas-Cezanne, T., et al. (2009). Control of autophagy initiation by phosphoinositide 3-phosphatase Jumpy. *EMBO J.* 28, 2244–2258. doi:10.1038/emboj.2009.159

Willmann, R., Possekel, S., Dubach-Powell, J., Meier, T., and Ruegg, M. A. (2009). Mammalian animal models for Duchenne muscular dystrophy. *Neuromuscul. Disord.* 19, 241–249. doi:10.1016/j.nmd.2008.11.015

Wong, P. M., Puente, C., Ganley, I. G., and Jiang, X. (2013). The ULK1 complex: sensing nutrient signals for autophagy activation. *Autophagy* 9, 124–137. doi:10.4161/auto.23323

Zhao, J., Brault, J. J., Schild, A., Cao, P., Sandri, M., Schiaffino, S., et al. (2007). FoxO3 coordinately activates protein degradation by the autophagic/lysosomal and proteasomal pathways in atrophying muscle cells. *Cell Metab.* 6, 472–483. doi:10.1016/j.cmet.2007.11.004

14

Shorter telomeres in peripheral blood mononuclear cells from older persons with sarcopenia: results from an exploratory study

Emanuele Marzetti[1]*, Maria Lorenzi[1], Manuela Antocicco[1], Stefano Bonassi[2], Michela Celi[1], Simona Mastropaolo[1], Silvana Settanni[1], Vanessa Valdiglesias[3], Francesco Landi[1], Roberto Bernabei[1] and Graziano Onder[1]

[1] *Department of Geriatrics, Neurosciences and Orthopedics, Teaching Hospital "Agostino Gemelli," Catholic University of the Sacred Heart School of Medicine, Rome, Italy*
[2] *Unit of Clinical and Molecular Epidemiology, IRCCS San Raffaele Pisana, Rome, Italy*
[3] *DICOMOSA Group, Department of Psychology, Area of Psychobiology, University of A Coruña, A Coruña, Spain*

Correspondence:
Emanuele Marzetti, Biogerontology Laboratory, Department of Geriatrics, Neurosciences and Orthopedics, Catholic University of the Sacred Heart School of Medicine, L.go F. Vito 1, Rome 00168, Italy
e-mail: emarzetti@live.com

Background: Telomere shortening in peripheral blood mononuclear cells (PBMCs) has been associated with biological age and several chronic degenerative diseases. However, the relationship between telomere length and sarcopenia, a hallmark of the aging process, is unknown. The aim of the present study was therefore to determine whether PBMC telomeres obtained from sarcopenic older persons were shorter relative to non-sarcopenic peers. We further explored if PBMC telomere length was associated with frailty, a major clinical correlate of sarcopenia.

Methods: Analyses were conducted in 142 persons aged ≥65 years referred to a geriatric outpatient clinic (University Hospital). The presence of sarcopenia was established according to the European Working Group on Sarcopenia in Older People criteria, with bioelectrical impedance analysis used for muscle mass estimation. The frailty status was determined by both the Fried's criteria (physical frailty, PF) and a modified Rockwood's frailty index (FI). Telomere length was measured in PBMCs by quantitative real-time polymerase chain reaction according to the telomere/single-copy gene ratio (T/S) method.

Results: Among 142 outpatients (mean age 75.0 ± 6.5 years, 59.2% women), sarcopenia was diagnosed in 23 individuals (19.3%). The PF phenotype was detected in 74 participants (52.1%). The average FI score was 0.46 ± 0.17. PBMC telomeres were shorter in sarcopenic subjects ($T/S = 0.21$; 95% CI: 0.18–0.24) relative to non-sarcopenic individuals ($T/S = 0.26$; 95% CI: 0.24–0.28; $p = 0.01$), independent of age, gender, smoking habit, or comorbidity. No significant associations were determined between telomere length and either PF or the FI.

Conclusion: PBMC telomere length, expressed as T/S values, is shorter in older outpatients with sarcopenia. The cross-sectional assessment of PBMC telomere length is not sufficient at capturing the complex, multidimensional syndrome of frailty.

Keywords: frailty, biological age, muscle aging, oxidative stress, inflammation, bioelectrical impedance analysis

INTRODUCTION

The remarkable inter-individual variability in functional and health status observed in late life indicates that chronological age *per se* does not precisely reflect the actual biological age of an organism (Mitnitski et al., 2002). This has instigated a great deal of research aimed at identifying clinical and biological parameters that are able to provide an overview of the health status, predict the risk of age-related diseases, and help estimate the remaining lifespan of an individual (Vasto et al., 2010).

Telomere biology has gained a special interest in the field of aging biomarkers (Lehmann et al., 2013). Telomeres are specialized structures located at the termini of mammalian chromosomes and consist of protein-bound, non-coding tandem-repeated hexamers (Blackburn, 1991). They serve to protect genome integrity by camouflaging chromosome ends from the DNA damage-response machinery, which would otherwise sense them as double-stranded breaks (Blackburn, 1991). In somatic cells, each round of DNA replication causes a loss of telomere repeats at the lagging strand, due to the presence of a terminal gap after degradation of the most distal primer. This phenomenon limits the total number of divisions normal somatic cells can undergo (Allsopp et al., 1992).

The observation that telomeres shorten over the life course and are implicated in cellular senescence has led to the hypothesis that telomere attrition may be a mechanism driving the aging process (Mikhelson and Gamaley, 2012). Indeed, associations have been determined between telomere erosion and premature aging syndromes, several age-sensitive measures (e.g., blood pressure, lung function, cognition, bone mineral density), age-related conditions (e.g., insulin resistance, type II diabetes mellitus, coronary artery disease, chronic obstructive pulmonary disease, dementia, cancer), and mortality [reviewed by Blasco (2005)]. As such, telomere length is considered to be an indicator of health status and, more in general, of biological age (Fossel, 2012).

At the clinical level, the assessment of muscle mass and function has emerged as a possible biomarker for aging (Fisher, 2004). Notably, the age-related loss in muscle mass and strength (sarcopenia) fulfills virtually all of the criteria defining an aging biomarker (Sprott, 2010). Indeed, sarcopenia (1) is an aging trait shared across species (Augustin and Partridge, 2009), (2) begins in adulthood and worsens over the course of aging (Frontera et al., 1991), (3) develops as a consequence of aging itself rather than being a mere correlate of other diseases (Iannuzzi-Sucich et al., 2002), (4) is not directly lethal, albeit impacting the health and functional status of an individual (Rolland et al., 2008), (5) is measurable and reproducible (Cruz-Jentoft et al., 2010), and (6) shows a clinical evolution that can be followed over relatively short periods of time (Marzetti, 2012).

The relationship between telomere attrition and muscle aging is currently unknown. The purpose of the present investigation was therefore to explore whether telomere length, measured in peripheral blood mononuclear cells (PBMCs), was associated with sarcopenia in a sample of older adults referred to a geriatric outpatient clinic. We further evaluated if PBMC telomere length was related to frailty, a major clinical consequence of sarcopenia (Roubenoff, 2000) and a possible additional clinical indicator of biological age (Mitnitski et al., 2002; Goggins et al., 2005).

MATERIALS AND METHODS

PARTICIPANT RECRUITMENT AND SETTING

The study was conducted at the outpatient clinic of the Department of Geriatrics, Neurosciences and Orthopedics, Teaching Hospital "Agostino Gemelli," Catholic University of the Sacred Heart (Rome, Italy). All patients aged 65+ years, admitted between October 2012 and January 2013, were invited to take part in the investigation. Exclusion criteria were: presence of disease conditions with an estimated life expectancy <6 months, inability to walk for 4 m, peripheral edema, presence of pacemaker or implantable cardioverter defibrillator, and unwillingness or inability to provide informed consent. The study was approved by the Institutional Review Board of the Catholic University of the Sacred Heart, and all participants signed a written consent. Study visits for physical function testing, body composition assessment, and blood sampling were scheduled within a week of enrollment.

DATA COLLECTION

Demographic, clinical data, and lifestyle habits were collected at the time of enrollment through a dedicated questionnaire. Disability status was evaluated by the Katz's Activities of the Daily Living (ADL) (Katz and Akpom, 1976). Cognition was assessed using the mini-mental state examination (MMSE) (Folstein et al., 1975), while mood was evaluated by the 15-item Geriatric Depression Scale (GDS) (Sheikh and Yesavage, 1986). Diagnoses were gathered from the patient, attending physicians, and the careful review of medical charts. Finally, the comorbidity burden was calculated via the Cumulative Illness Rating Scale (CIRS) (Linn et al., 1968).

IDENTIFICATION OF SARCOPENIA

The presence of sarcopenia was established according to the European Working Group on Sarcopenia in Older People (EWGSOP) criteria (Cruz-Jentoft et al., 2010). Whole-body fat-free mass was measured by bioelectrical impedance analysis (BIA) using a Quantum/S Bioelectrical Body Composition Analyzer (Akern Srl, Florence, Italy) with an operating frequency of 50 kHz at 800 μA. Measurements were taken under standard conditions, with the subject in a supine position and surface electrodes placed on the right wrist and ankle (NIH Expert Panel, 1996). Muscle mass was estimated using the equation developed by Janssen et al. (2000). The skeletal muscle index [SMI (kg/m^2)] was obtained dividing absolute muscle mass by squared height. According to the EWGSOP indications, low SMI was defined based on the following cut-offs: $<8.87\ kg/m^2$ in men and $<6.42\ kg/m^2$ in women (Cruz-Jentoft et al., 2010).

DEFINITION OF FRAILTY STATUS

The frailty status of participants was assessed according to both the Fried's criteria (physical frailty, PF) (Fried et al., 2001) and a modified Rockwood's frailty index (FI) (Searle et al., 2008). The following indicators were considered to define PF: (1) unintentional weight loss in prior 12 months; (2) poor endurance and energy; (3) weakness, defined by poor grip strength; (4) slowness, assessed via timed 4-m walk speed; and (5) low physical activity level according to the Physical Activity Scale for the Elderly (PASE) (Washburn et al., 1993) (**Table 1**).

The participant frailty status was further evaluated by constructing a FI based on the summation of "health deficits" principle (Rockwood et al., 2005), according to the procedure described by Searle et al. (2008). A total of 30 deficits were used for the construction of the FI, which is expressed as the ratio of deficits observed to the total number of deficits considered. The variables used for the computation of the FI and their corresponding cut-points are listed in **Table 2**.

BLOOD SAMPLING AND PROCESSING

Blood samples were obtained by Vacutainer™ venipuncture of the median cubital vein after overnight fasting. Blood samples (10 mL) were diluted 1:1 in phosphate-buffered saline (PBS) and PBMCs separated within 1 h of blood draw by Ficoll-Hypaque (Comercial RAFER, Zaragoza, Spain) density gradient following the manufacturer's instructions. Cells were washed twice with PBS and cryopreserved at -80°C in RPMI 1640 containing 50% fetal bovine serum and 10% dimethylsulfoxide.

MEASUREMENT OF TELOMERE LENGTH BY QUANTITATIVE REAL-TIME POLYMERASE CHAIN REACTION

Genomic DNA was extracted from isolated PBMCs using a commercial DNA isolation kit (Norgen Biotek, Thorold, Canada) as

Table 1 | Indicators of physical frailty.

Frailty criteria	Parameters
Weight loss	Loss of ≥5 kg in prior 12 months, unintentional
Exhaustion	Response of "a moderate amount of the time (3–4 days)" or "most of the time" to the CES-D scale item: "I felt that everything I did was an effort" during the past week
Weakness	Low grip strength assessed by a North Coast handheld dynamometer. Gender- and BMI-specific cutoff points provided by Fried et al. (2001) were adopted
Slowness	Time in seconds to complete a 4-m walk at usual pace. Gender- and height-specific cutoff points provided by Fried et al. (2001) were adopted
Low physical activity levels	Physical Activity Scale for the Elderly (PASE); cut-points: Men < 64, women < 52 (Rothman et al., 2008)
Frailty status	**Number of criteria**
Robust	0
Pre-frail	1–2
Frail	≥3

BMI, body mass index; CES-D, Center for Epidemiologic Studies-Depression.

per the manufacturer's instructions. Relative telomere length was measured by quantitative real-time polymerase chain reaction (qRT-PCR) according to the telomere/single-copy gene ratio (T/S) method (Cawthon, 2002) with minor modifications. Briefly, the method measures the ratio between the copy number of telomere repeats (T) and that of the single-copy gene 36B4 (S) used as a quantitative control, relative to a calibrator sample (human genomic DNA; Roche Diagnostic, Indianapolis, IN). qRT-PCR was performed using an Applied Biosystems 7300 RT-PCR System (ABI, Foster City, CA) with the following cycling conditions: 95°C for 10 min, 40 cycles at 95°C for 5 s, 56°C for 30 s, 72°C for 30 s. T and S were analyzed in duplicate within the same plate. The same calibrator sample was included in all plates to allow comparisons across runs. A no-template control was also included for quality control. The relative T/S values were calculated according to the $2^{-\Delta\Delta CT}$ method (Livak and Schmittgen, 2001).

STATISTICAL ANALYSES

All data are expressed as proportions (%) or mean ± SD. Given the non-normal distribution of T/S values, analyses were run using log-transformed values to ensure equality of variances and render the errors approximately normally distributed. Analysis of covariance (ANCOVA) was used to compare adjusted means of log T/S values according to sarcopenia, SMI categories, and frailty. Geometric means of T/S values are shown in tables and text. Analyses were adjusted for age, gender, smoking habit, presence of diabetes, and CIRS score. The Spearman's rank correlation coefficient was used to calculate the strength of association between variables. All analyses were performed using the SPSS software (version 18, SPSS Inc., Chicago, IL, USA).

Table 2 | Health variables and cut-points used for the computation of a modified Rockwood's frailty index.

Health variables	Condition or variable cut-points	Score
Marital status	Married or single	0
	Widow or divorced	1
Social involvement	Yes	0
	No	1
Impaired ADL	None	0
	1	0.25
	2	0.5
	3–4	0.75
	4–6	1
Impaired IADL	None	0
	1–2	0.25
	3–4	0.5
	5–6	0.75
	7–8	1
Walk speed (4 m)	≥0.8	0
	<0.8	1
Grip strength[a]	Normal	0
	Low	1
Cognition (MMSE)	>24	0
	20–24	0.25
	18–20	0.50
	11–17	0.75
	<10	1
Mood (GDS)	0–2	0
	3–5	0.25
	6–8	0.5
	9–11	0.75
	>11	1
Sedentarism (PASE)	Men ≥ 64, women ≥ 52	0
	Men < 64, women < 52	1
Hospital admission(s) in prior 12 months	No	0
	Yes	1
BMI	18.5–24.9	0
	25–30	0.5
	>30 or <18.5	1
Nutrition (MNA)	≥23.5	0
	≥17 < 23.5	0.5
	<17	1
Unintentional weight loss (>5 kg in prior 12 months)	No	0
	Yes	1
Chronic pain	No	0
	Yes	1
Fall(s) in prior 12 months	No	0
	Yes	1

(Continued)

Table 2 | Continued

Health variables	Condition or variable cut-points	Score
Cancer or active cancer treatment	No Yes	0 1
Cardiovascular disease	No Yes	0 1
Chronic lung diseases	No Yes	0 1
Hematological diseases	No Yes	0 1
Renal diseases	No Yes	0 1
Central nervous system diseases	No Yes	0 1
Peripheral nervous system diseases	No Yes	0 1
Gastrointestinal diseases	No Yes	0 1
Ear, nose, and throat diseases	No Yes	0 1
Orthopedic diseases	No Yes	0 1
Psychiatric disorders	No Yes	0 1
Diabetes mellitus	No Yes	0 1
Endocrine disorders	No Yes	0 1
Sarcopenia	No Yes	0 1
Polypharmacy (≥6 drugs)	No Yes	0 1

[a]Men: 1, BMI ≤ 24, grip strength ≤ 29 kg; BMI 24.1–28, grip strength ≤30 kg; BMI > 28, grip strength ≤ 32 kg. Women: 1, BMI ≤ 23, grip strength ≤ 17 kg; BMI 23.1–26, grip strength ≤ 17.3 kg; BMI 26.1–29, grip strength ≤ 18 kg; BMI > 29, grip strength ≤ 21 kg.

ADL, activities of daily living; BMI, body mass index; IADL, instrumental activities of daily living; GDS, Geriatric Depression Scale; MMSE, mini-mental state examination; MNA, Mini nutritional assessment; PASE, physical activity scale for the elderly.

RESULTS

A total of 142 subjects were enrolled in the study. The main characteristics of the study sample are shown in **Table 3**. Sarcopenia was identified in 23 participants (19.3%). The prevalence of sarcopenia was uniform across ages and genders. Frailty, as determined by the Fried's criteria (PF), was detected in 74 participants (52.1%). Individuals classified as frail according to PF were older relative to non-frail subjects (76.6 ± 6.7 vs. 73.1 ± 6.0 years; $p = 0.001$), with no differences between genders. An identical prevalence of frailty was observed using 0.44 as the cutoff for the FI, as recommended by Rockwood et al. (2007). Similar to PF, participants with a FI score ≥0.44 were older than those with lower scores (76.4 ± 6.6 vs. 73.2 ± 6.2 years; $p = 0.004$), with an equal gender distribution. Sixty-one participants were identified as frail based on both PF and the FI score, and the two measures of frailty were significantly correlated with each other ($r = 0.63$; $p < 0.0001$). The strength of this correlation is comparable to that reported using the original version of the FI (Rockwood et al., 2007). Hence, the modified FI constructed for the present study was able to capture the condition of interest. The coexistence of sarcopenia and PF was observed in 21 subjects (91.3%), whereas 15 (65.2%) participants with sarcopenia were classified as frail according to the FI.

Table 3 | Study sample characteristics.

	Whole sample ($n = 142$) n (%)
Age, years (mean ± SD)	74.9 ± 6.5
Female gender	84 (59.2)
Smokers	11 (7.7)
Education, years (mean ± SD)	10.0 ± 5.0
Hospital admission in prior 12 months	41 (29.0)
MMSE score (mean ± SD)	26.2 ± 3.4
CIRS (mean ± SD)	3.0 ± 2.2
GDS (mean ± SD)	10.8 ± 7.6
ADL scale (mean ± SD)	5.0 ± 1.3
IADL scale (mean ± SD)	5.9 ± 2.4
Fall in prior 12 months	66 (46.5)
BMI (mean ± SD)	27.7 ± 4.7
Number of drugs (mean ± SD)	6.1 ± 3.3
Frail (Fried's criteria, PF)	74 (52.1)
Number of frailty criteria (mean ± SD)	2.3 ± 1.8
Frail (modified Rockwood's frailty index, FI)	74 (52.1)
FI (mean ± SD)	0.46 ± 0.17
Sarcopenia (EWGSOP criteria)	23 (19.3)
PBMC telomere length (T/S)	0.27 ± 0.10

ADL, activities of daily living; BMI, body mass index; CIRS, Cumulative Illness Rating Scale; EWGSOP, European Working Group on Sarcopenia in Older People; FI, frailty index; GDS, Geriatric Depression Scale; IADL, instrumental activities of daily living; MMSE, mini-mental state examination; PBMC, peripheral blood mononuclear cell; PF, physical frailty.

PBMC telomeres were shorter in sarcopenic subjects ($T/S = 0.21$; 95% CI: 0.18–0.24) relative to non-sarcopenic individuals ($T/S = 0.26$; 95%: CI: 0.24–0.28; $p = 0.01$), independent of age, gender, smoking habit, presence of diabetes, and comorbidity (**Table 4**). Of the three parameters considered for the definition of sarcopenia (i.e., muscle mass, gait speed, and handgrip strength), T/S was only correlated with SMI (**Figure 1**).

PBMC telomeres showed a trend toward lower T/S values in frail subjects relative non-frail participants, but the difference did not reach the statistical significance in either unadjusted or

Table 4 | Mean telomere/single-copy gene ratio (*T/S*) values according to sarcopenia, skeletal muscle index, and frailty status.

	Mean telomere/single-copy gene ratio (*T/S*)			
	Unadjusted mean[a] (95% CI)	*p*	Adjusted[b] mean[a] (95% CI)	*p*
SARCOPENIA (EWGSOP DEFINITION)				
No sarcopenia ($n = 119$)	0.26 (0.25–0.28)	0.004	0.26 (0.24–0.28)	0.01
Sarcopenia ($n = 23$)	0.21 (0.17–0.24)		0.21 (0.18–0.24)	
SKELETAL MUSCLE INDEX (SMI)				
Normal SMI ($n = 116$)	0.26 (0.24–0.28)	0.003	0.26 (0.24–0.28)	0.008
Low SMI ($n = 26$)	0.21 (0.17–0.24)		0.21 (0.18–0.24)	
FRAILTY, PF				
No frailty ($n = 68$)	0.27 (0.24–0.29)	0.11	0.26 (0.24–0.29)	0.31
Frailty ($n = 74$)	0.24 (0.22–0.26)		0.24 (0.22–0.27)	
FRAILTY, FI ≥ 0.44				
No frailty ($n = 68$)	0.27 (0.24–0.29)	0.12	0.26 (0.24–0.29)	0.38
Frailty ($n = 74$)	0.23 (0.22–0.26)		0.24 (0.22–0.27)	

Low SMI was defined as SMI < 8.87 kg/m² for men and SMI < 6.42 kg/m² for women.

[a] *Geometric means were calculated from log-transformed values.*

[b] *Adjusted for age, gender, smoking habit, diabetes, and Cumulative Illness Rating Scale score.*

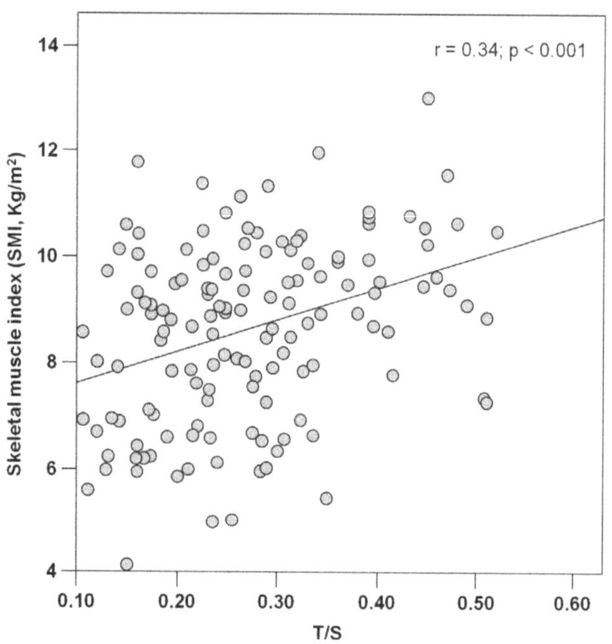

FIGURE 1 | Scatter plot of telomere/single-copy gene ratio (*T/S*) and the skeletal muscle index ($n = 142$).

adjusted analyses, regardless of the frailty assessment tool adopted (**Table 4**). Finally, no significant correlations were determined between *T/S* values and any of the five domains defining PF (data not shown).

DISCUSSION

Previous studies have shown that telomere attrition and dysfunction are implicated in a host of age-related disorders, including cancer, cardiovascular disease, type 2 diabetes mellitus, osteoarthritis, chronic obstructive pulmonary disease, dementia, and immunosenescence [reviewed by Xi et al. (2013)]. However, the literature is void of investigations concerning the relationship between telomere length and sarcopenia, a hallmark of the aging process (Fisher, 2004). Furthermore, only sparse reports exist that have examined the association between telomere length and frailty (Woo et al., 2008; Collerton et al., 2012), an additional clinical indicator of biological age (Mitnitski et al., 2002; Goggins et al., 2005) and a major consequence of sarcopenia (Roubenoff, 2000). The present investigation was therefore undertaken to explore whether a popular senescence biomarker (PBMC telomere length) was related to clinical measures of biological age (sarcopenia and frailty). Our results indicate that PBMC telomere length, expressed as *T/S* values, is associated with sarcopenia, but not frailty, in a sample of older outpatients.

These findings are supportive of the proposition that sarcopenia may serve as a clinical biomarker for aging (Fisher, 2004). The inverse association detected between PBMC telomere length and muscle mass could be reflective of a common pathogenic ground underlying age-related telomere shortening and muscle atrophy. Indeed, oxidative stress and chronic inflammation are involved both in telomere erosion (Aviv, 2004; Bayne and Liu, 2005) and sarcopenia (Marzetti et al., 2013). The exposure to high levels of free radicals has been identified as a causative factor for telomere shortening both *in vitro* (Richter and von Zglinicki, 2007) and in disease conditions characterized by enhanced oxidant generation, such as diabetes mellitus, dementia, cardiovascular disease, and cancer [reviewed by Aubert and Lansdorp (2008)]. Likewise, oxidative stress is a major culprit in the development of sarcopenia through irreversible damage to myocyte macromolecules, bioenergetic failure, and induction of apoptosis [reviewed by Marzetti et al. (2009) and Calvani et al. (2013)].

A major consequence of oxidative stress is the activation of redox-sensitive mediators, including nuclear factor-κB (NF-κB) (Chung et al., 2009). The latter, in turn, regulates the transcription of several pro-inflammatory cytokines (Chung et al., 2009). Under normal conditions, NF-κB activation in response to oxidative stimuli is short-lived, and the inflammatory reaction ceases with resolution. However, the long-term exposure to high levels of oxidants, as it seems to occur during aging, results in a chronic activation of NF-κB-mediated inflammatory response and cellular damage (Chung et al., 2006). Notably, increases in circulating levels of C-reactive protein (CRP) and serum amyloid A (SAA) were associated with proportional decreases in PBMC telomere length in a cohort of middle-aged workers exposed to occupational environmental pollution over 2 years of follow-up (Wong et al., 2014). In addition, cross-sectional analyses in a population of 1,962 older adults ranging in age between 70 and 79 years showed that individuals with elevated circulating levels of either interleukin-6 (IL-6) or tumor necrosis factor-alpha (TNF-α) had significantly higher odds for short PBMC telomeres, after adjustment for potential confounders (O'Donovan et al., 2011). Remarkably, the highest odds for short PBMC telomeres were found in older persons with high levels of both IL-6 and TNF-α (O'Donovan et al., 2011).

It is noteworthy that IL-6 (Payette et al., 2003), TNF-α (Pedersen et al., 2003), CRP (Cesari et al., 2005), and SAA (Zhang et al., 2009) have all been implicated in the pathogenesis of muscle atrophy in the context of sarcopenia or other muscle-wasting disorders. Similar to telomere attrition, the concomitant elevation of multiple inflammatory markers seems to play a synergistic role in age-related muscle loss (Visser et al., 2002).

The association between telomere length and sarcopenia was mainly driven by the relationship between *T/S* values and muscle mass. Indeed, of the three parameters indicated by the EWGSOP for the definition of sarcopenia (Cruz-Jentoft et al., 2010), PBMC telomere length was only correlated with SMI (**Figure 1**). The reasons for the absence of significant associations between *T/S* values and measures of muscle performance (handgrip strength and walk speed) are multifold. First, it is well known that losses in muscle mass and function follow different temporal trajectories during the course of aging, with steeper declines in strength relative to mass (Delmonico et al., 2009). Hence, at any given time point, PBMC telomere length may not necessarily correlate with all of the components of the sarcopenia syndrome. In addition, while SMI is intrinsic to muscle, force generation and ambulation depend on the coordinated function of multiple organ systems (i.e., musculoskeletal, cardiorespiratory, and central and peripheral nervous systems). Since the rate of aging varies across organs and tissues (Finkel et al., 1995), a single biological marker may not be equally effective at tracking the multitude of intrinsic and extrinsic factors responsible for muscle aging. A similar reasoning may explain the inability of PBMC telomere length measurements to capture the complex inter-organ interactions regulating muscle performance.

Since frailty has been proposed as a clinical meter for biological age (Mitnitski et al., 2002; Goggins et al., 2005) and represents a major consequence of sarcopenia (Roubenoff, 2000), one could have expected a relationship existed between PBMC telomere length and the frailty status. However, the lack of a significant association between *T/S* values and measures of frailty is in keeping with previous reports on the topic (Woo et al., 2008; Collerton et al., 2012). Similar to the present study, PBMC telomere length was indeed unrelated to either PF (Collerton et al., 2012) or the FI (Woo et al., 2008; Collerton et al., 2012). As previously reasoned with regard to muscle function, it is conceivable that the "snapshot" assessment of a single biological marker may not be sufficient at capturing a complex, multidimensional syndrome, such as frailty.

Although reporting novel findings, the present work presents some limitations that deserve further discussion. First of all, the study is exploratory in nature, evident by the relatively small sample size. For this reason, robust and pre-frail participants were considered as a single group, which prevented us from observing a possible gradient of *T/S* values across the frailty spectrum. Nevertheless, this approach allowed adjusting the analyses for a number of potential confounders, which adds further relevance to our findings. Second, the cross-sectional design of the study does not allow inferring about the temporal relationship among PBMC telomere length, frailty, and sarcopenia. Moreover, although BIA is an established technique for the estimation of lean body mass (Kyle et al., 2003), it does not represent the gold standard for the quantification of muscle mass. Nevertheless, BIA is safe, inexpensive, easy to use, and readily reproducible. This technique is indeed recommended by the EWGSOP for the estimation of muscle mass in ambulatory patients (Cruz-Jentoft et al., 2010), such as those enrolled in the present study. Furthermore, following the recommendations by the NIH Expert Panel (1996), BIA measurements were obtained under standard conditions to limit the possible variability arising from body position, hydration status, consumption of food and beverages, ambient air and skin temperature, recent physical activity, and conductance of the examining table. Finally, telomere length was estimated from *T/S* values, as determined by qRT-PCR, in place of absolute quantification by classic Southern blot methods on terminal restriction fragments. However, the *T/S* method has proven to be highly consistent with Southern blot (Epel et al., 2004; Grabowski et al., 2005).

CONCLUSION

Findings from this exploratory study indicate that PBMC telomeres are shorter in sarcopenic geriatric outpatients, after adjustment for potential confounders. The relationship between telomere length and sarcopenia appears to be mainly driven by muscle mass, which may be indicative of a common pathogenic ground for telomere erosion and muscle atrophy. The lack of a significant association between PBMC telomere length and measures of muscle performance or the frailty status reinforces the notion that telomere shortening may not suffice as a biomarker for complex, multidimensional age-related conditions (Woo et al., 2008; Collerton et al., 2012). Future studies are necessary to assess the relationship among telomere shortening, sarcopenia, and frailty over time as well as in response to interventions, such as physical exercise and nutrition, proven effective against muscle aging and its clinical correlates.

ACKNOWLEDGMENTS

This study was partly supported by the "Centro studi Achille e Linda Lorenzon" grants of the Ministry of Education, Universities and Research (MIUR – linea D1 2012 and linea D3.2 2013) and the Innovative Medicines Initiative Joint Undertaking (IMI–JU 115621). The authors wish to thank Dr. Riccardo Calvani (Catholic University of the Sacred Heart, Rome) for his critical review of the manuscript.

REFERENCES

Allsopp, R. C., Vaziri, H., Patterson, C., Goldstein, S., Younglai, E. V., Futcher, A. B., et al. (1992). Telomere length predicts replicative capacity of human fibroblasts. *Proc. Natl. Acad. Sci. U.S.A.* 89, 10114–10118. doi:10.1073/pnas.89.21.10114

Aubert, G., and Lansdorp, P. M. (2008). Telomeres and aging. *Physiol. Rev.* 88, 557–579. doi:10.1152/physrev.00026.2007

Augustin, H., and Partridge, L. (2009). Invertebrate models of age-related muscle degeneration. *Biochim. Biophys. Acta* 1790, 1084–1094. doi:10.1016/j.bbagen.2009.06.011

Aviv, A. (2004). Telomeres and human aging: facts and fibs. *Sci. Aging Knowledge Environ.* 2004, e43. doi:10.1126/sageke.2004.51.pe43

Bayne, S., and Liu, J. P. (2005). Hormones and growth factors regulate telomerase activity in ageing and cancer. *Mol. Cell. Endocrinol.* 240, 11–22. doi:10.1016/j.mce.2005.05.009

Blackburn, E. H. (1991). Structure and function of telomeres. *Nature* 350, 569–573. doi:10.1038/350569a0

Blasco, M. A. (2005). Telomeres and human disease: ageing, cancer and beyond. *Nat. Rev. Genet.* 6, 611–622. doi:10.1038/nrg1656

Calvani, R., Joseph, A. M., Adhihetty, P. J., Miccheli, A., Bossola, M., Leeuwenburgh, C., et al. (2013). Mitochondrial pathways in sarcopenia of aging and disuse muscle atrophy. *Biol. Chem.* 394, 393–414. doi:10.1515/hsz-2012-0247

Cawthon, R. M. (2002). Telomere measurement by quantitative PCR. *Nucleic Acids Res.* 30, e47. doi:10.1093/nar/30.10.e47

Cesari, M., Kritchevsky, S. B., Baumgartner, R. N., Atkinson, H. H., Penninx, B. W., Lenchik, L., et al. (2005). Sarcopenia, obesity, and inflammation – results from the Trial of Angiotensin Converting Enzyme Inhibition and Novel Cardiovascular Risk Factors Study. *Am. J. Clin. Nutr.* 82, 428–434.

Chung, H. Y., Cesari, M., Anton, S., Marzetti, E., Giovannini, S., Seo, A. Y., et al. (2009). Molecular inflammation: underpinnings of aging and age-related diseases. *Ageing Res. Rev.* 8, 18–30. doi:10.1016/j.arr.2008.07.002

Chung, H. Y., Sung, B., Jung, K. J., Zou, Y., and Yu, B. P. (2006). The molecular inflammatory process in aging. *Antioxid. Redox Signal.* 8, 572–581. doi:10.1089/ars.2006.8.572

Collerton, J., Martin-Ruiz, C., Davies, K., Hilkens, C. M., Isaacs, J., Kolenda, C., et al. (2012). Frailty and the role of inflammation, immunosenescence and cellular ageing in the very old: cross-sectional findings from the Newcastle 85+ study. *Mech. Ageing Dev.* 133, 456–466. doi:10.1016/j.mad.2012.05.005

Cruz-Jentoft, A. J., Baeyens, J. P., Bauer, J. M., Boirie, Y., Cederholm, T., Landi, F., et al. (2010). Sarcopenia: European consensus on definition and diagnosis: report of the European Working Group on Sarcopenia in Older People. *Age Ageing* 39, 412–423. doi:10.1093/ageing/afq034

Delmonico, M. J., Harris, T. B., Visser, M., Park, S. W., Conroy, M. B., Velasquez-Mieyer, P., et al. (2009). Longitudinal study of muscle strength, quality, and adipose tissue infiltration. *Am. J. Clin. Nutr.* 90, 1579–1585. doi:10.3945/ajcn.2009.28047

Epel, E. S., Blackburn, E. H., Lin, J., Dhabhar, F. S., Adler, N. E., Morrow, J. D., et al. (2004). Accelerated telomere shortening in response to life stress. *Proc. Natl. Acad. Sci. U.S.A.* 101, 17312–17315. doi:10.1073/pnas.0407162101

Finkel, D., Whitfield, K., and McGue, M. (1995). Genetic and environmental influences on functional age: a twin study. *J. Gerontol. B Psychol. Sci. Soc. Sci.* 50, 104–113. doi:10.1093/geronb/50B.2.P104

Fisher, A. L. (2004). Of worms and women: sarcopenia and its role in disability and mortality. *J. Am. Geriatr. Soc.* 52, 1185–1190. doi:10.1111/j.1532-5415.2004.52320.x

Folstein, M. F., Folstein, S. E., and McHugh, P. R. (1975). "Mini-mental state". A practical method for grading the cognitive state of patients for the clinician. *J. Psychiatr. Res.* 12, 189–198. doi:10.1016/0022-3956(75)90026-6

Fossel, M. (2012). Use of telomere length as a biomarker for aging and age-related disease. *Curr. Transl. Geriatr. Exp. Gerontol. Rep.* 1, 121–127. doi:10.1007/s13670-012-0013-6

Fried, L. P., Tangen, C. M., Walston, J., Newman, A. B., Hirsch, C., Gottdiener, J., et al. (2001). Cardiovascular Health Study Collaborative Research Group. Frailty in older adults: evidence for a phenotype. *J. Gerontol. A Biol. Sci. Med. Sci.* 56, M146–M156. doi:10.1093/gerona/56.3.M146

Frontera, W. R., Hughes, V. A., Lutz, K. J., and Evans, W. J. (1991). A cross-sectional study of muscle strength and mass in 45- to 78-yr-old men and women. *J. Appl. Physiol.* 71, 644–650.

Goggins, W. B., Woo, J., Sham, A., and Ho, S. C. (2005). Frailty index as a measure of biological age in a Chinese population. *J. Gerontol. A Biol. Sci. Med. Sci.* 60, 1046–1051. doi:10.1093/gerona/60.8.1046

Grabowski, P., Hultdin, M., Karlsson, K., Tobin, G., Aleskog, A., Thunberg, U., et al. (2005). Telomere length as a prognostic parameter in chronic lymphocytic leukemia with special reference to VH gene mutation status. *Blood* 105, 4807–4812. doi:10.1182/blood-2004-11-4394

Iannuzzi-Sucich, M., Prestwood, K. M., and Kenny, A. M. (2002). Prevalence of sarcopenia and predictors of skeletal muscle mass in healthy, older men and women. *J. Gerontol. A Biol. Sci. Med. Sci.* 57, M772–M777. doi:10.1093/gerona/57.12.M772

Janssen, I., Heymsfield, S. B., Baumgartner, R. N., and Ross, R. (2000). Estimation of skeletal muscle mass by bioelectrical impedance analysis. *J. Appl. Physiol.* 89, 465–471.

Katz, S., and Akpom, C. A. (1976). A measure of primary sociobiological functions. *Int. J. Health Serv.* 6, 493–508. doi:10.2190/UURL-2RYU-WRYD-EY3K

Kyle, U. G., Genton, L., Hans, D., and Pichard, C. (2003). Validation of a bioelectrical impedance analysis equation to predict appendicular skeletal muscle mass (ASMM). *Clin. Nutr.* 22, 537–543. doi:10.1016/S0261-5614(03)00048-7

Lehmann, G., Muradian, K. K., and Fraifeld, V. E. (2013). Telomere length and body temperature-independent determinants of mammalian longevity? *Front. Genet.* 4:111. doi:10.3389/fgene.2013.00111

Linn, B. S., Linn, M. W., and Gurel, L. (1968). Cumulative illness rating scale. *J. Am. Geriatr. Soc.* 16, 622–626.

Livak, K. J., and Schmittgen, T. D. (2001). Analysis of relative gene expression data using real-time quantitative PCR and the 2(-Delta Delta C(T)) method. *Methods* 25, 402–408. doi:10.1006/meth.2001.1262

Marzetti, E. (2012). Imaging, functional and biological markers for sarcopenia: the pursuit of the golden ratio. *J. Frailty Aging* 1, 97–98.

Marzetti, E., Calvani, R., Cesari, M., Buford, T. W., Lorenzi, M., Behnke, B. J., et al. (2013). Mitochondrial dysfunction and sarcopenia of aging: from signaling pathways to clinical trials. *Int. J. Biochem. Cell Biol.* 45, 2288–2301. doi:10.1016/j.biocel.2013.06.024

Marzetti, E., Lees, H. A., Wohlgemuth, S. E., and Leeuwenburgh, C. (2009). Sarcopenia of aging: underlying cellular mechanisms and protection by calorie restriction. *Biofactors* 35, 28–35. doi:10.1002/biof.5

Mikhelson, V. M., and Gamaley, I. A. (2012). Telomere shortening is a sole mechanism of aging in mammals. *Curr. Aging Sci.* 5, 203–208. doi:10.2174/1874609811205030006

Mitnitski, A. B., Graham, J. E., Mogilner, A. J., and Rockwood, K. (2002). Frailty, fitness and late-life mortality in relation to chronological and biological age. *BMC Geriatr.* 2:1. doi:10.1186/1471-2318-2-1

NIH Expert Panel, X. (1996). Bioelectrical impedance analysis in body composition measurement: National Institutes of Health Technology Assessment Conference Statement. *Am. J. Clin. Nutr.* 64, 524S–532S.

O'Donovan, A., Pantell, M. S., Puterman, E., Dhabhar, F. S., Blackburn, E. H., Yaffe, K., et al. (2011). Cumulative inflammatory load is associated with short leukocyte telomere length in the Health, Aging and Body Composition Study. *PLoS ONE* 6:e19687. doi:10.1371/journal.pone.0019687

Payette, H., Roubenoff, R., Jacques, P. F., Dinarello, C. A., Wilson, P. W., Abad, L. W., et al. (2003). Insulin-like growth factor-1 and interleukin 6 predict sarcopenia in very old community-living men and women: the Framingham Heart Study. *J. Am. Geriatr. Soc.* 51, 1237–1243. doi:10.1046/j.1532-5415.2003.51407.x

Pedersen, M., Bruunsgaard, H., Weis, N., Hendel, H. W., Andreassen, B. U., Eldrup, E., et al. (2003). Circulating levels of TNF-alpha and IL-6-relation to truncal fat mass and muscle mass in healthy elderly individuals and in patients with type-2 diabetes. *Mech. Ageing Dev.* 124, 495–502. doi:10.1016/S0047-6374(03)00027-7

Richter, T., and von Zglinicki, T. (2007). A continuous correlation between oxidative stress and telomere shortening in fibroblasts. *Exp. Gerontol.* 42, 1039–1042. doi:10.1016/j.exger.2007.08.005

Rockwood, K., Andrew, M., and Mitnitski, A. (2007). A comparison of two approaches to measuring frailty in elderly people. *J. Gerontol. A Biol. Sci. Med. Sci.* 62, 738–743. doi:10.1093/gerona/62.7.738

Rockwood, K., Song, X., MacKnight, C., Bergman, H., Hogan, D. B., McDowell, I., et al. (2005). A global clinical measure of fitness and frailty in elderly people. *CMAJ* 173, 489–495. doi:10.1503/cmaj.050051

Rolland, Y., Czerwinski, S., Abellan Van Kan, G., Morley, J. E., Cesari, M., Onder, G., et al. (2008). Sarcopenia: its assessment, etiology, pathogenesis, consequences and future perspectives. *J. Nutr. Health Aging* 12, 433–450. doi:10.1007/BF02982704

Rothman, M. D., Leo-Summers, L., and Gill, T. M. (2008). Prognostic significance of potential frailty criteria. *J. Am. Geriatr. Soc.* 56, 2211–2116. doi:10.1111/j.1532-5415.2008.02008.x

Roubenoff, R. (2000). Sarcopenia: a major modifiable cause of frailty in the elderly. *J. Nutr. Health Aging* 4, 140–142.

Searle, S. D., Mitnitski, A., Gahbauer, E. A., Gill, T. M., and Rockwood, K. (2008). A standard procedure for creating a frailty index. *BMC Geriatr.* 8:24. doi:10.1186/1471-2318-8-24

Sheikh, J. I., and Yesavage, J. A. (1986). "Geriatric Depression Scale (GDS) recent evidence and development of a shorter version," in *Clinical Gerontology: A Guide to Assessment and Intervention*, ed. T. L. Brink (New York, NY: The Haworth Press), 165–173.

Sprott, R. L. (2010). Biomarkers of aging and disease: introduction and definitions. *Exp. Gerontol.* 45, 2–4. doi:10.1016/j.exger.2009.07.008

Vasto, S., Scapagnini, G., Bulati, M., Candore, G., Castiglia, L., Colonna-Romano, G., et al. (2010). Biomarkes of aging. *Front. Biosci. (Schol. Ed.)* 2:392–402. doi:10.2741/72

Visser, M., Pahor, M., Taaffe, D. R., Goodpaster, B. H., Simonsick, E. M., Newman, A. B., et al. (2002). Relationship of interleukin-6 and tumor necrosis factor-alpha with muscle mass and muscle strength in elderly men and women: the Health ABC Study. *J. Gerontol. A Biol. Sci. Med. Sci.* 57, M326–M332. doi:10.1093/gerona/57.5.M326

Washburn, R. A., Smith, K. W., Jette, A. M., and Janney, C. A. (1993). The Physical Activity Scale for the Elderly (PASE): development and evaluation. *J. Clin. Epidemiol.* 46, 153–162. doi:10.1016/0895-4356(93)90053-4

Wong, J. Y., De Vivo, I., Lin, X., Fang, S. C., and Christiani, D. C. (2014). The relationship between inflammatory biomarkers and telomere length in an occupational prospective cohort study. *PLoS ONE* 9:e87348. doi:10.1371/journal.pone.0087348

Woo, J., Tang, N. L., Suen, E., Leung, J. C., and Leung, P. C. (2008). Telomeres and frailty. *Mech. Ageing Dev.* 129, 642–648. doi:10.1016/j.mad.2008.08.003

Xi, H., Li, C., Ren, F., Zhang, H., and Zhang, L. (2013). Telomere, aging and age-related diseases. *Aging Clin. Exp. Res.* 25, 139–146. doi:10.1007/s40520-013-0021-1

Zhang, L., Du, J., Hu, Z., Han, G., Delafontaine, P., Garcia, G., et al. (2009). IL-6 and serum amyloid A synergy mediates angiotensin II-induced muscle wasting. *J. Am. Soc. Nephrol.* 20, 604–612. doi:10.1681/ASN.2008060628

15

Laminin α2 chain-deficiency is associated with microRNA deregulation in skeletal muscle and plasma

Johan Holmberg*, Azra Alajbegovic, Kinga Izabela Gawlik, Linda Elowsson and Madeleine Durbeej

Muscle Biology Unit, Department of Experimental Medical Science, University of Lund, Lund, Sweden

Correspondence:
Johan Holmberg, Muscle Biology Unit, Department of Experimental Medical Science, University of Lund, BMC B12, Lund 221 84, Sweden
e-mail: johan_k.holmberg@med.lu.se

microRNAs (miRNAs) are widespread regulators of gene expression, but little is known of their potential roles in congenital muscular dystrophy type 1A (MDC1A). MDC1A is a severe form of muscular dystrophy caused by mutations in the gene encoding laminin α2 chain. To gain insight into the pathophysiological roles of miRNAs associated with MDC1A pathology, laminin α2 chain-deficient mice were evaluated by quantitative PCR. We demonstrate that expression of muscle-specific miR-1, miR-133a, and miR-206 is deregulated in laminin α2 chain-deficient muscle. Furthermore, expression of miR-223 and miR-21, associated with immune cell infiltration and fibrosis, respectively, is altered. Finally, we show that plasma levels of muscle-specific miRNAs are markedly elevated in laminin α2 chain-deficient mice and partially normalized in response to proteasome inhibition therapy. Altogether, our data suggest important roles for miRNAs in MDC1A pathology and we propose plasma levels of muscle-specific miRNAs as promising biomarkers for the progression of MDC1A.

Keywords: fibrosis, inflammation, laminin, MDC1A, microRNA, muscular dystrophy

INTRODUCTION

Muscular dystrophy encompasses a group of inherited disorders mainly affecting skeletal muscle. Different types of muscular dystrophy are genetically diverse but share common phenotypic features including progressive myofiber degeneration, muscle weakness, and declined muscle function (Cohn and Campbell, 2000). Mutations in the human *LAMA2* gene, encoding the laminin α2 chain, lead to congenital muscular dystrophy type 1A (MDC1A). MDC1A is a severe form of muscular dystrophy characterized by hypotonia at birth, muscle weakness, delayed motor development, and joint contractures (Tome et al., 1994). Laminins are cruciform or T-shaped heterotrimeric molecules composed of one α, one β, and one γ subunit. To date, at least 18 different laminin isoforms have been identified. However, the most abundant laminin isoform in the skeletal muscle basement membrane is laminin-211 (α2, β1, and γ1) (Ehrig et al., 1990). Together with the dystrophin–glycoprotein complex laminin-211 forms a link between the basement membrane and the intracellular cytoskeleton protecting the muscle fiber from contraction-induced damage (Ervasti and Campbell, 1993).

Despite considerable research efforts there is currently no cure for MDC1A. Hence, the discovery that microRNAs (miRNAs) are deregulated in muscle diseases makes them attractive therapeutic targets (Eisenberg et al., 2007). miRNAs are small non-protein-coding RNAs, which regulate gene expression at the post-transcriptional level (Chen and Rajewsky, 2007). Investigations of miRNA expression and function in dystrophic muscles have identified a large number of deregulated miRNAs. Among the best characterized are three muscle-specific miRNAs: miR-1, miR-133a, and miR-206 (Chen et al., 2006; Yuasa et al., 2008). Moreover, miRNAs associated with specific features of muscular dystrophy such as infiltration of inflammatory cells (miR-223) and fibrogenesis (miR-21 and miR-29), are also altered in dystrophic muscles (Eisenberg et al., 2007; Greco et al., 2009). In addition, miRNAs are released into the blood stream of muscular dystrophy patients and mouse models, indicating that they represent biomarkers for disease progression and experimental therapies (Cacchiarelli et al., 2011; Mizuno et al., 2011).

An extended analysis of miRNA expression in MDC1A patients or mouse models has never been performed. Hence, in this study, we have analyzed expression of six miRNAs (miR-1, miR-133a, miR-206, miR-21, miR-29c, and miR-223) in muscle and plasma from two different MDC1A mouse models (dy^{3K}/dy^{3K} and dy^{2J}/dy^{2J}). The dy^{3K}/dy^{3K} mouse is completely deficient for laminin α2 and displays very severe muscle pathology whereas the dy^{2J}/dy^{2J} mouse, which expresses reduced levels of a truncated laminin α2, displays a milder muscular phenotype. Together, these mouse models are representative of the complexity of the MDC1A pathology.

Finally, our research group recently observed increased proteasomal activity in skeletal muscle from dy^{3K}/dy^{3K} mice, an observation that seems to be specific for muscular dystrophy caused by loss of laminin-211. Here, we have taken advantage of a proteasome inhibitor that reduces the dy^{3K}/dy^{3K} pathology (Körner et al., 2014), to investigate whether reduction in muscle pathology correlates with levels of muscle-specific miRNAs in plasma.

MATERIALS AND METHODS

ANIMAL MODELS

Laminin α2 chain-deficient dy^{3K}/dy^{3K} mice have been described (Miyagoe et al., 1997). Wild-type and dy^{2J}/dy^{2J} (B6.WK-$Lama^{2dy\text{-}2J}$/J) (Xu et al., 1994; Sunada et al., 1995) were purchased from Jackson laboratory and bred in the Biomedical Center vivarium in accordance with the animal care guidelines set by the Malmö/Lund (Sweden) ethical committee for animal research. Mice were analyzed at 6 weeks of age (dy^{2J}/dy^{2J}), 3 weeks of age

(dy^{3K}/dy^{3K}), or at 9 days of age (young dy^{3K}/dy^{3K}). All comparisons were made against age-matched wild-type mice.

RNA ISOLATION

Skeletal muscle total RNA was extracted from quadriceps muscles snap-frozen in liquid nitrogen using the miRCURY RNA Isolation Kit following the manufacturer's instructions (Exiqon). Blood was collected from heart puncture and transferred to anticoagulant tubes (EDTA) and centrifuged at 1100 × *g* for 10 min. Total RNA from blood plasma was extracted following the manufacturer's instructions (Qiagen miRNeasy® Mini Kit). Briefly, plasma was thawed on ice and centrifuged at 3000 × *g* for 5 min in a 4°C centrifuge. Fifty microliters of plasma per sample was transferred to a new microcentrifuge tube and 190 μl of QIAzol mixture containing 0.8 μg/μl MS2 bacteriophage RNA (Roche Applied Science) was added to each tube. Fifty microliters of chloroform was added to each tube followed by centrifugation at 12000 × *g* for 15 min in a 4°C microcentrifuge. The supernatant was transferred to a new microcentrifuge tube and 435 μl ethanol was added to each sample. A rinse step was performed with 1 × 500 μl RWT buffer and 3 × 500 μl RPE buffer. Total RNA was eluted by adding 50 μl RNase-free water to the membrane of the Qiagen RNeasy Mini spin column followed by centrifugation at 15000 × *g* for 1 min. The RNA was stored at −80°C.

QUANTITATIVE RT-PCR

Twenty nanograms of muscle RNA was reverse transcribed using the miRCURY LNA Universal RT cDNA Synthesis Kit (Exiqon). The cDNA was diluted 80× and assayed in 10 μl PCR reactions according to the protocol for the miRCURY LNA Universal RT miRNA PCR system. The amplification was performed in a LightCycler 480 Real-Time PCR System (Roche) in 96-well plates. Primers were designed by Exiqon. Delta–delta Ct values were calculated relative to let-7a and miR-16 (Roberts et al., 2012).

One microliter of RNA blood plasma eluate was reverse transcribed in a 10 μl reaction using the miRCURY LNA Universal RT cDNA Synthesis Kit (Exiqon). The cDNA was diluted 40× and assayed in a 10 μl reaction according to the protocol for the miRCURY LNA™ Universal RT miRNA PCR system (Exiqon). miRNA plasma levels were calculated relative to miR-21a and miR-223 (Roberts et al., 2012).

No-RT control reactions were performed to ensure no DNA carryover. All amplifications were performed in triplicate on a LightCycler 480 Real-Time PCR System (Roche) in 96-well plates. The amplification curves were analyzed using the Roche LC software for determination of Cp (by second derivate method) and for melting curve analysis. The miRCURY RNA spike-in kit (synthetic control template) was used to control for the quality of the cDNA synthesis reaction. All oligonucleotide sequences were designed by and ordered from Exiqon with the following product numbers: hsa-miR-1, 204344; hsa-let-7a-5p, 204775; hsa-miR-16-5p, 204409; hsa-miR-21-5p, 204230; hsa-miR-29c-3p, 204729; hsa-miR-133a, 204788; hsa-miR-206, 204616; and hsa-miR-223-3p, 204256.

HISTOLOGY

Quadriceps muscles were isolated and frozen in OCT (Tissue Tek) in liquid nitrogen. Transverse cryosections of 8 μm were transferred to positively charged glass slides and stored in −80°C. Sections were stained with hematoxylin and eosin (H&E) for quantification of centrally nucleated fibers or with Sirius red and Fast green (Sigma-Aldrich) for visualization of collagenous and non-collagenous tissue, respectively. Central nucleation is represented as a percentage of the total number of fibers counted in entire transverse quadriceps sections. For Sirius red and Fast green staining, sections were acclimated to RT for 15 min and fixated in Bouin's solution at 55°C for 1 h, incubated in 0.1% Fast green for 10 min followed by incubation in 0.1% Picro Sirius red for 30 min. Sections were then dehydrated in ethanol and cleared in xylene.

IMMUNOFLUORESCENCE ASSAYS

Transverse sections of 8 μm were fixed in ice-cold acetone for 8 min. For CD11b (rat monoclonal M1/70, 1:300, BD Pharmingen), CD68 (rat monoclonal FA-11, 1:100, AbD Serotec), and laminin γ1 chain (rabbit polyclonal 1083 + E1, 1:100, kindly provided by Dr. T. Sasaki), sections were blocked in 3% BSA in PBS at RT for 30 min followed by incubation in primary antibody at RT for 1 h. For embryonic myosin heavy chain (mouse monoclonal F1.652, 1:10, Developmental Studies Hybridoma Bank), sections were blocked in 4% goat serum and 0.05% Triton-X in PBS at RT for 40 min followed by incubation in primary antibody at RT for 90 min. Primary antibodies were incubated with appropriate secondary antibodies for 60 or 45 min (embryonic myosin heavy chain). Antibody stained sections were analyzed using a Zeiss Axioplan fluorescent microscope using Openlab 3 and an ORCA 1394 ER digital camera. The percentage of embryonic myosin heavy chain–positive fibers was obtained by counting the number of fibers positive for embryonic myosin heavy chain in a whole quadriceps section and dividing by the total number of myofibers.

HYDROXYPROLINE ASSAY (COLLAGEN CONTENT IN MUSCLE)

Quadriceps muscles were isolated and frozen in liquid nitrogen. Samples were weighed and incubated overnight in 200 μl concentrated HCl (12 M) at 95°C. Twenty five microliters of hydrolyzate was neutralized with 25 μl NaOH (0.6 M) and incubated with 450 μl Chloramine-T reagent (0.056 M) at RT for 25 min. A volume of 500 μl freshly prepared Ehrlich's reagent [1 M 4-(dimethylamino)benzaldehyde] was added to each sample and incubated at 65°C for 1 h. After cooling on ice, 100 μl in duplicates was transferred to a 96-well plate and absorbance was read at 560 nm. Standards from 4-hydroxyproline at concentrations (microgram per milliliter); 0, 0.05, 0.1, 0.15, 0.2, 0.25, 0.4 were treated the same way as the samples. Absorbance (A_{560}) of standards was plotted against amount of hydroxyproline (microgram) and a linear regression was performed to determine slope and intercept. All absorbance values were subtracted with blank (0 μg/ml hydroxyproline). Content of hydroxyproline in samples was calculated by equation:

$$x\ (\mu g) = \left(A_{560} - Y_{\text{axis intercept}}\right)/\text{slope}$$

Collagen conversion factor = 13.5 (Neuman and Logan, 1950). Values are presented as relative amount of collagen.

CREATINE KINASE ASSAY

Blood was collected from heart puncture and transferred to anticoagulant tubes (EDTA) and centrifuged at 1100 × g for 10 min at 4°C. Plasma was analyzed at Clinical Chemistry Laboratory at Skåne University Hospital. The CK_P_S Cobas method was used to quantify enzyme activity.

BORTEZOMIB TREATMENT

Briefly, dy^{3K}/dy^{3K} mice were administered 0.4 mg/kg bortezomib (LC Laboratories) via tail vein injection at 2.5 and 3.5 weeks of age. Mice were analyzed 14 days after injection (Körner et al., 2014).

STATISTICAL ANALYSES

Data shown in qRT-PCR analyses are the result of at least three independent experiments. Statistical significance of differences between means was assessed by one-way analysis of variance. Multiple comparisons were performed using the Holm–Sidak method. Unpaired t-test was used when two groups were compared. $P < 0.05$ was considered significant. All statistical analysis was performed using PRISM 6.0b software (GraphPad).

RESULTS

ALTERED EXPRESSION OF MUSCLE-SPECIFIC miRNAs IN dy^{3K}/dy^{3K} AND dy^{2J}/dy^{2J} QUADRICEPS MUSCLE

To determine whether miRNAs previously shown to be differentially expressed in dystrophic muscle (Eisenberg et al., 2007; Greco et al., 2009) are deregulated in MDC1A, we investigated miRNA expression in two different mouse models: dy^{3K}/dy^{3K} (completely devoid of laminin α2 chain) and dy^{2J}/dy^{2J} mice (expressing slightly reduced levels of a truncated laminin α2 chain) (Xu et al., 1994; Miyagoe et al., 1997). The dy^{3K}/dy^{3K} mice were analyzed at 3 weeks of age due to lethality between 4 and 5 weeks of age. The dy^{2J}/dy^{2J} mice however do not display any obvious signs of muscle pathology at that time point. Hence, these mice were instead analyzed at 6 weeks of age correlating with clear signs of muscle pathology.

We observed a decreased expression of miR-1 and miR-133a and an increase in miR-206 expression in dy^{3K}/dy^{3K} and dy^{2J}/dy^{2J} quadriceps muscle compared with wild-type controls (**Figure 1A**). Moreover, both miR-1 and miR-206 were differentially expressed in dy^{3K}/dy^{3K} and dy^{2J}/dy^{2J} mice, which may reflect differences in disease development. The observation that miR-206 expression was significantly higher in muscle from dy^{3K}/dy^{3K} mice compared with dy^{2J}/dy^{2J}, together with the established role of miR-206 in muscle regeneration prompted us to investigate the number of myofibers with central nuclei (reflecting overall muscle regeneration) and the number of fibers expressing embryonic myosin heavy chain (eMHC, reflecting the initial phase of myofiber regeneration) in dy^{3K}/dy^{3K} and dy^{2J}/dy^{2J} mice (Yuasa et al., 2008; Liu et al., 2012). We observed a significant increase in overall myofiber regeneration in dy^{3K}/dy^{3K} compared with dy^{2J}/dy^{2J} mice, closely resembling miR-206 expression (**Figures 1A–C**). However, staining against eMHC, which is transiently expressed in nascent myofibers revealed a low number of positive fibers, both in dy^{3K}/dy^{3K} and dy^{2J}/dy^{2J} mice, indicating that miR-206 expression reflects the overall regenerative status of the muscle rather than the initial stages of regeneration (**Figures 1B,C**). These findings are consistent with the effect of induced muscle damage on miR-206 expression, which increased markedly on day 5 post-injury (Yuasa et al., 2008).

Taken together, miR-1 and miR-133a are significantly downregulated in dy^{3K}/dy^{3K} and dy^{2J}/dy^{2J} muscle while miR-206 expression is upregulated, reflecting the overall regenerative status of the dystrophic muscle.

EXPRESSION OF miR-21 IS DEREGULATED IN dy^{3K}/dy^{3K} AND dy^{2J}/dy^{2J} QUADRICEPS MUSCLE

Dystrophic myofibers are progressively replaced by adipose and fibrotic tissue leading to irreversible loss of muscle (Mann et al., 2011). Laminin α2 chain-deficient muscles display extensive fibrosis, both in MDC1A patients and in dy^{3K}/dy^{3K} and dy^{2J}/dy^{2J} mice as shown by Fast green and Sirius red staining (visualizing non-collagenous and collagenous tissue, respectively) and biochemical collagen quantification (**Figure 2A**). Newly published data demonstrate a role of miR-21 and miR-29 as regulators of fibrogenesis (Ardite et al., 2012; Wang et al., 2012).

Based on these observations we analyzed the expression of miR-21 and miR-29c in muscle from dy^{3K}/dy^{3K} and dy^{2J}/dy^{2J} mice. We noticed a significant upregulation of miR-21 in both dy^{3K}/dy^{3K} and dy^{2J}/dy^{2J} mice compared with wild-type controls (**Figure 2B**). However, we did not observe any significant difference in miR-29c expression. Previous data suggest that miR-29c expression in dystrophic muscle depends on muscle group and age (Greco et al., 2009; Roberts et al., 2012). It may be that the effect of laminin α2 chain-deficiency on miR-29c expression is influenced by similar factors.

Dystrophic muscles are characterized by infiltration of inflammatory cells (Mann et al., 2011). This is also true for laminin α2 chain-deficient muscle (Pegoraro et al., 1996). miR-223 has been shown to be involved in granulocyte production and several studies report increased expression of miR-223 in dystrophic muscle (Eisenberg et al., 2007; Johnnidis et al., 2008). We did not observe any significant upregulation of miR-223 in quadriceps muscles from dy^{3K}/dy^{3K} or dy^{2J}/dy^{2J} mice at 3 and 6 weeks of age, respectively (**Figure 2B**). This is consistent with the relatively low number of CD11b- and CD68-positive immune cells (monocytes/macrophages) at the indicated time points (**Figure 2C**).

CIRCULATING MUSCLE-SPECIFIC miRNAs ARE ENRICHED IN dy^{3K}/dy^{3K} AND dy^{2J}/dy^{2J} MICE

In addition to aberrant miRNA expression in skeletal muscle, muscular dystrophy patients and mice display altered levels of miRNAs in the blood (Cacchiarelli et al., 2011; Mizuno et al., 2011; Vignier et al., 2013). Hence, we investigated levels of muscle-specific miR-1, miR-133a, and miR-206 in plasma from 3-week-old dy^{3K}/dy^{3K} and 6-week-old dy^{2J}/dy^{2J} mice. We observed a significant increase in miR-1 (~7-fold), miR-133a (~15-fold), and miR-206 (~15-fold) compared with wild-type controls, however no significant differences were observed between dy^{3K}/dy^{3K} and dy^{2J}/dy^{2J} mice (**Figure 3A**).

Recent data suggest that extra-cellular miRNAs is the result of selective rather than uncontrolled release from damaged myofibers (Roberts et al., 2013). To investigate this further we analyzed

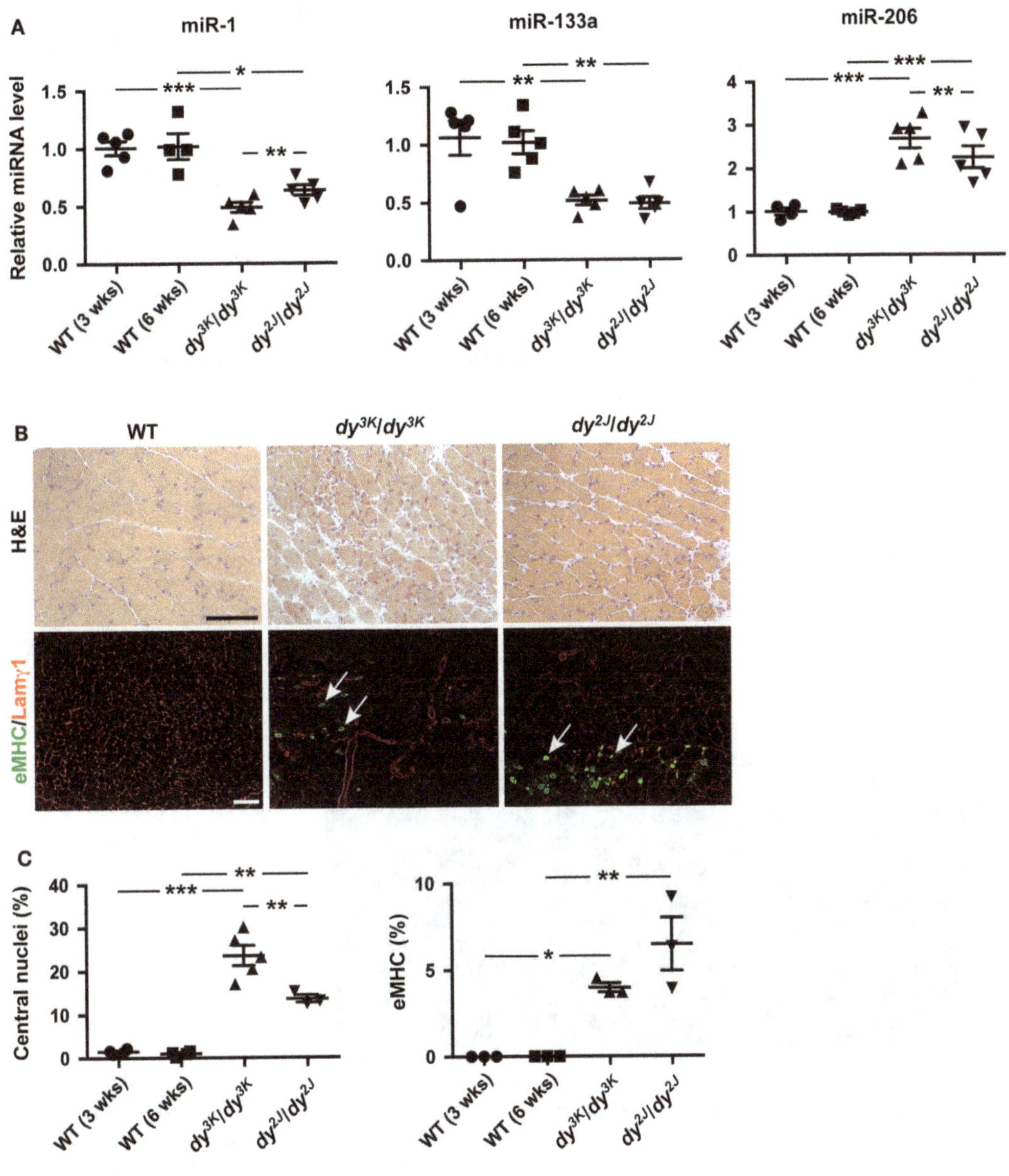

FIGURE 1 | Laminin α2 chain-deficiency results in altered expression of muscle-specific miRNAs. (A) RT-qPCR analysis of indicated miRNAs in muscles from 3-week-old dy^{3K}/dy^{3K} and 6-week-old dy^{2J}/dy^{2J} mice ($n \geq 4$). **(B)** Transverse sections of muscles from WT, dy^{3K}/dy^{3K}, and dy^{2J}/dy^{2J} mice stained for H&E to visualize histopathology and eMHC/Lamγ1 to identify early regenerating fibers. Arrows indicate eMHC positive cells (green). Bar, 100 μm. **(C)** Percentage of fibers with centralized nuclei or positive for eMHC in muscles from WT, dy^{3K}/dy^{3K}, and dy^{2J}/dy^{2J} mice ($n \geq 3$). WT, wild-type; H&E, hematoxylin/eosin; eMHC, embryonic myosin heavy chain; Lamγ1, laminin γ1 chain. Error bars represent SEM, $^{*}P < 0.05$, $^{**}P < 0.01$, $^{***}P < 0.001$.

plasma creatine kinase (CK) levels, a classical index of sarcolemmal integrity. Significant increase in CK levels was observed only in dy^{3K}/dy^{3K} mice (**Figure 3B**). Notably, the degree of sarcolemmal damage between dy^{3K}/dy^{3K} and dy^{2J}/dy^{2J} mice is in sharp contrast to levels of muscle-specific miRNAs in circulation, supporting the observation that release of miRNAs into circulation is a regulated process rather than simple leakage from damaged fibers. Taken together, the abundance of circulating muscle-specific miRNAs is significantly increased upon laminin α2 chain-deficiency.

Increased proteasomal activity is a feature of MDC1A and recent studies demonstrated that proteasome inhibition partially improves muscle integrity in dy^{3K}/dy^{3K} mice accompanied by increased expression of miR-1 and miR-133a (Carmignac et al., 2011; Körner et al., 2014). To determine if reduced muscle pathology had an impact on plasma levels of dysregulated miRNAs, dy^{3K}/dy^{3K} mice were given bortezomib (a proteasome inhibitor). Notably, administration of bortezomib resulted in a partial normalization of plasma levels of miR-1 and miR-133a in dy^{3K}/dy^{3K} mice (**Figure 3C**). However, bortezomib did not affect miR-206 plasma levels. This is consistent with observations that bortezomib does not significantly reduce myofiber regeneration in dy^{3K}/dy^{3K} mice (Körner et al., 2014). In summary, the partial normalization

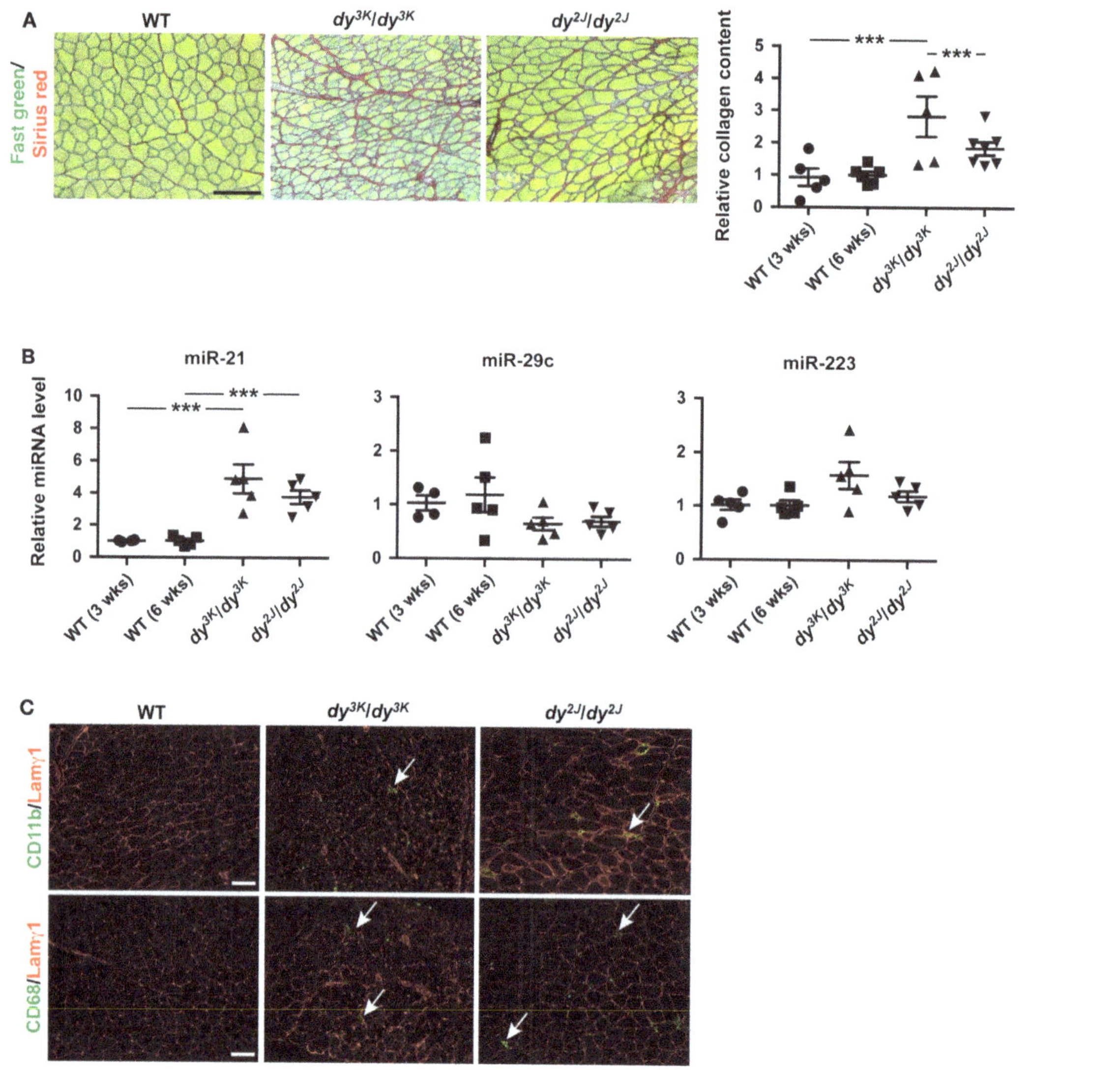

FIGURE 2 | Fibrosis in laminin α2 chain-deficient muscle is associated with increased expression of miR-21. (A) Left: transverse sections of muscles from WT, dy^{3K}/dy^{3K}, and dy^{2J}/dy^{2J} mice stained for Fast green/Sirius red to visualize non-collagenous and collagenous tissue, respectively. Bar, 100 μm. Right: quantification of relative collagen content (fibrosis) in dy^{3K}/dy^{3K} and dy^{2J}/dy^{2J} mice ($n \geq 5$). **(B)** RT-qPCR analysis of indicated miRNAs in muscles from dy^{3K}/dy^{3K} and dy^{2J}/dy^{2J} mice ($n \geq 4$). **(C)** CD11b/CD68/Lamγ1 stained sections of muscles from WT, dy^{3K}/dy^{3K}, and dy^{2J}/dy^{2J} mice. Arrows indicate CD11b and CD68-positive cells (green). Bar, 100 μm. WT, wild-type; Lamγ1, laminin γ1 chain. Error bars represent SEM, $^{***}P < 0.001$.

of miR-1 and miR-133a in response to bortezomib administration indicates that these miRNAs are promising disease biomarkers for MDC1A.

miRNA EXPRESSION IN dy^{3K}/dy^{3K} MICE CHANGES DYNAMICALLY OVER TIME

microRNA expression is a dynamic process possibly reflecting the development of the underlying dystrophic pathology (Roberts et al., 2013). Hence, we analyzed the expression of miRNAs in dy^{3K}/dy^{3K} muscles and plasma at an early age (9 days of age). At this time point, the number of regenerating fibers positive for eMHC is high while the level of overall myofiber regeneration is low, reflected in unaltered expression of miR-206 in muscle (**Figures 4A–C**). In addition, at 9 days of age dy^{3K}/dy^{3K} mice display extensive infiltration of inflammatory cells and accumulation of extra-cellular matrix components (**Figure 4A**). Accordingly, we noticed a significant increase in miR-223 (immune cells) and miR-21 expression (fibrosis) in muscle from dy^{3K}/dy^{3K} mice compared with wild-type controls (**Figure 4C**). Notably, expression of muscle-specific miR-1 and miR-133a were unaffected at young ages (**Figure 4C**).

We also investigated levels of circulating muscle-specific miRNAs in young dy^{3K}/dy^{3K} mice. Extra-cellular levels of miR-1 and miR-133a were unaltered whereas levels of miR-206 were significantly increased compared with wild-type controls (in contrast to muscle) (**Figures 4C,D**). The discrepancy between muscle and plasma levels of miR-206 could be due to plasma levels preceding the increase in miR-206 expression in muscle. It is also possible that

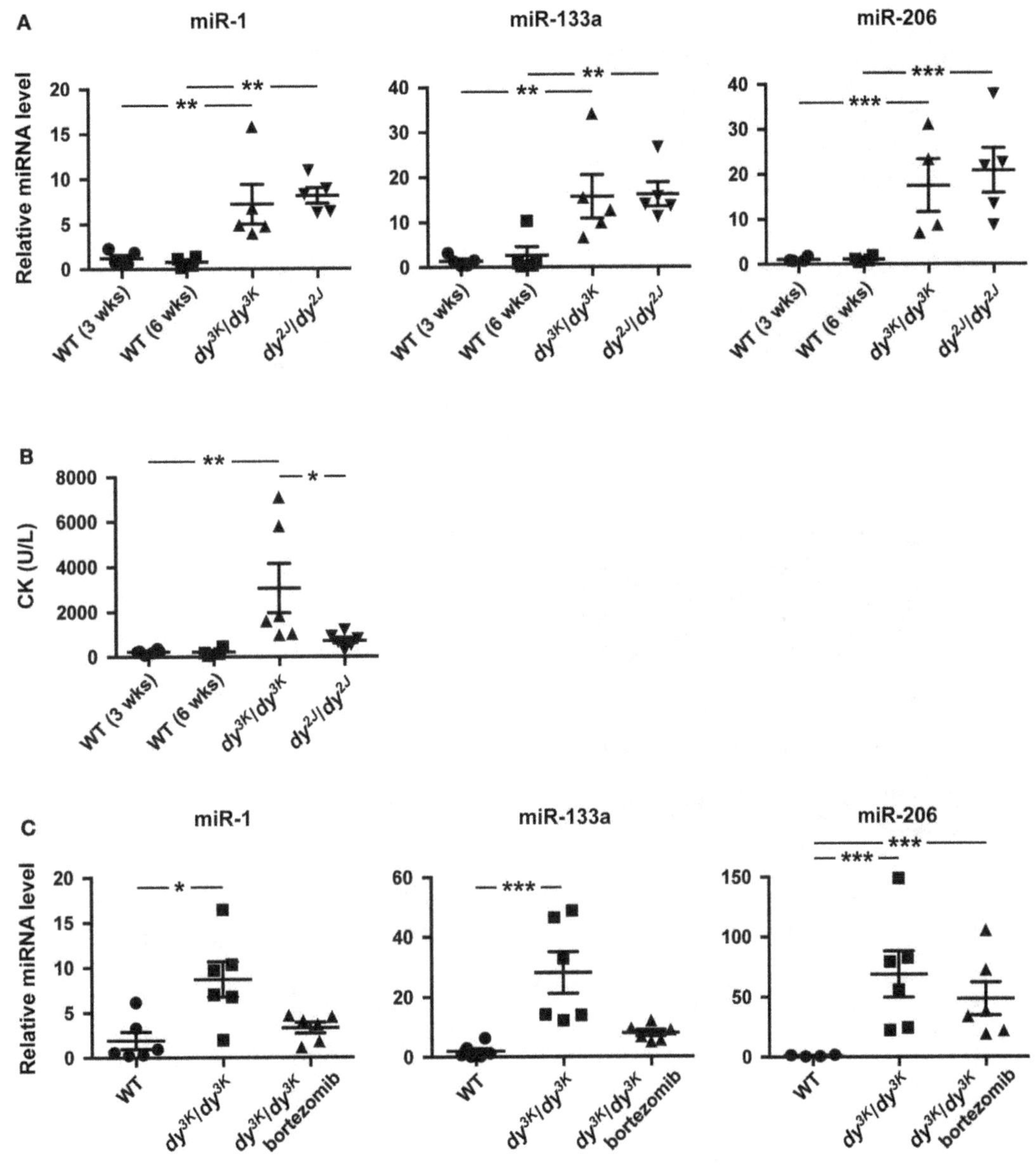

FIGURE 3 | Enrichment of muscle-specific miRNAs in plasma upon laminin α2-deficiency. (A) RT-qPCR analysis of plasma levels of indicated miRNAs in 3-week-old dy^{3K}/dy^{3K} and 6-week-old dy^{2J}/dy^{2J} mice ($n \geq 4$). **(B)** Analysis of CK levels in plasma from WT, dy^{3K}/dy^{3K}, and dy^{2J}/dy^{2J} mice ($n \geq 4$). **(C)** RT-qPCR analysis of plasma levels of indicated miRNAs in WT, dy^{3K}/dy^{3K}, and bortezomib injected dy^{3K}/dy^{3K} mice ($n \geq 4$). WT, wild-type; CK, creatine kinase. Error bars represent SEM, $*P < 0.05$, $**P < 0.01$, $***P < 0.001$.

additional muscle groups contribute to the increase in miR-206 plasma levels (Roberts et al., 2013). Taken together, abundance of miRNAs in dy^{3K}/dy^{3K} mice is dynamic and changes as the muscular dystrophy develops.

DISCUSSION

In the current study, we present evidences that MDC1A physiopathology is associated with altered expression of miRNAs, both in muscle and plasma. Specifically, we demonstrate that loss of laminin α2 chain leads to downregulation of muscle-specific miR-1 and miR-133a together with increased expression of miR-206 in muscle, consistent with data on other types of muscular dystrophy. The role of miR-206 in myofiber regeneration is well characterized and loss of miR-206 leads to delayed regeneration upon induced muscle damage (Liu et al., 2012). In contrast, the precise function of miR-1 and miR-133a in skeletal muscle is less clear. Studies on C2C12 myoblasts suggest that miR-133a and miR-1 promote proliferation and differentiation, respectively (Chen et al., 2006). However, mice deficient for miR-133a do not display any skeletal muscle anomalies until they are adult and skeletal muscle from miR-1-deficient mice is grossly normal (Zhao et al., 2007; Liu et al., 2011). These observations make it difficult to draw any firm conclusions regarding the impact of miR-133a and miR-1 dysregulation on the MDC1A pathology.

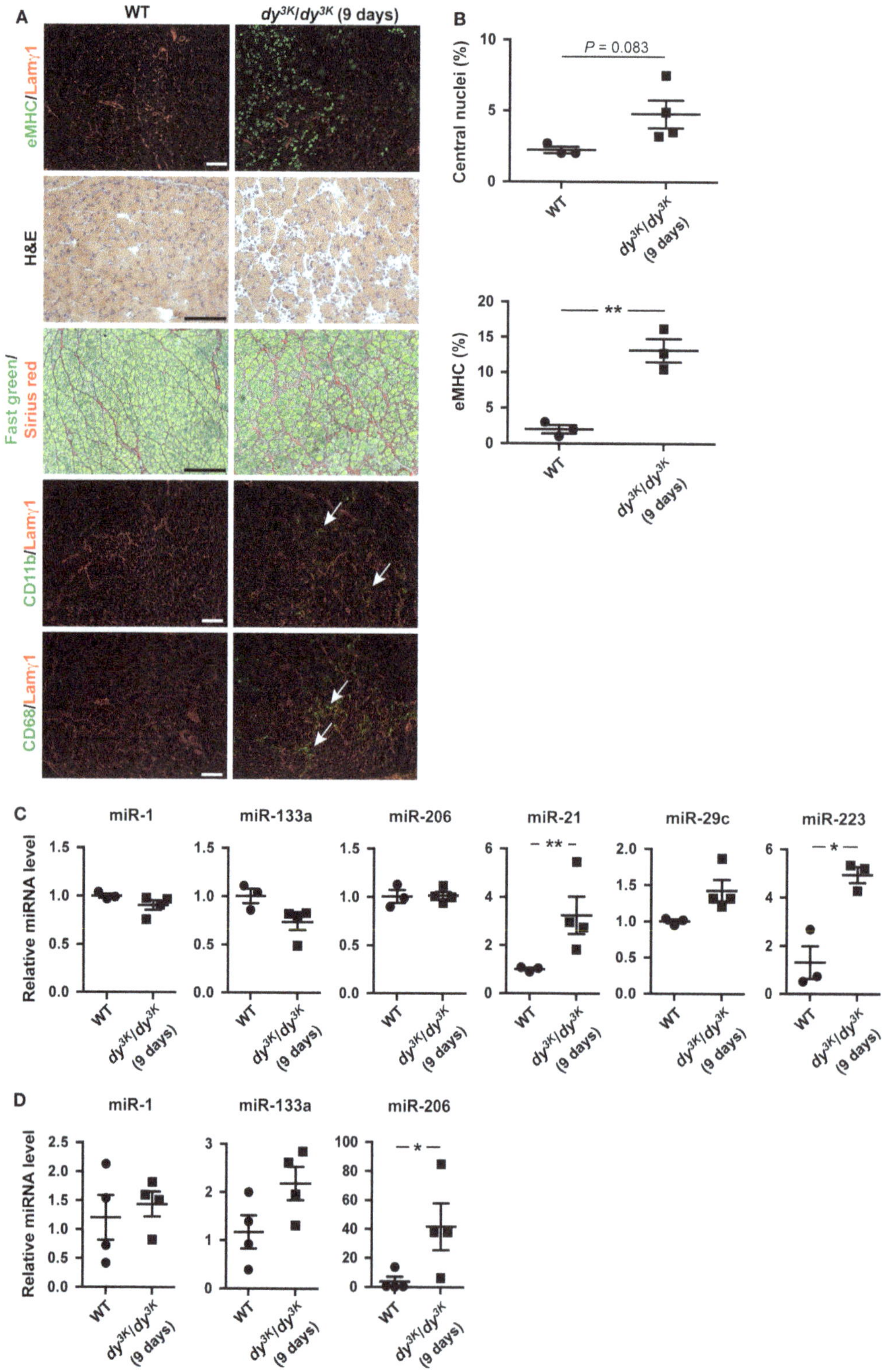

FIGURE 4 | Dynamic miRNA expression in laminin α2-deficient mice over time. (A) Transverse sections of muscles from 9-day-old WT and dy^{3K}/dy^{3K} mice stained for eMHC/Lamγ1, H&E, Fast green/Sirius red, and CD11b/CD68/Lamγ1. Arrows indicate CD11b and CD68-positive cells (green). Bar, 100 μm. **(B)** Percentage of fibers with centralized nuclei or positive for eMHC in muscles from WT and dy^{3K}/dy^{3K} mice ($n \geq 3$). **(C)** RT-qPCR analysis of indicated miRNAs in muscles from 9-day-old WT and dy^{3K}/dy^{3K} mice ($n \geq 3$). **(D)** RT-qPCR analysis of plasma levels of indicated miRNAs in 9-day-old WT and dy^{3K}/dy^{3K} mice ($n = 4$). WT, wild-type; H&E, hematoxylin/eosin; eMHC, embryonic myosin heavy chain; Lamγ1, laminin γ1 chain. Error bars represent SEM, $*P < 0.05$, $**P < 0.01$.

In this report, we also describe that miR-223 and miR-21 expression is positively associated with inflammation and fibrosis, respectively, in dy^{3K}/dy^{3K} and dy^{2J}/dy^{2J} muscle. Inflammation in MDC1A muscles ultimately results in progressive and irreversible replacement of muscle by adipose and fibrotic tissue. Severe inflammation in muscle from dy^{3K}/dy^{3K} mice is evident already at 7 days of age (Gawlik et al., 2014). However, inflammation appears arrested in older muscles (**Figures 2C** and **4A**) (Gawlik et al., 2014). Importantly, we show that miR-223 expression reflects the degree of immune cell infiltration in muscle from dy^{3K}/dy^{3K} mice and could therefore be involved in modulating the inflammatory response in MDC1A. The importance of immune cells in chronic myopathic conditions is emphasized by experiments on dystrophin-deficient *mdx* mice lacking functional B and/or T lymphocytes. These mice displayed reduced levels of the profibrotic cytokine transforming growth factor (TGF)-β and less diaphragm fibrosis (Morrison et al., 2000; Farini et al., 2007).

Furthermore, muscle fibrosis is associated with disease progression in MDC1A. Despite efforts to combat fibrogenesis in laminin α2-deficient mice, clinical applications for MDC1A remain years away (Elbaz et al., 2012; Meinen et al., 2012). Hence, the recent discovery that miR-21 and miR-29c can function as antifibrotic molecules in dystrophic muscles suggests miRNAs as attractive therapeutic candidates (Cacchiarelli et al., 2010; Ardite et al., 2012; Wang et al., 2012). In contrast to miR-21, we did not observe altered expression of miR-29c in dy^{3K}/dy^{3K} and dy^{2J}/dy^{2J} muscle. Expression of miR-29c is downregulated by TGF-β signaling, which is increased in dystrophic skeletal muscle (Bernasconi et al., 1995, 1999). However, TGF-β signaling seems to be less pronounced in MDC1A muscle, which may explain the unaltered expression of miR-29c in dy^{3K}/dy^{3K} and dy^{2J}/dy^{2J} muscle (Bernasconi et al., 1999). Collectively, these data suggest that fibrosis in MDC1A may be driven by other molecules than TGF-β.

It should be noted that Roberts and colleagues demonstrated important differences in miRNA expression between individual muscle groups in the *mdx* mouse (Roberts et al., 2012). In this report, miRNA expression analysis was limited to quadriceps muscles. Future studies on miRNA expression in laminin α2-deficient mice should include additional skeletal muscle groups.

Finally, we demonstrate that MDC1A is accompanied by increased levels of circulating muscle-specific miRNAs, which are partially normalized upon reduction of the dystrophic pathology. The precise biological function for extra-cellular miRNA remains largely unknown. However, we and others have demonstrated that expression of muscle-specific miRNAs in muscle does not reflect miRNA abundance in plasma or serum, indicating that miRNAs could enter circulation by exocytosis or be released in vesicles rather than by uncontrolled leakage. Moreover, the enrichment of circulating muscle-specific miRNAs in laminin α2-deficient mice is similar to observations in the *mdx* mouse, despite significantly more sarcolemmal damage in the latter (Straub et al., 1997; Roberts et al., 2012).

We also demonstrate that levels of plasma miRNAs in dy^{3K}/dy^{3K} change over time. These observations are consistent with data from other muscle disorders and suggest that levels of circulating miRNAs could serve as biomarkers for monitoring treatment strategies and diagnosis of MDC1A. Current methods are largely based on muscle biopsies and CK assays. In contrast to CK, extra-cellular miRNAs are resistant to stress and more accurately reflects disease severity (Cacchiarelli et al., 2011; Mizuno et al., 2011). In addition, miRNAs are present in numerous biological fluids easily accessible for analysis, including saliva and urine (De Guire et al., 2013). However, we observed a significant variability in levels of muscle-specific miRNAs in plasma from dy^{3K}/dy^{3K} and dy^{2J}/dy^{2J} mice, similar to studies on *mdx* mice (Cacchiarelli et al., 2011; Roberts et al., 2012).

A possible reason is that dystrophic muscles typically enter cycles of myofiber degeneration/regeneration, which lead to irreversible muscle wasting over time. Variation in onset of these regeneration cycles between mice could at least explain the variability in miR-206 levels in circulation. To establish miRNAs as biomarkers in MDC1A pathology, additional studies identifying and coupling miRNA levels in biofluids to pathology markers need to be performed. Moreover, global analysis of extra-cellular miRNA levels in laminin α2-deficient animals should facilitate the identification of miRNA profiles that correlate well with degree of muscle pathology.

Taken together, the discovery that miRNA expression is altered in MDC1A mouse models opens new strategies to combat this devastating disorder. Despite several challenges, recent refinements in delivery carriers, miRNA mimic molecules, and anti-miRs have improved delivery, specificity, and stability of miRNA therapeutics. Currently, one miRNA drug (miravirsen) has reached clinical trials and additional miRNA drugs are likely to enter clinical trials soon (Gebert et al., 2014).

AUTHOR CONTRIBUTIONS

Johan Holmberg and Madeleine Durbeej designed the experiments. Johan Holmberg and Azra Alajbegovic performed most of the experiments. Kinga Izabela Gawlik designed and analyzed immunofluorescence assays. Linda Elowsson performed and analyzed hydroxyproline assays. Johan Holmberg wrote the paper and other authors commented on the manuscript.

ACKNOWLEDGMENTS

This work was supported by grants from the Swedish Research Council, Association Française contre les Myopathies, Crafoord Foundation, Kock Foundation, Alfred Österlund Foundation, the Royal Physiographic Society in Lund, and Olle Engkvist Byggmästare. The authors thank Z. Körner and A. Aspberg for technical expertise.

REFERENCES

Ardite, E., Perdiguero, E., Vidal, B., Gutarra, S., Serrano, A. L., and Munoz-Canoves, P. (2012). PAI-1-regulated miR-21 defines a novel age-associated fibrogenic pathway in muscular dystrophy. *J. Cell Biol.* 196, 163–175. doi:10.1083/jcb.201105013

Bernasconi, P., Di Blasi, C., Mora, M., Morandi, L., Galbiati, S., Confalonieri, P., et al. (1999). Transforming growth factor-beta1 and fibrosis in congenital muscular dystrophies. *Neuromuscul. Disord.* 9, 28–33. doi:10.1016/S0960-8966(98)00093-5

Bernasconi, P., Torchiana, E., Confalonieri, P., Brugnoni, R., Barresi, R., Mora, M., et al. (1995). Expression of transforming growth factor-beta 1 in dystrophic patient muscles correlates with fibrosis. Pathogenetic role of a fibrogenic cytokine. *J. Clin. Invest.* 96, 1137–1144. doi:10.1172/JCI118101

Cacchiarelli, D., Legnini, I., Martone, J., Cazzella, V., D'Amico, A., Bertini, E., et al. (2011). miRNAs as serum biomarkers for Duchenne muscular dystrophy. *EMBO Mol. Med.* 3, 258–265. doi:10.1002/emmm.201100133

Cacchiarelli, D., Martone, J., Girardi, E., Cesana, M., Incitti, T., Morlando, M., et al. (2010). microRNAs involved in molecular circuitries relevant for the Duchenne muscular dystrophy pathogenesis are controlled by the dystrophin/nNOS pathway. *Cell Metab.* 12, 341–351. doi:10.1016/j.cmet.2010.07.008

Carmignac, V., Quere, R., and Durbeej, M. (2011). Proteasome inhibition improves the muscle of laminin alpha2 chain-deficient mice. *Hum. Mol. Genet.* 20, 541–552. doi:10.1093/hmg/ddq499

Chen, J. F., Mandel, E. M., Thomson, J. M., Wu, Q., Callis, T. E., Hammond, S. M., et al. (2006). The role of microRNA-1 and microRNA-133 in skeletal muscle proliferation and differentiation. *Nat. Genet.* 38, 228–233. doi:10.1038/ng1725

Chen, K., and Rajewsky, N. (2007). The evolution of gene regulation by transcription factors and microRNAs. *Nat. Rev. Genet.* 8, 93–103. doi:10.1038/nrg1990

Cohn, R. D., and Campbell, K. P. (2000). Molecular basis of muscular dystrophies. *Muscle Nerve* 23, 1456–1471. doi:10.1002/1097-4598(200010)23:10<1456::AID-MUS2>3.0.CO;2-T

De Guire, V., Robitaille, R., Tetreault, N., Guerin, R., Menard, C., Bambace, N., et al. (2013). Circulating miRNAs as sensitive and specific biomarkers for the diagnosis and monitoring of human diseases: promises and challenges. *Clin. Biochem.* 46, 846–860. doi:10.1016/j.clinbiochem.2013.03.015

Ehrig, K., Leivo, I., Argraves, W. S., Ruoslahti, E., and Engvall, E. (1990). Merosin, a tissue-specific basement membrane protein, is a laminin-like protein. *Proc. Natl. Acad. Sci. U.S.A.* 87, 3264–3268. doi:10.1073/pnas.87.9.3264

Eisenberg, I., Eran, A., Nishino, I., Moggio, M., Lamperti, C., Amato, A. A., et al. (2007). Distinctive patterns of microRNA expression in primary muscular disorders. *Proc. Natl. Acad. Sci. U.S.A.* 104, 17016–17021. doi:10.1073/pnas.0708115104

Elbaz, M., Yanay, N., Aga-Mizrachi, S., Brunschwig, Z., Kassis, I., Ettinger, K., et al. (2012). Losartan, a therapeutic candidate in congenital muscular dystrophy: studies in the dy(2J)/dy(2J) mouse. *Ann. Neurol.* 71, 699–708. doi:10.1002/ana.22694

Ervasti, J. M., and Campbell, K. P. (1993). A role for the dystrophin-glycoprotein complex as a transmembrane linker between laminin and actin. *J. Cell Biol.* 122, 809–823. doi:10.1083/jcb.122.4.809

Farini, A., Meregalli, M., Belicchi, M., Battistelli, M., Parolini, D., D'Antona, G., et al. (2007). T and B lymphocyte depletion has a marked effect on the fibrosis of dystrophic skeletal muscles in the scid/mdx mouse. *J. Pathol.* 213, 229–238. doi:10.1002/path.2213

Gawlik, K. I., Holmberg, J., and Durbeej, M. (2014). Loss of dystrophin and beta-sarcoglycan, respectively, significantly exacerbates the phenotype of laminin alpha2 chain-deficient animals. *Am. J. Pathol.* 184, 740–752. doi:10.1016/j.ajpath.2013.11.017

Gebert, L. F., Rebhan, M. A., Crivelli, S. E., Denzler, R., Stoffel, M., and Hall, J. (2014). Miravirsen (SPC3649) can inhibit the biogenesis of miR-122. *Nucleic Acids Res.* 42, 609–621. doi:10.1093/nar/gkt852

Greco, S., De Simone, M., Colussi, C., Zaccagnini, G., Fasanaro, P., Pescatori, M., et al. (2009). Common micro-RNA signature in skeletal muscle damage and regeneration induced by Duchenne muscular dystrophy and acute ischemia. *FASEB J.* 23, 3335–3346. doi:10.1096/fj.08-128579

Johnnidis, J. B., Harris, M. H., Wheeler, R. T., Stehling-Sun, S., Lam, M. H., Kirak, O., et al. (2008). Regulation of progenitor cell proliferation and granulocyte function by microRNA-223. *Nature* 451, 1125–1129. doi:10.1038/nature06607

Körner, Z., Holmberg, J., Fontes-Oliveira, C. C., Carmignac, V., and Durbeej, M. (2014). Bortezomib partially improves laminin α2 chain-deficient muscular dystrophy. *Am. J. Pathol.* 184, 1518–1528. doi:10.1016/j.ajpath.2014.01.019

Liu, N., Bezprozvannaya, S., Shelton, J. M., Frisard, M. I., Hulver, M. W., McMillan, R. P., et al. (2011). Mice lacking microRNA 133a develop dynamin 2-dependent centronuclear myopathy. *J. Clin. Invest.* 121, 3258–3268. doi:10.1172/JCI46267

Liu, N., Williams, A. H., Maxeiner, J. M., Bezprozvannaya, S., Shelton, J. M., Richardson, J. A., et al. (2012). microRNA-206 promotes skeletal muscle regeneration and delays progression of Duchenne muscular dystrophy in mice. *J. Clin. Invest.* 122, 2054–2065. doi:10.1172/JCI62656

Mann, C. J., Perdiguero, E., Kharraz, Y., Aguilar, S., Pessina, P., Serrano, A. L., et al. (2011). Aberrant repair and fibrosis development in skeletal muscle. *Skelet. Muscle* 1, 21. doi:10.1186/2044-5040-1-21

Meinen, S., Lin, S., and Ruegg, M. A. (2012). Angiotensin II type 1 receptor antagonists alleviate muscle pathology in the mouse model for laminin-alpha2-deficient congenital muscular dystrophy (MDC1A). *Skelet. Muscle* 2, 18. doi:10.1186/2044-5040-2-18

Miyagoe, Y., Hanaoka, K., Nonaka, I., Hayasaka, M., Nabeshima, Y., Arahata, K., et al. (1997). Laminin alpha2 chain-null mutant mice by targeted disruption of the Lama2 gene: a new model of merosin (laminin 2)-deficient congenital muscular dystrophy. *FEBS Lett.* 415, 33–39. doi:10.1016/S0014-5793(97)01007-7

Mizuno, H., Nakamura, A., Aoki, Y., Ito, N., Kishi, S., Yamamoto, K., et al. (2011). Identification of muscle-specific microRNAs in serum of muscular dystrophy animal models: promising novel blood-based markers for muscular dystrophy. *PLoS ONE* 6:e18388. doi:10.1371/journal.pone.0018388

Morrison, J., Lu, Q. L., Pastoret, C., Partridge, T., and Bou-Gharios, G. (2000). T-cell-dependent fibrosis in the mdx dystrophic mouse. *Lab. Invest.* 80, 881–891. doi:10.1038/labinvest.3780092

Neuman, R. E., and Logan, M. A. (1950). The determination of hydroxyproline. *J. Biol. Chem.* 184, 299–306.

Pegoraro, E., Mancias, P., Swerdlow, S. H., Raikow, R. B., Garcia, C., Marks, H., et al. (1996). Congenital muscular dystrophy with primary laminin alpha2 (merosin) deficiency presenting as inflammatory myopathy. *Ann. Neurol.* 40, 782–791. doi:10.1002/ana.410400515

Roberts, T. C., Blomberg, K. E., McClorey, G., Andaloussi, S. E., Godfrey, C., Betts, C., et al. (2012). Expression analysis in multiple muscle groups and serum reveals complexity in the microRNA transcriptome of the mdx mouse with implications for therapy. *Mol. Ther. Nucleic Acids* 1, e39. doi:10.1038/mtna.2012.26

Roberts, T. C., Godfrey, C., McClorey, G., Vader, P., Briggs, D., Gardiner, C., et al. (2013). Extracellular microRNAs are dynamic non-vesicular biomarkers of muscle turnover. *Nucleic Acids Res.* 41, 9500–9513. doi:10.1093/nar/gkt724

Straub, V., Rafael, J. A., Chamberlain, J. S., and Campbell, K. P. (1997). Animal models for muscular dystrophy show different patterns of sarcolemmal disruption. *J. Cell Biol.* 139, 375–385. doi:10.1083/jcb.139.2.375

Sunada, Y., Bernier, S. M., Utani, A., Yamada, Y., and Campbell, K. P. (1995). Identification of a novel mutant transcript of laminin alpha 2 chain gene responsible for muscular dystrophy and dysmyelination in dy2J mice. *Hum. Mol. Genet.* 4, 1055–1061. doi:10.1093/hmg/4.6.1055

Tome, F. M., Evangelista, T., Leclerc, A., Sunada, Y., Manole, E., Estournet, B., et al. (1994). Congenital muscular dystrophy with merosin deficiency. *C. R. Acad. Sci. III, Sci. Vie* 317, 351–357.

Vignier, N., Amor, F., Fogel, P., Duvallet, A., Poupiot, J., Charrier, S., et al. (2013). Distinctive serum miRNA profile in mouse models of striated muscular pathologies. *PLoS ONE* 8:e55281. doi:10.1371/journal.pone.0055281

Wang, L., Zhou, L., Jiang, P., Lu, L., Chen, X., Lan, H., et al. (2012). Loss of miR-29 in myoblasts contributes to dystrophic muscle pathogenesis. *Mol. Ther.* 20, 1222–1233. doi:10.1038/mt.2012.35

Xu, H., Wu, X. R., Wewer, U. M., and Engvall, E. (1994). Murine muscular dystrophy caused by a mutation in the laminin alpha 2 (Lama2) gene. *Nat. Genet.* 8, 297–302. doi:10.1038/ng1194-297

Yuasa, K., Hagiwara, Y., Ando, M., Nakamura, A., Takeda, S., and Hijikata, T. (2008). microRNA-206 is highly expressed in newly formed muscle fibers: implications regarding potential for muscle regeneration and maturation in muscular dystrophy. *Cell Struct. Funct.* 33, 163–169. doi:10.1247/csf.08022

Zhao, Y., Ransom, J. F., Li, A., Vedantham, V., von Drehle, M., Muth, A. N., et al. (2007). Dysregulation of cardiogenesis, cardiac conduction, and cell cycle in mice lacking miRNA-1-2. *Cell* 129, 303–317. doi:10.1016/j.cell.2007.03.030

16

Fetal stem cells and skeletal muscle regeneration: a therapeutic approach

Michela Pozzobon[1], Chiara Franzin[1], Martina Piccoli[1] and Paolo De Coppi[2]*

[1] Fondazione Istituto di Ricerca Pediatrica Città della Speranza, Padova, Italy
[2] UCL Institute of Child Health and Great Ormond Street Hospital, London, UK

***Correspondence:**
Paolo De Coppi, UCL Institute of Child Health and Great Ormond Street Hospital, 30 Guilford Street, London WC1N 1EH, UK
e-mail: paolo.decoppi@gosh.nhs.uk

More than 40% of the body mass is represented by muscle tissue, which possesses the innate ability to regenerate after damage through the activation of muscle-specific stem cells, namely satellite cells. Muscle diseases, in particular chronic degenerative states of skeletal muscle such as dystrophies, lead to a perturbation of the regenerative process, which causes the premature exhaustion of satellite cell reservoir due to continuous cycles of degeneration/regeneration. Nowadays, the research is focused on different therapeutic approaches, ranging from gene and cell to pharmacological therapy, but still there is no definitive cure in particular for genetic muscle disease. Keeping this in mind, in this article, we will give special consideration to muscle diseases and the use of fetal derived stem cells as a new approach for therapy. Cells of fetal origin, from cord blood to placenta and amniotic fluid, can be easily obtained without ethical concern, expanded and differentiated in culture, and possess immune-modulatory properties. The *in vivo* approach in animal models can be helpful to study the mechanism underneath the operating principle of the stem cell reservoir, namely the niche, which holds great potential to understand the onset of muscle pathologies.

Keywords: fetal cells, muscle dystrophies, cell therapy, placenta, cord blood, amniotic fluid

INTRODUCTION

The muscular dystrophies are heterogeneous genetic diseases that strongly impair skeletal muscle structure and function. These disorders are caused by mutations in genes encoding for structural proteins essential for muscle integrity, and depending on the alteration, it is possible to distinguish dystrophies due to (i) mutations on a specific gene, such as Duchenne muscular dystrophy (DMD) or on distinct genes, e.g., limb-girdle muscular dystrophies (LGMD); (ii) epigenetic alterations, for instance facioscapulohumeral muscular dystrophy; and (iii) repeat expansion, such as myotonic dystrophy. The primary genetic defect results in a wide range of pathological phenotypes, different for fashion of inheritance, age of onset, severity and distribution of muscle weakness, and speed of progression (Leung and Wagner, 2013).

In particular, DMD is the most prevalent and severe dystrophy that affects skeletal muscle. It is an X-linked recessive disease due to mutations on dystrophin gene, which determines the production of a truncated and non-functional protein. Dystrophin functions as a muscle fiber stabilizer by linking the cytoplasmic actin filaments with the extracellular matrix. The DMD muscle is characterized by continuous fiber damage, which results in an altered regenerative turnover thus leading to the premature exhaustion of muscle stem cell compartment, the development of chronic inflammation, and the infiltration of adipose and fibrotic tissues. In DMD patients, the muscle loss begins very early in childhood starting from lower extremities and leading to progressive difficulty with walking, and finally, up to the confinement in a wheelchair. In addition to loss of mobility, the major disabling co-morbidities are represented by heart disease and respiratory failure that are the most common causes of death (Wilschut et al., 2012; Kharraz et al., 2014). In 1984, Bulfield and co-workers described an X chromosome-linked mutant mouse, also called *mdx*, which mimics the human DMD showing elevated plasma levels of muscle creatine kinase and pyruvate kinase and histological lesions characteristic of muscular dystrophies, although with a milder phenotype (Bulfield et al., 1984). In 2010, Sacco et al. (2010) created a new mouse model where *mdx* mutation was associated with the loss of telomerase (mTR) activity. Indeed, these double-knockout mice display a more severe as well as rapidly progressing phenotype and a greatly reduced life span. In order to allow human cell transplantation for preclinical studies, immunocompromised *mdx* mouse strains have been created, such as *mdx* nude mice (Partridge et al., 1989) and NOD/$Rag1^{null}mdx5^{cv}$ mice (Lapan et al., 2012).

Limb-girdle muscular dystrophies are a family of diseases affecting mainly proximal muscle, in particular shoulders, upper arms, pelvic area, and thighs. These disorders are caused by mutation in various genes encoding muscle structural proteins and present different inheritance patterns; therefore, they consistently differ in terms of age of onset, progress, and severity of disease (Mitsuhashi and Kang, 2012). There are many mouse models for LGMD, according to the variety of involved genes and genetic defects that result in this family of muscle dystrophies. For example, knockout mice for α-sarcoglycan gene accurately resemble the LGMD-2D phenotype (Duclos et al., 1998), a deletion on dysferlin gene produces a LGMD-2B phenotype in SJL-Dysf mice (Bittner et al., 1999), while mice carrying mutations on myotilin gene develop the autosomal dominant LGMD-1A (Liu et al., 2014).

Beside these muscle-specific diseases, there are pathologies that arise from other tissues and consequently affect skeletal muscle. Since the close interplay between nervous system and skeletal muscle compartment, many of these disorders are related to neural degeneration, which causes muscle loss. One example is spinal muscular atrophy (SMA), an autosomal recessive disorder characterized by degeneration of anterior horn neurons and consequent muscle weakness and atrophy. The incidence of SMA is about one in 10,000 live births. It was first described at the end of nineteenth century and only 100 years later the genetic defect was found and localized in the chromosome 5 cared by survival motor neuron (*SMN*) gene (Gilliam et al., 1990; Lefebvre et al., 1995). In humans, there are normally two copies of *SMN* gene, *SMN1* is essential to the pathogenesis, while the number of copies of *SMN2* determines the severity of the disease (Lorson et al., 1998; Feldkotter et al., 2002). Different strategies have been deployed to create murine model of SMA, and using the cre-loxP system the loss of function of *Smn* gene has been directed toward specific tissues, in particular to skeletal muscle. The mouse model *HSA-Cre, $Smn^{F7/F7}$* allows to evaluate the effect of *Smn* knockout on muscle since the Cre-recombinase is placed under the control of alpha skeletal actin (Nicole et al., 2003). For this reason, mutant mice display pathological features that mimic a muscle dystrophy phenotype, such as muscle weakness and atrophy and chest deformation with consequent respiratory failure (Cifuentes-Diaz et al., 2001; Salah-Mohellibi et al., 2006).

The research is currently focused on three main therapeutic approaches for muscle diseases. Gene therapy aims to restore the dystrophin protein complex through different strategies, ranging from the development of new vectors capable of delivering efficiently the missing gene to the postmitotic nuclei of the muscle fibers, to exon skipping and the enhancement of the synthesis of proteins such as utrophin. The pharmacological approach is mainly focused on the attenuation of the inflammation (corticosteroids administration) and the treatment of co-morbidities (cardiomyopathy, osteoporosis, respiratory failure). Nowadays, new compounds modulating muscle-specific neuronal nitric oxide synthase (nNOSμ) pathway and TGFβ pathway are under investigation (Berardi et al., 2014). The cell therapy approach is devoted to functionally rescue the tissue through cell delivery; so far, in place of muscle satellite cells, other cells isolated from embryonic (Filareto et al., 2013) and adult [pericytes, bone marrow, mesangioblasts (Ferrari et al., 1998; Gussoni et al., 1999; Sampaolesi et al., 2006; Dellavalle et al., 2011)] sources or induced pluripotent stem (iPS) cells (Darabi et al., 2012; Tedesco et al., 2012) have been shown to contribute to muscle regeneration. However, except for embryonic cells, a real integration of administered cells in muscle niche has barely been observed. Recently, mesenchymal stem cells (MSCs) from human fetal blood (Chang et al., 2006) and skeletal muscle progenitors from mouse embryo (Sakai et al., 2013) have been used in muscle regeneration. Several studies demonstrated that fetal tissues are abundant sources of MSCs, including term placenta, fetal bone marrow, blood, lung, liver, and spleen (in 't Anker et al., 2003; Fukuchi et al., 2004), but the most available and easy sources to obtain fetal stem cells are placenta, cord blood, Wharton's jelly, and amniotic fluid (AF).

FETAL STEM CELLS AND MUSCLE REGENERATION

Research on fetal stem cells and muscle is quite recent. Placenta, cord blood, and AF represent an easy source of stem cells without ethical concerns and are immune-privileged tissues (Toda et al., 2007; Wang et al., 2009; Di Trapani et al., 2013). Placenta has been primarily used as a membrane to treat burns, injuries, and skin ulcers (Bujang-Safawi et al., 2010) and it has been studied also to treat lung fibrosis (Cargnoni et al., 2009) and inflammatory corneal diseases (Dekaris and Gabric, 2009). Cord blood has been considered mainly as a source of hematopoietic cells (Cairo and Wagner, 1997), although new field of applications such as diabetes are open (Zhao et al., 2012). Amniotic fluid stem (AFS) cells recently found applications from the heart (Bollini et al., 2011) to the kidney (Rota et al., 2011) and the lung (Carraro et al., 2008).

This review will evaluate the use of cells from the above mentioned sources in muscle regeneration (**Table 1**), focusing on both the limits and future potential for therapy.

CORD BLOOD AND WHARTON'S JELLY CELLS

Umbilical cord connects the fetus to the placenta; it develops from the body stalk of the embryo and contains blood vessels and Wharton's jelly, surrounded by the amnion. Umbilical cord blood (UCB) supplies the developing fetus of nutrients and oxygen through the umbilical vein.

Umbilical cord blood possesses three main types of stem cells that are of interest in regenerative medicine: (1) hematopoietic stem cells, (2) MSCs, and (3) non-hematopoietic multipotent stem cells characterized by the expression of SSEA-4, the transcription factors OCT4, SOX2, and NANOG usually expressed by pluripotent stem cells (McGuckin et al., 2005, 2008; Kucia et al., 2007; Zuba-Surma et al., 2009). The blood vessels of the cord blood are insulated with the gelatinous connective tissue called Wharton's jelly that prevents vein compression (Ferguson and Dodson, 2009). The cells isolated from this biological source share properties with MSCs from UCB such as differentiation ability (Anzalone et al., 2010). Upon *in vitro* muscle differentiation, $CD105^+$ cells form Wharton's jelly have been injected in injured rat *Tibialis anterior* muscle and after 15 days a mild muscle regeneration has been detected (Conconi et al., 2006).

The involvement of UCB in therapeutic application was reported since 1972, when clinicians treated one case of lymphoblastic leukemia (Ende and Ende, 1972). Nowadays, the translational potential of the clinical applications of UCB stem cells is increased due to important advantages such as the ease to recover the cells right after birth without any risk for the donor, the lack of ethical issues, the low onset of graft-versus-host disease (GVHD) (Broxmeyer et al., 1989; Ballen, 2005; Schoemans et al., 2006; Brunstein et al., 2007; Hwang et al., 2007; Broxmeyer, 2010), and finally the high proliferation rate and long telomere maintenance (Kim et al., 1999; Pipes et al., 2006). Starting from 2003, Pesce and co-workers demonstrated muscle amelioration after injection of $CD34^+$ UCB cells in injured adductor muscle and new $MYOD^+$ cells of UCB origin (Pesce et al., 2003) in a CD1 mouse model of hindlimb ischemia. Later, in 2007, Koponen and colleagues, using ischemia damage in the immunocompromised BALB/cA-nu mouse, analyzed both endothelium and muscle after local injection of several cell types, namely UCB $CD133^+$, $CD34^+$, MSCs,

Table 1 | Different fetal stem cells displayed myogenic differentiation ability.

Perinatal sources	Mouse model/injury	Engraftment	Reference
HUMAN ORIGIN			
UCB ($CD34^+$)	Sjl-Disf	Yes, 12 weeks post injection	Kong et al. (2004)
UCB (MSCs, $CD133^+$)	Balb/cA-nu: hindlimb ischemia damage	No	Koponen et al. (2007)
UCB (MSCs)	Mdx	Yes, Dys^+ fibers 45 days post local injection	Nunes et al. (2007)
UCB ($CD34^+$)	CD1: hindlimb ischemia damage	$MyoD^+$ cells	Pesce et al. (2003)
Wharton's jelly	Lewis rat: bupivacaine injury	Yes, 15 days post local injection	Conconi et al. (2006)
Placenta	*In vitro* only	Lentiviral transfection with MyoD	Akizawa et al. (2013)
Placenta	SCID/mdx	Yes, 4 weeks post injection	Kawamichi et al. (2010)
Placenta ($CD146^+$, $CD34^+$, $CD146^-$ $CD34^-$)	SCID/mdx	Yes, 4 weeks post injection	Park et al. (2010)
AF c-Kit cells	SCID	No	Gekas et al. (2010)
AFS cells	BALB/cSlc-nu	Yes, 21 days post injection	Kim et al. (2013)
AFS cells	NOD/SCID	Yes, 4 weeks post injection	Ma et al. (2012)
MOUSE ORIGIN			
AFS cells	HSA-Cre, $Smn^{F7/F7}$	Yes, 1 and 15 month post injection and after secondary transplant	Piccoli et al. (2012)

VEGF-D, or eGFP transduced cells, highlighting that the skeletal muscle regeneration was an indirect effect of cytokines, such as VEGF and FGF, released by the injected progenitor cells (Koponen et al., 2007).

In the *mdx* mouse, Nunes and colleagues were able to find a small number of human dystrophin-positive fibers 45 days after injection of $CD34^+$ UCB cells in quadriceps muscle. In the murine model of LGMD-2B, the SJL-Dysf mouse, whole UCB, and $CD34^\pm$ subgroups are engrafted in muscles after systemic injection (Nunes et al., 2007), and expression of dysferlin and human dystrophin was detected 12 weeks post injection of different subpopulation of UCB cells, although in a small amount (Kong et al., 2004).

PLACENTA STEM CELLS

The placenta develops at the feto-maternal interface and is a temporary organ that grows during pregnancy. It is formed by fetal (amnion and chorionic plate) and maternal (decidua) portions and contains different types of cells. Indeed, the placenta is rich in stem/progenitor cells. While in the amnion human amniotic epithelial cells, which express embryonic stem cell markers, have been isolated (epiblast-derived pluripotent/multipotent stem cells) (Prusa and Hengstschlager, 2002; Miki et al., 2005, 2007), the placenta MSCs have been separated not only from amnion, but also chorion and decidua (Huang et al., 2009; Pozzobon et al., 2014). These cells share with the adult MSCs the spindle-shape appearance and the property to adhere to plastic and to expand. Moreover, placenta MSCs expand faster *in vitro* and are more immunosuppressive and less immunogenic than the adult MSCs (Battula et al., 2008; Brooke et al., 2008). Recently, a specific subgroup of cells isolated from the human placenta villi and relevant for muscle regeneration, namely the perivascular multipotent mesenchymal progenitor cells, have been characterized by Park et al. (2010). In this research, they studied the angiogenic and myogenic potential of the $CD146^+$ $CD45^-$ $CD34^-$ $CD56^-$ cells (pericytes fraction) and $CD146^-$ $CD45^-$ $CD34^-$ $CD56^-$ cells (non-pericytes fraction). When these cell populations were intramuscularly implanted into damaged *Gastrocnemius* of immunodeficient dystrophic mice, fibers positive for human dystrophin were found at the periphery of the damaged area. The combination of perivascular progenitors together with the multipotent MSCs isolated from the placenta enhanced the migration and regeneration capacity of the placenta stem cells demonstrating that this extra-embryonic tissue is a reservoir of stem/progenitor cells with myogenic potential. The *in vitro* myogenic differentiation of cells from chorionic plate has been recently documented (Kawamichi et al., 2010) using a standard chemical treatment of inducing myoblasts formation (5-azacytidine) and also forcing *MYOD* expression through a lentiviral vector (Akizawa et al., 2013). Kawamichi and colleagues proved also the *in vivo* ability of placenta-derived cells to ameliorate the dystrophic phenotype of *mdx* mice inducing the appearance of newly formed fibers expressing human dystrophin.

AMNIOTIC FLUID STEM CELLS

Amniotic fluid contains a heterogeneous population of cells displaying a wide range of morphologies. Most of these cells are epithelial in nature and have a limited capacity to proliferate in culture. Traditionally, AF has been used for decades as a tool for prenatal diagnosis, but recent studies provided important evidences about the potential of AF as an alternative source of stem cells. Many works have characterized putative stem cell populations isolated from AF, such as Prusa et al. (2003) that showed the expression of OCT4 within a subset of AF cells. Moreover, demonstration of proliferation within this population suggests that pluripotent stem cells can be isolated and propagated from the human AF.

Employing immunoselection technique, AF cells expressing the cell surface antigen c-Kit were purified from primary amniocentesis cultures (De Coppi et al., 2007). Isolated cells, called AFS cells, grew rapidly in culture, display a normal karyotype and maintain telomere length during long-term culture. This latter attribute facilitated the establishment of clonal lines from AFS cells, necessary to establish the "stemness" of a population. Clonal AFS cell lines differentiated *in vitro* to putative adipocytes, endothelial cells, hepatocytes, osteocytes, myocytes, and neurons, derivatives of all germ layers. This broad plasticity appeared to be a general attribute of the selected cells: 19 different amniocentesis cultures yielded multipotent AFS cell clonal lines. A subsequent report demonstrated the AFS cells *in vitro* chondrogenic differentiation thus providing further evidence of the plasticity and clinical potential of cells isolated from the AF (Preitschopf et al., 2012). Moreover, these cells displayed the ability to reconstitute the depleted bone marrow of $Rag1^{-/-}$ mice after systemic injection and secondary transplantation (Ditadi et al., 2009).

Another peculiar characteristic of AFS cells is indeed the ability to pass through the endothelial barrier, thus they can be administered locally or systemically, which represents a great advantage in treating whole body diseases such as muscle dystrophies. Considering this important aspect, mouse AFS cells were used in the *HSA-Cre*, $Smn^{F7/F7}$ mouse model by transplantation via tail vein (Piccoli et al., 2012). After injection, AFS cells demonstrated remarkable ability to differentiate directly *in vivo* into myogenic cells but most importantly were able to generate new muscle fibers after cardiotoxin injury or secondary transplant, suggesting the idea that AFS cells are capable of differentiating also in skeletal muscle stem cells repopulating the muscle niche. In this work, the use of freshly isolated or expanded murine AFS cells generated similar results, but it is worth noticing that, with human AFS cells, muscle lineage differentiation becomes difficult to obtain after *in vitro* expansion. Gekas and colleagues indeed, did not find any myogenic differentiation of human AF c-Kit^{+} cells after transplantation into the skeletal muscle of SCID mice (Gekas et al., 2010). Myogenic differentiation of AF cells can be induced *in vitro* by DNA demethylation (e.g., using chemicals such as 5-aza-2′-deoxycytidine), co-culture with myoblasts or myogenic cell lines, or directly with *in vivo* muscle transplantation (De Coppi et al., 2007; Gekas et al., 2010; Ma et al., 2012; Yang et al., 2012), but all these approaches result in the induction of MYOD expression. In fact, by transfecting human AFS cells with *MYOD* lentivirus, Kim and co-workers demonstrated that human cells also were able to differentiate into myogenic lineage *in vitro* and *in vivo*, after injection into injured muscles of immunodeficient BALB/cSlc-nu mice (Kim et al., 2013). All these data indicate that stem cells obtained from discarded AF could be considered good candidates for deeper research and investigation on their ability to differentiate into myogenic cells. Further analyses must be performed to make these cells more committed and at the same time safe for future clinical applications using, for instance, non-viral system such as Piggy Bac or Sleeping Beauty transposons (Izsvak et al., 2009). These tools allow modifying cells by inserting new genes, ensuring a constitutive genetic integration of the insertion and opening possible way to cure genetic defects.

CONCLUSION

Muscle pathologies are devastating diseases and nowadays researchers still make efforts to find a cure and not a therapy alone. It has been demonstrated that, after injection in injured or diseased muscle, fetal stem cells act through a mechanism that is mostly due to a bystander effect rather than a direct differentiation. The indirect action is mainly supposed to enhance the production of cytokines, such as VEGF, that stimulate the temporary restoring of the tissue function. To obtain a long lasting action due to efficient cell integration and tissue repopulation, fetal stem cells need to be genetically modified, forcing their differentiation in tissue-specific cells. Nevertheless, the development of safe genetic manipulation methods could make cells of fetal origin appealing for therapeutic application.

Conversely, the long-term positive effect observed using freshly isolated murine AFS cells, highlights that they could have a decisive role in replenishing the muscle stem cell niche, which represent the reservoir of cells able to rescue the defect. Indeed, AFS cells are a safe and immune-privileged cell source prone to integrate in muscle tissue. This knowledge opens the challenge to improve the culture protocol for the AFS cells of human origin, which, so far, is still a limit to overcome for future clinical application to treat genetic and non-genetic muscle dysfunctions (dystrophies, skeletal muscle malformations, traumatic injuries).

ACKNOWLEDGMENTS

We would like to thank Anilkumar Dave for helpful comments. Michela Pozzobon, Martina Piccoli, and Chiara Franzin are supported by Fondazione Istituto di Ricerca Pediatrica Città della Speranza, Padova, Italy. Paolo De Coppi is funded by the Great Ormond Street Hospital Charity.

REFERENCES

Akizawa, Y., Kanno, H., Kawamichi, Y., Matsuda, Y., Ohta, H., Fujii, H., et al. (2013). Enhanced expression of myogenic differentiation factors and skeletal muscle proteins in human amnion-derived cells via the forced expression of MYOD1. *Brain Dev.* 35, 349–355. doi:10.1016/j.braindev.2012.05.012

Anzalone, R., Lo Iacono, M., Corrao, S., Magno, F., Loria, T., Cappello, F., et al. (2010). New emerging potentials for human Wharton's jelly mesenchymal stem cells: immunological features and hepatocyte-like differentiative capacity. *Stem Cells Dev.* 19, 423–438. doi:10.1089/scd.2009.0299

Ballen, K. K. (2005). New trends in umbilical cord blood transplantation. *Blood* 105, 3786–3792. doi:10.1182/blood-2004-10-4125

Battula, V. L., Treml, S., Abele, H., and Buhring, H. J. (2008). Prospective isolation and characterization of mesenchymal stem cells from human placenta using a frizzled-9-specific monoclonal antibody. *Differentiation* 76, 326–336. doi:10.1111/j.1432-0436.2007.00225.x

Berardi, E., Annibali, D., Cassano, M., Crippa, S., and Sampaolesi, M. (2014). Molecular and cell-based therapies for muscle degenerations: a road under construction. *Front. Physiol.* 5:119. doi:10.3389/fphys.2014.00119

Bittner, R. E., Anderson, L. V., Burkhardt, E., Bashir, R., Vafiadaki, E., Ivanova, S., et al. (1999). Dysferlin deletion in SJL mice (SJL-Dysf) defines a natural model for limb girdle muscular dystrophy 2B. *Nat. Genet.* 23, 141–142. doi:10.1038/13770

Bollini, S., Cheung, K. K., Riegler, J., Dong, X., Smart, N., Ghionzoli, M., et al. (2011). Amniotic fluid stem cells are cardioprotective following acute myocardial infarction. *Stem Cells Dev.* 20, 1985–1994. doi:10.1089/scd.2010.0424

Brooke, G., Tong, H., Levesque, J. P., and Atkinson, K. (2008). Molecular trafficking mechanisms of multipotent mesenchymal stem cells derived from human bone marrow and placenta. *Stem Cells Dev.* 17, 929–940. doi:10.1089/scd.2007.0156

Broxmeyer, H. E. (2010). Will iPS cells enhance therapeutic applicability of cord blood cells and banking? *Cell Stem Cell* 6, 21–24. doi:10.1016/j.stem.2009.12.008

Broxmeyer, H. E., Douglas, G. W., Hangoc, G., Cooper, S., Bard, J., English, D., et al. (1989). Human umbilical cord blood as a potential source of transplantable hematopoietic stem/progenitor cells. *Proc. Natl. Acad. Sci. U.S.A.* 86, 3828–3832. doi:10.1073/pnas.86.10.3828

Brunstein, C. G., Baker, K. S., and Wagner, J. E. (2007). Umbilical cord blood transplantation for myeloid malignancies. *Curr. Opin. Hematol.* 14, 162–169. doi:10.1097/MOH.0b013e32802f7da4

Bujang-Safawi, E., Halim, A. S., Khoo, T. L., and Dorai, A. A. (2010). Dried irradiated human amniotic membrane as a biological dressing for facial burns – a 7-year case series. *Burns* 36, 876–882. doi:10.1016/j.burns.2009.07.001

Bulfield, G., Siller, W. G., Wight, P. A., and Moore, K. J. (1984). X chromosome-linked muscular dystrophy (mdx) in the mouse. *Proc. Natl. Acad. Sci. U.S.A.* 81, 1189–1192. doi:10.1073/pnas.81.4.1189

Cairo, M. S., and Wagner, J. E. (1997). Placental and/or umbilical cord blood: an alternative source of hematopoietic stem cells for transplantation. *Blood* 90, 4665–4678.

Cargnoni, A., Gibelli, L., Tosini, A., Signoroni, P. B., Nassuato, C., Arienti, D., et al. (2009). Transplantation of allogeneic and xenogeneic placenta-derived cells reduces bleomycin-induced lung fibrosis. *Cell Transplant.* 18, 405–422. doi:10.3727/096368909788809857

Carraro, G., Perin, L., Sedrakyan, S., Giuliani, S., Tiozzo, C., Lee, J., et al. (2008). Human amniotic fluid stem cells can integrate and differentiate into epithelial lung lineages. *Stem Cells* 26, 2902–2911. doi:10.1634/stemcells.2008-0090

Chang, Y. J., Shih, D. T., Tseng, C. P., Hsieh, T. B., Lee, D. C., and Hwang, S. M. (2006). Disparate mesenchyme-lineage tendencies in mesenchymal stem cells from human bone marrow and umbilical cord blood. *Stem Cells* 24, 679–685. doi:10.1634/stemcells.2004-0308

Cifuentes-Diaz, C., Frugier, T., Tiziano, F. D., Lacene, E., Roblot, N., Joshi, V., et al. (2001). Deletion of murine SMN exon 7 directed to skeletal muscle leads to severe muscular dystrophy. *J. Cell Biol.* 152, 1107–1114. doi:10.1083/jcb.152.5.1107

Conconi, M. T., Burra, P., Di Liddo, R., Calore, C., Turetta, M., Bellini, S., et al. (2006). CD105(+) cells from Wharton's jelly show in vitro and in vivo myogenic differentiative potential. *Int. J. Mol. Med.* 18, 1089–1096. doi:10.3892/ijmm.18.6.1089

Darabi, R., Arpke, R. W., Irion, S., Dimos, J. T., Grskovic, M., Kyba, M., et al. (2012). Human ES- and iPS-derived myogenic progenitors restore DYSTROPHIN and improve contractility upon transplantation in dystrophic mice. *Cell Stem Cell* 10, 610–619. doi:10.1016/j.stem.2012.02.015

De Coppi, P., Bartsch, G. Jr., Siddiqui, M. M., Xu, T., Santos, C. C., Perin, L., et al. (2007). Isolation of amniotic stem cell lines with potential for therapy. *Nat. Biotechnol.* 25, 100–106. doi:10.1038/nbt1274

Dekaris, I., and Gabric, N. (2009). Preparation and preservation of amniotic membrane. *Dev. Ophthalmol.* 43, 97–104. doi:10.1159/000223842

Dellavalle, A., Maroli, G., Covarello, D., Azzoni, E., Innocenzi, A., Perani, L., et al. (2011). Pericytes resident in postnatal skeletal muscle differentiate into muscle fibres and generate satellite cells. *Nat. Commun.* 2, 499. doi:10.1038/ncomms1508

Di Trapani, M., Bassi, G., Ricciardi, M., Fontana, E., Bifari, F., Pacelli, L., et al. (2013). Comparative study of immune regulatory properties of stem cells derived from different tissues. *Stem Cells Dev.* 22, 2990–3002. doi:10.1089/scd.2013.0204

Ditadi, A., De Coppi, P., Picone, O., Gautreau, L., Smati, R., Six, E., et al. (2009). Human and murine amniotic fluid c-Kit+Lin- cells display hematopoietic activity. *Blood* 113, 3953–3960. doi:10.1182/blood-2008-10-182105

Duclos, F., Straub, V., Moore, S. A., Venzke, D. P., Hrstka, R. F., Crosbie, R. H., et al. (1998). Progressive muscular dystrophy in alpha-sarcoglycan-deficient mice. *J. Cell Biol.* 142, 1461–1471. doi:10.1083/jcb.142.6.1461

Ende, M., and Ende, N. (1972). Hematopoietic transplantation by means of fetal (cord) blood. A new method. *Va. Med. Mon. (1918)* 99, 276–280.

Feldkotter, M., Schwarzer, V., Wirth, R., Wienker, T. F., and Wirth, B. (2002). Quantitative analyses of SMN1 and SMN2 based on real-time lightCycler PCR: fast and highly reliable carrier testing and prediction of severity of spinal muscular atrophy. *Am. J. Hum. Genet.* 70, 358–368. doi:10.1086/338627

Ferguson, V. L., and Dodson, R. B. (2009). Bioengineering aspects of the umbilical cord. *Eur. J. Obstet. Gynecol. Reprod. Biol.* 144(Suppl. 1), S108–S113. doi:10.1016/j.ejogrb.2009.02.024

Ferrari, G., Cusella-De Angelis, G., Coletta, M., Paolucci, E., Stornaiuolo, A., Cossu, G., et al. (1998). Muscle regeneration by bone marrow-derived myogenic progenitors. *Science* 279, 1528–1530. doi:10.1126/science.279.5356.1528

Filareto, A., Darabi, R., and Perlingeiro, R. C. (2013). Engraftment of ES-derived myogenic progenitors in a severe mouse model of muscular dystrophy. *J. Stem Cell Res. Ther.* 10, 1–13. doi:10.4172/2157-7633.S10-001

Fukuchi, Y., Nakajima, H., Sugiyama, D., Hirose, I., Kitamura, T., and Tsuji, K. (2004). Human placenta-derived cells have mesenchymal stem/progenitor cell potential. *Stem Cells* 22, 649–658. doi:10.1634/stemcells.22-5-649

Gekas, J., Walther, G., Skuk, D., Bujold, E., Harvey, I., and Bertrand, O. F. (2010). In vitro and in vivo study of human amniotic fluid-derived stem cell differentiation into myogenic lineage. *Clin. Exp. Med.* 10, 1–6. doi:10.1007/s10238-009-0060-2

Gilliam, T. C., Brzustowicz, L. M., Castilla, L. H., Lehner, T., Penchaszadeh, G. K., Daniels, R. J., et al. (1990). Genetic homogeneity between acute and chronic forms of spinal muscular atrophy. *Nature* 345, 823–825. doi:10.1038/345823a0

Gussoni, E., Soneoka, Y., Strickland, C. D., Buzney, E. A., Khan, M. K., Flint, A. F., et al. (1999). Dystrophin expression in the mdx mouse restored by stem cell transplantation. *Nature* 401, 390–394. doi:10.1038/43919

Huang, Y. C., Yang, Z. M., Chen, X. H., Tan, M. Y., Wang, J., Li, X. Q., et al. (2009). Isolation of mesenchymal stem cells from human placental decidua basalis and resistance to hypoxia and serum deprivation. *Stem Cell. Rev.* 5, 247–255. doi:10.1007/s12015-009-9069-x

Hwang, W. Y., Samuel, M., Tan, D., Koh, L. P., Lim, W., and Linn, Y. C. (2007). A meta-analysis of unrelated donor umbilical cord blood transplantation versus unrelated donor bone marrow transplantation in adult and pediatric patients. *Biol. Blood Marrow Transplant.* 13, 444–453. doi:10.1016/j.bbmt.2006.11.005

in 't Anker, P. S., Noort, W. A., Scherjon, S. A., Kleijburg-Van Der Keur, C., Kruisselbrink, A. B., Van Bezooijen, R. L., et al. (2003). Mesenchymal stem cells in human second-trimester bone marrow, liver, lung, and spleen exhibit a similar immunophenotype but a heterogeneous multilineage differentiation potential. *Haematologica* 88, 845–852. doi:10.1016/S0301-472X(03)00202-9

Izsvak, Z., Chuah, M. K., Vandendriessche, T., and Ivics, Z. (2009). Efficient stable gene transfer into human cells by the sleeping beauty transposon vectors. *Methods* 49, 287–297. doi:10.1016/j.ymeth.2009.07.001

Kawamichi, Y., Cui, C. H., Toyoda, M., Makino, H., Horie, A., Takahashi, Y., et al. (2010). Cells of extraembryonic mesodermal origin confer human dystrophin in the mdx model of Duchenne muscular dystrophy. *J. Cell. Physiol.* 223, 695–702. doi:10.1002/jcp.22076

Kharraz, Y., Guerra, J., Pessina, P., Serrano, A. L., and Munoz-Canoves, P. (2014). Understanding the process of fibrosis in Duchenne muscular dystrophy. *Biomed Res. Int.* 2014, 965631. doi:10.1155/2014/965631

Kim, D. K., Fujiki, Y., Fukushima, T., Ema, H., Shibuya, A., and Nakauchi, H. (1999). Comparison of hematopoietic activities of human bone marrow and umbilical cord blood CD34 positive and negative cells. *Stem Cells* 17, 286–294. doi:10.1002/stem.170286

Kim, J. A., Shon, Y. H., Lim, J. O., Yoo, J. J., Shin, H. I., and Park, E. K. (2013). MYOD mediates skeletal myogenic differentiation of human amniotic fluid stem cells and regeneration of muscle injury. *Stem Cell Res Ther.* 4, 147. doi:10.1186/scrt358

Kong, K. Y., Ren, J., Kraus, M., Finklestein, S. P., and Brown, R. H. Jr. (2004). Human umbilical cord blood cells differentiate into muscle in sjl muscular dystrophy mice. *Stem Cells* 22, 981–993. doi:10.1634/stemcells.22-6-981

Koponen, J. K., Kekarainen, T., E Heinonen, S., Laitinen, A., Nystedt, J., Laine, J., et al. (2007). Umbilical cord blood-derived progenitor cells enhance muscle regeneration in mouse hindlimb ischemia model. *Mol. Ther.* 15, 2172–2177. doi:10.1038/sj.mt.6300302

Kucia, M., Halasa, M., Wysoczynski, M., Baskiewicz-Masiuk, M., Moldenhawer, S., Zuba-Surma, E., et al. (2007). Morphological and molecular characterization of novel population of CXCR4+ SSEA-4+ Oct-4+ very small embryonic-like cells purified from human cord blood: preliminary report. *Leukemia* 21, 297–303. doi:10.1038/sj.leu.2404470

Lapan, A. D., Rozkalne, A., and Gussoni, E. (2012). Human fetal skeletal muscle contains a myogenic side population that expresses the melanoma cell-adhesion molecule. *Hum. Mol. Genet.* 21, 3668–3680. doi:10.1093/hmg/dds196

Lefebvre, S., Burglen, L., Reboullet, S., Clermont, O., Burlet, P., Viollet, L., et al. (1995). Identification and characterization of a spinal muscular atrophy-determining gene. *Cell* 80, 155–165. doi:10.1016/0092-8674(95)90460-3

Leung, D. G., and Wagner, K. R. (2013). Therapeutic advances in muscular dystrophy. *Ann. Neurol.* 74, 404–411. doi:10.1002/ana.23989

Liu, J., Wallace, L. M., Garwick-Coppens, S. E., Sloboda, D. D., Davis, C. S., Hakim, C. H., et al. (2014). RNAi-mediated gene silencing of mutant myotilin improves myopathy in LGMD1A mice. *Mol Ther Nucleic Acids* 3, e160. doi:10.1038/mtna.2014.13

Lorson, C. L., Strasswimmer, J., Yao, J. M., Baleja, J. D., Hahnen, E., Wirth, B., et al. (1998). SMN oligomerization defect correlates with spinal muscular atrophy severity. *Nat. Genet.* 19, 63–66. doi:10.1038/ng0598-63

Ma, X., Zhang, S., Zhou, J., Chen, B., Shang, Y., Gao, T., et al. (2012). Clone-derived human AF-amniotic fluid stem cells are capable of skeletal myogenic differentiation in vitro and in vivo. *J. Tissue Eng. Regen. Med.* 6, 598–613. doi:10.1002/term.462

McGuckin, C., Jurga, M., Ali, H., Strbad, M., and Forraz, N. (2008). Culture of embryonic-like stem cells from human umbilical cord blood and onward differentiation to neural cells in vitro. *Nat. Protoc.* 3, 1046–1055. doi:10.1038/nprot.2008.69

McGuckin, C. P., Forraz, N., Baradez, M. O., Navran, S., Zhao, J., Urban, R., et al. (2005). Production of stem cells with embryonic characteristics from human umbilical cord blood. *Cell Prolif.* 38, 245–255. doi:10.1111/j.1365-2184.2005.00346.x

Miki, T., Lehmann, T., Cai, H., Stolz, D. B., and Strom, S. C. (2005). Stem cell characteristics of amniotic epithelial cells. *Stem Cells* 23, 1549–1559. doi:10.1634/stemcells.2004-0357

Miki, T., Mitamura, K., Ross, M. A., Stolz, D. B., and Strom, S. C. (2007). Identification of stem cell marker-positive cells by immunofluorescence in term human amnion. *J. Reprod. Immunol.* 75, 91–96. doi:10.1016/j.jri.2007.03.017

Mitsuhashi, S., and Kang, P. B. (2012). Update on the genetics of limb girdle muscular dystrophy. *Semin. Pediatr. Neurol.* 19, 211–218. doi:10.1016/j.spen.2012.09.008

Nicole, S., Desforges, B., Millet, G., Lesbordes, J., Cifuentes-Diaz, C., Vertes, D., et al. (2003). Intact satellite cells lead to remarkable protection against Smn gene defect in differentiated skeletal muscle. *J. Cell Biol.* 161, 571–582. doi:10.1083/jcb.200210117

Nunes, V. A., Cavacana, N., Canovas, M., Strauss, B. E., and Zatz, M. (2007). Stem cells from umbilical cord blood differentiate into myotubes and express dystrophin in vitro only after exposure to in vivo muscle environment. *Biol. Cell* 99, 185–196. doi:10.1042/BC20060075

Park, T. S., Gavina, M., Chen, C. W., Sun, B., Teng, P. N., Huard, J., et al. (2010). Placental perivascular cells for human muscle regeneration. *Stem Cells Dev.* 20, 451–463. doi:10.1089/scd.2010.0354

Partridge, T. A., Morgan, J. E., Coulton, G. R., Hoffman, E. P., and Kunkel, L. M. (1989). Conversion of mdx myofibres from dystrophin-negative to -positive by injection of normal myoblasts. *Nature* 337, 176–179. doi:10.1038/337176a0

Pesce, M., Orlandi, A., Iachininoto, M. G., Straino, S., Torella, A. R., Rizzuti, V., et al. (2003). Myoendothelial differentiation of human umbilical cord blood-derived stem cells in ischemic limb tissues. *Circ. Res.* 93, e51–e62. doi:10.1161/01.RES.0000090624.04507.45

Piccoli, M., Franzin, C., Bertin, E., Urbani, L., Blaauw, B., Repele, A., et al. (2012). Amniotic fluid stem cells restore the muscle cell niche in a HSA-Cre, Smn(F7/F7) mouse model. *Stem Cells* 30, 1675–1684. doi:10.1002/stem.1134

Pipes, B. L., Tsang, T., Peng, S. X., Fiederlein, R., Graham, M., and Harris, D. T. (2006). Telomere length changes after umbilical cord blood transplant. *Transfusion* 46, 1038–1043. doi:10.1111/j.1537-2995.2006.00839.x

Pozzobon, M., Piccoli, M., and De Coppi, P. (2014). Stem cells from fetal membranes and amniotic fluid: markers for cell isolation and therapy. *Cell Tissue Bank.* 15, 199–211. doi:10.1007/s10561-014-9428-y

Preitschopf, A., Zwickl, H., Li, K., Lubec, G., Joo, G., Rosner, M., et al. (2012). Chondrogenic differentiation of amniotic fluid stem cells and their potential for regenerative therapy. *Stem Cell. Rev.* 8, 1267–1274. doi:10.1007/s12015-012-9405-4

Prusa, A. R., and Hengstschlager, M. (2002). Amniotic fluid cells and human stem cell research: a new connection. *Med. Sci. Monit.* 8, RA253–RA257.

Prusa, A. R., Marton, E., Rosner, M., Bernaschek, G., and Hengstschlager, M. (2003). Oct-4-expressing cells in human amniotic fluid: a new source for stem cell research? *Hum. Reprod.* 18, 1489–1493. doi:10.1093/humrep/deg279

Rota, C., Imberti, B., Pozzobon, M., Piccoli, M., De Coppi, P., Atala, A., et al. (2011). Human amniotic fluid stem cell preconditioning improves their regenerative potential. *Stem Cells Dev.* 21, 1911–1923. doi:10.1089/scd.2011.0333

Sacco, A., Mourkioti, F., Tran, R., Choi, J., Llewellyn, M., Kraft, P., et al. (2010). Short telomeres and stem cell exhaustion model Duchenne muscular dystrophy in mdx/mTR mice. *Cell* 143, 1059–1071. doi:10.1016/j.cell.2010.11.039

Sakai, H., Sato, T., Sakurai, H., Yamamoto, T., Hanaoka, K., Montarras, D., et al. (2013). Fetal skeletal muscle progenitors have regenerative capacity after intramuscular engraftment in dystrophin deficient mice. *PLoS ONE* 8:e63016. doi:10.1371/journal.pone.0063016

Salah-Mohellibi, N., Millet, G., Andre-Schmutz, I., Desforges, B., Olaso, R., Roblot, N., et al. (2006). Bone marrow transplantation attenuates the myopathic phenotype of a muscular mouse model of spinal muscular atrophy. *Stem Cells* 24, 2723–2732. doi:10.1634/stemcells.2006-0170

Sampaolesi, M., Blot, S., D'Antona, G., Granger, N., Tonlorenzi, R., Innocenzi, A., et al. (2006). Mesoangioblast stem cells ameliorate muscle function in dystrophic dogs. *Nature* 444, 574–579. doi:10.1038/nature05282

Schoemans, H., Theunissen, K., Maertens, J., Boogaerts, M., Verfaillie, C., and Wagner, J. (2006). Adult umbilical cord blood transplantation: a comprehensive review. *Bone Marrow Transplant.* 38, 83–93. doi:10.1038/sj.bmt.1705403

Tedesco, F. S., Gerli, M. F., Perani, L., Benedetti, S., Ungaro, F., Cassano, M., et al. (2012). Transplantation of genetically corrected human iPSC-derived progenitors in mice with limb-girdle muscular dystrophy. *Sci. Transl. Med.* 4, 140ra189. doi:10.1126/scitranslmed.3003541

Toda, A., Okabe, M., Yoshida, T., and Nikaido, T. (2007). The potential of amniotic membrane/amnion-derived cells for regeneration of various tissues. *J. Pharmacol. Sci.* 105, 215–228. doi:10.1254/jphs.CR0070034

Wang, M., Yang, Y., Yang, D., Luo, F., Liang, W., Guo, S., et al. (2009). The immunomodulatory activity of human umbilical cord blood-derived mesenchymal stem cells in vitro. *Immunology* 126, 220–232. doi:10.1111/j.1365-2567.2008.02891.x

Wilschut, K. J., Ling, V. B., and Bernstein, H. S. (2012). Concise review: stem cell therapy for muscular dystrophies. *Stem Cells Transl Med* 1, 833–842. doi:10.5966/sctm.2012-0071

Yang, D. Y., Sheu, M. L., Su, H. L., Cheng, F. C., Chen, Y. J., Chen, C. J., et al. (2012). Dual regeneration of muscle and nerve by intravenous administration of human amniotic fluid-derived mesenchymal stem cells regulated by stromal cell-derived factor-1alpha in a sciatic nerve injury model. *J. Neurosurg.* 116, 1357–1367. doi:10.3171/2012.2.JNS111360

Zhao, Y., Jiang, Z., Zhao, T., Ye, M., Hu, C., Yin, Z., et al. (2012). Reversal of type 1 diabetes via islet beta cell regeneration following immune modulation by cord blood-derived multipotent stem cells. *BMC Med.* 10:3. doi:10.1186/1741-7015-10-3

Zuba-Surma, E. K., Klich, I., Greco, N., Laughlin, M. J., Ratajczak, J., and Ratajczak, M. Z. (2009). Optimization of isolation and further characterization of umbilical-cord-blood-derived very small embryonic/epiblast-like stem cells (VSELs). *Eur. J. Haematol.* 84, 34–46. doi:10.1111/j.1600-0609.2009.01352.x

17

Pathogenic mechanisms in centronuclear myopathies

Heinz Jungbluth[1,2,3] * and Mathias Gautel[3]

[1] *Neuromuscular Service, Department of Paediatric Neurology, Evelina Children's Hospital, St Thomas' Hospital, London, UK*
[2] *Department of Basic and Clinical Neuroscience, Institute of Psychiatry, Psychology and Neuroscience (IoPPN), King's College London, London, UK*
[3] *Randall Division of Cell and Molecular Biophysics and Cardiovascular Division, King's College London BHF Centre of Research Excellence, London, UK*

***Correspondence:**
Heinz Jungbluth, Children's Neuroscience Centre, St Thomas' Hospital, Floor 01 – Staircase D South Wing, London SE1 7EH, UK
e-mail: heinz.jungbluth@gstt.nhs.uk

Centronuclear myopathies (CNMs) are a genetically heterogeneous group of inherited neuromuscular disorders characterized by clinical features of a congenital myopathy and abundant central nuclei as the most prominent histopathological feature. The most common forms of congenital myopathies with central nuclei have been attributed to X-linked recessive mutations in the *MTM1* gene encoding myotubularin ("X-linked myotubular myopathy"), autosomal-dominant mutations in the *DNM2* gene encoding dynamin-2 and the *BIN1* gene encoding amphiphysin-2 (also named bridging integrator-1, BIN1, or SH3P9), and autosomal-recessive mutations in *BIN1*, the *RYR1* gene encoding the skeletal muscle ryanodine receptor, and the *TTN* gene encoding titin. Models to study and rescue the affected cellular pathways are now available in yeast, *C. elegans*, drosophila, zebrafish, mouse, and dog. Defects in membrane trafficking have emerged as a key pathogenic mechanisms, with aberrant T-tubule formation, abnormalities of triadic assembly, and disturbance of the excitation–contraction machinery the main downstream effects studied to date. Abnormal autophagy has recently been recognized as another important collateral of defective membrane trafficking in different genetic forms of CNM, suggesting an intriguing link to primary disorders of defective autophagy with overlapping histopathological features. The following review will provide an overview of clinical, histopathological, and genetic aspects of the CNMs in the context of the key pathogenic mechanism, outline unresolved questions, and indicate promising future lines of enquiry.

Keywords: centronuclear myopathy, myotubular myopathy, *MTM1* myotubularin gene, *DNM2* dynamin-2 gene, *BIN1* bridging integrator-1/amphiphysin-2 gene, *RYR1* ryanodine receptor-1 gene, *TTN titin* gene, autophagy

INTRODUCTION

Centronuclear myopathies (CNMs) are a genetically heterogeneous group of inherited neuromuscular disorders characterized by clinical features of a congenital myopathy and abundant central nuclei as the most prominent histopathological feature [for review, see Jungbluth et al. (2008)]. CNMs are genetically widely heterogeneous and have been attributed to X-linked recessive mutations in *MTM1* encoding myotubularin ["X-linked myotubular myopathy (XLMTM)"] (Laporte et al., 1996), autosomal-dominant mutations in *DNM2* encoding dynamin-2 (Bitoun et al., 2005) and the *BIN1* gene encoding amphiphysin-2 (also named bridging integrator-1, BIN1, or SH3P9) (Bohm et al., 2014), and autosomal-recessive mutations in *BIN1* (Nicot et al., 2007), *RYR1* encoding the skeletal muscle ryanodine receptor (Wilmshurst et al., 2010), and *TTN* encoding titin (Ceyhan-Birsoy et al., 2013).

Whilst histopathological abnormalities other than abundant central nuclei are not typically observed in association with *MTM1* and *BIN1* mutations, the common occurrence of central nuclei, marked variability in fiber size and cores with some of the other genetic backgrounds, in particular recessive *RYR1* (Bevilacqua et al., 2011) and *TTN* mutations (Ceyhan-Birsoy et al., 2013; Chauveau et al., 2014a), have challenged the concept of CNM as a "pure" entity (Romero, 2010) and have suggested a continuum with other congenital myopathies, in particular the core myopathies [for review, see Jungbluth et al. (2011)] and congenital fiber type disproportion (CFTD) (Clarke et al., 2010). The neuromuscular disorder due to dominant mutations in the *CCDC78* gene encoding Coiled-Coil Domain-Containing 78 (Majczenko et al., 2012) is another example of a congenital myopathy difficult to classify on histopathological grounds due to the common occurrence of internalized nuclei and cores, containing sarcoplasmic aggregated CCDC78, desmin (DES), actin (ACTA1), and RYR1.

Models to study and rescue the cellular pathways affected in various forms of CNM are now available in yeast (Parrish et al., 2004; Cebollero et al., 2012), *C. elegans* (Dang et al., 2004; Zou et al., 2009; Neukomm et al., 2011), drosophila (Velichkova et al., 2010), zebrafish (Dowling et al., 2009; Gibbs et al., 2013), mouse (Buj-Bello et al., 2002; Durieux et al., 2010b; Pierson et al., 2012; Fetalvero et al., 2013; Reifler et al., 2014), and dog (Beggs et al., 2010; Bohm et al., 2013). Based on observations in these models, several pathogenic mechanisms have now been suggested, including abnormalities of triads and calcium handling (Al-Qusairi et al., 2009; Dowling et al., 2009; Bohm et al., 2014), as well as defects of the neuromuscular junction (Robb et al., 2011; Dowling et al., 2012), satellite cells (Lawlor et al., 2012), mitochondria, and the DES cytoskeleton (Hnia et al., 2011).

Alterations of the autophagy pathway have recently emerged as a pathogenic mechanism common to different genetic forms of CNM (Al-Qusairi et al., 2013; Fetalvero et al., 2013). Autophagy is a fundamental cellular degradation pathway conserved throughout evolution with important roles in the removal of defective proteins and organelles, defense against infections and adaptation to changing metabolic demands (Mizushima, 2007; Sandri et al., 2013; Wang and Robbins, 2013). Autophagy is physiologically enhanced in neurons and muscle, and in conjunction with the ubiquitin–proteasome pathway, plays a major role in the pathogenesis of muscle atrophy (Sandri, 2013). The autophagy pathway involves several tightly regulated steps, evolving from the initial formation of phagophores to autophagosomes, whose fusion with lysosomes results in the final structures of degradation, autolysosomes [for review, see Mizushima (2007)]. The recent implication of defective autophagy in CNM corresponds to the recognition of its increasing role in a wide range of neuromuscular disorders with both primary and secondary autophagy defects (Merlini and Nishino, 2014). The observation of histopathological features closely resembling CNM in Vici syndrome (McClelland et al., 2010), a severe human multisystem disorders due to recessive mutations affecting the key autophagy regulator epg5 (Cullup et al., 2013), provides additional support for a link between the CNMs and the autophagy pathway.

The majority of the defective proteins implicated in the CNMs to date – myotubularin, dynamin-2, and amphiphysin-2 – are involved in various aspects of membrane trafficking and remodeling relevant to essential cellular processes including endocytosis, intracellular vesicle trafficking, and autophagy [for review, see Cowling et al. (2012)], suggesting a pathogenic "master mechanism" upstream of the more specific downstream pathogenic mechanisms outlined above. However, a link between membrane trafficking and other genes implicated in the CNMs is not immediately obvious, and the communality of clinico-pathological features between *MTM1*, *DNM2*, and *BIN1*-related CNM on one hand and the more recently reported forms due to recessive mutations in *RYR1* and *TTN* on the other hand remains currently unaccounted for on the molecular level.

The following review will give an overview of the key clinical, histopathological, and genetic aspects of the different forms of CNM, outline pathogenic mechanisms where already known, with a particular emphasis on defects in membrane trafficking and autophagy, and summarize unresolved questions and future lines of enquiry. **Table 1** summarizes the genes and proteins implicated in the CNMs and outlines their main function(s) where known. **Figure 1** illustrates tentative links between the different pathways implicated in the CNMs.

MTM1-RELATED CNM ("X-LINKED MYOTUBULAR MYOPATHY")

Centronuclear myopathy due to X-linked recessive mutations in the myotubularin *(MTM1)* gene (also commonly referred to as XLMTM) is a rare congenital myopathy that affects approximately 2/100000 male births per year [for review, see Jungbluth et al. (2008)].

X-linked myotubular myopathy is characterized by a severe phenotype in males with often antenatal onset, profound hypotonia, and weakness at birth with associated severe respiratory and bulbar involvement necessitating invasive ventilation and nasogastric tube feeds. Extraocular muscle involvement is common. The condition is usually fatal within the first year of life but a proportion of more mildly affected males may survive into adolescence or adulthood, sometimes even without requiring constant ventilatory support. Although profound muscle involvement is the most dramatic and earliest feature of myotubularin deficiency, long-term survivors show additional organ manifestations such as hepatic peliosis suggestive of a multisystem disorder (Herman et al., 1999), indicating that myotubularin does play a vital role in tissues other than muscle. Moreover, despite muscle atrophy and weakness, males with XLMTM typically exhibit signs of macrosomia consistent with an overgrowth syndrome (Leguennec et al., 1988; Joseph et al., 1995), suggesting a differential effect of myotubularin deficiency on muscle and other growth pathways. A dilated cardiomyopathy has been reported in two adult brothers with a mild form of XLMTM (Yu et al., 2003), raising the possibility of a cardiac phenotype in long-term survivors that remains to be systematically evaluated. Histopathological features in addition to numerous central nuclei include type 1 predominance and hypotrophy, a region devoid of myofibrils surrounding the central nucleus and necklace fibers (Romero and Bitoun, 2011), but additional sarcomeric disorganization or overt cores are unusual in contrast to the *DNM2*-, *RYR1*- and *TTN*-related forms.

More than 300 *MTM1* mutations have been identified to date (Laporte et al., 2000; Herman et al., 2002; Biancalana et al., 2003; Tsai et al., 2005), distributed throughout the entire coding sequence and with only few recurrent substitutions. Genotype–phenotype studies have been limited due to the private nature of many *MTM1* mutations, however, not unexpectedly truncating mutations usually give rise to the more severe phenotype whilst non-truncating mutations outside the myotubularin catalytic domain have been associated with milder presentations. Markedly skewed X-inactivation in manifesting females (Jungbluth et al., 2003), as well as complex rearrangements involving the *MTM1* locus have also been recently reported (Trump et al., 2011; Amburgey et al., 2013).

Myotubularin defines a family of 14 phosphoinositide phosphatases in mammals [for review, see Laporte et al. (1998, 2001, 2003), Begley and Dixon (2005), Clague and Lorenzo (2005), Robinson and Dixon (2006), and Amoasii et al. (2012)], two of which, MTMR2 and MTMR13, have also been implicated in different forms of Charcot-Marie-Tooth (CMT) disease, CMT4B1 (Berger et al., 2002) and CMT4B2 (Azzedine et al., 2003), respectively. In addition to the catalytic and enzymatically active domain, myotubularin contains four other domains, including a coiled–coiled domain involved in homo- and heterodimer formation. Apart from the recognized interaction with DES, only little is known about interactions with other proteins in skeletal muscle.

Myotubularin dephosphorylates phosphatidylinositol 3-phosphate [PI(3)P] and phosphatidylinositol 3,5-phosphate [PI(3,5)P] [(Blondeau et al., 2000; Taylor et al., 2000; Tronchere et al., 2004); for review, see Tronchere et al. (2003), Robinson and Dixon (2006), and Rohde et al. (2009)], second messengers with a crucial role in membrane trafficking whose production is under the control of specific phosphatidylinositide

Table 1 | Genes and proteins implicated in various forms of centronuclear myopathy (CNM).

Gene	Inheritance	Protein	Principal function(s)	Main pathogenic effects in muscle
MTM1	XL	Myotubularin	PI3P regulation Membrane formation/trafficking Endocytosis Endo(lyso)some formation	Abnormal nuclear positioning Abnormalities of triad positioning and function Abnormal autophagy Abnormal cytoskeletal architecture Abnormal mitochondrial positioning Autophagosome formation
DNM2	AD	Dynamin-2	Membrane formation/trafficking Vesicle formation and fission	Abnormal nuclear positioning Abnormalities of triad positioning and function Abnormal autophagy Abnormal cytoskeletal architecture Abnormal mitochondrial positioning
BIN1	AR, AD	Amphiphysin-2	Membrane remodeling	Abnormalities of nuclear positioning, triad assembly and function
RYR1	AR	Skeletal muscle ryanodine receptor	Sarcoplasmic reticulum calcium release	Abnormal nuclear positioning Abnormalities of triad assembly and function Abnormal SR calcium release
TTN	AR	Titin	Elastic link between actin and myosin filaments Organizer of Z-disk and M-band assembly Organizer of myosin filament, possibly by regulating myosin motor domains Mechanosensor Signaling scaffold organizing ubiquitin–proteasome and autophagy–lysosomal protein turnover	Abnormal sarcomere assembly and turnover Disrupted force transmission Abnormal myosin force generation Abnormal transcriptional regulation
MTMR14	AR? Digenic?	hJUMPY	PI3P regulation Membrane formation/trafficking	Abnormal nuclear positioning Abnormal excitation–contraction coupling Abnormal autophagy
CCDC78	AD	Coiled-coil domain-containing protein 78	Centriole biogenesis?	Abnormal nuclear positioning Core formation?

kinases. In skeletal muscle, the main generator of PI(3)P is the PI3 kinase PIK3C3 (Backer, 2008; Meijer and Klionsky, 2011), a key regulator of a wide range of cellular processes including autophagy, in particular formation and maturation of autophagosomes (Funderburk et al., 2010).

The fundamental role of myotubularin and its orthologs in PI3P regulation, endocytosis, and endo(lyso)somal function has been documented in drosophila, *C. elegans*, zebrafish, mouse, and higher mammalian models of myotubularin deficiency [for review, see Cowling et al. (2012)]. Zebrafish morphants following mtm1 morpholino knockdown show abnormal motor behavior and reproduce some of the histopathological features also seen in human XLMTM, associated with increased PI3P levels in muscle (Dowling et al., 2009). In contrast to human XLMTM, the mtm1 knockout mouse develops muscle weakness and atrophy only in the postnatal period, suggesting an effect of myotubularin deficiency on muscle maintenance rather than muscle development (Buj-Bello et al., 2002). Secondary abnormalities of T-tubules, sarcoplasmic reticulum (SR) and the triads (Al-Qusairi et al., 2009; Dowling et al., 2009; Beggs et al., 2010; Toussaint et al., 2011) and, less frequently, abnormalities of intermediate filaments and mitochondrial dynamics (Hnia et al., 2011) have been reported as an important common downstream effect of myotubularin deficiency in zebrafish, mouse, dog, and humans.

Initiation of autophagy, in particular formation of autophagosomes and autophagosome–lysosome fusion, depends on PI3P synthesis (Vergne and Deretic, 2010; Cebollero et al., 2012), and the concerted interaction of autophagy-related (Atg) proteins at the phagophore assembly site (PAS) (Lamb et al., 2013; Ge et al., 2014); considering the important role of myotubularin in regulating PI3P levels in muscle, it is not surprising that alterations of muscle autophagy have now been reported in animal models of XLMTM: In particular, a marked disturbance of autophagy has been reported in zebrafish following double knockdown of the myotubularin family members *MTM1* and *MTMR14* (Dowling et al., 2010), the latter also known as Jumpy and implicated in very rare digenic forms of CNM (Tosch et al., 2006). Mytotubularin deficiency has also been associated with increased mTORC1 activity, disconnection between starvation and autophagy induction (Fetalvero et al., 2013), increased IGF1R/Akt signaling, upregulation of atrogenes and an increase in autophagy markers in the mtm1 knockout mouse (Al-Qusairi et al., 2013), indicating both up- and downstream effects of murine myotubularin deficiency on the autophagy pathway that are potentially amenable

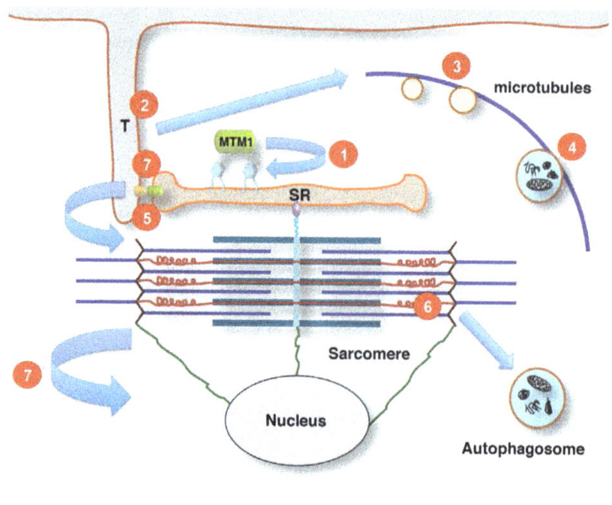

FIGURE 1 | Tentative links between membrane signaling, sarcomere activity, and nuclear positioning. T-tubules (T) link the sarcolemma to the sarcoplasmic reticulum (SR) at the triads by contacts between dihydropyridine receptors (small orange oval) and ryanodine receptors (small green oval). Phosphoinositol phosphates (PIP; blue hexagonal symbols at SR membrane) are turned over by the lipid phosphatase myotubularin, regulating membrane dynamics, and PIP-dependent downstream signaling. This affects multiple pathways, including autophagy. Altered membrane remodeling and microtubular transport will converge on these pathways. Defects affecting Titin's scaffolding role concerning multiple components of the protein quality control machinery impinge on contractile function, sarcomere turnover and possibly sarcomere-nuclear links. Nuclei and sarcomeres are joined by peripheral cytoskeletal networks, including desmin intermediate filaments and nesprin via "transmembrane actin-associated nuclear links" (Luxton et al., 2011). **1**, Mutations affecting lipid phosphatase activity of myotubularin (MTM1 and MTMR14); **2**, mutations in components of the membrane remodeling machinery (BIN1); **3**, defects in vesicular traffic or microtubule dynamics (DNM2); **4**, mutations in the endosomal–autophagosomal–lysosomal pathway (EPG5); **5**, defective calcium homeostasis and excitation–contraction coupling (RYR1); **6**, defective sarcomeric maintenance and protein quality control (TTN); **7**, disrupted nuclear cytoskeleton links, abnormal nuclear positioning and possibly impaired triad function via impaired microtubule/centriole function (CCDC78).

to mTOR inhibition with Rapamycin (Fetalvero et al., 2013) and adeno-associated virus (AAV)-mediated delivery of functional myotubularin (Al-Qusairi et al., 2013). Interestingly, a recent study reporting a muscle-specific conditional knockout of PIK3C3, the phosphatidylinositide 3-kinase critical for PI3P levels in muscle, indicates marked autophagolysosomal abnormalities with histopathological features more suggestive of a muscular dystrophy rather than CNM (Reifler et al., 2014). These observations suggest the autophagy pathway and its upstream regulators as potential therapeutic targets in CNM and, possibly, other forms of neuromuscular disorders.

DNM2-RELATED CNM

Dominantly inherited *DNM2*-related CNM is usually much milder than X-linked and recessive forms of CNM although more severe presentations have been reported [for review, see Jungbluth et al. (2008)]. Onset is typically in adolescence or early adulthood, featuring predominant proximal weakness with additional distal involvement particularly in the lower limbs, ptosis with external ophthalmoplegia, and a stable or slowly progressive course. Exertional myalgia may be the presenting feature before the evolution of overt weakness and muscle hypertrophy, occasionally localized, has been observed (Liewluck et al., 2010). Specific dominant intermediate (CMTDIB) and axonal forms of CMT disease (CMT2), respectively, are allelic conditions (Zuchner et al., 2005; Fabrizi et al., 2007). In addition to myopathic changes, EMG and nerve conduction studies may show mild signs of axonal peripheral nerve involvement also in *DNM2*-related CNM patients (Fischer et al., 2006; Echaniz-Laguna et al., 2007), suggesting a clinical continuum between myopathic and neuropathic manifestations of *DNM2* mutations. Other *DNM2*-mutated patients may feature additional neutropenia (Liewluck et al., 2010) or cataracts (Jungbluth et al., 2010), suggesting a role of dynamin-2 in tissues other than muscle, as well as clinical overlap with multisystem disorders due to primary autophagy defects such as *EPG5*-related Vici syndrome (Cullup et al., 2013), where cataracts and hematological abnormalities are common. Homozygosity for the *DNM2* Phe379Val missense mutation has been recently associated with a congenital lethal syndrome in humans (Koutsopoulos et al., 2013). Histopathological features in addition to centralized nuclei may include type 1 predominance, typical sarcoplasmic radial strands surrounding the central nuclei, increases in connective tissues and cores (Fischer et al., 2006; Schessl et al., 2007; Jeub et al., 2008; Hanisch et al., 2011; Bohm et al., 2012a; Catteruccia et al., 2013).

The *DNM2* gene is one of three members of the dynamin family (Praefcke and McMahon, 2004) and ubiquitously expressed, in contrast to *DNM1* that is mainly expressed in the brain, and *DNM3* expressed in brain and testes. *DNM2* encodes a large GTPase protein organized in five functional domains, an N-terminal GTPase domain, a middle domain (MD), a pleckstrin homology (PH) domain, a GTPase effector domain, and a C-terminal proline rich domain (PRD) (McNiven, 2005). Through its PH and PRD domains, dynamin-2 binds to phosphoinositides and SH3 domain proteins such as amphiphysin, respectively. Dominant mutations affecting the dynamin-2 MD have been associated with a mild phenotype of CNM (Bitoun et al., 2005), whilst more severe presentations with neonatal onset have been attributed to heterozygous *de novo* dominant mutations affecting the PH domain (Bitoun et al., 2007; Jungbluth et al., 2010). The dynamin-2 PH domain is also predominantly affected by *DNM2* mutations causing primary neuropathic phenotypes. A recurrent *DNM2* mutation (c.1393C > T; p.Arg465Trp) has been identified in a number of unrelated autosomal-dominant pedigrees with a mild form of CNM.

Dynamins are involved in membrane fission, and the role of various isoforms including dynamin-2 in clathrin-dependent and independent endocytosis, vesicle formation and processing (Jones et al., 1998; Praefcke and McMahon, 2004; Durieux et al., 2010a) has been documented in various models of dynamin deficiency. Additional roles have been proposed in the microtubule network, actin cytoskeleton assembly (Gu et al., 2010), and centrosome cohesion (Thompson et al., 2004), the latter of potential relevance for the nuclear abnormalities observed in *DNM2*-related CNM.

Murine models of the common human *DNM2* R465W dominant CNM mutation do replicate aspects of the human phenotype, and not unexpected considering the close links between endocytic and autophagic pathways, show variable abnormalities of autophagy: Durieux et al. (2010b, 2012) demonstrated a slowly progressive myopathy with upregulation of genes involved in ubiquitin–proteosome (UPS) and autophagy pathways in a heterozygous knock-in mouse model of the common CMT-associated heterozygous *DNM2* mutation R465W. Mice homozygous for the R465W mutation showed a severe phenotype similar to what has been observed in other mouse models of dysregulated autophagy (Durieux et al., 2012), characterized by increased glycogen storage, hepatomegaly, hypoglycemia, and early lethality. The same mice showed microscopic evidence of delayed autophagosome maturation and of reduced autophagic flux on *in vitro* studies. Another mouse model generated by intramuscular AAV injection of mutant R465W–DNM2 generated histopathological abnormalities and T-tubule defects similar to those observed in humans and animal models of other forms of CNM, suggesting a muscle maintenance defect as the principal abnormality also in *DNM2*-related CNM. An intriguing and potentially therapeutically exploitable link between *DNM2*- and *MTM1*-related pathways has been recently indicated by demonstrating rescue of the XLMTM phenotype through dynamin-2 reduction in mice (Cowling et al., 2014).

BIN1-RELATED CNM

Autosomal-recessive *BIN1*-related CNM has only been reported in a small number of families associated with a mild to moderate phenotype characterized by early-childhood onset, extraocular muscle involvement and slowly progressive muscle weakness, and atrophy (Nicot et al., 2007; Claeys et al., 2010). However, more severe, early-onset lethal (Nicot et al., 2007) and rapidly progressive presentations due to homozygous *BIN1* mutations affecting splicing have been reported (Bohm et al., 2010, 2013). Dominant inheritance of *BIN1* mutations has also been recently recognized (Bohm et al., 2014). In addition to central nuclei, type 1 fiber-type predominance may be an additional feature, but sarcomeric disorganization and core-like areas are uncommon [for review, see Jungbluth et al. (2008)].

BIN1 encodes amphiphysin-2, a protein belonging to the BAR (Bin/Amphiphysin/Rvs) domain-containing family of proteins (Peter et al., 2004) involved in various key cellular processes including membrane recycling and endocyotosis [for review, see Prokic et al. (2014)]. Corresponding to other proteins implicated in the CNMs, BIN1 also contains a phosphoinositide-binding domain and is involved in T-tubule formation. Mutations affecting the *BIN1* BAR domain impair membrane tubulation and result in structural abnormalities (Wu et al., 2014). *BIN1* is ubiquitously expressed but subject to tissue-specific alternative splicing, whereas amphiphysin 1, the other member of the amphiphysin family, is mainly expressed in brain. *BIN1* downregulation has been associated with cancer progression and cardiac disease, whereas *BIN1* overexpression has been linked to an increased risk for late-onset Alzheimer disease [for review, see Prokic et al. (2014)].

The essential role of amphiphysins and their orthologs in endocytosis, membrane remodeling and recycling has been documented in drosophila and *C. elegans* models of amphiphysin deficiency [for review, see Cowling et al. (2012)]. A recent Bin1-deficient zebrafish model of *BIN1*-related CNM reproduces the histopathological features of the human phenotype, and indicates abnormal calcium release resulting from aberrant triad formation as an important pathogenic mechanism downstream of the principal membrane remodeling abnormality (Smith et al., 2014). The T-tubule and triadic abnormalities observed in the Bin1-deficient zebrafish model are similar to those observed in *MTM1*- and *DNM2*-related CNM (Toussaint et al., 2011), indicating a shared pathogenic mechanism due to implication of the defective proteins in the same pathway. *BIN1*-deficient mice show early lethality (Muller et al., 2003), but murine skeletal muscle has not yet been thoroughly analyzed. A recent mouse model of Bin1 depletion in the heart shows abnormalities of T-tubule folding resulting in free diffusion of local extracellular calcium and potassium ions, prolonged action-potential duration and increased susceptibility to ventricular arrhythmias (Hong et al., 2014).

BIN1 deficiency has not yet been associated with defects in the autophagy pathway, however, it is of note that structurally related BAR domain-containing proteins such as SH3P2 translocate to the PAS following autophagy induction and appear to play a role in autophagosome formation (Zhuang et al., 2013).

RYR1-RELATED CNM

Recessive mutations in *RYR1* are another cause of congenital myopathies with central nuclei (Wilmshurst et al., 2010). *RYR1* mutations are one of the most common causes of inherited neuromuscular disorders, ranging from the malignant hyperthermia susceptibility (MHS) trait without any associated weakness to various congenital myopathies, including mainly dominantly inherited Central Core Disease (CCD) as well as mainly recessively inherited Multi-minicore Disease (MmD) [for review, see Jungbluth et al. (2011)], CFTD (Clarke et al., 2010), and CNM (Wilmshurst et al., 2010). The genetics of *RYR1*-related myopathies are not infrequently complex, occasionally with two clearly pathogenic *RYR1* mutations occurring on the same allele or running independently in the same family, possibly accounting for the wide phenotypical variability and variable penetrance (Klein et al., 2012). There is substantial clinical and pathological overlap between MmD, CFTD, and CNM due to recessive *RYR1* mutations, and it appears appropriate to view these conditions as part of a recessive *RYR1*-related continuum rather than completely distinct entities.

Clinically, *RYR1*-related CNM is of intermediate severity compared to other genetic forms, with facial weakness, external ophthalmoplegia, predominantly proximal muscle involvement but less pronounced bulbar or respiratory impairment (Wilmshurst et al., 2010). There is however, a more severe end of the spectrum, with some profoundly affected males showing clinical presentations indistinguishable from the XLMTM phenotype. Patients with *RYR1*-related CNM show a marked tendency to improve over time, even following an initially severe presentation, a feature also in other recessive *RYR1*-related myopathies (Bohm et al., 2012b) that remains currently unexplained.

On the pathological level, central and multiple internalized nuclei are often the principal histopathological feature when muscle biopsy is performed early in life (Jungbluth et al., 2007), but other histopathological features typically associated with recessive *RYR1*-related myopathies – marked type 1 predominance or uniformity, fiber type disproportion and cores – may evolve over time (Bevilacqua et al., 2011).

In contrast to dominantly inherited MHS and CCD where most features can be explained by abnormal calcium release from the mutant RyR1 channel [for review, see Treves et al. (2005)], the pathogenesis of recessive *RYR1*-related myopathies is currently only partly understood and probably more complex. Recessive *RYR1* genotypes, often featuring compound heterozygosity for *RYR1* missense and truncating mutations, result in reduced expression of the RyR1 protein and secondary reduction of the DHPR receptor, its principal ligand (Wilmshurst et al., 2010; Bevilacqua et al., 2011; Zhou et al., 2013). Additional upregulation of the IP3R receptor may be found in some cases, an observation currently of uncertain significance (Zhou et al., 2013). Whilst the concomitant reduction of RyR1 and DHPR and the resulting excitation–contraction (EC) coupling defect are likely to explain the weakness, muscle atrophy as well as histopathological features of fiber-type disproportion and centralized nuclei are not readily explained by alterations of calcium release in recessive *RYR1*-related myopathies.

In contrast to other genetic forms of CNM, defects in membrane trafficking and autophagy have not been implicated in recessive *RYR1*-related CNM. However, it is of note that marked autophagy abnormalities have been observed in mice following induced reduction of the DHPR receptor (Pietri-Rouxel et al., 2010), a secondary feature also in recessive *RYR1*-related myopathies. In addition, the recent implication of annexin-1 and annexin-5, members of the annexin family of proteins that bind to phospholipid membranes in a calcium-dependent manner, in autophagosome maturation (Ghislat and Knecht, 2012) suggests a potential link between disturbed calcium homeostasis and autophagy regulation that may warrant further investigation. Effect of altered calcium release on autophagic pathways have been previously considered but with conflicting conclusions (East and Campanella, 2013).

TTN-RELATED CNM

Recessive mutations in *TTN* encoding the giant sarcomeric ruler protein titin have recently been identified by next generation sequencing in five individuals selected from a cohort of 29 unrelated and genetically unresolved patients with a clinicopathological diagnosis of CNM (Ceyhan-Birsoy et al., 2013). *TTN* mutations have recently also been indicated as one of the most common identifiable genetic causes of dilated cardiomyopathy (Herman et al., 2012), and have been implicated in a wide range of neuromuscular disorders, including late-onset tibial muscular dystrophy, limb girdle muscular dystrophy type 2J (LGMD2J), hereditary myopathy with early respiratory failure (HMERF), and early-onset myopathy with fatal cardiomyopathy [reviewed recently in Chauveau et al. (2014b)]. Although the functional relevance and clear genotype–phenotype correlations have been established for many unequivocally pathogenic *TTN* mutations, it is also important to bear in mind that truncating *TTN* variants are exceedingly common [over 6000 in the December 2014 release of the 1000 genomes database, and ca. 3% of controls reported in Herman et al. (2012)] and that pathogenicity is not always immediately evident even if those variants are truncating. This might be due to tissue-specific and developmentally regulated exon usage, especially in the extensively differentially spliced I-band region of titin (Bang et al., 2001), making some truncating variants penetrant in only a small subset of titin isoforms. But also, truncating mutations near the C-terminus appear, on the whole, to be recessive without an adult phenotype (Carmignac et al., 2007; Ceyhan-Birsoy et al., 2013; Chauveau et al., 2014a). The reasons for the recessive inheritance of truncating variants in constitutively expressed exons remains to be understood.

Clinical features of the five patients with *TTN*-related CNM in the study by Ceyhan-Birsoy et al. (2013) were characterized by early-childhood onset, generalized weakness, and respiratory impairment, but without evidence of cardiac involvement at the time of the last follow-up in childhood or late adolescence (5–19 years). In contrast to other genetic forms of CNM, extraocular muscles were spared and in one case CK levels were increased >1000 IU/l. Histopathological features included increases in connective tissue, fiber type disproportion, and type 1 predominance and hypotrophy. In contrast to *MTM1*-related CNM, but corresponding to findings in the *RYR1*-related form, central and internalized nuclei were typically multiple rather than single. Similar observations were made in the seminal paper on the recessive truncating *TTN*-linked early-onset Salih myopathy (Carmignac et al., 2007) and in four families with compound heterozygous *TTN* variants in Autosomal-Recessive Multi-minicore Disease with Heart Disease (AR MmD-HD) (Chauveau et al., 2014a). Patients with AR MmD-HD show marked centronucleation with additional morphological changes, notably the formation of protein aggregates and Z-disk streaming that show ultrastructural similarities to those found in myofibrillar myopathy. Patients also display various cardiac phenotypes, from left-ventricular non-compaction to septal defects (ASD and VSD) and dilated cardiomyopathy, in some instances requiring transplantation (Chauveau et al., 2014a). Additional findings of core-like areas on oxidative stain and myofibrillar disruption on EM, in particular Z-disk streaming and sarcomere disruption, suggest that *TTN*-related CNM and AR MmD-HD may be part of a *TTN*-related histopathological spectrum rather than a pure entity, again corresponding to observations in the *RYR1*-related form.

The pathogenesis of *TTN*-related CNM and in particular its association with pathways affected in other forms of CNM, if any, remains currently uncertain. Most mutations identified in *TTN*-related CNM give rise to significant C-terminal truncations, with or without the expression of disruptive missense variants, resulting in secondary reduction of interacting proteins such as nebulin and calpain-3 that may contribute to the phenotype. Calpain-3 is required for the normal recruitment of RyR1 receptors to the triad, a function that, if disturbed, may give rise to similar abnormalities of triad assembly and EC coupling as seen in other genetic forms of CNM. A common feature of *TTN*-linked AR MmD-HD and CNM is, however, the disruption of titin M-band linked interactions; of these, three are possibly mechanistically related to pathways linked to the "classical" CNM variants. Firstly, M-band titin links the sarcomere to the SR via its interactions with the giant protein obscurin (Bagnato et al., 2003; Kontrogianni-Konstantopoulos et al., 2003; Fukuzawa et al., 2008) and thus contributes to the organized integration of the EC-coupling machinery of T-tubules, junctional SR, and sarcomeres. Intriguingly, obscurin knockout mice also develop a myopathic phenotype with centralized nuclei and disordered SR (Lange et al., 2009). Secondly, the M-band associated kinase domain of titin is linked to the control of protein turnover via the autophagy cargo adaptors Nbr1 and SQSTM1 [reviewed in Gautel (2011)]. Lastly, mutations in the C-terminus of titin are linked to secondary calpain-3 deficiency also in the case of adult titinopathies (Udd, 2012), likely due to the abrogation of a calpain-3 binding site near the C-terminus of titin (Charton et al., 2010). While the connections between titin mutations, protein turnover, and abnormal nuclear positioning in titin-associated CNM-like myopathies are currently unclear, accumulating evidence suggests that protein turnover via autophagy and calpain-mediated turnover converge on M-band titin and that these connections are concerted with physical links to the SR and triad systems. If such links exist, it seems plausible that the ablation or functional disruption of titin-linked autophagy functions in M-band titinopathies (Chauveau et al., 2014a) result in partial phenotypic overlap with membrane-associated components of the autophagy machinery.

RARE CONGENITAL MYOPATHIES WITH CENTRAL NUCLEI

Congenital myopathies with features of CNM with or without additional histopathological abnormalities due to uncommon genetic backgrounds have been observed in isolated families.

Tosch and colleagues reported single heterozygous missense variants in hJUMPY (also known as MTMR14, a member of the myotubularin family) in two sporadic cases with features of CNM and uncertain inheritance (Tosch et al., 2006). Although both variants were demonstrated to reduce the enzymatic activity of hJUMPY, identification of an additional *DNM2* mutation in one patient suggests that a second mutation may be required for full manifestation of clinical features; this is also in keeping with the observation of a more severe phenotype in the MTM1–MTMR14 zebrafish double knockout compared to knockout of each single gene (Dowling et al., 2010).

Autosomal-dominant mutations in CCDC78 have also recently been identified in a single family characterized by core-like areas and increased internalized nuclei (Majczenko et al., 2012); CCDC78 encodes a skeletal muscle protein enriched in the perinuclear region and at the sarcolemma and possibly triad (Majczenko et al., 2012), suggesting a possible link with a pathogenic mechanism, abnormal triad assembly, and resulting disturbance of EC coupling, common to other forms of CNM. CCDC78 plays a key role in centriole biogenesis (Klos Dehring et al., 2013); the impaired function in CNM4 and the link to potential triad malfunction or abnormal nuclear positioning via impaired microtubule function is currently elusive.

CONCLUSION AND OUTLOOK

Recent years have seen substantial advances in our understanding of the CNMs, in particular those due to mutations in *MTM1*, *DNM2*, and *BIN1*, encoding proteins intricately linked in various aspects of phosphoinositide metabolism and membrane trafficking, with aberrant T-tubule formation, abnormalities of triad assembly and disturbance of the EC machinery as the most important downstream effects studied to date. Abnormal autophagy has recently been recognized as another important pathogenic mechanism in different genetic forms of CNM, suggesting an intriguing link to primary disorders of defective autophagy with overlapping histopathological features. These findings have illustrated the role of defective pathways common to several genetic forms of CNM that may be potentially amenable to therapeutic intervention. It remains currently uncertain if the proteins encoded by genes more recently implicated in the CNMs, in particular *RYR1* and *TTN*, are involved with the same pathways or linked with altogether different mechanisms. The functional links between the genetic mechanisms implicated in CNM are tentative at the moment, and it has to be seen whether all myopathies clinically classified as CNM indeed join into a common pathomechanistic pathway. Although the mechanisms outlined above may at least partially explain the muscle weakness and atrophy observed in different forms of CNM, other aspects such as the consistent abnormality of nuclear positioning remain currently unaccounted for. The molecular machinery involved in nuclear positioning is currently only partially understood [for review, see Osorio and Gomes (2014)], but emerging evidence suggests that normal positioning of the nucleus is a prerequisite for its normal functioning (Metzger et al., 2012). Recent work has already suggested a link between N-WASP and BIN1-related nuclear positioning and triad organization (Falcone et al., 2014). Further investigation of the CNMs as a paradigm of disorders with nuclear positioning as the most prominent pathological hallmark will advance our understanding of the intricate interaction between the nucleus, microtubules and the actomyosin cytoskeleton (Luxton et al., 2011; Cadot et al., 2012), and delineate the importance of the interplay of these structures for cellular function in health and disease.

ACKNOWLEDGMENTS

Grant support from the Myotubular Trust/Sparks (Grant Ref. 12KCL01-MT) is gratefully acknowledged. Mathias Gautel holds the British Heart Foundation Chair of Molecular Cardiology.

REFERENCES

Al-Qusairi, L., Prokic, I., Amoasii, L., Kretz, C., Messaddeq, N., Mandel, J. L., et al. (2013). Lack of myotubularin (MTM1) leads to muscle hypotrophy through unbalanced regulation of the autophagy and ubiquitin-proteasome pathways. *FASEB J.* 27, 3384–3394. doi:10.1096/fj.12-220947

Al-Qusairi, L., Weiss, N., Toussaint, A., Berbey, C., Messaddeq, N., Kretz, C., et al. (2009). T-tubule disorganization and defective excitation-contraction coupling in muscle fibers lacking myotubularin lipid phosphatase. *Proc. Natl. Acad. Sci. U. S. A.* 106, 18763–18768. doi:10.1073/pnas.0900705106

Amburgey, K., Lawlor, M. W., Del Gaudio, D., Cheng, Y. W., Fitzpatrick, C., Minor, A., et al. (2013). Large duplication in MTM1 associated with myotubular myopathy. *Neuromuscul. Disord.* 23, 214–218. doi:10.1016/j.nmd.2012.11.010

Amoasii, L., Hnia, K., and Laporte, J. (2012). Myotubularin phosphoinositide phosphatases in human diseases. *Curr. Top. Microbiol. Immunol.* 362, 209–233. doi:10.1007/978-94-007-5025-8_10

Azzedine, H., Bolino, A., Taieb, T., Birouk, N., Di Duca, M., Bouhouche, A., et al. (2003). Mutations in MTMR13, a new pseudophosphatase homologue of MTMR2 and Sbf1, in two families with an autosomal recessive demyelinating form of Charcot-Marie-Tooth disease associated with early-onset glaucoma. *Am. J. Hum. Genet.* 72, 1141–1153. doi:10.1086/375034

Backer, J. M. (2008). The regulation and function of class III PI3Ks: novel roles for Vps34. *Biochem. J.* 410, 1–17. doi:10.1042/BJ20071427

Bagnato, P., Barone, V., Giacomello, E., Rossi, D., and Sorrentino, V. (2003). Binding of an ankyrin-1 isoform to obscurin suggests a molecular link between the sarcoplasmic reticulum and myofibrils in striated muscles. *J. Cell Biol.* 160, 245–253. doi:10.1083/jcb.200208109

Bang, M. L., Centner, T., Fornoff, F., Geach, A. J., Gotthardt, M., McNabb, M., et al. (2001). The complete gene sequence of titin, expression of an unusual approximately 700-kDa titin isoform, and its interaction with obscurin identify a novel Z-line to I-band linking system. *Circ. Res.* 89, 1065–1072. doi:10.1161/hh2301.100981

Beggs, A. H., Bohm, J., Snead, E., Kozlowski, M., Maurer, M., Minor, K., et al. (2010). MTM1 mutation associated with X-linked myotubular myopathy in labrador retrievers. *Proc. Natl. Acad. Sci. U. S. A.* 107, 14697–14702. doi:10.1073/pnas.1003677107

Begley, M. J., and Dixon, J. E. (2005). The structure and regulation of myotubularin phosphatases. *Curr. Opin. Struct. Biol.* 15, 614–620. doi:10.1016/j.sbi.2005.10.016

Berger, P., Bonneick, S., Willi, S., Wymann, M., and Suter, U. (2002). Loss of phosphatase activity in myotubularin-related protein 2 is associated with Charcot-Marie-Tooth disease type 4B1. *Hum. Mol. Genet.* 11, 1569–1579. doi:10.1093/hmg/11.13.1569

Bevilacqua, J. A., Monnier, N., Bitoun, M., Eymard, B., Ferreiro, A., Monges, S., et al. (2011). Recessive RYR1 mutations cause unusual congenital myopathy with prominent nuclear internalization and large areas of myofibrillar disorganization. *Neuropathol. Appl. Neurobiol.* 37, 271–284. doi:10.1111/j.1365-2990.2010.01149.x

Biancalana, V., Caron, O., Gallati, S., Baas, F., Kress, W., Novelli, G., et al. (2003). Characterisation of mutations in 77 patients with X-linked myotubular myopathy, including a family with a very mild phenotype. *Hum. Genet.* 112, 135–142. doi:10.1007/s00439-002-0869-1

Bitoun, M., Bevilacqua, J. A., Prudhon, B., Maugenre, S., Taratuto, A. L., Monges, S., et al. (2007). Dynamin 2 mutations cause sporadic centronuclear myopathy with neonatal onset. *Ann. Neurol.* 62, 666–670. doi:10.1002/ana.21235

Bitoun, M., Maugenre, S., Jeannet, P. Y., Lacene, E., Ferrer, X., Laforet, P., et al. (2005). Mutations in dynamin 2 cause dominant centronuclear myopathy. *Nat. Genet.* 37, 1207–1209. doi:10.1038/ng1657

Blondeau, F., Laporte, J., Bodin, S., Superti-Furga, G., Payrastre, B., and Mandel, J. L. (2000). Myotubularin, a phosphatase deficient in myotubular myopathy, acts on phosphatidylinositol 3-kinase and phosphatidylinositol 3-phosphate pathway. *Hum. Mol. Genet.* 9, 2223–2229. doi:10.1093/oxfordjournals.hmg.a018913

Bohm, J., Biancalana, V., Dechene, E. T., Bitoun, M., Pierson, C. R., Schaefer, E., et al. (2012a). Mutation spectrum in the large GTPase dynamin 2, and genotype-phenotype correlation in autosomal dominant centronuclear myopathy. *Hum. Mutat.* 33, 949–959. doi:10.1002/humu.22067

Bohm, J., Leshinsky-Silver, E., Vassilopoulos, S., Le Gras, S., Lerman-Sagie, T., Ginzberg, M., et al. (2012b). Samaritan myopathy, an ultimately benign congenital myopathy, is caused by a RYR1 mutation. *Acta Neuropathol.* 124, 575–581. doi:10.1007/s00401-012-1007-3

Bohm, J., Biancalana, V., Malfatti, E., Dondaine, N., Koch, C., Vasli, N., et al. (2014). Adult-onset autosomal dominant centronuclear myopathy due to BIN1 mutations. *Brain* 137, 3160–3170. doi:10.1093/brain/awu272

Bohm, J., Vasli, N., Maurer, M., Cowling, B., Shelton, G. D., Kress, W., et al. (2013). Altered splicing of the BIN1 muscle-specific exon in humans and dogs with highly progressive centronuclear myopathy. *PLoS Genet.* 9:e1003430. doi:10.1371/journal.pgen.1003430

Bohm, J., Yis, U., Ortac, R., Cakmakci, H., Kurul, S. H., Dirik, E., et al. (2010). Case report of intrafamilial variability in autosomal recessive centronuclear myopathy associated to a novel BIN1 stop mutation. *Orphanet J. Rare Dis.* 5, 35. doi:10.1186/1750-1172-5-35

Buj-Bello, A., Laugel, V., Messaddeq, N., Zahreddine, H., Laporte, J., Pellissier, J. F., et al. (2002). The lipid phosphatase myotubularin is essential for skeletal muscle maintenance but not for myogenesis in mice. *Proc. Natl. Acad. Sci. U. S. A.* 99, 15060–15065. doi:10.1073/pnas.212498399

Cadot, B., Gache, V., Vasyutina, E., Falcone, S., Birchmeier, C., and Gomes, E. R. (2012). Nuclear movement during myotube formation is microtubule and dynein dependent and is regulated by Cdc42, Par6 and Par3. *EMBO Rep.* 13, 741–749. doi:10.1038/embor.2012.89

Carmignac, V., Salih, M. A., Quijano-Roy, S., Marchand, S., Al Rayess, M. M., Mukhtar, M. M., et al. (2007). C-terminal titin deletions cause a novel early-onset myopathy with fatal cardiomyopathy. *Ann. Neurol.* 61, 340–351. doi:10.1002/ana.21089

Catteruccia, M., Fattori, F., Codemo, V., Ruggiero, L., Maggi, L., Tasca, G., et al. (2013). Centronuclear myopathy related to dynamin 2 mutations: clinical, morphological, muscle imaging and genetic features of an Italian cohort. *Neuromuscul. Disord.* 23, 229–238. doi:10.1016/j.nmd.2012.12.009

Cebollero, E., Van Der Vaart, A., Zhao, M., Rieter, E., Klionsky, D. J., Helms, J. B., et al. (2012). Phosphatidylinositol-3-phosphate clearance plays a key role in autophagosome completion. *Curr. Biol.* 22, 1545–1553. doi:10.1016/j.cub.2012.06.029

Ceyhan-Birsoy, O., Agrawal, P. B., Hidalgo, C., Schmitz-Abe, K., Dechene, E. T., Swanson, L. C., et al. (2013). Recessive truncating titin gene, TTN, mutations presenting as centronuclear myopathy. *Neurology* 81, 1205–1214. doi:10.1212/WNL.0b013e3182a6ca62

Charton, K., Daniele, N., Vihola, A., Roudaut, C., Gicquel, E., Monjaret, F., et al. (2010). Removal of the calpain 3 protease reverses the myopathology in a mouse model for titinopathies. *Hum. Mol. Genet.* 19, 4608–4624. doi:10.1093/hmg/ddq388

Chauveau, C., Bonnemann, C., Julien, C., Kho, A. L., Marks, H., Talim, B., et al. (2014a). Recessive TTN truncating mutations define novel forms of core myopathy with heart disease. *Hum. Mol. Genet.* 23, 980–991. doi:10.1093/hmg/ddt494

Chauveau, C., Rowell, J., and Ferreiro, A. (2014b). A rising titan: TTN review and mutation update. *Hum. Mutat.* 35, 1046–1059. doi:10.1002/humu.22611

Claeys, K. G., Maisonobe, T., Bohm, J., Laporte, J., Hezode, M., Romero, N. B., et al. (2010). Phenotype of a patient with recessive centronuclear myopathy and a novel BIN1 mutation. *Neurology* 74, 519–521. doi:10.1212/WNL.0b013e3181cef7f9

Clague, M. J., and Lorenzo, O. (2005). The myotubularin family of lipid phosphatases. *Traffic* 6, 1063–1069. doi:10.1111/j.1600-0854.2005.00338.x

Clarke, N. F., Waddell, L. B., Cooper, S. T., Perry, M., Smith, R. L., Kornberg, A. J., et al. (2010). Recessive mutations in RYR1 are a common cause of congenital fiber type disproportion. *Hum. Mutat.* 31, E1544–E1550. doi:10.1002/humu.21278

Cowling, B. S., Chevremont, T., Prokic, I., Kretz, C., Ferry, A., Coirault, C., et al. (2014). Reducing dynamin 2 expression rescues X-linked centronuclear myopathy. *J. Clin. Invest.* 124, 1350–1363. doi:10.1172/JCI71206

Cowling, B. S., Toussaint, A., Muller, J., and Laporte, J. (2012). Defective membrane remodeling in neuromuscular diseases: insights from animal models. *PLoS Genet.* 8:e1002595. doi:10.1371/journal.pgen.1002595

Cullup, T., Kho, A. L., Dionisi-Vici, C., Brandmeier, B., Smith, F., Urry, Z., et al. (2013). Recessive mutations in EPG5 cause Vici syndrome, a multisystem disorder with defective autophagy. *Nat. Genet.* 45, 83–87. doi:10.1038/ng.2497

Dang, H., Li, Z., Skolnik, E. Y., and Fares, H. (2004). Disease-related myotubularins function in endocytic traffic in *Caenorhabditis elegans*. *Mol. Biol. Cell* 15, 189–196. doi:10.1091/mbc.E03-08-0605

Dowling, J. J., Joubert, R., Low, S. E., Durban, A. N., Messaddeq, N., Li, X., et al. (2012). Myotubular myopathy and the neuromuscular junction: a novel therapeutic approach from mouse models. *Dis. Model Mech.* 5, 852–859. doi:10.1242/dmm.009746

Dowling, J. J., Low, S. E., Busta, A. S., and Feldman, E. L. (2010). Zebrafish MTMR14 is required for excitation-contraction coupling, developmental motor function and the regulation of autophagy. *Hum. Mol. Genet.* 19, 2668–2681. doi:10.1093/hmg/ddq153

Dowling, J. J., Vreede, A. P., Low, S. E., Gibbs, E. M., Kuwada, J. Y., Bonnemann, C. G., et al. (2009). Loss of myotubularin function results in T-tubule disorganization in zebrafish and human myotubular myopathy. *PLoS Genet.* 5:e1000372. doi:10.1371/journal.pgen.1000372

Durieux, A. C., Prudhon, B., Guicheney, P., and Bitoun, M. (2010a). Dynamin 2 and human diseases. *J. Mol. Med.* 88, 339–350. doi:10.1007/s00109-009-0587-4

Durieux, A. C., Vignaud, A., Prudhon, B., Viou, M. T., Beuvin, M., Vassilopoulos, S., et al. (2010b). A centronuclear myopathy-dynamin 2 mutation impairs skeletal muscle structure and function in mice. *Hum. Mol. Genet.* 19, 4820–4836. doi:10.1093/hmg/ddq413

Durieux, A. C., Vassilopoulos, S., Laine, J., Fraysse, B., Brinas, L., Prudhon, B., et al. (2012). A centronuclear myopathy – dynamin 2 mutation impairs autophagy in mice. *Traffic* 13, 869–879. doi:10.1111/j.1600-0854.2012.01348.x

East, D. A., and Campanella, M. (2013). Ca2+ in quality control: an unresolved riddle critical to autophagy and mitophagy. *Autophagy* 9, 1710–1719. doi:10.4161/auto.25367

Echaniz-Laguna, A., Nicot, A. S., Carre, S., Franques, J., Tranchant, C., Dondaine, N., et al. (2007). Subtle central and peripheral nervous system abnormalities in a family with centronuclear myopathy and a novel dynamin 2 gene mutation. *Neuromuscul. Disord.* 17, 955–959. doi:10.1016/j.nmd.2007.06.467

Fabrizi, G. M., Ferrarini, M., Cavallaro, T., Cabrini, I., Cerini, R., Bertolasi, L., et al. (2007). Two novel mutations in dynamin-2 cause axonal Charcot-Marie-Tooth disease. *Neurology* 69, 291–295. doi:10.1212/01.wnl.0000265820.51075.61

Falcone, S., Roman, W., Hnia, K., Gache, V., Didier, N., Laine, J., et al. (2014). N-WASP is required for Amphiphysin-2/BIN1-dependent nuclear positioning and triad organization in skeletal muscle and is involved in the pathophysiology of centronuclear myopathy. *EMBO Mol. Med.* 6, 1455–1475. doi:10.15252/emmm.201404436

Fetalvero, K. M., Yu, Y., Goetschkes, M., Liang, G., Valdez, R. A., Gould, T., et al. (2013). Defective autophagy and mTORC1 signaling in myotubularin null mice. *Mol. Cell. Biol.* 33, 98–110. doi:10.1128/MCB.01075-12

Fischer, D., Herasse, M., Bitoun, M., Barragan-Campos, H. M., Chiras, J., Laforet, P., et al. (2006). Characterization of the muscle involvement in dynamin 2-related centronuclear myopathy. *Brain* 129, 1463–1469. doi:10.1093/brain/awl071

Fukuzawa, A., Lange, S., Holt, M. R., Vihola, A., Carmignac, V., Ferreiro, A., et al. (2008). Interactions with titin and myomesin target obscurin and its small homologue, obscurin-like 1, to the sarcomeric M-band: implications for hereditary myopathies. *J. Cell. Sci.* 121, 1841–1851. doi:10.1242/jcs.028019

Funderburk, S. F., Wang, Q. J., and Yue, Z. (2010). The Beclin 1-VPS34 complex – at the crossroads of autophagy and beyond. *Trends Cell Biol.* 20, 355–362. doi:10.1016/j.tcb.2010.03.002

Gautel, M. (2011). Cytoskeletal protein kinases: titin and its relations in mechanosensing. *Pflugers Arch.* 462, 119–134. doi:10.1007/s00424-011-0946-1

Ge, L., Baskaran, S., Schekman, R., and Hurley, J. H. (2014). The protein-vesicle network of autophagy. *Curr. Opin. Cell Biol.* 29C, 18–24. doi:10.1016/j.ceb.2014.02.005

Ghislat, G., and Knecht, E. (2012). New Ca(2+)-dependent regulators of autophagosome maturation. *Commun. Integr. Biol.* 5, 308–311. doi:10.4161/cib.20076

Gibbs, E. M., Clarke, N. F., Rose, K., Oates, E. C., Webster, R., Feldman, E. L., et al. (2013). Neuromuscular junction abnormalities in DNM2-related centronuclear myopathy. *J. Mol. Med.* 91, 727–737. doi:10.1007/s00109-013-0994-4

Gu, C., Yaddanapudi, S., Weins, A., Osborn, T., Reiser, J., Pollak, M., et al. (2010). Direct dynamin-actin interactions regulate the actin cytoskeleton. *EMBO J.* 29, 3593–3606. doi:10.1038/emboj.2010.249

Hanisch, F., Muller, T., Dietz, A., Bitoun, M., Kress, W., Weis, J., et al. (2011). Phenotype variability and histopathological findings in centronuclear myopathy due to DNM2 mutations. *J. Neurol.* 258, 1085–1090. doi:10.1007/s00415-010-5889-5

Herman, D. S., Lam, L., Taylor, M. R., Wang, L., Teekakirikul, P., Christodoulou, D., et al. (2012). Truncations of titin causing dilated cardiomyopathy. *N. Engl. J. Med.* 366, 619–628. doi:10.1056/NEJMoa1110186

Herman, G. E., Finegold, M., Zhao, W., De Gouyon, B., and Metzenberg, A. (1999). Medical complications in long-term survivors with X-linked myotubular myopathy. *J. Pediatr.* 134, 206–214. doi:10.1016/S0022-3476(99)70417-8

Herman, G. E., Kopacz, K., Zhao, W., Mills, P. L., Metzenberg, A., and Das, S. (2002). Characterization of mutations in fifty North American patients with X-linked myotubular myopathy. *Hum. Mutat.* 19, 114–121. doi:10.1002/humu.10033

Hnia, K., Tronchere, H., Tomczak, K. K., Amoasii, L., Schultz, P., Beggs, A. H., et al. (2011). Myotubularin controls desmin intermediate filament architecture and mitochondrial dynamics in human and mouse skeletal muscle. *J. Clin. Invest.* 121, 70–85. doi:10.1172/JCI44021

Hong, T., Yang, H., Zhang, S. S., Cho, H. C., Kalashnikova, M., Sun, B., et al. (2014). Cardiac BIN1 folds T-tubule membrane, controlling ion flux and limiting arrhythmia. *Nat. Med.* 20, 624–632. doi:10.1038/nm.3543

Jeub, M., Bitoun, M., Guicheney, P., Kappes-Horn, K., Strach, K., Druschky, K. F., et al. (2008). Dynamin 2-related centronuclear myopathy: clinical, histological and genetic aspects of further patients and review of the literature. *Clin. Neuropathol.* 27, 430–438. doi:10.5414/NPP27430

Jones, S. M., Howell, K. E., Henley, J. R., Cao, H., and McNiven, M. A. (1998). Role of dynamin in the formation of transport vesicles from the trans-Golgi network. *Science* 279, 573–577. doi:10.1126/science.279.5350.573

Joseph, M., Pai, G. S., Holden, K. R., and Herman, G. (1995). X-linked myotubular myopathy: clinical observations in ten additional cases. *Am. J. Med. Genet.* 59, 168–173. doi:10.1002/ajmg.1320590211

Jungbluth, H., Cullup, T., Lillis, S., Zhou, H., Abbs, S., Sewry, C., et al. (2010). Centronuclear myopathy with cataracts due to a novel dynamin 2 (DNM2) mutation. *Neuromuscul. Disord.* 20, 49–52. doi:10.1016/j.nmd.2009.10.005

Jungbluth, H., Sewry, C. A., Buj-Bello, A., Kristiansen, M., Orstavik, K. H., Kelsey, A., et al. (2003). Early and severe presentation of X-linked myotubular myopathy in a girl with skewed X-inactivation. *Neuromuscul. Disord.* 13, 55–59. doi:10.1016/S0960-8966(02)00194-3

Jungbluth, H., Sewry, C. A., and Muntoni, F. (2011). Core myopathies. *Semin. Pediatr. Neurol.* 18, 239–249. doi:10.1016/j.spen.2011.10.005

Jungbluth, H., Wallgren-Pettersson, C., and Laporte, J. (2008). Centronuclear (myotubular) myopathy. *Orphanet J. Rare Dis.* 3, 26. doi:10.1186/1750-1172-3-26

Jungbluth, H., Zhou, H., Sewry, C. A., Robb, S., Treves, S., Bitoun, M., et al. (2007). Centronuclear myopathy due to a de novo dominant mutation in the skeletal muscle ryanodine receptor (RYR1) gene. *Neuromuscul. Disord.* 17, 338–345. doi:10.1016/j.nmd.2007.01.016

Klein, A., Lillis, S., Munteanu, I., Scoto, M., Zhou, H., Quinlivan, R., et al. (2012). Clinical and genetic findings in a large cohort of patients with ryanodine receptor 1 gene-associated myopathies. *Hum. Mutat.* 33, 981–988. doi:10.1002/humu.22056

Klos Dehring, D. A., Vladar, E. K., Werner, M. E., Mitchell, J. W., Hwang, P., and Mitchell, B. J. (2013). Deuterosome-mediated centriole biogenesis. *Dev. Cell* 27, 103–112. doi:10.1016/j.devcel.2013.08.021

Kontrogianni-Konstantopoulos, A., Jones, E. M., Van Rossum, D. B., and Bloch, R. J. (2003). Obscurin is a ligand for small ankyrin 1 in skeletal muscle. *Mol. Biol. Cell* 14, 1138–1148. doi:10.1091/mbc.E02-07-0411

Koutsopoulos, O. S., Kretz, C., Weller, C. M., Roux, A., Mojzisova, H., Bohm, J., et al. (2013). Dynamin 2 homozygous mutation in humans with a lethal congenital syndrome. *Eur. J. Hum. Genet.* 21, 637–642. doi:10.1038/ejhg.2012.226

Lamb, C. A., Yoshimori, T., and Tooze, S. A. (2013). The autophagosome: origins unknown, biogenesis complex. *Nat. Rev. Mol. Cell Biol.* 14, 759–774. doi:10.1038/nrm3696

Lange, S., Ouyang, K., Meyer, G., Cui, L., Cheng, H., Lieber, R. L., et al. (2009). Obscurin determines the architecture of the longitudinal sarcoplasmic reticulum. *J. Cell. Sci.* 122, 2640–2650. doi:10.1242/jcs.046193

Laporte, J., Bedez, F., Bolino, A., and Mandel, J. L. (2003). Myotubularins, a large disease-associated family of cooperating catalytically active and inactive phosphoinositides phosphatases. *Hum. Mol. Genet.* 2, R285–R292. doi:10.1093/hmg/ddg273

Laporte, J., Biancalana, V., Tanner, S. M., Kress, W., Schneider, V., Wallgren-Pettersson, C., et al. (2000). MTM1 mutations in X-linked myotubular myopathy. *Hum. Mutat.* 15, 393–409. doi:10.1002/(SICI)1098-1004(200005)15:5<393::AID-HUMU1>3.0.CO;2-R

Laporte, J., Blondeau, F., Buj-Bello, A., and Mandel, J. L. (2001). The myotubularin family: from genetic disease to phosphoinositide metabolism. *Trends Genet.* 17, 221–228. doi:10.1016/S0168-9525(01)02245-4

Laporte, J., Blondeau, F., Buj-Bello, A., Tentler, D., Kretz, C., Dahl, N., et al. (1998). Characterization of the myotubularin dual specificity phosphatase gene family from yeast to human. *Hum. Mol. Genet.* 7, 1703–1712. doi:10.1093/hmg/7.11.1703

Laporte, J., Hu, L. J., Kretz, C., Mandel, J. L., Kioschis, P., Coy, J. F., et al. (1996). A gene mutated in X-linked myotubular myopathy defines a new putative tyrosine phosphatase family conserved in yeast. *Nat. Genet.* 13, 175–182. doi:10.1038/ng0696-175

Lawlor, M. W., Alexander, M. S., Viola, M. G., Meng, H., Joubert, R., Gupta, V., et al. (2012). Myotubularin-deficient myoblasts display increased apoptosis, delayed proliferation, and poor cell engraftment. *Am. J. Pathol.* 181, 961–968. doi:10.1016/j.ajpath.2012.05.016

Leguennec, J. C., Bernier, J. P., and Lamarche, J. (1988). High stature in neonatal myotubular myopathy. *Acta Paediatr. Scand.* 77, 610–611. doi:10.1111/j.1651-2227.1988.tb10714.x

Liewluck, T., Lovell, T. L., Bite, A. V., and Engel, A. G. (2010). Sporadic centronuclear myopathy with muscle pseudohypertrophy, neutropenia, and necklace fibers due to a DNM2 mutation. *Neuromuscul. Disord.* 20, 801–804. doi:10.1016/j.nmd.2010.07.273

Luxton, G. W., Gomes, E. R., Folker, E. S., Worman, H. J., and Gundersen, G. G. (2011). TAN lines: a novel nuclear envelope structure involved in nuclear positioning. *Nucleus* 2, 173–181. doi:10.1073/pnas.1000824108

Majczenko, K., Davidson, A. E., Camelo-Piragua, S., Agrawal, P. B., Manfready, R. A., Li, X., et al. (2012). Dominant mutation of CCDC78 in a unique congenital myopathy with prominent internal nuclei and atypical cores. *Am. J. Hum. Genet.* 91, 365–371. doi:10.1016/j.ajhg.2012.06.012

McClelland, V., Cullup, T., Bodi, I., Ruddy, D., Buj-Bello, A., Biancalana, V., et al. (2010). Vici syndrome associated with sensorineural hearing loss and evidence of neuromuscular involvement on muscle biopsy. *Am. J. Med. Genet. A* 152A, 741–747. doi:10.1002/ajmg.a.33296

McNiven, M. A. (2005). Dynamin in disease. *Nat. Genet.* 37, 215–216. doi:10.1038/ng0305-215

Meijer, A. J., and Klionsky, D. J. (2011). Vps34 is a phosphatidylinositol 3-kinase, not a phosphoinositide 3-kinase. *Autophagy* 7, 563–564. doi:10.4161/auto.7.6.14873

Merlini, L., and Nishino, I. (2014). 201st ENMC international workshop: autophagy in muscular dystrophies – translational approach, 1-3 November 2013, Bussum, The Netherlands. *Neuromuscul. Disord.* 24, 546–561. doi:10.1016/j.nmd.2014.03.009

Metzger, T., Gache, V., Xu, M., Cadot, B., Folker, E. S., Richardson, B. E., et al. (2012). MAP and kinesin-dependent nuclear positioning is required for skeletal muscle function. *Nature* 484, 120–124. doi:10.1038/nature10914

Mizushima, N. (2007). Autophagy: process and function. *Genes Dev.* 21, 2861–2873. doi:10.1101/gad.1599207

Muller, A. J., Baker, J. F., Duhadaway, J. B., Ge, K., Farmer, G., Donover, P. S., et al. (2003). Targeted disruption of the murine Bin1/Amphiphysin II gene does not disable endocytosis but results in embryonic cardiomyopathy with aberrant myofibril formation. *Mol. Cell. Biol.* 23, 4295–4306. doi:10.1128/MCB.23.12.4295-4306.2003

Neukomm, L. J., Nicot, A. S., Kinchen, J. M., Almendinger, J., Pinto, S. M., Zeng, S., et al. (2011). The phosphoinositide phosphatase MTM-1 regulates apoptotic cell corpse clearance through CED-5-CED-12 in *C. elegans*. *Development* 138, 2003–2014. doi:10.1242/dev.060012

Nicot, A. S., Toussaint, A., Tosch, V., Kretz, C., Wallgren-Pettersson, C., Iwarsson, E., et al. (2007). Mutations in amphiphysin 2 (BIN1) disrupt interaction with dynamin 2 and cause autosomal recessive centronuclear myopathy. *Nat. Genet.* 39, 1134–1139. doi:10.1038/ng2086

Osorio, D. S., and Gomes, E. R. (2014). Connecting the nucleus to the cytoskeleton for nuclear positioning and cell migration. *Adv. Exp. Med. Biol.* 773, 505–520. doi:10.1007/978-1-4899-8032-8_23

Parrish, W. R., Stefan, C. J., and Emr, S. D. (2004). Essential role for the myotubularin-related phosphatase Ymr1p and the synaptojanin-like phosphatases Sjl2p and Sjl3p in regulation of phosphatidylinositol 3-phosphate in yeast. *Mol. Biol. Cell* 15, 3567–3579. doi:10.1091/mbc.E04-03-0209

Peter, B. J., Kent, H. M., Mills, I. G., Vallis, Y., Butler, P. J., Evans, P. R., et al. (2004). BAR domains as sensors of membrane curvature: the amphiphysin BAR structure. *Science* 303, 495–499. doi:10.1126/science.1092586

Pierson, C. R., Dulin-Smith, A. N., Durban, A. N., Marshall, M. L., Marshall, J. T., Snyder, A. D., et al. (2012). Modeling the human MTM1 p.R69C mutation in murine Mtm1 results in exon 4 skipping and a less severe myotubular myopathy phenotype. *Hum. Mol. Genet.* 21, 811–825. doi:10.1093/hmg/ddr512

Pietri-Rouxel, F., Gentil, C., Vassilopoulos, S., Baas, D., Mouisel, E., Ferry, A., et al. (2010). DHPR alpha1S subunit controls skeletal muscle mass and morphogenesis. *EMBO J.* 29, 643–654. doi:10.1038/emboj.2009.366

Praefcke, G. J., and McMahon, H. T. (2004). The dynamin superfamily: universal membrane tubulation and fission molecules? *Nat. Rev. Mol. Cell Biol.* 5, 133–147. doi:10.1038/nrm1313

Prokic, I., Cowling, B. S., and Laporte, J. (2014). Amphiphysin 2 (BIN1) in physiology and diseases. *J. Mol. Med.* 92, 453–463. doi:10.1007/s00109-014-1138-1

Reifler, A., Li, X., Archambeau, A. J., McDade, J. R., Sabha, N., Michele, D. E., et al. (2014). Conditional knockout of pik3c3 causes a murine muscular dystrophy. *Am. J. Pathol.* 184, 1819–1830. doi:10.1016/j.ajpath.2014.02.012

Robb, S. A., Sewry, C. A., Dowling, J. J., Feng, L., Cullup, T., Lillis, S., et al. (2011). Impaired neuromuscular transmission and response to acetylcholinesterase inhibitors in centronuclear myopathies. *Neuromuscul. Disord.* 21, 379–386. doi:10.1016/j.nmd.2011.02.012

Robinson, F. L., and Dixon, J. E. (2006). Myotubularin phosphatases: policing 3-phosphoinositides. *Trends Cell Biol.* 16, 403–412. doi:10.1016/j.tcb.2006.06.001

Rohde, H. M., Tronchere, H., Payrastre, B., and Laporte, J. (2009). Detection of myotubularin phosphatases activity on phosphoinositides in vitro and ex vivo. *Methods Mol. Biol.* 462, 265–278. doi:10.1007/978-1-60327-115-8_18

Romero, N. B. (2010). Centronuclear myopathies: a widening concept. *Neuromuscul. Disord.* 20, 223–228. doi:10.1016/j.nmd.2010.01.014

Romero, N. B., and Bitoun, M. (2011). Centronuclear myopathies. *Semin. Pediatr. Neurol.* 18, 250–256. doi:10.1016/j.spen.2011.10.006

Sandri, M. (2013). Protein breakdown in muscle wasting: role of autophagy-lysosome and ubiquitin-proteasome. *Int. J. Biochem. Cell Biol.* 45, 2121–2129. doi:10.1016/j.biocel.2013.04.023

Sandri, M., Coletto, L., Grumati, P., and Bonaldo, P. (2013). Misregulation of autophagy and protein degradation systems in myopathies and muscular dystrophies. *J. Cell. Sci.* 126, 5325–5333. doi:10.1242/jcs.114041

Schessl, J., Medne, L., Hu, Y., Zou, Y., Brown, M. J., Huse, J. T., et al. (2007). MRI in DNM2-related centronuclear myopathy: evidence for highly selective muscle involvement. *Neuromuscul. Disord.* 17, 28–32. doi:10.1016/j.nmd.2006.09.013

Smith, L. L., Gupta, V. A., and Beggs, A. H. (2014). Bridging integrator 1 (Bin1) deficiency in zebrafish results in centronuclear myopathy. *Hum. Mol. Genet.* 23, 3566–3578. doi:10.1093/hmg/ddu067

Taylor, G. S., Maehama, T., and Dixon, J. E. (2000). Myotubularin, a protein tyrosine phosphatase mutated in myotubular myopathy, dephosphorylates the lipid second messenger, phosphatidylinositol 3-phosphate. *Proc. Natl. Acad. Sci. U. S. A.* 97, 8910–8915. doi:10.1073/pnas.160255697

Thompson, H. M., Cao, H., Chen, J., Euteneuer, U., and McNiven, M. A. (2004). Dynamin 2 binds gamma-tubulin and participates in centrosome cohesion. *Nat. Cell Biol.* 6, 335–342. doi:10.1038/ncb1112

Tosch, V., Rohde, H. M., Tronchere, H., Zanoteli, E., Monroy, N., Kretz, C., et al. (2006). A novel PtdIns3P and PtdIns(3,5)P2 phosphatase with an inactivating variant in centronuclear myopathy. *Hum. Mol. Genet.* 15, 3098–3106. doi:10.1093/hmg/ddl250

Toussaint, A., Cowling, B. S., Hnia, K., Mohr, M., Oldfors, A., Schwab, Y., et al. (2011). Defects in amphiphysin 2 (BIN1) and triads in several forms of centronuclear myopathies. *Acta Neuropathol.* 121, 253–266. doi:10.1007/s00401-010-0754-2

Treves, S., Anderson, A. A., Ducreux, S., Divet, A., Bleunven, C., Grasso, C., et al. (2005). Ryanodine receptor 1 mutations, dysregulation of calcium homeostasis and neuromuscular disorders. *Neuromuscul. Disord.* 15, 577–587. doi:10.1016/j.nmd.2005.06.008

Tronchere, H., Buj-Bello, A., Mandel, J. L., and Payrastre, B. (2003). Implication of phosphoinositide phosphatases in genetic diseases: the case of myotubularin. *Cell. Mol. Life Sci.* 60, 2084–2099. doi:10.1007/s00018-003-3062-3

Tronchere, H., Laporte, J., Pendaries, C., Chaussade, C., Liaubet, L., Pirola, L., et al. (2004). Production of phosphatidylinositol 5-phosphate by the phosphoinositide 3-phosphatase myotubularin in mammalian cells. *J. Biol. Chem.* 279, 7304–7312. doi:10.1074/jbc.M311071200

Trump, N., Cullup, T., Verheij, J. B., Manzur, A., Muntoni, F., Abbs, S., et al. (2011). X-linked myotubular myopathy due to a complex rearrangement involving a duplication of MTM1 exon 10. *Neuromuscul. Disord.* 22, 384–388. doi:10.1016/j.nmd.2011.11.004

Tsai, T. C., Horinouchi, H., Noguchi, S., Minami, N., Murayama, K., Hayashi, Y. K., et al. (2005). Characterization of MTM1 mutations in 31 Japanese families with myotubular myopathy, including a patient carrying 240 kb deletion in Xq28 without male hypogenitalism. *Neuromuscul. Disord.* 15, 245–252. doi:10.1016/j.nmd.2004.12.005

Udd, B. (2012). Distal myopathies – new genetic entities expand diagnostic challenge. *Neuromuscul. Disord.* 22, 5–12. doi:10.1016/j.nmd.2011.10.003

Velichkova, M., Juan, J., Kadandale, P., Jean, S., Ribeiro, I., Raman, V., et al. (2010). Drosophila Mtm and class II PI3K coregulate a PI(3)P pool with cortical and endolysosomal functions. *J. Cell Biol.* 190, 407–425. doi:10.1083/jcb.200911020

Vergne, I., and Deretic, V. (2010). The role of PI3P phosphatases in the regulation of autophagy. *FEBS Lett.* 584, 1313–1318. doi:10.1016/j.febslet.2010.02.054

Wang, X., and Robbins, J. (2013). Proteasomal and lysosomal protein degradation and heart disease. *J. Mol. Cell. Cardiol.* 71, 16–24. doi:10.1016/j.yjmcc.2013.11.006

Wilmshurst, J. M., Lillis, S., Zhou, H., Pillay, K., Henderson, H., Kress, W., et al. (2010). RYR1 mutations are a common cause of congenital myopathies with central nuclei. *Ann. Neurol.* 68, 717–726. doi:10.1002/ana.22119

Wu, T., Shi, Z., and Baumgart, T. (2014). Mutations in BIN1 associated with centronuclear myopathy disrupt membrane remodeling by affecting protein density and oligomerization. *PLoS ONE* 9:e93060. doi:10.1371/journal.pone.0093060

Yu, S., Manson, J., White, S., Bourne, A., Waddy, H., Davis, M., et al. (2003). X-linked myotubular myopathy in a family with three adult survivors. *Clin. Genet.* 64, 148–152. doi:10.1034/j.1399-0004.2003.00118.x

Zhou, H., Rokach, O., Feng, L., Munteanu, I., Mamchaoui, K., Wilmshurst, J. M., et al. (2013). RyR1 deficiency in congenital myopathies disrupts excitation-contraction coupling. *Hum. Mutat.* 34, 986–996. doi:10.1002/humu.22326

Zhuang, X., Wang, H., Lam, S. K., Gao, C., Wang, X., Cai, Y., et al. (2013). A BAR-domain protein SH3P2, which binds to phosphatidylinositol 3-phosphate and ATG8, regulates autophagosome formation in Arabidopsis. *Plant Cell* 25, 4596–4615. doi:10.1105/tpc.113.118307

Zou, W., Lu, Q., Zhao, D., Li, W., Mapes, J., Xie, Y., et al. (2009). *Caenorhabditis elegans* myotubularin MTM-1 negatively regulates the engulfment of apoptotic cells. *PLoS Genet.* 5:e1000679. doi:10.1371/journal.pgen.1000679

Zuchner, S., Noureddine, M., Kennerson, M., Verhoeven, K., Claeys, K., De Jonghe, P., et al. (2005). Mutations in the pleckstrin homology domain of dynamin 2 cause dominant intermediate Charcot-Marie-Tooth disease. *Nat. Genet.* 37, 289–294. doi:10.1038/ng1514

18

Pompe disease: from pathophysiology to therapy and back again

***Jeong-A Lim*[†]*, Lishu Li*[†] *and Nina Raben* ***

Laboratory of Muscle Stem Cells and Gene Regulation, National Institute of Arthritis and Musculoskeletal and Skin Diseases (NIAMS), National Institutes of Health, Bethesda, MD, USA

Correspondence:
Nina Raben, Laboratory of Muscle Stem Cells and Gene Regulation, National Institute of Arthritis and Musculoskeletal and Skin Diseases (NIAMS), National Institutes of Health, 50 South Drive, Bld. 50/Room 1345, Bethesda, MD 20892, USA
e-mail: rabenn@mail.nih.gov

[†] These authors have contributed equally to this work.

Pompe disease is a lysosomal storage disorder in which acid alpha-glucosidase (GAA) is deficient or absent. Deficiency of this lysosomal enzyme results in progressive expansion of glycogen-filled lysosomes in multiple tissues, with cardiac and skeletal muscle being the most severely affected. The clinical spectrum ranges from fatal hypertrophic cardiomyopathy and skeletal muscle myopathy in infants to relatively attenuated forms, which manifest as a progressive myopathy without cardiac involvement. The currently available enzyme replacement therapy (ERT) proved to be successful in reversing cardiac but not skeletal muscle abnormalities. Although the overall understanding of the disease has progressed, the pathophysiology of muscle damage remains poorly understood. Lysosomal enlargement/rupture has long been considered a mechanism of relentless muscle damage in Pompe disease. In past years, it became clear that this simple view of the pathology is inadequate; the pathological cascade involves dysfunctional autophagy, a major lysosome-dependent intracellular degradative pathway. The autophagic process in Pompe skeletal muscle is affected at the termination stage—impaired autophagosomal-lysosomal fusion. Yet another abnormality in the diseased muscle is the accelerated production of large, unrelated to ageing, lipofuscin deposits—a marker of cellular oxidative damage and a sign of mitochondrial dysfunction. The massive autophagic buildup and lipofuscin inclusions appear to cause a greater effect on muscle architecture than the enlarged lysosomes outside the autophagic regions. Furthermore, the dysfunctional autophagy affects the trafficking of the replacement enzyme and interferes with its delivery to the lysosomes. Several new therapeutic approaches have been tested in Pompe mouse models: substrate reduction therapy, lysosomal exocytosis following the overexpression of transcription factor EB and a closely related but distinct factor E3, and genetic manipulation of autophagy.

Keywords: autophagy, lysosome, Pompe disease, lipofuscin, enzyme replacement therapy

BACKGROUND AND HISTORY

Pompe disease, also known as glycogen storage disease type II (GSDII) or "acid maltase deficiency", is caused by the absence or deficiency of acid alpha-glucosidase (GAA), a lysosomal enzyme that is responsible for the cleavage of the α-1,4- and α-1,6-glycosidic bonds of glycogen to glucose. The deficiency of the enzyme leads to the accumulation of glycogen in the lysosomes in numerous tissues, but clinical symptoms are primarily due to cardiac and skeletal muscles involvement. The disease is characterized by a wide variety of manifestations ranging from severe infantile-onset muscle weakness, hypotonia, and hypertrophic cardiomyopathy to a relatively mild slowly progressive skeletal muscle myopathy in adults (Hirschhorn and Reuser, 2001). Pompe disease is a rare disorder with an estimated frequency of 1:40,000 (Martiniuk et al., 1998; Ausems et al., 1999). The neonatal screening program for lysosomal storage diseases (LSDs) in Taiwan and Austria using dried blood spots revealed a higher than expected frequency of the disease in these populations (Chien et al., 2008; Mechtler et al., 2012).

In 1932, Johannes Cassianus Pompe, a Dutch pathologist, described the disease in a 7-month-old infant who died of idiopathic hypertrophy of the heart; in addition to the cardiac problems, the infant had generalized muscle weakness. Dr. Pompe made the crucial observation that the baby's symptoms were associated with massive "vacuolar" glycogen storage in virtually all tissues; reports of similar cases appeared in literature the same year (Bischoff, 1932; Putschar, 1932) as well as in the following years. In 1954 the disease was classified as glycogen storage disease type II to reflect the abnormal metabolism of glycogen (Cori, 1954). However, at that time, the cause of the disease, the "vacuolar" nature of the storage, and the apparent normal molecular structure of the accumulated glycogen all remained a mystery. The connection between lysosomes, the enzyme defect, and Pompe disease was made much later, in 1963, by a Belgian biochemist Henri-Gery Hers. He discovered a new enzyme (maltase) that carried out the hydrolysis of glycogen to glucose at an acidic pH, and he demonstrated that the enzyme was absent in patients with Pompe disease (Hers, 1963). By a fortunate coincidence, Dr. Hers had been previously working in the laboratory of Christian de Duve, who in 1955 postulated the existence of a new group of intracellular organelles, lysosomes. Dr. Hers realized that his new enzyme resides in the lysosomes, and that this is the only glycogen-degrading enzyme present in the lysosomes. Based on this research, the concept of LSDs has been established, and the search for other missing lysosomal enzymes began. Pompe disease became the first in a diverse group of more than 50 currently recognized lysosomal storage disorders. The cause of Pompe disease became known 30 years after its initial description, and it would take even longer to develop the first therapy.

GENETIC DEFECTS AND CLINICAL MANIFESTATIONS

Pompe disease comes at different ages and with different degrees of severity. The severity of the clinical presentations, the tissue involvement, and the age of onset generally correlate well with the nature of the mutation and the degree of residual enzyme activity. A database containing all the reported mutations and polymorphisms of the *GAA* gene on chromosome 17 q25 (Hoefsloot et al., 1988, 1990; Martiniuk et al., 1990; Kuo et al., 1996) (>300 variants) may be accessed at http://www.pompecenter.nl. The majority of mutations are private—found only in a single family or a small population—and most patients are compound heterozygotes. The mutations are spread throughout the gene and affect one of the multiple steps involved in synthesis, post-translational modifications, lysosomal trafficking, and proteolytic processing of GAA (see below).

The most common mutation among Caucasian children and adults is c.-32-13T>G (IVS1), a splicing defect which allows for the synthesis of low levels (~10–20%) of normal enzyme (Huie et al., 1994; Boerkoel et al., 1995; Raben et al., 1996). A study of a large cohort of patients with a similar genotype—IVS1 in combination with a second null mutation—unexpectedly showed a significant variability in the age at disease onset, suggesting the role of secondary modifying factors on the clinical course (Kroos et al., 2012). One of the possible factors responsible for the wide clinical variability has recently come to light: the deletion/deletion polymorphism in the gene coding for the angiotensin-converting enzyme (ACE), which is known to increase the number of type II fibers and influence muscle properties, is associated with earlier onset, higher creatine kinase (CK) levels, muscle pain, and more severe progression of the disease in patients with adult form (de Filippi et al., 2010).

Two mutations—c.del525T and exon18 deletion—are frequent in the Netherlands (Hermans et al., 1994; Hirschhorn and Huie, 1999), and a common defect, c.1935C>A (p.Asp645Glu), is shared by Chinese patients in Taiwan (Shieh and Lin, 1998). The most common mutation in African-Americans, c.2560C>T (p.Arg854Ter), most likely originated in their ancestral population from north-central Africa and was brought to the Americas during the slave trade (Becker et al., 1998).

The most severe end of the phenotypic continuum is the disease in which symptoms begin within the first months of life, and include profound muscle weakness, hypotonia ("floppy baby"), and hypertrophic cardiomyopathy. Massive cardiomegaly, which is easily detectable by chest X-rays, is one of the leading manifestations of the disease in infants. The weakness of respiratory muscle and cardiomegaly often lead to diminished ventilation and frequent infections. Macroglossia, mild hepatomegaly, feeding difficulties, and significantly delayed motor milestones are also typical manifestations of this rapidly progressive form; most patients do not survive beyond the first year of life and die from cardiac failure. This severe subtype, described by Dr. Pompe, is called the classic infantile form, and is caused by complete or near complete loss of GAA activity (van den Hout et al., 2003; Kishnani et al., 2006). Similar clinical presentations in infants with less severe cardiomyopathy, absence of left ventricular outflow obstruction, and somewhat longer survival have been classified as a non-classical infantile form (Slonim et al., 2000).

Partial loss of enzyme activity (residual enzyme activity between 1 and 30%) manifests as progressive muscle dysfunction and respiratory insufficiency without cardiac involvement. A spectrum of phenotypic variation and genotypic heterogeneity is characteristic of this less dismal form of the disease. The lower limbs and paraspinal muscles are frequently affected first, followed by the respiratory muscle, particularly the diaphragm, intercostal, and accessory muscles. As the disease progresses, patients may develop severe scoliosis and lumbar hyperlordosis and many become wheelchair dependent and require assisted ventilation. Respiratory failure is the main cause of increased morbidity and mortality (Herzog et al., 2012; Schuller et al., 2012). Although skeletal muscle weakness dominates the clinical picture, there is increasing evidence of the involvement of non-muscle tissues in this group of patients (Filosto et al., 2013).

A variety of scientific terms are used in literature to describe these different forms of the disease, such as typical and atypical infantile, non-infantile, muscular, childhood-, juvenile-, and adult-onset, etc.; the broad term, late-onset Pompe disease (LOPD), is often used to describe patients with muscle weakness without cardiac involvement and the onset of symptoms after 12 months of age. However, the continuum of phenotypes often defies categorization. Recently, the Pompe community accepted the following proposed nomenclature: (1) "classic infantile", as described above; (2) "childhood" form with onset of symptoms from birth till adolescence without persisting and progressive cardiac hypertrophy; and (3) "adult" form with onset of symptoms from adolescence to late adulthood (Güngör and Reuser, 2013).

ACID ALPHA-GLUCOSIDASE AND ENZYME REPLACEMENT THERAPY (ERT)

Like many other lysosomal enzymes, GAA is synthesized in the rough endoplasmic reticulum (ER), where high mannose oligosaccharides are added to the 110 kDa precursor molecules, a process known as glycosylation (Hermans et al., 1993). The glycosylation and proper folding in the ER are essential for the trafficking of the enzyme through the Golgi complex to the lysosomes. On the way to the lysosomes, the protein undergoes sugar chain modifications and proteolytic cleavage (Wisselaar et al., 1993). In the Golgi, the addition of the mannose-6-phosphate (M6P) moiety (phosphorylation) allows for the recognition of the enzyme by (M6P) receptors, which transport the enzyme to early and late endosomes. The Golgi is also a site for the first proteolytic cleavage of the precursor followed by the additional cleavage at both the amino- and carboxyl-terminal ends before and after entry to the lysosomes (Wisselaar et al., 1993; Moreland et al., 2005). The posttranslational modifications of the precursor protein, a process called maturation, increase its activity of the enzyme for glycogen (Wisselaar et al., 1993). GAA along with other lysosomal enzymes leaves the Golgi complex in a vesicle which delivers its content to early/late endosomes and lysosomes. Once inside the late endosomes, the receptor-ligand complexes dissociate due to the low pH in these vesicles, and the enzyme is delivered to the lysosome, whereas the receptors recycle back for the next round of sorting (Kornfeld, 1992). A portion of the GAA precursor is secreted, and can be taken up by neighboring cells via cation independent mannose 6-phosphate receptor (CI-MPR) on the plasma membrane, which directs the endocytosis and transport of the enzyme to the lysosome. The ability of cells to secrete and internalize lysosomal enzymes, first demonstrated in cross-correction experiments, in which normal cells rescued the nearby deficient cells (Neufeld and Fratantoni, 1970), became the fundamental basis of enzyme replacement therapy (ERT) for lysosomal storage diseases, including Pompe disease.

In Pompe disease, the CHO-produced recombinant human GAA (rhGAA; alglucosidase alpha, Myozyme®, Genzyme Corporation, Framingham, MA) is a 110 kDa precursor containing M6P groups that enable the enzyme to bind the receptor on the cell surface. Once inside the cell, the rhGAA, like the endogenous precursor, is cleaved to yield intermediate and fully mature 76 and 70 kDa lysosomal forms. In 2006 the drug received broad-label marketing approval in Europe, and later in the U.S. This is the first therapy for GSDII, and the first attempt to direct recombinant enzyme to skeletal muscle. This therapy is based on a straightforward hypothesis to explain the disease pathogenesis, namely that the progressive enlargement of glycogen-filled lysosomes, lysosomal rupture (due to mechanical pressure in muscle fibers), and release of glycogen and toxic substances into the cytosol would ultimately result in organ dysfunctions (Griffin, 1984a; Thurberg et al., 2006). The stages and progression of skeletal muscle damage have been described for the classical infantile form: small glycogen-filled lysosomes in between intact myofibrils are typical for stage 1; an increase in cytoplasmic glycogen and the size and number of lysosomes combined with fragmentation of myofibrils constitute stage 2; after that, glycogen-filled lysosomes are tightly packed, some show membrane rupture, and only few myofibril fragments remain in stage 3; finally, in stages 4 and 5, most glycogen is cytoplasmic, the contractile elements of muscle cells are completely lost, and the cells bloat due to the influx of water (Thurberg et al., 2006).

The assumption was that early treatment, initiated before lysosomal integrity was compromised, would reverse this pathogenic cascade and cure the disease. The outcome, however, was somewhat unexpected—cardiac muscle responded remarkably well to therapy, but skeletal muscle did not. Even with extremely high dosages of the drug (20–40 mg/kg body weight, which is significantly higher than in other LSDs), patients with the childhood and adult forms of the disease experience limited clinical benefit, such as modest improvements in walking distance and respiratory function, but skeletal muscle weakness often persists, and some show signs of disease progression (Van den Hout et al., 2004; Kishnani et al., 2007; Schoser et al., 2008; Strothotte et al., 2010; Van der Ploeg et al., 2010; Angelini and Semplicini, 2012).

The reversal of cardiac abnormalities dramatically changed the natural course of the disease in infants; most survive significantly longer compared with untreated group analyzed by retrospective studies (Kishnani et al., 2007; Nicolino et al., 2009). However, the great success of ERT in Pompe disease comes with unintended consequences: many long-term survivors suffer from debilitating skeletal muscle myopathy and develop new previously unrecognized symptoms such as ptosis, hypernasal speech, osteopenia, hearing loss and gastroesophageal reflux. Although the response to therapy varies significantly in this group of patients, an emerging pattern—initial improvement followed by a decline and chronic disability—indicates that even at a very high doses, the drug does not halt the progression of the disease (Chakrapani et al., 2010; Prater et al., 2012, 2013).

One thing appears to be clear: treatment of the infants should start within days after birth, not months (Chien et al., 2009, 2013; Prater et al., 2013). The effect of therapy in pre-symptomatic infants who were diagnosed through a newborn screening program (in Taiwan) was better than in those who were diagnosed later based on clinical symptoms (Chien et al., 2009). It is also clear that sustained high antibody titers on ERT, particularly in infants with cross-reactive immunological material (CRIM)-negative status, are associated with poor outcome (Banugaria et al., 2011).

The neonatal screening program, which allows for the early diagnosis and timely initiation of therapy in infants, would also identify patients with mutations that are associated with onset of symptoms in the second, fourth or six decade of life. The appropriate age for the initiation of therapy in patients with milder forms of the disease is not clear, thus adding to the complexity of ethical issues related to such a program. The argument in favor of such a program for Pompe disease comes from our own experience (however limited), which indicates that the best morphological results are achieved when the therapy is initiated in asymptomatic patients. A case in point is a normal muscle biopsy after only 6 months of therapy, in an infant who was diagnosed through the newborn screening program, but whose genetic makeup was consistent with the childhood form of the disease; the baseline biopsy of this asymptomatic patient with slightly elevated CK level showed well-preserved fibers with minimally enlarged lysosomes and no autophagic buildup (Raben et al., 2010a).

The limitations of current therapy stimulated research on more effective second-generation drugs. The evolving new therapies are designed to improve the delivery of the recombinant enzyme to skeletal muscle. The poor capacity of the current drug to reach skeletal muscle (most of the administered enzyme is taken by liver) has been attributed to the low number of M6P receptors on the plasma membrane of skeletal muscle cells. Therefore, the development of chemically modified recombinant human GAA with high affinity for the receptor and enhanced targeting properties is currently being pursued by academic institutions and pharmaceutical companies (Zhu et al., 2009; Tiels et al., 2012; Maga et al., 2013). Albuterol, a drug that enhances the M6P receptor expression, is also in clinical trial in combination with ERT (Koeberl et al., 2014). Another therapeutic approach includes the use of pharmacological chaperones to increase the stability and half-life of the current drug (Porto et al., 2009, 2012). It is, however, unclear how much enzyme is needed to reverse the established pathology in Pompe skeletal muscle, and this uncertainty remains a concern with these new approaches. It is widely believed that the levels of ~30% of average normal activity would be sufficient, since the disease manifests when the acid α-glucosidase activity drops below this critical threshold. However, our data in transgenic mice expressing human GAA in skeletal muscle of the GAA knockout mice (see Models of Pompe disease) suggest that much higher levels might be needed for the reversal of the advanced disease (Raben et al., 2005). The benefits of these new strategies for enzyme delivery are beyond the scope of this review.

GENE THERAPY

A major development in the field is the commencement of the first phase I/II clinical trial of rAAV1-hGAA intramuscular gene transfer. Five children with chronic ventilator dependence (full-time mechanical ventilation despite ERT) and severe phrenic neuromuscular dysfunction were enrolled in the trial. All patients were on ERT, which was continued throughout the study. The outcome of the 180-day safety and ventilatory outcomes following intradiaphragmatic delivery of AAV-mediated *GAA* gene therapy has been reported (Smith et al., 2013). The results indicated that rAAV1-hGAA was safe and led to a modest improvement in ventilatory function. This trial is the first critical step in the development of a successful AAV-based gene therapy for Pompe disease. Extensive preclinical studies (both *in vitro* and *in vivo* in the mouse model) by a number of groups established the basis and feasibility of gene therapy for this disorder; the reader is referred to a review on this subject (Byrne et al., 2011). Here, we will focus on the pathogenesis of skeletal muscle damage in Pompe disease, which turned out to be more complex than previously thought, and involves a profound disturbance of autophagy.

MODELS OF POMPE DISEASE

Naturally occurring animal models of Pompe disease include cattle, dogs, cats, sheep, and Japanese quails. The underlying genetic defects have been identified in Brahman and Shorthorn cattle breeds in Australia, in quails (AMD quails), and Finnish and Swedish Lapphunds. Curiously, the two Scandinavian dog breeds, which share a common origin and physical appearance, have been recently shown (Seppala et al., 2013) to contain a frameshift mutation similar to that found in patients with the infantile form of the disease (the finding points to a "hot spot" in the *GAA* gene). The presence of residual GAA activity in quails (due to the expression of other alpha-glucosidases) accounts for the milder form of the disease, which mimics human childhood or adult forms without cardiac dysfunction; the birds show progressive muscle weakness, difficulty in lifting their wings or turning from the supine position. With the development of the knockout mouse models, the usefulness of this model became outdated, but AMD quails deserve a special mention because they were the first to be used for testing ERT (Kikuchi et al., 1998).

Genotypically and phenotypically more accurate models were made in mice by targeted disruption of exon 6 and exon 13 of the *GAA* gene [GAA-KO (Raben et al., 1998) and AGLU-/- (Bijvoet et al., 1998)]. These two models have features of both infantile and adult forms: the animals develop cardiomegaly, cardiomyopathy (Bijvoet et al., 1998) and skeletal muscle myopathy, but obvious clinical signs of the disease, such as kyphosis and muscle wasting manifest late relative to their lifespan—at ~7–9 months. Both strains are widely used for testing different therapeutic approaches. Several transgenic lines and double knockouts on the GAA-KO background are available: GFP- LC3:GAA-KO, in which autophagosomes are labeled with green fluorescent protein; GAA-KO:SCID, which do not produce antibody following administration of recombinant human GAA (Xu et al., 2004); and muscle-specific autophagy-deficient GAA-KO, which will be discussed below.

In addition, GAA-KO crosses to H-$2K^b$-tsA58 transgenic mice (also called Immortomouse; Charles River Laboratories) allowed for the generation of an *in vitro* model of Pompe disease—GAA-deficient immortalized mouse muscle cell lines. The transgene contains the temperature-sensitive immortalizing SV40 large T antigen tsA58 (tsA58 TAg) under the control of the interferon-inducible H-$2K^b$ promoter; the SV40 large T antigen is functional at permissive temperature (33°C plus interferon-γ), but is inactivated at 37° in the absence of interferon. The advantage of this system is that myoblasts derived from the GAA-KO: H-$2K^b$-tsA58 mice proliferate and undergo immortalization when the oncogene is expressed, but the differentiation of the cells to myotubes proceeds under "normal" condition when the oncogene is silenced (Jat et al., 1991). Unlike primary myoblasts with their limited proliferation capacity, the immortalized cells can undergo multiple passages without losing the ability to differentiate. The *in vitro* model replicates lysosomal, but not autophagic pathology (see below) (**Figure 1**; Spampanato et al., 2013), and as such can be used to decipher the early events which precede the development of autophagic buildup—a hallmark of the disease in Pompe muscle fibers.

PATHOGENESIS

AUTOPHAGY

At least three autophagic pathways have been described based on the route by which the cargo enters the lysosomes. Microautophagy is a direct engulfment of cytoplasmic components into the lysosomal lumen; in chaperone-mediated autophagy (CMA), a subset of soluble cytosolic proteins with a particular pentapeptide motif are recognized by molecular chaperones and directly translocated into lysosomes through a receptor (LAMP-2A) on the lysosomal membrane; the major third form, most relevant to Pompe disease, is macroautophagy, which fulfils the role of supplying amino acids and energy under starvation by "self-digestion" of intracellular components (Klionsky, 2007; He and Klionsky, 2009; Yang and Klionsky, 2010; Kaushik et al., 2011). Macroautophagy also operates at a low level under a nutrient-rich environment to rid the cells of misfolded proteins, protein

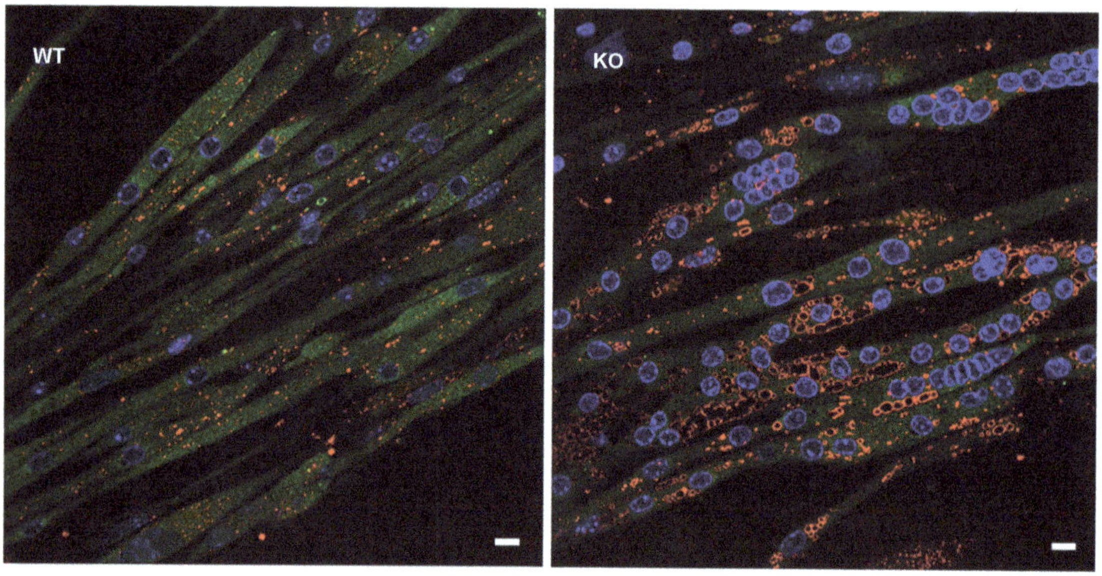

FIGURE 1 | *In vitro* model of Pompe disease replicates lysosomal, but not autophagic pathology. The images show wild type (**WT**) and GAA-KO (**KO**) myotubes. Immortalized myoblasts were used for the differentiation into multinucleated myotubes. WT myoblasts were derived from mice generated by crosses of GFP-LC3:WT to Immortomice; GAA-KO myoblasts were derived from mice generated by crosses of GFP-LC3:GAA-KO to Immortomice. LC3 (green) is a specific autophagosomal marker. No autophagosomal accumulation is seen in the GAA-KO cells. Myotubes were fixed and stained for lysosomal marker LAMP1 (red). Enlarged lysosomes are seen in the GAA-KO, but not in control WT muscle cells. Bars: 10 μm.

aggregates, and worn-out organelles such as mitochondria. Upon induction, the process of macroautophagy (often referred to simply as autophagy) begins with the development of a double membrane, which engulfs part of the cytoplasm, resulting in the formation of the double-membrane structure called autophagosome. Autophagosomes fuses with the lysosome, where the inner membrane and the content of the autophagosome are degraded and recycled. The two pathways, autophagic and endocytic, by which the recombinant human GAA traffics to the lysosomes are interconnected; autophagosomes can fuse with early/late endosomes before fusion with the lysosome, giving rise to an intermediate structure, called amphisome (Berg et al., 1998).

AUTOPHAGY IN POMPE MOUSE MODELS

The morphological evidence for abnormal autophagy in muscle biopsies from adult Pompe patients was first reported by Andrew Engel in 1970 (Engel, 1970), at the time when the field of autophagy was still in its infancy. Perhaps not surprisingly, this pathology and its contribution to the pathogenesis of Pompe disease have been largely ignored until recently. Studies in a GAA-KO model developed in our lab (Raben et al., 1998) clearly demonstrated that abnormalities in Pompe muscle cells were not limited to the enlargement of lysosomes. Analysis of myoblasts derived from GAA-KO mice showed an acidification defect in a subset of late endosomes/lysosomes, a dramatic expansion of all vesicles of the endocytic/autophagic pathways, and a slowdown in the vesicular trafficking in the overcrowded cells (Fukuda et al., 2006).

Electron microscopy (EM) of skeletal muscle from the KO mice revealed large areas of autophagic accumulation containing vesicular structures at different stages of a stalled autophagic process: small and large double-membrane autophagosomes with undigested cytosolic material or glycogen particles, multivesicular bodies, multimembrane structures, autofluorescent material, as well other cellular debris (**Figure 2**). EM established the presence of autophagic accumulation of Pompe muscle, but the extent of this pathology became clear when single muscle fibers were immunostained for lysosomal marker, LAMP1, and autophagosomal marker, LC3, followed by confocal microscopy—an approach best-suited for the detection of autophagic accumulation within the fibers (Raben et al., 2009). Two forms of LC3 are documented: the soluble cytosolic LC3I and lipidated LC3II; the latter remains on the autophagosomal membrane during autophagic process and serves as a highly specific marker of autophagosomes (Kabeya et al., 2000). LAMP1/LC3-double staining showed that the core of the fibers was filled with clusters of densely packed late endosomes/lysosomes and autophagosomes, collectively called autophagic buildup. This buildup often spans the entire length of the fibers, and in many fibers the enlarged lysosomes in the periphery of the fibers look inconsequential (Raben et al., 2007a).

Autophagy is a dynamic multi-step process which encompasses autophagosome formation, maturation, fusion with lysosomes, and breakdown and recycling of autophagic substrates. The term "autophagic flux" refers to the whole process—the flux is complete if the formation of autophagosomes is followed by their fusion with lysosomes and degradation of the cargo. The failure of a downstream step of autophagy, fusion between autophagosomes and lysosomes, would result in incomplete flux, a condition known as autophagic block (Mizushima et al., 2010). Therefore, the increase in the number of autophagosomes (as shown by a significant increase in the LC3II levels) in Pompe

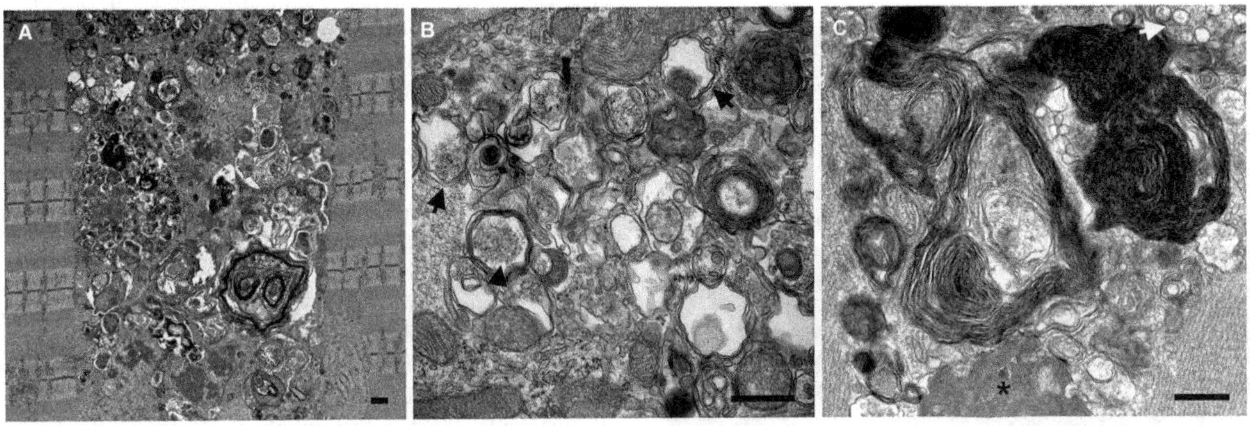

FIGURE 2 | Electron microscopy images show the presence and the extent (A) of autophagic buildup in skeletal muscle from a 5 month-old GAA-KO mouse. Larger magnification images **(B and C)** show classical double membrane autophagosomes with undigested cytosolic material (black arrows) or glycogen particles (arrowhead), multimembrane structures (most prominent in **C**), multivesicular body (white arrow), electron dense material (asterisk), as well other cellular debris of unknown origin. Bars: 0.5 μm.

muscle fibers could indicate an upregulation of autophagy or defects in autophagosome-lysosome fusion. An ubiquitin-binding scaffold protein, p62, also known as sequestosome 1 (SQSTM1), is commonly used as a marker of autophagic flux. The protein accumulates in cells from autophagy-deficient mice (Komatsu et al., 2007), and an increase in the level of p62 is an indication of a functional deficiency of autophagy. The protein itself is a substrate for autophagy-mediated degradation; in addition, p62 can directly bind to LC3, thus connecting ubiquitinated (Ub) proteins which are destined for degradation and autophagic machinery (Pankiv et al., 2007; Bjørkøy et al., 2009).

The levels of potentially toxic high molecular mass Ub-proteins in Pompe muscle were significantly increased suggesting a failure of autophagosomal–lysosomal fusion and a block in autophagosomal turnover. The accumulation of Ub-proteins in the GAA-KO muscle, particularly in the non-soluble fraction, preceded the development of clinical symptoms and increased with age. In addition, immunostaining of isolated muscle fibers showed that both the Ub-proteins and p62/SQSTM1 were seen within the autophagic areas, again indicating that the recycling process is inefficient in Pompe skeletal muscle (Raben et al., 2008; Shea and Raben, 2009). A direct evidence of the impaired autophagosomal-lysosomal fusion came from time-lapse microscopy of muscle fibers in which autophagosomes were labeled with GFP-LC3 and lysosomes were labeled with mCherry-LAMP1. These fibers were derived from transgenic GFP-LC3:GAA-KO mice, in which muscles had been *in vivo* transfected with mCherry-LAMP1 (**Figure 3**). The autophagosomal-lysosomal fusion events were essentially non-existent in the autophagic areas over the course of several hours of time-lapse microscopy (Spampanato et al., 2013).

The autophagic buildup containing cellular debris represents a huge non-contractile inclusion in the diseased muscle fibers. Studies in a different mouse model of Pompe disease, AGLU-/- (Bijvoet et al., 1998), have shown that the enlarged lysosomes in skeletal muscle cannot adequately account for the reduction in mechanical performance, and that the presence of large inclusions greatly contributes to the impairment of muscle function (Hesselink et al., 2003; Drost et al., 2005). Unlike sarcomeres, these inclusions are unable to generate force leading to a significant loss of force per unit of muscle mass. It has also been shown that skeletal muscle weakness in old AGLU-/- mice is caused by both loss of contractility and muscle mass (Hesselink et al., 2003; Drost et al., 2005).

Furthermore, our data demonstrated that the autophagic buildup affects the trafficking and delivery of the recombinant enzyme. The fate of the therapeutic enzyme was analyzed by monitoring the trafficking of the labeled rhGAA (Alexa-Fluor 546) in GFP-LC3:GAA-KO mice. The recombinant enzyme was detected almost exclusively within autophagosomes clustered in the buildup areas (Spampanato et al., 2013). This finding is not unexpected, considering the relationship between the autophagic pathway and the endocytic pathway; as mentioned above, the autophagic and endocytic pathways converge not only at the lysosome, but also at other steps along the way. It appears that the therapeutic drug is diverted away from its intended destination, the lysosome, and instead ends up in the autophagic area, which becomes a sink for the recombinant enzyme (Fukuda et al., 2006; Spampanato et al., 2013). Thus, in Pompe disease, a profoundly disordered intracellular recycling system appears to be an important contributor to the muscle weakness and to the incomplete response to treatment. The autophagic dead-end found in the muscle of Pompe mice is largely limited to muscles rich in glycolytic type II muscle fibers, which are most resistant to therapy, thus confirming the link between the defective autophagy, and the unresponsiveness to ERT with recombinant human enzyme. Abnormal autophagy and toxicity from accumulated Ub material may also be a general mechanism of cellular damage in other lysosomal storage disorders (Lieberman et al., 2012).

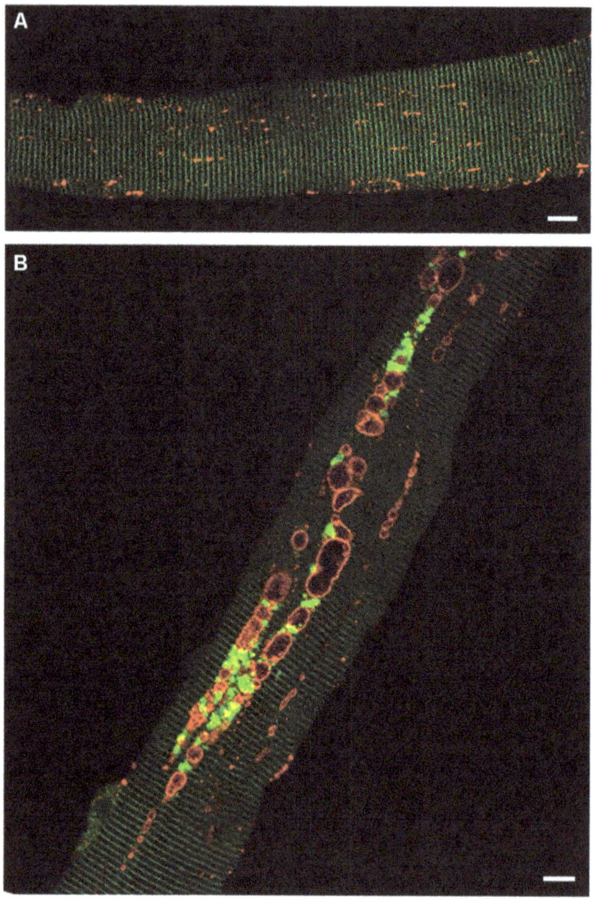

FIGURE 3 | Confocal microscopy images of fibers from GFP-LC3:WT (A) and GFP-LC3:GAA-KO (B) mice. In these strains autophagosomes are labeled with green fluorescent protein. Accumulation of autophagosomes (green) can be seen in live unstained muscle fibers derived from GAA-KO, but not from WT mice. Muscle was transfected *in vivo* by electroporation with mCherry-LAMP1 to visualize lysosomes (red); fibers were isolated 6 days after the procedure. **(A)** Autophagosomes are not detectable in the control muscle. **(B)** This still image shows autophagic buildup in the core of a fiber from the diseased muscle. Time-lapse microscopy of mCherry-LAMP1 transfected fibers demonstrated that there is little, if any, fusion between lysosomes and autophagosomes in the areas of autophagic buildup. Bar: 10 μm.

AUTOPHAGY IN POMPE PATIENTS

The apparent disconnect between the findings in Pompe mice, in which dysfunctional autophagy seemed to be a prominent feature of skeletal muscle pathology, and the morphological data (described above) on the stages of the disease progression in infants (Thurberg et al., 2006) raised some skepticism regarding the relevance of mouse studies to human disease. A closer look at muscle biopsies of untreated patients with severe classic infantile form aimed specifically to detect autophagy (namely, immunostaining of isolated fibers for lysosomal and autophagosomal markers) showed that, indeed, the overwhelming characteristic of muscle fibers in infants was the presence of hugely expanded lysosomes often without clear borders, a feature consistent with the long-held hypothesis of lysosomal rupture and the release of glycogen and lytic enzymes into the cytoplasm as a cause of muscle destruction (Griffin, 1984b; Thurberg et al., 2006).

However, analyses of muscle biopsies from patients with milder childhood/juvenile and adult forms of the disease justified the role of autophagy as a critical player in the pathogenesis of Pompe disease in this subset of patients. The pathological changes in many muscle fibers from these patients, even more so than in mice, reflected the autophagic abnormalities leading to muscle destruction. Large autophagic buildup often dwarfs the enlarged glycogen-filled lysosomes that lie outside the autophagic region, and in some fibers the buildup appears to be the only pathology (Raben et al., 2007b; Lewandowska et al., 2008; Raben et al., 2010a); unlike in mice, there is no selective involvement of the different histochemical fiber types. Similar to the findings in the murine model, the defective autophagic flux in muscle of patients with these forms impinges on the maturation of GAA and the uptake of recombinant enzyme during ERT (Nascimbeni et al., 2012a,b).

Notably, autophagic accumulation, closely resembling that in children and adults, becomes prominent (although limited in size) in infants who benefit most from ERT and survive beyond infancy (Raben et al., 2010a). The autophagic buildup in muscle biopsies from these patients is usually seen in fibers with minimal or no lysosomal enlargement outside the autophagic area, suggesting that the therapeutic enzyme reached these lysosomes, and digested the accumulated glycogen. The emergence of autophagic buildup on therapy is clearly not a "side effect" of the treatment, but rather an indication that the drug reverses the pathology only partially, and leaves a subset of lysosomes that are unable to fuse with the autophagosomes. It remains unclear to what extent this autophagic buildup could grow in size in patients on therapy; it is also not clear whether the clinical decline is caused by this emerging pathology.

LIPOFUSCINOSIS

There is yet another abnormality in both untreated and treated children and adults as well as in treated infants which recently came to light: muscle biopsies in the majority of patients contain large, irregularly shaped autofluorescent inclusions (**Figure 4**). In some patients, more than 75% of fibers contained these structures, which can span up to several hundred microns along the length of the fiber. These structures are usually located in the area of autophagic buildup within LAMP-positive lysosomes or LAMP/LC3-double positive autolysosomes (vesicles formed by autophagosomal-lysosomal fusion) or free in the cytoplasm. Their characteristics—electron density, contrast in transmitted light, a wide-spectrum of autofluorescence, which is quenched by Sudan Black B, and positive staining for lipid markers—unequivocally identify the particles as lipofuscin (Schoser et al., 2007; Feeney et al., 2014). Similar inclusions, although much smaller in size, have been found in muscle of old knockout mice.

Lipofuscin is an autofluorescent lipopigment, which is composed of highly cross-linked undegradable protein aggregates, lipids, carbohydrates, and metals (particularly iron) (Terman et al., 2010). Gradual intralysosomal accumulation of lipofuscin, particularly in terminally differentiated cells (i.e., neurons, retinal pigment epithelium, cardiac myocytes, and muscle cells) is a

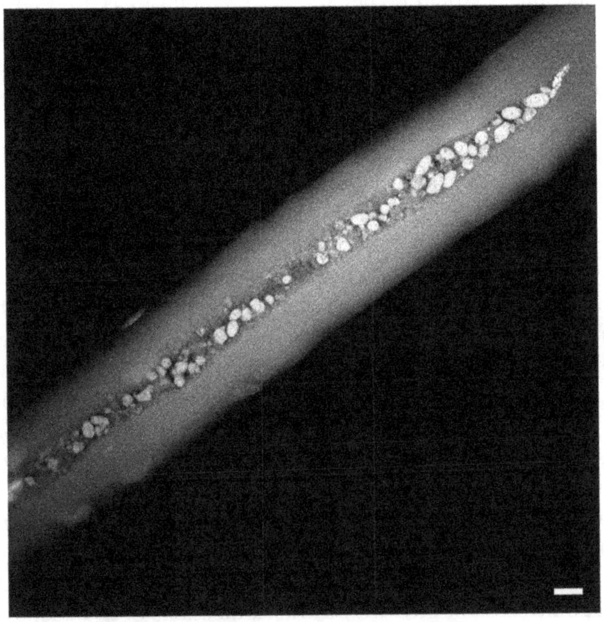

FIGURE 4 | Autofluorescent lipofuscin inclusions in a muscle biopsy from a patient (NBSL9a) with a childhood form of Pompe disease. The patient was diagnosed during a family study and began therapy at 7 years of age. The biopsy was taken prior to the initiation of ERT. Bar: 10 μm.

characteristic sign of cellular oxidative damage and aging (Brunk and Terman, 2002; Terman and Brunk, 2006; Terman et al., 2006). Given the unique role of autophagy and lysosomes in mitochondrial degradation, the diminished degradative capacity of lysosomes due to the progressive deposition of lipofuscin in these organelles would lead to a decrease in the autophagic turnover of damaged mitochondria, which in turn would result in the generation of reactive oxygen species and formation of oxidized proteins and aggregates, thus perpetuating the production of lipofuscin. In addition, intralysosomal accumulation of lipofuscin affects the trafficking of the newly synthesized lysosomal enzymes, thus further diminishing the degrading capacity of the lysosomes. This "vicious circle" of mitochondrial oxidative damage and lysosomal deposition of lipofuscin is at the heart of a well-known "mitochondrial-lysosomal axis theory of ageing", which was put forward by Ulf Brunk and Alexei Terman (Brunk and Terman, 2002). According to this model, accumulation of "biological garbage" results from the natural decline in the ability of the cellular degradative machinery to efficiently clear the cells from damaged structures (Terman et al., 2010).

The view of lysosomes as the only site for lipofuscin formation has been recently challenged; it was shown that inhibition of autophagy and reduced lysosomal uptake of protein aggregates did not prevent the formation of lipofuscin, suggesting that lipofuscin can be formed in the cytoplasm (Höhn et al., 2012). If lysosomes are not required for the formation of lipofuscin, then their engulfment by autophagosomes may serve as a protective mechanism designed to mitigate the toxicity (Höhn et al., 2014). In Pompe skeletal muscle, lipofuscin deposits are seen both inside and outside of lysosomes/autophagosomes; the presence of free cytoplasmic lipofuscin may reflect its extralysosomal formation or release into cytoplasm due to lysosomal rupture. Whatever the origin, these deposits are strikingly large in size (**Figure 4**) and are not associated with advanced age; they are seen in muscle biopsies from patients at different ages, including very young children (Schoser et al., 2007; Raben et al., 2010a; Feeney et al., 2014).

In retrospect, the reported in literature abnormal inclusions in muscle biopsies from Pompe patients—called "reducing body-like inclusions", "peculiar globular inclusions", "autofluorescent balloon-like structures", "acid phosphatase-positive globular inclusions"—all represent lipofuscin (Jay et al., 1992; Sharma et al., 2005; Raben et al., 2010a; Tsuburaya et al., 2012). Given the reduced autophagic activity and a failure of autophagosomal turnover, the presence of lipofuscin in the diseased muscle is not unexpected, but the magnitude of this pathology is. Interestingly, lipofuscin inclusions are often seen in otherwise normal looking fibers. It was suggested that these acid phosphatase-positive/periodic acid Schiff (PAS)-negative inclusions may be a hallmark of the disease and a diagnostic marker, particularly in adult form, which every so often represent the diagnostic challenge (Tsuburaya et al., 2012; Fujimoto et al., 2013).

Thus, our view of the pathogenesis of skeletal muscle damage in Pompe disease (at least in milder childhood and adult forms) evolved from a simple idea of gradual glycogen accumulation and lysosomal expansion to a much more complex picture, which involves a profound dysregulation of autophagy, accumulation of potentially toxic undegradable materials and non-contractile inclusion, as well as oxidative stress. Mitochondrial abnormalities, no doubt, contribute to the pathogenic cascade (our unpublished data). The disease has the characteristics of autophagic myopathy, premature "muscle ageing" or "muscle lipofuscinosis".

The evolution of our understanding of the pathogenesis of muscle destruction in Pompe disease reflects to a large degree the expansion of the role of the lysosomes themselves. The days of looking at the lysosomes as cellular "garbage disposal unit" or "suicide bags" [the latter term used by Christian de Duve who discovered this organelle (Appelmans et al., 1955)] are long gone. Lysosomes are now viewed more like "the center of cellular universe" (Walkley, 2008). In addition to their role in the digestion and recycling of various extra- and intracellular materials, lysosomes carry multiple tasks—they are implicated in cholesterol homeostasis, plasma membrane repair, tissue remodeling, pathogen defense, MHC class II antigen presentation, down-regulation of surface receptors, and cell death and proliferation (Saftig and Klumperman, 2009). Furthermore, recent studies indicate that lysosomes control their own biogenesis and provide a platform for both activation and deactivation of mTORC1 (mechanistic target of rapamycin complex1), a powerful anabolic regulator of cell growth and metabolism (Zoncu et al., 2011; Bar-Peled and Sabatini, 2014; Demetriades et al., 2014; Menon et al., 2014; Settembre and Ballabio, 2014).

EXPERIMENTAL APPROACHES TO THERAPY

SUBSTRATE REDUCTION THERAPY (SRT)

Successful application of SRT to other lysosomal diseases (Hollak and Wijburg, 2014) stimulated efforts to test a similar approach in Pompe disease. Inhibition of the two major enzymes involved in glycogen synthesis, glycogenin (GYG) and glycogen synthase (GYS), in primary myoblasts from GAA-KO mice by shRNAs resulted in a decrease in cytoplasmic and lysosomal glycogen accumulation and a reduction in the lysosomal size. A single intramuscular injection of recombinant AAV-1 vectors expressing shGYS into newborn knockout mice led to a significant reduction of glycogen accumulation in skeletal muscle (Douillard-Guilloux et al., 2008). Furthermore, genetic inactivation of GYS1 in the GAA-KO mice reversed cardiac abnormalities, reduced glycogen storage and autophagic buildup, and improved exercise capacity (Douillard-Guilloux et al., 2010). Of note, the disruption of GYS1 (muscle form) in the wild type mice (known as MGSKO) leads to abnormal cardiac development and a severe early perinatal mortality; 90% of GYS1-null pups die due to impaired cardiac function (Pederson et al., 2004). However, the lack of glycogen in skeletal muscle in the surviving 10% mice does not affect either the morphology of this tissues or the animals' ability to exercise. A severe deficiency of muscle glycogen synthase (mutations in the *GYS1* gene; glycogen storage disease type 0), leading to cardiac arrest, has been described in several families (Kollberg et al., 2007; Cameron et al., 2009; Sukigara et al., 2012), thus highlighting the risk of GYS1 suppression in Pompe disease—only muscle-targeted inhibition of GYS1 can be considered.

FIBER TYPE CONVERSION

A selective resistance of glycolytic type II muscle fibers (fast muscle) to ERT in the GAA-KO mice combined with massive accumulation of autophagic debris in these fibers suggested that a switch from fast to slow fibers may be beneficial in Pompe disease. A successful fiber type conversion was achieved by transgenic expression of PGC-1α—a transcription factor that promotes mitochondrial biogenesis and muscle remodeling (Lin et al., 2002)—in skeletal muscle of the GAA-KO mice. The conversion of fast muscle into muscle with slow metabolic profile restored autophagic flux, reduced the amount of accumulated Ub-proteins, and completely eliminated autophagic buildup. The absence of buildup was unexpectedly associated with induction rather than suppression of autophagy, as shown by a significant upregulation of several autophagy-related proteins, such as LC3II, GABARAP, Beclin-1, and BNIP3. A concomitant dramatic increase in the number of lysosomes in the PGC-1α-overexpressing muscle accounts for this apparent paradox. However, overexpression of PGC-1α in the diseased muscle failed to improve the ERT, mainly because of the considerable increase in the lysosomal glycogen load (Takikita et al., 2010). Although disappointing, these results are interesting in two respects: (1) a slight PGC-1α-induced increase in the levels of cytoplasmic glycogen (seen in wild type muscle) leads to a massive accumulation of lysosomal glycogen in GAA-deficient muscle, suggesting a high rate of lysosomal glycogen disposal in skeletal muscle. This may explain a much higher requirement for the therapeutic drug in skeletal muscle than in the heart; and (2) the biogenesis of lysosomes and autophagosomes is regulated coordinately.

SUPPRESSION OF AUTOPHAGY IN SKELETAL MUSCLE

The association between autophagic buildup and resistance to therapy in Pompe skeletal muscle suggested that suppression of autophagy would be helpful. Since autophagy is a presumed mechanism of glycogen transport to the lysosomes (Schiaffino and Hanzlikova, 1972; Kotoulas et al., 2006; Schiaffino et al., 2008), this approach also had a potential to reduce or even eliminate lysosomal glycogen accumulation. The genetic suppression of autophagy in GAA-KO mice was achieved by selective inactivation of a critical autophagic gene, Atg7, in skeletal muscles (Atg7/GAA double knockout). Indeed, inactivation of autophagy resulted in a significant decrease in the amount of accumulated glycogen, supporting the idea that autophagic pathway is at least partially responsible for the delivery of glycogen to the lysosomes; microautophagy could be another route by which glycogen enters the lysosome. As expected, autophagic buildup was not observed in the double knockout mice, although small clusters of double-membrane vesicles were detected by electron microscopy. In our experience, the phenotype of these muscle-specific autophagy-deficient GAA-KO mice is not worse (if not better) compared to that of the GAA-KO; however, an assessment of muscle strength by functional tests are needed to clarify this point (Raben et al., 2010b). The loss of autophagy alone in skeletal muscle of wild type mice is associated with the accumulations of dysfunctional mitochondria, mild atrophy, and age-dependent decrease in muscle strength (Masiero et al., 2009; Wu et al., 2009; Masiero and Sandri, 2010). The negative effects of suppression of autophagy in the GAA-KO mice are likely balanced by the beneficial effect of glycogen reduction.

Inactivation of a different autophagic gene, Atg5, in skeletal muscle of the GAA-KO mice, led to a modest glycogen reduction and worsening of clinical manifestations: these Atg5/GAA double knockouts develop early signs of muscle wasting and do not survive beyond 9–12 months of age (both GAA-KO and Atg7/GAA-KO have near normal lifespan) (Raben et al., 2008). The reason for the difference between the two double knockouts (expected to be indistinguishable), is not clear; a various degree of autophagy inactivation due to the difference in the promoters, which were used to excise the autophagic genes (human skeletal actin for the Atg5 and myosin light chain for the Atg7), may explain the discrepancy. However, both autophagy-deficient GAA-KO strains responded remarkably well to ERT—a near complete removal of stored lysosomal glycogen was observed in skeletal muscle—an outcome never seen in the ERT-treated GAA-KO mice. These data established the rational for autophagy-targeted therapy (Raben et al., 2010b).

STIMULATION OF LYSOSOMAL EXOCYTOSIS

Perhaps the most intriguing approach is that which exploits the intrinsic property of lysosomes to undergo regulated exocytosis. The process involves translocation and docking of lysosomes to the plasma membrane, followed by fusion with the membrane and release of the lysosomal content into the extracellular space. Initially ascribed to a subset of secretory lysosome-related organelles in hematopoietic cells or melanocytes, this calcium-dependent process is now attributed to all conventional lysosomes—a finding that changed the view of lysosomes as a terminal, dead-end degradation compartment (Andrews, 2000). Furthermore, this ability of lysosomes to exocytose is now seen as an integral part of the lysosomal function—to accomplish cellular clearance by degrading the cargo or by discharging it (Settembre and Ballabio, 2014). However, it was not until the discovery of transcription factor EB (TFEB) that the induction of lysosomal exocytosis became a therapeutic strategy in a variety of lysosomal storage disease and disorders with accumulation of abnormal proteins (Sardiello et al., 2009; Medina et al., 2011; Settembre and Ballabio, 2011).

The bHLH-leucine zipper TFEB, a master regulator of lysosomal biogenesis and autophagy, has been shown to stimulate the generation of new lysosomes and autophagosomes, and to promote fusion of lysosomes with autophagosomes and plasma membrane in a variety of cell types (Sardiello et al., 2009; Settembre and Ballabio, 2011; Settembre et al., 2011). The mechanism of TFEB-mediated gene regulation involves its ability to directly bind a 10-base pair sequence (called CLEAR: Coordinated Lysosomal Expression and Regulation) in the promoter regions of many lysosomal and autophagic genes (Sardiello et al., 2009).

Indeed, overexpression of TFEB in both GAA-KO mice and cultured Pompe muscle cells reduced glycogen load and lysosomal size, improved autophagosome processing, and alleviated excessive accumulation of autophagic vacuoles, thus establishing TFEB as a valid therapeutic target in Pompe disease. Lysosomal docking/fusion with the plasma membrane was visualized during time-lapse microscopy of live muscle fibers isolated from TFEB-treated GAA-KO mice (Feeney et al., 2013; Spampanato et al., 2013). More recent studies showed that a closely related but distinct transcription factor E3 (TFE3) is another target (perhaps even more attractive) since it is abundant in skeletal muscle, whereas TFEB is not. Similar to TFEB, TFE3 binds to the CLEAR elements in the promoter region of multiple lysosomal genes (Martina et al., 2014a,b). Furthermore, mapping TFE3 binding sites across the genome in the wild type muscle cells by ChIP-seq analysis showed similarity to known TFEB binding locations (our unpublished data). Overexpression of TFE3 induced lysosomal exocytosis and promoted glycogen clearance in Pompe muscle cells (Martina et al., 2014b).

The appeal of TFEB or TFE3 modulation as a therapeutic option in Pompe disease is twofold: (1) this approach circumvents the major hurdle of the current therapy—inefficient enzyme delivery to skeletal muscle; and (2) unlike other efforts, it restores autophagic flux and addresses both lysosomal and autophagic pathologies.

CONCLUSION AND FUTURE STUDIES

The limitations of enzyme replacement therapy in Pompe disease have led to reassessment of the basic skeletal muscle pathology, which in turn uncovered new pathogenic mechanisms, in particular the role of autophagy. This new understanding allowed for the identification of novel therapeutic targets that hopefully will guide us toward the development of fresh strategies independent of or complementary to ERT.

In spite of all the advances, many questions still remain. The signaling pathways which are linked to the lysosomes are still an unexplored area in Pompe disease. Recent findings have positioned the lysosome at the center of the mTORC1 signaling pathway; mTORC1 is a protein kinase complex that functions as a central regulator of cellular growth and metabolism by integrating signals from nutrients, energy, and growth factors (Zoncu et al., 2011; Bar-Peled and Sabatini, 2014). A skeleton explanation of the activation and inhibition of the mTORC1 is as follows. Accumulation of amino acids in the lysosomal lumen initiates a signal to a multiprotein lysosome-based complex, which culminates in the mTORC1 recruitment to the lysosome where it is activated by Rheb (Ras homolog enriched in brain). The recruitment and activation of mTORC1 depends on the nucleotide-bound state of the Rags (Bar-Peled and Sabatini, 2014). The inhibition of lysosomal function or depletion of amino acids from the lysosome results in the release of mTORC1 from the lysosome and its inactivation (Zoncu et al., 2011). Perhaps even more relevant to Pompe disease is the data indicating that the Rag family also signals glucose concentration to mTOR; in other words, glucose, like amino acids, controls mTORC1 recruitment to the lysosomal surface and its activation (Efeyan et al., 2013).

Activation of mTORC1 also induces phosphorylation of TFEB and TFE3 and their retention in the cytosol where these transcription factors remain inactive; inhibition of phosphorylation (for example, by nutrient deprivation) stimulates their nuclear translocation and activation leading to the induction of multiple target gens including lysosomal genes (Settembre et al., 2011; Martina et al., 2012; Settembre et al., 2012; Martina et al., 2014b). Thus, the lysosome regulates its own biogenesis by a lysosome-to-nucleus signaling mechanism (Settembre et al., 2012). Therefore, pharmacological inhibition of TFE3 phosphorylation would promote cellular clearance in Pompe disease as well as in other lysosomal storage disorders. The regulation of TFEB and TFE3 in skeletal muscle in general and in Pompe disease in particular remains an open question. This is a rewarding field for future studies.

FUNDING

This research was supported in part by the Intramural Research Program of the National Institute of Arthritis and Musculoskeletal and Skin diseases of the National Institutes of Health. Dr. Lim and Dr. Li are supported in part by a CRADA between NIH and Genzyme Corporation and by the Acid Maltase Deficiency Association.

REFERENCES

Andrews, N. W. (2000). Regulated secretion of conventional lysosomes. *Trends Cell Biol.* 10, 316–321. doi: 10.1016/s0962-8924(00)01794-3

Angelini, C., and Semplicini, C. (2012). Enzyme replacement therapy for Pompe disease. *Curr. Neurol. Neurosci. Rep.* 12, 70–75. doi: 10.1007/s11910-011-0236-5

Appelmans, F., Wattiaux, R., and De Duve, C. (1955). Tissue fractionation studies. 5. The association of acid phosphatase with a special class of cytoplasmic granules in rat liver. *Biochem. J.* 59, 438–445.

Ausems, M. G., Verbiest, J., Hermans, M. P., Kroos, M. A., Beemer, F. A., Wokke, J. H., et al. (1999). Frequency of glycogen storage disease type II in the Netherlands: implications for diagnosis and genetic counselling. *Eur. J. Hum. Genet.* 7, 713–716. doi: 10.1038/sj.ejhg.5200367

Banugaria, S. G., Prater, S. N., Ng, Y. K., Kobori, J. A., Finkel, R. S., Ladda, R. L., et al. (2011). The impact of antibodies on clinical outcomes in diseases treated with therapeutic protein: lessons learned from infantile Pompe disease. *Genet. Med.* 13, 729–736. doi: 10.1097/gim.0b013e3182174703

Bar-Peled, L., and Sabatini, D. M. (2014). Regulation of mTORC1 by amino acids. *Trends Cell Biol.* 24, 400–406. doi: 10.1016/j.tcb.2014.03.003

Becker, J. A., Vlach, J., Raben, N., Nagaraju, K., Adams, E. M., Hermans, M. M., et al. (1998). The African origin of the common mutation in African American patients with glycogen-storage disease type II. *Am. J. Hum. Genet.* 62, 991–994. doi: 10.1086/301788

Berg, T. O., Fengsrud, M., Stromhaug, P. E., Berg, T., and Seglen, P. O. (1998). Isolation and characterization of rat liver amphisomes. Evidence for fusion of autophagosomes with both early and late endosomes. *J. Biol. Chem.* 273, 21883–21892. doi: 10.1074/jbc.273.34.21883

Bijvoet, A. G., Van De Kamp, E. H., Kroos, M. A., Ding, J. H., Yang, B. Z., Visser, P., et al. (1998). Generalized glycogen storage and cardiomegaly in a knockout mouse model of Pompe disease. *Hum. Mol. Genet.* 7, 53–62. doi: 10.1093/hmg/7.1.53

Bischoff, G. (1932). Zum klinischen bild der glykogen-speicherungs-krankheit (glykogenose). *Z. Kinderheilkd.* 52, 722–726. doi: 10.1007/BF02248461

Bjørkøy, G., Lamark, T., Pankiv, S., Overvatn, A., Brech, A., and Johansen, T. (2009). Monitoring autophagic degradation of p62/SQSTM1. *Methods Enzymol.* 452, 181–197. doi: 10.1016/s0076-6879(08)03612-4

Boerkoel, C. F., Exelbert, R., Nicastri, C., Nichols, R. C., Miller, F. W., Plotz, P. H., et al. (1995). Leaky splicing mutation in the acid maltase gene is associated with delayed onset of glycogenosis type II. *Am. J. Hum. Genet.* 56, 887–897.

Brunk, U. T., and Terman, A. (2002). Lipofuscin: mechanisms of age-related accumulation and influence on cell function. *Free Radic. Biol. Med.* 33, 611–619. doi: 10.1016/s0891-5849(02)00959-0

Byrne, B. J., Falk, D. J., Pacak, C. A., Nayak, S., Herzog, R. W., Elder, M. E., et al. (2011). Pompe disease gene therapy. *Hum. Mol. Genet.* 20, R61–R68. doi: 10.1093/hmg/ddr174

Cameron, J. M., Levandovskiy, V., Mackay, N., Utgikar, R., Ackerley, C., Chiasson, D., et al. (2009). Identification of a novel mutation in GYS1 (muscle-specific glycogen synthase) resulting in sudden cardiac death, that is diagnosable from skin fibroblasts. *Mol. Genet. Metab.* 98, 378–382. doi: 10.1016/j.ymgme.2009.07.012

Chakrapani, A., Vellodi, A., Robinson, P., Jones, S., and Wraith, J. E. (2010). Treatment of infantile Pompe disease with alglucosidase alpha: the UK experience. *J. Inherit. Metab. Dis.* 33, 747–750. doi: 10.1007/s10545-010-9206-3

Chien, Y. H., Chiang, S. C., Zhang, X. K., Keutzer, J., Lee, N. C., Huang, A. C., et al. (2008). Early detection of Pompe disease by newborn screening is feasible: results from the Taiwan screening program. *Pediatrics* 122, e39–e45. doi: 10.1542/peds.2007-2222

Chien, Y. H., Hwu, W. L., and Lee, N. C. (2013). Pompe disease: early diagnosis and early treatment make a difference. *Pediatr. Neonatol.* 54, 219–227. doi: 10.1016/j.pedneo.2013.03.009

Chien, Y. H., Lee, N. C., Thurberg, B. L., Chiang, S. C., Zhang, X. K., Keutzer, J., et al. (2009). Pompe disease in infants: improving the prognosis by newborn screening and early treatment. *Pediatrics* 124, e1116–e1125. doi: 10.1542/peds.2008-3667

Cori, G. T. (1954). Enzymes and glycogen structure in glycogenosis. *Osterr. Z. Kinderheilkd. Kinderfuersorge* 10, 38–42.

de Filippi, P., Ravaglia, S., Bembi, B., Costa, A., Moglia, A., Piccolo, G., et al. (2010). The angiotensin-converting enzyme insertion/deletion polymorphism modifies the clinical outcome in patients with Pompe disease. *Genet. Med.* 12, 206–211. doi: 10.1097/gim.0b013e3181d2900e

Demetriades, C., Doumpas, N., and Teleman, A. A. (2014). Regulation of TORC1 in response to amino acid starvation via lysosomal recruitment of TSC2. *Cell* 156, 786–799. doi: 10.1016/j.cell.2014.01.024

Douillard-Guilloux, G., Raben, N., Takikita, S., Batista, L., Caillaud, C., and Richard, E. (2008). Modulation of glycogen synthesis by RNA interference: towards a new therapeutic approach for glycogenosis type II. *Hum. Mol. Genet.* 17, 3876–3886. doi: 10.1093/hmg/ddn290

Douillard-Guilloux, G., Raben, N., Takikita, S., Ferry, A., Vignaud, A., Guillet-Deniau, I., et al. (2010). Restoration of muscle functionality by genetic suppression of glycogen synthesis in a murine model of Pompe disease. *Hum. Mol. Genet.* 19, 684–696. doi: 10.1093/hmg/ddp535

Drost, M. R., Hesselink, R. P., Oomens, C. W., and Van Der Vusse, G. J. (2005). Effects of non-contractile inclusions on mechanical performance of skeletal muscle. *J. Biomech.* 38, 1035–1043. doi: 10.1016/j.jbiomech.2004.05.040

Efeyan, A., Zoncu, R., Chang, S., Gumper, I., Snitkin, H., Wolfson, R. L., et al. (2013). Regulation of mTORC1 by the Rag GTPases is necessary for neonatal autophagy and survival. *Nature* 493, 679–683. doi: 10.1038/nature11745

Engel, A. G. (1970). Acid maltase deficiency in adults: studies in four cases of a syndrome which may mimic muscular dystrophy or other myopathies. *Brain* 93, 599–616. doi: 10.1093/brain/93.3.599

Feeney, E. J., Austin, S., Chien, Y. H., Mandel, H., Schoser, B., Prater, S., et al. (2014). The value of muscle biopsies in Pompe disease: identifying lipofuscin inclusions in juvenile- and adult-onset patients. *Acta Neuropathol. Commun.* 2, 2–17. doi: 10.1186/2051-5960-2-2

Feeney, E. J., Spampanato, C., Puertollano, R., Ballabio, A., Parenti, G., and Raben, N. (2013). What else is in store for autophagy? Exocytosis of autolysosomes as a mechanism of TFEB-mediated cellular clearance in Pompe disease. *Autophagy* 9, 1117–1118. doi: 10.4161/auto.24920

Filosto, M., Todeschini, A., Cotelli, M. S., Vielmi, V., Rinaldi, F., Rota, S., et al. (2013). Non-muscle involvement in late-onset glycogenosis II. *Acta Myol.* 32, 91–94.

Fujimoto, S., Manabe, Y., Fujii, D., Kozai, Y., Matsuzono, K., Takahashi, Y., et al. (2013). A novel mutation of the GAA gene in a patient with adult-onset Pompe disease lacking a disease-specific pathology. *Intern. Med.* 52, 2461–2464. doi: 10.2169/internalmedicine.52.0311

Fukuda, T., Ahearn, M., Roberts, A., Mattaliano, R. J., Zaal, K., Ralston, E., et al. (2006). Autophagy and mistargeting of therapeutic enzyme in skeletal muscle in Pompe disease. *Mol. Ther.* 14, 831–839. doi: 10.1016/j.ymthe.2006.08.009

Griffin, J. L. (1984a). Infantile acid maltase deficiency. I. Muscle fiber destruction after lysosomal rupture4. *Virchows Arch. B Cell Pathol. Incl. Mol. Pathol.* 45, 23–36. doi: 10.1007/bf02889849

Griffin, J. L. (1984b). Infantile acid maltase deficiency. II. Muscle fiber hypertrophy and the ultrastructure of end-stage fibers3. *Virchows Arch. B Cell Pathol. Incl. Mol. Pathol.* 45, 37–50. doi: 10.1007/bf02889850

Güngör, D., and Reuser, A. J. (2013). How to describe the clinical spectrum in Pompe disease. *Am. J. Med. Genet. A* 161A, 399–400. doi: 10.1002/ajmg.a.35662

He, C., and Klionsky, D. J. (2009). Regulation mechanisms and signaling pathways of autophagy. *Annu. Rev. Genet.* 43, 67–93. doi: 10.1146/annurev-genet-102808-114910

Hermans, M. M., De Graaff, E., Kroos, M. A., Mohkamsing, S., Eussen, B. J., Joosse, M., et al. (1994). The effect of a single base pair deletion (delta T525) and a C1634T missense mutation (pro545leu) on the expression of lysosomal alpha-glucosidase in patients with glycogen storage disease type II. *Hum. Mol. Genet.* 3, 2213–2218. doi: 10.1093/hmg/3.12.2213

Hermans, M. M., Wisselaar, H. A., Kroos, M. A., Oostra, B. A., and Reuser, A. J. (1993). Human lysosomal alpha-glucosidase: functional characterization of the glycosylation sites. *Biochem. J.* 289, 681–686.

Hers, H. G. (1963). Alpha-glucosidase deficiency in generalize glycogen storage disease (Pompe's disease). *Biochem. J.* 86, 11–16.

Herzog, A., Hartung, R., Reuser, A. J., Hermanns, P., Runz, H., Karabul, N., et al. (2012). A cross-sectional single-centre study on the spectrum of Pompe disease, German patients: molecular analysis of the GAA gene, manifestation and genotype-phenotype correlations. *Orphanet J. Rare Dis.* 7:35. doi: 10.1186/1750-1172-7-35

Hesselink, R. P., Wagenmakers, A. J., Drost, M. R., and Van Der Vusse, G. J. (2003). Lysosomal dysfunction in muscle with special reference to glycogen storage disease type II. *Biochim. Biophys. Acta* 1637, 164–170. doi: 10.1016/s0925-4439(02)00229-6

Hirschhorn, R., and Huie, M. L. (1999). Frequency of mutations for glycogen storage disease type II in different populations: the delta525T and deltaexon 18 mutations are not generally "common" in white populations. *J. Med. Genet.* 36, 85–86.

Hirschhorn, R., and Reuser, A. J. (2001). "Glycogen storage disease type II: acid alpha-glucosidase (acid maltase) deficiency," in *The Metabolic and Molecular Basis of Inherited Disease,* eds C. R. Scriver, A. Beaudet, W. S. Sly and D. Valle (New York, NY: McGraw-Hill), 3389–3420.

Hoefsloot, L. H., Hoogeveen-Westerveld, M., Kroos, M. A., Van Beeumen, J., Reuser, A. J., and Oostra, B. A. (1988). Primary structure and processing of lysosomal alpha-glucosidase; homology with the intestinal sucrase-isomaltase complex. *EMBO J.* 7, 1697–1704.

Hoefsloot, L. H., Hoogeveen-Westerveld, M., Reuser, A. J., and Oostra, B. A. (1990). Characterization of the human lysosomal alpha-glucosidase gene. *Biochem. J.* 272, 493–497.

Höhn, A., Jung, T., and Grune, T. (2014). Pathophysiological importance of aggregated damaged proteins. *Free Radic. Biol. Med.* 71C, 70–89. doi: 10.1016/j.freeradbiomed.2014.02.028

Höhn, A., Sittig, A., Jung, T., Grimm, S., and Grune, T. (2012). Lipofuscin is formed independently of macroautophagy and lysosomal activity in stress-induced prematurely senescent human fibroblasts. *Free Radic. Biol. Med.* 53, 1760–1769. doi: 10.1016/j.freeradbiomed.2012.08.591

Hollak, C. E., and Wijburg, F. A. (2014). Treatment of lysosomal storage disorders: successes and challenges. *J. Inherit. Metab. Dis.* doi: 10.1007/s10545-014-9718-3. [Epub ahead of print].

Huie, M. L., Chen, A. S., Tsujino, S., Shanske, S., Dimauro, S., Engel, A. G., et al. (1994). Aberrant splicing in adult onset glycogen storage disease type II (GSDII): molecular identification of an IVS1 (-13T->G) mutation in a majority of patients and a novel IVS10 (+1GT->CT) mutation. *Hum. Mol. Genet.* 3, 2231–2236. doi: 10.1093/hmg/3.12.2231

Jay, V., Christodoulou, J., Mercer-Connolly, A., and Mcinnes, R. R. (1992). "Reducing body"-like inclusions in skeletal muscle in childhood-onset acid maltase deficiency. *Acta Neuropathol.* 85, 111–115. doi: 10.1007/bf00304641

Jat, P. S., Noble, M. D., Ataliotis, P., Tanaka, Y., Yannoutsos, N., Larsen, L., et al. (1991). Direct derivation of conditionally immortal cell lines from an H-2Kb-tsA58 transgenic mouse. *Proc. Natl. Acad. Sci. U S A* 88, 5096–5100. doi: 10.1073/pnas.88.12.5096

Kabeya, Y., Mizushima, N., Ueno, T., Yamamoto, A., Kirisako, T., Noda, T., et al. (2000). LC3, a mammalian homologue of yeast Apg8p, is localized in autophagosome membranes after processing. *EMBO J.* 19, 5720–5728. doi: 10.1093/emboj/19.21.5720

Kaushik, S., Bandyopadhyay, U., Sridhar, S., Kiffin, R., Martinez-Vicente, M., Kon, M., et al. (2011). Chaperone-mediated autophagy at a glance. *J. Cell Sci.* 124, 495–499. doi: 10.1242/jcs.073874

Kikuchi, T., Yang, H. W., Pennybacker, M., Ichihara, N., Mizutani, M., Van Hove, J. L., et al. (1998). Clinical and metabolic correction of pompe disease by enzyme therapy in acid maltase-deficient quail. *J. Clin. Invest.* 101, 827–833. doi: 10.1172/jci1722

Kishnani, P. S., Corzo, D., Nicolino, M., Byrne, B., Mandel, H., Hwu, W. L., et al. (2007). Recombinant human acid [alpha]-glucosidase: major clinical benefits in infantile-onset Pompe disease. *Neurology* 68, 99–109. doi: 10.1212/01.wnl.0000251268.41188.04

Kishnani, P. S., Hwu, W. L., Mandel, H., Nicolino, M., Yong, F., and Corzo, D. (2006). A retrospective, multinational, multicenter study on the natural history of infantile-onset Pompe disease. *J. Pediatr.* 148, 671–676. doi: 10.1016/j.jpeds.2005.11.033

Klionsky, D. J. (2007). Autophagy: from phenomenology to molecular understanding in less than a decade. *Nat. Rev. Mol. Cell Biol.* 8, 931–937. doi: 10.1038/nrm2245

Koeberl, D. D., Austin, S., Case, L. E., Smith, E. C., Buckley, A. F., Young, S. P., et al. (2014). Adjunctive albuterol enhances the response to enzyme replacement therapy in late-onset Pompe disease. *FASEB J.* 28, 2171–2176. doi: 10.1096/fj.13-241893

Kollberg, G., Tulinius, M., Gilljam, T., Ostman-Smith, I., Forsander, G., Jotorp, P., et al. (2007). Cardiomyopathy and exercise intolerance in muscle glycogen storage disease 0. *N. Engl. J. Med.* 357, 1507–1514. doi: 10.1056/nejmoa066691

Komatsu, M., Waguri, S., Koike, M., Sou, Y. S., Ueno, T., Hara, T., et al. (2007). Homeostatic levels of p62 control cytoplasmic inclusion body formation in autophagy-deficient mice. *Cell* 131, 1149–1163. doi: 10.1016/j.cell.2007.10.035

Kornfeld, S. (1992). Structure and function of the mannose 6-phosphate/insulinlike growth factor II receptors. *Annu. Rev. Biochem.* 61, 307–330. doi: 10.1146/annurev.biochem.61.1.307

Kotoulas, O. B., Kalamidas, S. A., and Kondomerkos, D. J. (2006). Glycogen autophagy in glucose homeostasis. *Pathol. Res. Pract.* 202, 631–638. doi: 10.1016/j.prp.2006.04.001

Kroos, M., Hoogeveen-Westerveld, M., Van Der Ploeg, A., and Reuser, A. J. (2012). The genotype-phenotype correlation in Pompe disease. *Am. J. Med. Genet. C Semin. Med. Genet.* 160, 59–68. doi: 10.1002/ajmg.c.31318

Kuo, W. L., Hirschhorn, R., Huie, M. L., and Hirschhorn, K. (1996). Localization and ordering of acid alpha-glucosidase (GAA) and thymidine kinase (TK1) by fluorescence in situ hybridization. *Hum. Genet.* 97, 404–406. doi: 10.1007/bf02185782

Lewandowska, E., Wierzba-Bobrowicz, T., Rola, R., Modzelewska, J., Stepien, T., Lugowska, A., et al. (2008). Pathology of skeletal muscle cells in adult-onset glycogenosis type II (Pompe disease): ultrastructural study. *Folia Neuropathol.* 46, 123–133.

Lieberman, A. P., Puertollano, R., Raben, N., Slaugenhaupt, S., Walkley, S. U., and Ballabio, A. (2012). Autophagy in lysosomal storage disorders. *Autophagy* 8, 719–730. doi: 10.4161/auto.19469

Lin, J., Wu, H., Tarr, P. T., Zhang, C. Y., Wu, Z., Boss, O., et al. (2002). Transcriptional co-activator PGC-1 alpha drives the formation of slow-twitch muscle fibres. *Nature* 418, 797–801. doi: 10.1038/nature00904

Maga, J. A., Zhou, J., Kambampati, R., Peng, S., Wang, X., Bohnsack, R. N., et al. (2013). Glycosylation-independent lysosomal targeting of acid alpha-glucosidase enhances muscle glycogen clearance in Pompe mice. *J. Biol. Chem.* 288, 1428–1438. doi: 10.1074/jbc.M112.438663

Martina, J. A., Chen, Y., Gucek, M., and Puertollano, R. (2012). MTORC1 functions as a transcriptional regulator of autophagy by preventing nuclear transport of TFEB. *Autophagy* 8, 903–914. doi: 10.4161/auto.19653

Martina, J. A., Diab, H. I., Li, H., and Puertollano, R. (2014a). Novel roles for the MiTF/TFE family of transcription factors in organelle biogenesis, nutrient sensing and energy homeostasis. *Cell. Mol. Life Sci.* 71, 2483–2497. doi: 10.1007/s00018-014-1565-8

Martina, J. A., Diab, H. I., Lishu, L., Jeong-A, L., Patange, S., Raben, N., et al. (2014b). The nutrient-responsive transcription factor TFE3 promotes autophagy, lysosomal biogenesis and clearance of cellular debris. *Sci. Signal.* 7:ra9. doi: 10.1126/scisignal.2004754

Martiniuk, F., Chen, A., Mack, A., Arvanitopoulos, E., Chen, Y., Rom, W. N., et al. (1998). Carrier frequency for glycogen storage disease type II in New York and estimates of affected individuals born with the disease. *Am. J. Med. Genet.* 79, 69–72. doi: 10.1002/(sici)1096-8628(19980827)79:1<69::aid-ajmg16>3.0.co;2-k

Martiniuk, F., Mehler, M., Tzall, S., Meredith, G., and Hirschhorn, R. (1990). Sequence of the cDNA and 5'-flanking region for human acid alpha-glucosidase, detection of an intron in the 5' untranslated leader sequence, definition of 18-bp polymorphisms and differences with previous cDNA and amino acid sequences. *DNA Cell Biol.* 9, 85–94. doi: 10.1089/dna.1990.9.85

Masiero, E., Agatea, L., Mammucari, C., Blaauw, B., Loro, E., Komatsu, M., et al. (2009). Autophagy is required to maintain muscle mass. *Cell Metab.* 10, 507–515. doi: 10.1016/j.cmet.2009.10.008

Masiero, E., and Sandri, M. (2010). Autophagy inhibition induces atrophy and myopathy in adult skeletal muscles. *Autophagy* 6, 307–309. doi: 10.4161/auto.6.2.11137

Mechtler, T. P., Stary, S., Metz, T. F., De Jesus, V. R., Greber-Platzer, S., Pollak, A., et al. (2012). Neonatal screening for lysosomal storage disorders: feasibility and incidence from a nationwide study in Austria. *Lancet* 379, 335–341. doi: 10.1016/S0140-6736(11)61266-X

Medina, D. L., Fraldi, A., Bouche, V., Annunziata, F., Mansueto, G., Spampanato, C., et al. (2011). Transcriptional activation of lysosomal exocytosis promotes cellular clearance. *Dev. Cell* 21, 421–430. doi: 10.1016/j.devcel.2011.07.016

Menon, S., Dibble, C. C., Talbott, G., Hoxhaj, G., Valvezan, A. J., Takahashi, H., et al. (2014). Spatial control of the TSC complex integrates insulin and nutrient regulation of mTORC1 at the lysosome. *Cell* 156, 771–785. doi: 10.1016/j.cell.2013.11.049

Mizushima, N., Yoshimori, T., and Levine, B. (2010). Methods in mammalian autophagy research. *Cell* 140, 313–326. doi: 10.1016/j.cell.2010.01.028

Moreland, R. J., Jin, X., Zhang, X. K., Decker, R. W., Albee, K. L., Lee, K. L., et al. (2005). Lysosomal acid alpha-glucosidase consists of four different peptides processed from a single chain precursor. *J. Biol. Chem.* 280, 6780–6791. doi: 10.1074/jbc.m404008200

Nascimbeni, A. C., Fanin, M., Masiero, E., Angelini, C., and Sandri, M. (2012a). Impaired autophagy contributes to muscle atrophy in glycogen storage disease type II patients. *Autophagy* 8, 1697–1700. doi: 10.4161/auto.21691

Nascimbeni, A. C., Fanin, M., Masiero, E., Angelini, C., and Sandri, M. (2012b). The role of autophagy in the pathogenesis of glycogen storage disease type II (GSDII). *Cell Death Differ.* 19, 1698–1708. doi: 10.1038/cdd.2012.52

Neufeld, E. F., and Fratantoni, J. C. (1970). Inborn errors of mucopolysaccharide metabolism. *Science* 169, 141–146. doi: 10.1126/science.169.3941.141

Nicolino, M., Byrne, B., Wraith, J. E., Leslie, N., Mandel, H., Freyer, D. R., et al. (2009). Clinical outcomes after long-term treatment with alglucosidase alfa in infants and children with advanced Pompe disease. *Genet. Med.* 11, 210–219. doi: 10.1097/GIM.0b013e31819d0996

Pankiv, S., Clausen, T. H., Lamark, T., Brech, A., Bruun, J. A., Outzen, H., et al. (2007). p62/SQSTM1 binds directly to Atg8/LC3 to facilitate degradation of ubiquitinated protein aggregates by autophagy. *J. Biol. Chem.* 282, 24131–24145. doi: 10.1074/jbc.m702824200

Pederson, B. A., Chen, H., Schroeder, J. M., Shou, W., Depaoli-Roach, A. A., and Roach, P. J. (2004). Abnormal cardiac development in the absence of heart glycogen. *Mol. Cell. Biol.* 24, 7179–7187. doi: 10.1128/mcb.24.16.7179-7187.2004

Porto, C., Cardone, M., Fontana, F., Rossi, B., Tuzzi, M. R., Tarallo, A., et al. (2009). The pharmacological chaperone N-butyldeoxynojirimycin enhances enzyme replacement therapy in Pompe disease fibroblasts. *Mol. Ther.* 17, 964–971. doi: 10.1038/mt.2009.53

Porto, C., Ferrara, M. C., Meli, M., Acampora, E., Avolio, V., Rosa, M., et al. (2012). Pharmacological enhancement of alpha-glucosidase by the allosteric chaperone N-acetylcysteine. *Mol. Ther.* 20, 2201–2211. doi: 10.1038/mt.2012.152

Prater, S. N., Banugaria, S. G., Dearmey, S. M., Botha, E. G., Stege, E. M., Case, L. E., et al. (2012). The emerging phenotype of long-term survivors with infantile Pompe disease. *Genet. Med.* 14, 800–810. doi: 10.1038/gim.2012.44

Prater, S. N., Patel, T. T., Buckley, A. F., Mandel, H., Vlodavski, E., Banugaria, S. G., et al. (2013). Skeletal muscle pathology of infantile Pompe disease during long-term enzyme replacement therapy. *Orphanet J. Rare Dis.* 8:90. doi: 10.1186/1750-1172-8-90. [Epub ahead of print].

Putschar, M. (1932). Uber angeborene Glykogenspeicher-Krankheit des herzens. *Beitr. Pathol. Anat. Allg. Pathol.* 90:222.

Raben, N., Fukuda, T., Gilbert, A. L., De Jong, D., Thurberg, B. L., Mattaliano, R. J., et al. (2005). Replacing acid alpha-glucosidase in Pompe disease: recombinant and transgenic enzymes are equipotent, but neither completely clears glycogen from type II muscle fibers. *Mol. Ther.* 11, 48–56. doi: 10.1016/j.ymthe.2004.09.017

Raben, N., Hill, V., Shea, L., Takikita, S., Baum, R., Mizushima, N., et al. (2008). Suppression of autophagy in skeletal muscle uncovers the accumulation of ubiquitinated proteins and their potential role in muscle damage in Pompe disease. *Hum. Mol. Genet.* 17, 3897–3908. doi: 10.1093/hmg/ddn292

Raben, N., Nagaraju, K., Lee, E., Kessler, P., Byrne, B., Lee, L., et al. (1998). Targeted disruption of the acid alpha-glucosidase gene in mice causes an illness with critical features of both infantile and adult human glycogen storage disease type II. *J. Biol. Chem.* 273, 19086–19092. doi: 10.1074/jbc.273.30.19086

Raben, N., Nichols, R. C., Martiniuk, F., and Plotz, P. H. (1996). A model of mRNA splicing in adult lysosomal storage disease (glycogenosis type II). *Hum. Mol. Genet.* 5, 995–1000. doi: 10.1093/hmg/5.7.995

Raben, N., Ralston, E., Chien, Y. H., Baum, R., Schreiner, C., Hwu, W. L., et al. (2010a). Differences in the predominance of lysosomal and autophagic pathologies between infants and adults with Pompe disease: implications for therapy. *Mol. Genet. Metab.* 101, 324–331. doi: 10.1016/j.ymgme.2010.08.001

Raben, N., Roberts, A., and Plotz, P. H. (2007a). Role of autophagy in the pathogenesis of Pompe disease. *Acta Myol.* 26, 45–48.

Raben, N., Schreiner, C., Baum, R., Takikita, S., Xu, S., Xie, T., et al. (2010b). Suppression of autophagy permits successful enzyme replacement therapy in a lysosomal storage disorder–murine Pompe disease. *Autophagy* 6, 1078–1089. doi: 10.4161/auto.6.8.13378

Raben, N., Shea, L., Hill, V., and Plotz, P. (2009). Monitoring autophagy in lysosomal storage disorders. *Methods Enzymol.* 453, 417–449. doi: 10.1016/S0076-6879(08)04021-4

Raben, N., Takikita, S., Pittis, M. G., Bembi, B., Marie, S. K. N., Roberts, A., et al. (2007b). Deconstructing Pompe disease by analyzing single muscle fibers. *Autophagy* 3, 546–552.

Saftig, P., and Klumperman, J. (2009). Lysosome biogenesis and lysosomal membrane proteins: trafficking meets function. *Nat. Rev. Mol. Cell Biol.* 10, 623–635. doi: 10.1038/nrm2745

Sardiello, M., Palmieri, M., Di Ronza, A., Medina, D. L., Valenza, M., Gennarino, V. A., et al. (2009). A gene network regulating lysosomal biogenesis and function. *Science* 325, 473–477. doi: 10.1126/science.1174447

Schiaffino, S., and Hanzlikova, V. (1972). Autophagic degradation of glycogen in skeletal muscles of the newborn rat. *J. Cell Biol.* 52, 41–51. doi: 10.1083/jcb.52.1.41

Schiaffino, S., Mammucari, C., and Sandri, M. (2008). The role of autophagy in neonatal tissues: just a response to amino acid starvation? *Autophagy* 4, 727–730.

Schoser, B., Hill, V., and Raben, N. (2008). Therapeutic approaches in glycogen storage disease type II/Pompe disease. *Neurotherapeutics* 5, 569–578. doi: 10.1016/j.nurt.2008.08.009

Schoser, B. G., Muller-Hocker, J., Horvath, R., Gempel, K., Pongratz, D., Lochmuller, H., et al. (2007). Adult-onset glycogen storage disease type 2: clinico-pathological phenotype revisited. *Neuropathol. Appl. Neurobiol.* 33, 544–559. doi: 10.1111/j.1365-2990.2007.00839.x

Schuller, A., Wenninger, S., Strigl-Pill, N., and Schoser, B. (2012). Toward deconstructing the phenotype of late-onset Pompe disease. *Am. J. Med. Genet. C Semin. Med. Genet.* 160C, 80–88. doi: 10.1002/ajmg.c.31322

Seppala, E. H., Reuser, A. J., and Lohi, H. (2013). A nonsense mutation in the acid alpha-glucosidase gene causes Pompe disease in Finnish and Swedish Lapphunds. *PLoS One* 8:e56825. doi: 10.1371/journal.pone.0056825

Settembre, C., and Ballabio, A. (2011). TFEB regulates autophagy: an integrated coordination of cellular degradation and recycling processes. *Autophagy* 7, 1379–1381. doi: 10.4161/auto.7.11.17166

Settembre, C., and Ballabio, A. (2014). Lysosomal adaptation: how the lysosome responds to external cues. *Cold Spring Harb. Perspect. Biol.* 6:a016907. doi: 10.1101/cshperspect.a016907

Settembre, C., Di Malta, C., Polito, V. A., Garcia Arencibia, M., Vetrini, F., Erdin, S., et al. (2011). TFEB links autophagy to lysosomal biogenesis. *Science* 332, 1429–1433. doi: 10.1126/science.1204592

Settembre, C., Zoncu, R., Medina, D. L., Vetrini, F., Erdin, S., Huynh, T., et al. (2012). A lysosome-to-nucleus signalling mechanism senses and regulates the lysosome via mTOR and TFEB. *EMBO J.* 31, 1095–1108. doi: 10.1038/emboj.2012.32

Sharma, M. C., Schultze, C., Von Moers, A., Stoltenburg-Didinger, G., Shin, Y. S., Podskarbi, T., et al. (2005). Delayed or late-onset type II glycogenosis with globular inclusions. *Acta Neuropathol.* 110, 151–157. doi: 10.1007/s00401-005-1026-4

Shea, L., and Raben, N. (2009). Autophagy in skeletal muscle: implications for Pompe disease. *Int. J. Clin. Pharmacol. Ther.* 47(Suppl. 1), S42–S47. doi: 10.5414/cpp47042

Shieh, J. J., and Lin, C. Y. (1998). Frequent mutation in Chinese patients with infantile type of GSD II in Taiwan: evidence for a founder effect. *Hum. Mutat.* 11, 306–312. doi: 10.1002/(sici)1098-1004(1998)11:4<306::aid-humu8>3.3.co;2-j

Slonim, A. E., Bulone, L., Ritz, S., Goldberg, T., Chen, A., and Martiniuk, F. (2000). Identification of two subtypes of infantile acid maltase deficiency. *J. Pediatr.* 137, 283–285. doi: 10.1067/mpd.2000.107112

Smith, B. K., Collins, S. W., Conlon, T. J., Mah, C. S., Lawson, L. A., Martin, A. D., et al. (2013). Phase I/II trial of adeno-associated virus-mediated alpha-glucosidase gene therapy to the diaphragm for chronic respiratory failure in Pompe disease: initial safety and ventilatory outcomes. *Hum. Gene Ther.* 24, 630–640. doi: 10.1089/hum.2012.250

Spampanato, C., Feeney, E., Li, L., Cardone, M., Lim, J. A., Annunziata, F., et al. (2013). Transcription factor EB (TFEB) is a new therapeutic target for Pompe disease. *EMBO Mol. Med.* 5, 691–706. doi: 10.1002/emmm.201202176

Strothotte, S., Strigl-Pill, N., Grunert, B., Kornblum, C., Eger, K., Wessig, C., et al. (2010). Enzyme replacement therapy with alglucosidase alfa in 44 patients with late-onset glycogen storage disease type 2: 12-month results of an observational clinical trial. *J. Neurol.* 257, 91–97. doi: 10.1007/s00415-009-5275-3

Sukigara, S., Liang, W. C., Komaki, H., Fukuda, T., Miyamoto, T., Saito, T., et al. (2012). Muscle glycogen storage disease 0 presenting recurrent syncope with weakness and myalgia. *Neuromuscul. Disord.* 22, 162–165. doi: 10.1016/j.nmd.2011.08.008

Takikita, S., Schreiner, C., Baum, R., Xie, T., Ralston, E., Plotz, P. H., et al. (2010). Fiber type conversion by PGC-1alpha activates lysosomal and autophagosomal biogenesis in both unaffected and Pompe skeletal muscle. *PLoS One* 5:e15239. doi: 10.1371/journal.pone.0015239

Terman, A., and Brunk, U. T. (2006). Oxidative stress, accumulation of biological 'garbage' and aging. *Antioxid. Redox Signal.* 8, 197–204. doi: 10.1089/ars.2006.8.197

Terman, A., Gustafsson, B., and Brunk, U. T. (2006). The lysosomal-mitochondrial axis theory of postmitotic aging and cell death. *Chem. Biol. Interact.* 163, 29–37. doi: 10.1016/j.cbi.2006.04.013

Terman, A., Kurz, T., Navratil, M., Arriaga, E. A., and Brunk, U. T. (2010). Mitochondrial turnover and aging of long-lived postmitotic cells: the mitochondrial-lysosomal axis theory of aging. *Antioxid. Redox Signal.* 12, 503–535. doi: 10.1089/ars.2009.2598

Thurberg, B. L., Lynch, M. C., Vaccaro, C., Afonso, K., Tsai, A. C., Bossen, E., et al. (2006). Characterization of pre- and post-treatment pathology after enzyme replacement therapy for pompe disease. *Lab. Invest.* 86, 1208–1220. doi: 10.1038/labinvest.3700484

Tiels, P., Baranova, E., Piens, K., De Visscher, C., Pynaert, G., Nerinckx, W., et al. (2012). A bacterial glycosidase enables mannose-6-phosphate modification and improved cellular uptake of yeast-produced recombinant human lysosomal enzymes. *Nat. Biotechnol.* 30, 1225–1231. doi: 10.1038/nbt.2427

Tsuburaya, R. S., Monma, K., Oya, Y., Nakayama, T., Fukuda, T., Sugie, H., et al. (2012). Acid phosphatase-positive globular inclusions is a good diagnostic marker for two patients with adult-onset Pompe disease lacking disease specific pathology. *Neuromuscul. Disord.* 22, 389–393. doi: 10.1016/j.nmd.2011.11.003

van den Hout, H. M., Hop, W., van Diggelen, O. P., Smeitink, J. A., Smit, G. P., Poll-The, B. T., et al. (2003). The natural course of infantile Pompe's disease: 20 original cases compared with 133 cases from the literature. *Pediatrics* 112, 332–340. doi: 10.1542/peds.112.2.332

Van den Hout, J. M., Kamphoven, J. H., Winkel, L. P., Arts, W. F., De Klerk, J. B., Loonen, M. C., et al. (2004). Long-term intravenous treatment of Pompe disease with recombinant human alpha-glucosidase from milk. *Pediatrics* 113, e448–e457. doi: 10.1542/peds.113.5.e448

Van der Ploeg, A. T., Clemens, P. R., Corzo, D., Escolar, D. M., Florence, J., Groeneveld, G. J., et al. (2010). A randomized study of alglucosidase alfa in late-onset Pompe's disease. *N. Engl. J. Med.* 362, 1396–1406. doi: 10.1056/NEJMoa0909859

Walkley, S. U. (2008). "Pathogenesis of CNS disease in lysosomal storage disorders," in *10th International Symposium on Mucopolysaccharide and Related Diseases* (Vancouver, Canada).

Wisselaar, H. A., Kroos, M. A., Hermans, M. M., van Beeumen, J., and Reuser, A. J. (1993). Structural and functional changes of lysosomal acid alpha-glucosidase during intracellular transport and maturation. *J. Biol. Chem.* 268, 2223–2231.

Wu, J. J., Quijano, C., Chen, E., Liu, H., Cao, L., Fergusson, M. M., et al. (2009). Mitochondrial dysfunction and oxidative stress mediate the physiological impairment induced by the disruption of autophagy. *Aging (Albany NY)* 1, 425–437.

Xu, F., Ding, E., Liao, S. X., Migone, F., Dai, J., Schneider, A., et al. (2004). Improved efficacy of gene therapy approaches for Pompe disease using a new, immune-deficient GSD-II mouse model. *Gene Ther.* 11, 1590–1598. doi: 10.1038/sj.gt.3302314

Yang, Z., and Klionsky, D. J. (2010). Mammalian autophagy: core molecular machinery and signaling regulation. *Curr. Opin. Cell Biol.* 22, 124–131. doi: 10.1016/j.ceb.2009.11.014

Zhu, Y., Jiang, J. L., Gumlaw, N. K., Zhang, J., Bercury, S. D., Ziegler, R. J., et al. (2009). Glycoengineered acid alpha-glucosidase with improved efficacy at correcting the metabolic aberrations and motor function deficits in a mouse model of Pompe disease. *Mol. Ther.* 17, 954–963. doi: 10.1038/mt.2009.37

Zoncu, R., Bar-Peled, L., Efeyan, A., Wang, S., Sancak, Y., and Sabatini, D. M. (2011). mTORC1 senses lysosomal amino acids through an inside-out mechanism that requires the vacuolar H(+)-ATPase. *Science* 334, 678–683. doi: 10.1126/science.1207056

19

Regulation of satellite cell function in sarcopenia

Stephen E. Alway[1,2,3]*, Matthew J. Myers[1] and Junaith S. Mohamed[1]

[1] Laboratory of Muscle Biology and Sarcopenia, Department of Exercise Physiology, West Virginia University School of Medicine, Morgantown, WV, USA
[2] West Virginia Clinical and Translational Science Institute, Morgantown, WV, USA
[3] Center for Cardiovascular and Respiratory Sciences, Morgantown, WV, USA

***Correspondence:**
Stephen E. Alway, Laboratory of Muscle Biology and Sarcopenia, Department of Exercise Physiology, Robert C Byrd Health Sciences Center, West Virginia University School of Medicine, 1 Medical Center Drive, P.O. Box. 9227, Morgantown, WV 26506, USA
e-mail: salway@hsc.wvu.edu

The mechanisms contributing to sarcopenia include reduced satellite cell (myogenic stem cell) function that is impacted by the environment (niche) of these cells. Satellite cell function is affected by oxidative stress, which is elevated in aged muscles, and this along with changes in largely unknown systemic factors, likely contribute to the manner in which satellite cells respond to stressors such as exercise, disuse, or rehabilitation in sarcopenic muscles. Nutritional intervention provides one therapeutic strategy to improve the satellite cell niche and systemic factors, with the goal of improving satellite cell function in aging muscles. Although many elderly persons consume various nutraceuticals with the hope of improving health, most of these compounds have not been thoroughly tested, and the impacts that they might have on sarcopenia and satellite cell function are not clear. This review discusses data pertaining to the satellite cell responses and function in aging skeletal muscle, and the impact that three compounds: resveratrol, green tea catechins, and β-Hydroxy-β-methylbutyrate have on regulating satellite cell function and therefore contributing to reducing sarcopenia or improving muscle mass after disuse in aging. The data suggest that these nutraceutical compounds improve satellite cell function during rehabilitative loading in animal models of aging after disuse (i.e., muscle regeneration). While these compounds have not been rigorously tested in humans, the data from animal models of aging provide a strong basis for conducting additional focused work to determine if these or other nutraceuticals can offset the muscle losses, or improve regeneration in sarcopenic muscles of older humans via improving satellite cell function.

Keywords: aging, oxidative stress, apoptosis, rehabilitation, injury, disuse atrophy

INTRODUCTION

Sarcopenia is the age-associated reduction in muscle mass and function (Evans, 1995; Kim and Choi, 2013), which is particularly severe after the seventh decade of life (Dutta et al., 1997). Sarcopenia increases the susceptibility to muscle injury (Faulkner et al., 1995), serious falls (Tinetti, 2001), obesity (Stenholm et al., 2008), and diabetes (Kim et al., 2010; Ghosh et al., 2014). Furthermore, the deleterious effects of extended muscle disuse (e.g., prolonged bed rest in the elderly) on muscle mass, strength, and function is exacerbated with sarcopenia (Suetta et al., 2009; Marzetti et al., 2010; Hao et al., 2011; Calvani et al., 2013; Alway et al., 2014a). As a result, it is important to identify strategies that could slow or reverse sarcopenia. One area that has attracted recent attention is the area of myogenic stem cells or satellite cells, as a means to improve regeneration of old muscles and to offset the negative consequences of sarcopenia.

MECHANISMS THAT MAY CONTRIBUTE TO SARCOPENIA AND LOWER THE ABILITY TO REVERSE ATROPHY IN AGING

To mount an effective therapeutic strategy to treat sarcopenia, it becomes necessary to understand the components that contribute to this pathogenesis. While the mechanisms responsible for sarcopenia are not well understood, there are likely several factors that contribute to muscle loss in aging. These include but may not be limited to: reduced protein synthesis (Dickinson et al., 2013; Churchward-Venne et al., 2014), declines in neural function (Drey et al., 2013; Kwan, 2013; Mosole et al., 2014), hormonal deficits (Michalakis et al., 2013), chronic inflammation (Lee et al., 2007; Degens, 2010; Mavros et al., 2014), oxidative stress (Hiona and Leeuwenburgh, 2008; Jackson et al., 2010; Armand et al., 2011; Marzetti et al., 2013; Sullivan-Gunn and Lewandowski, 2013), loss of mitochondrial function (Chabi et al., 2008; Ljubicic et al., 2009; Calvani et al., 2013; Marzetti et al., 2013), inappropriate signaling in muscle due at least in part to inadequate nutrition (Burgos, 2012; Ghosh et al., 2014; Welch, 2014; Welch et al., 2014), nuclear apoptosis (Sjostrom et al., 1992; Alway et al., 2002, 2011; Leeuwenburgh, 2003; Dupont-Versteegden, 2005; Alway and Siu, 2008; Chabi et al., 2008), and reduced satellite cell function (Conboy and Rando, 2005; Snijders et al., 2009; Barberi et al., 2013). This review will focus on the potential impact that mediation of satellite cell function has in aging skeletal muscle.

SATELLITE CELL BIOLOGY

Satellite cells are a heterogeneous collection of adult muscle stem cells that are normally quiescent. They were first identified more than 50 years ago as a unique population of nuclei that were "sandwiched" between the sarcolemma and the basement membrane of the muscle fiber (Mauro, 1961). Utilization of unique cell surface markers and methods to identify satellite cell proliferation and differentiation have provided evidence to show that this cell is critically important in muscle growth and repair as well as the processes of adaptation to stresses including exercise, disease, injury, and aging. Satellite cell progression from proliferation through differentiation of their daughter cells is tightly regulated by muscle transcription factors. Adult quiescent satellite cells express the paired homeobox transcription factor Pax7 (Seale et al., 2000, 2004). Another transcription factor, Pax3, a paralog of Pax7, is also expressed in a subset of satellite cells of some but not all muscles (Relaix et al., 2006; Buckingham and Relaix, 2007; Day et al., 2007; Yablonka-Reuveni et al., 2008). Nevertheless, Pax7 appears to be necessary in satellite cells after birth as Pax7-null mice are viable but lack any functional satellite cells (Kuang et al., 2006; Seale et al., 2000; Seale et al., 2004).

Under basal conditions, adult satellite cells remain quiescent and reside (relatively) dormant within their niche adjacent to the myofiber (Schultz et al., 1978) (**Figure 1**). While satellite cells might be exposed to the changing cellular niche, they do not become activated until a major insult or stress (e.g., exercise loading) occurs. In response to injury, satellite cells proliferate and their Pax7-positive daughter cells either differentiate, by migrating through the sarcolemma and fusing with existing muscle fibers (**Figure 1**) during the growth and regeneration of muscle (Moss and Leblond, 1971; von et al., 2013), or they commit to a program of self-renew (Schmalbruch and Lewis, 2000; Collins et al., 2005). Myogenic regulator factor (MRF) genes provide myogenic specificity for activated satellite cells. The MRFs include myogenic differentiation 1 protein (MyoD), myogenic factor 5 (Myf5), myogenin, and muscle-specific regulatory factor 4 (Mrf4). Myf5 and/or MyoD expression are quickly increased at the point of satellite cell activation (Cornelison and Wold, 1997). Pax7 regulates Myf5 and MyoD expression levels (Parise et al., 2008; Rudnicki et al., 2008) in satellite cells. It is necessary for Pax7 to be down-regulated prior to terminal differentiation of the satellite cell derived daughter cells (Olguin and Olwin, 2004; Olguin et al., 2007). The satellite cell pool is repopulated by the fraction of activated satellite cells that maintain a high level of Pax7.

A number of studies using different Pax7 ablation strategies in mouse muscles, have clearly shown that satellite cells are indispensable for muscle regeneration (Lepper et al., 2011; Murphy et al., 2011; Sambasivan et al., 2011). Furthermore, when satellite cells are absent, injured skeletal muscle does not regenerate or regenerate very poorly in response to muscle injury (Seale and Rudnicki, 2000; Seale et al., 2000; Oustanina et al., 2004; Kuang et al., 2006). To make it worse, inflammatory and adipogenic cells replace injured regions of contractile tissue in muscles from Pax7-null animals (Sambasivan et al., 2011), and the increase in non-contractile tissue in repair or growth in the absence of Pax7 decreases the specific tension (force per cross sectional area) potential in skeletal muscle (Fry et al., 2014). It is also important to note that non-myogenic stem cells are unable to repair the injured muscle, suggesting that satellite cells are essential for skeletal muscle regeneration (Sambasivan et al., 2011). Furthermore, while some muscle hypertrophy that is induced via overload appears possible in the absence of

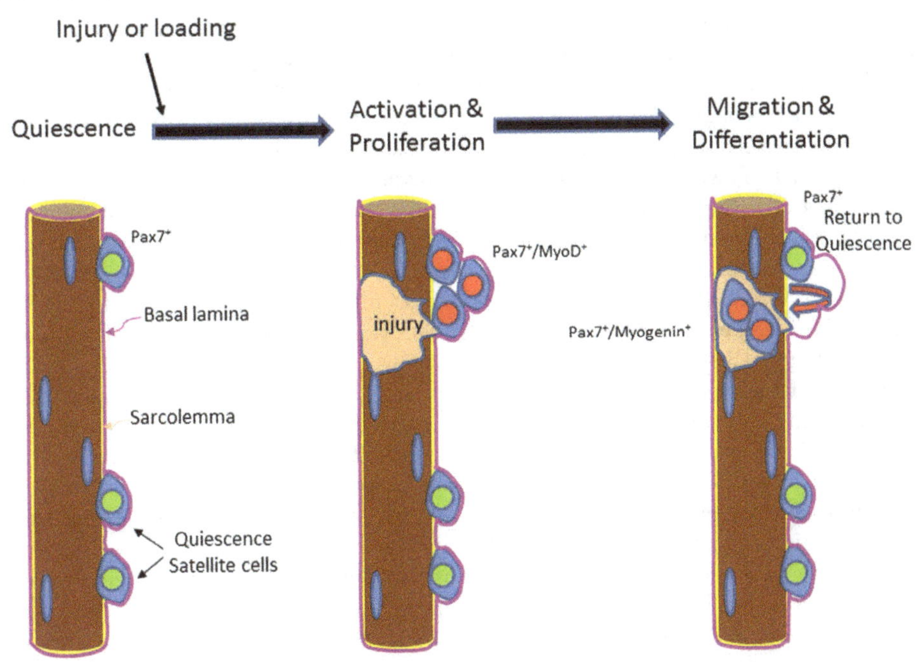

FIGURE 1 | Illustration of the activation and the differentiation of satellite cells in muscles of young or old hosts. Satellite cells are positioned anatomically between the basal lamina (purple) and the sarcolemma (yellow). Satellite cells express Pax7 in the quiescent (green) state. Upon injury or loading, satellite cells are activated and proliferate (red) and express Pax7 followed by both Pax7 and MyoD. Some of the proliferated daughter cells from the original satellite cells leave their position and pass through the sarcolemma and migrate to the site of injury, where they fuse with the existing fiber and engage in fiber repair and/or contribute to fiber growth/hypertrophy. In aging and sarcopenic muscles, satellite cell proliferation and/or differentiation may be impaired, which contribute to a lower regenerative potential.

satellite cells, long-term muscle adaptation to overload is diminished, as seen by smaller muscle fibers and a lower muscle mass and muscle strength. Thus, satellite cells are important not only in muscle repair but also in regulating muscle adaptations to hypertrophic growth (Fry et al., 2014). Thus, it is possible, or even likely that a diminished function in satellite cells plays an important role in mediating the long-term muscle reductions with sarcopenia.

SATELLITE CELL FUNCTION IN AGING

The potential mechanisms involved in the reduction of skeletal muscle mass during sarcopenia converge on satellite cells, and together they contribute to failure of satellite cells to replace and repair damaged muscle fibers (Jang et al., 2011; Garcia-Prat et al., 2013; Wang et al., 2013; Sousa-Victor et al., 2014). The lower regenerative potential of aged muscles is correlated nicely with the decline in satellite cell function (Jang et al., 2011; Chakkalakal and Brack, 2012; Collins-Hooper et al., 2012; Bernet et al., 2014) and a reduction in the Pax7 pool of myogenic stem cells (Collins et al., 2007). For example, the proliferation and differentiation potentials of satellite cells in both mammals and non-mammals are reduced with increasing age (Bortoli et al., 2005; Velleman et al., 2010; Barberi et al., 2013; Harthan et al., 2013). In addition, recent evidence by Sousa-Victor et al. (2014) suggest that a large portion of the aged (geriatric) satellite cells switch from the reversible quiescent state to a senescence state, which prevents proliferation and renewal of the satellite cell pool. Thus, this loss of satellite cell function likely contributes strongly to the reduced ability to repair or replace muscle that is lost in sarcopenia. Although satellite cells in the aged niche are not proliferative, they do express Sprouty1 (*spry1*), an inhibitor of fibroblast growth factor (FGF) signaling (Chakkalakal et al., 2012). It is thought that increasing FGF signaling in aged satellite cells under basal conditions by down regulating *spry1* would result in a loss of quiescence (Chakkalakal et al., 2012). Thus, aged satellite cells may actively promote quiescence through regulating *spry1* in their own niche, thereby making it more difficult to activate these cells for growth or repair.

Moreover, satellite cell content has been reported to decrease in muscles of old humans and animals as compared to their younger counter parts (Day et al., 2010; Verdijk et al., 2012, 2014). Furthermore, there is evidence that a decline in satellite cell number contributes to muscle fiber atrophy (Brack et al., 2005). Nevertheless, some studies have not found a loss of satellite cells in old muscles as compared to muscles from young animals (van der Meer et al., 2011b), but this is complicated by the fact that although muscle mass/bodyweight was lower in the old animals, the absolute muscle mass was similar in young and old animals.

Whether satellite cell number is lost or not, it appears more clear that satellite cell function is reduced in aging. However, it is likely that an important cause for reduced satellite cell function in aging may be a result of altered systemic factors that influence and/or regulate satellite cell activity and differentiation. Notably, important observations from Rando and colleagues using parabiotic pairs have shown that the regenerative potential of satellite cells can be improved in muscles from aged mice that share the circulation with young mice (Conboy and Rando, 2005; Conboy et al., 2005). Reductions in Notch signaling in muscles of aged rodents lead to a reduced satellite cell proliferation and an inability to produce myoblasts in response to muscle injury. In addition, restoring circulating levels of protein growth differentiation factor 11 (GDF11) in old mice has recently been shown to improve satellite cell and muscle function (Sinha et al., 2014). Other factors contributing to sarcopenia potentially through their actions on satellite cells could involve reduced IGF-I (Harridge, 2003), inflammation and pro-inflammatory cytokines (Degens, 2010), and altered muscle metabolism (Jang et al., 2011).

Although satellite cells appear to have important roles in regeneration of old or young muscles, their involvement in regulating muscle mass in response to atrophic or hypertrophic stimuli is quite complex. For example, rapid muscle loss occurring from denervation has been reported to result in a transient increase in satellite cells in muscles of old rats within 1 week after denervation (van der Meer et al., 2011b), presumably in an attempt to improve the transcriptional control of muscle proteins during this rapid period of atrophy. However, satellite cell numbers then decreased in old muscle in subsequent denervation from 2 to 4 weeks (although satellite cells/muscle cross sectional area were constant during this time) (van der Meer et al., 2011b). In contrast, muscles in young animals had an increase in satellite cell numbers over 4 weeks of denervation (van der Meer et al., 2011b), yet the increase in satellite cell numbers was unable to prevent muscle atrophy (van der Meer et al., 2011b). Clearly, there are age-induced differences in the responses of satellite cells to this atrophy stimulus by denervation, yet simply having the potential for greater transcriptional control by having more satellite cells and their daughter cells, fails to prevent the rapid muscle fiber atrophy caused by denervation.

The role that satellite cell number has in muscle growth is also complex. For example, there is evidence that at least some degree of hypertrophy can occur without the prerequisite to activate satellite cells to add new nuclei (McCarthy et al., 2011; van der Meer et al., 2011a; Jackson et al., 2012); however, larger fibers in old muscles appear to add more nuclei than smaller fibers in young animals to maintain a relatively constant nuclear domain size (van der Meer et al., 2011b), and more nuclei improve the potential for greater transcriptional control to presumably sustain their new larger muscle fiber size (Carson and Alway, 1996; Alway et al., 2003; van der Meer et al., 2011a). In addition, the extent of hypertrophy is suppressed in models where satellite cells are absent (Fry et al., 2014). Thus, satellite cells may have an important role in long-term modulating of muscle fiber size, but at least in some models of muscle wasting, increases in myonuclear number does not guarantee greater fiber sizes in denervation, and losses in satellite cells over time, follows, and does not determine, the reductions in muscle fiber size (van der Meer et al., 2011a,b). Nevertheless, it is clear that hypertrophic adaptations are suppressed when satellite cells are eliminated, and therefore, it is likely that satellite cells have a complex modulating effect on muscle mass, and in doing so, impacts muscle function. In addition, we would expect that loss of satellite cells or reduced satellite cell function by whatever means, would diminish the ability for aging muscle to both hypertrophy in response to a growth stimulus, and repair in response to an injury. Clearly, this area requires more work to fully understand the complex nature and responses of satellite cells in muscle remodeling in aging.

MODULATORS OF SATELLITE CELLS IN SARCOPENIA

METABOLIC REGULATION OF SATELLITE CELL FUNCTION

Metabolic regulators of the satellite cell niche are likely to be important modulators of satellite cell function. One potential mediator is Sirtuin 1 (Sirt1), a NAD^+ deacetylase that is activated by caloric restriction (Cohen et al., 2004) and resveratrol (Chen et al., 2009; Price et al., 2012), a compound found in abundance in grape skins and red wine. Sirt1 also works in concert with a number of transcription factors to exert a mostly catabolic effect in cellular metabolism. One subset of these activated transcription factors is the peroxisome proliferator-activated receptor (PPAR) family (Lin et al., 2005), including PPAR γ co-activator 1α (PGC1α). PGC1α is a transcriptional co-activator and a major regulator of mitochondrial biogenesis and metabolism (Spiegelman, 2007; Stepto et al., 2012). In muscle and other cell types, PGC1α regulates the activity of PPAR alpha (PPARα) and PPAR delta (PPARδ). PPARα, is expressed in the heart, liver, and skeletal muscle, regulates mitochondrial biogenesis and fatty acid uptake and oxidation. PPARδ is expressed in the intestines, liver, and skeletal muscle but notably, experiments that have eliminated PPARδ in muscle, have reported a decreased level of satellite cell proliferation, leading to reduced muscle regenerative capacity after injury, further establishing its link to satellite cell function (Angione et al., 2011). PGC1α induced mitochondrial biogenesis appears to be an important component that regulates satellite cell function in regenerating muscle following injury (Duguez et al., 2002). Supporting this finding, short-term caloric restriction has been found to increase satellite cell proliferation in young and old mice, presumably through a Sirt1-PGC1α mechanism (Cerletti et al., 2012). Furthermore, alterations in PGC1α through Sirt1 have been shown to reduce satellite cell-induced muscle regeneration during conditions of muscle wasting (Toledo et al., 2011). Thus, there appears to be a clear link between mitochondrial biogenesis/function and satellite cell function, and increasing mitochondrial function increases satellite cell proliferation in muscle regeneration (Jash and Adhya, 2012). However, the mechanisms that mediate this interaction are less clear and the impact that altering mitochondrial-mediated metabolic function will have on satellite cell function in muscles of old animals is less well known. Furthermore, it is not known if mitochondrially induced satellite cell modulation is fiber-type specific in aged muscles.

MITOCHONDRIAL FUNCTION AND OXIDATIVE STRESS REGULATE SATELLITE CELL FUNCTION IN AGING

In addition to metabolic function, mitochondria are key producers of reactive oxygen species (ROS). A low level of ROS is thought to be an important regulator of several cell signal transduction pathways in a variety of cellular functions including muscle (Frey et al., 2006, 2009; Powers et al., 2011). However, excessive ROS levels are believed to be key initiators and mediators of dysfunction in a variety of cells including muscle cells. This includes ROS mediated disruptions in cell signaling, metabolism, transcriptional activity, mitochondrial function, and increased activation of apoptotic pathways (Allen and Tresini, 2000; Marzetti et al., 2013; Sullivan-Gunn and Lewandowski, 2013). For example, aging is associated with excessive ROS levels, which increases mitochondrial damage, and in turn, contributes to mitochondrially mediated apoptotic signaling (Barberi et al., 2013; Bennett et al., 2013; Szczesny et al., 2013; Vasilaki and Jackson, 2013). This suggests that mitochondria might produce high ROS levels in muscle and in activated satellite cells, and this could contribute to impaired satellite cell function (or initiate pathways that could result in satellite cell death). However, this relationship is complex because human muscle satellite cells that were isolated from elderly human vastus lateralis muscles have reduced mitochondrial mass, and lower whole cell ATP levels, but when they were stimulated maximally, they appeared to have normal mitochondrial ATP production, increased mitochondrial membrane potential, and increased superoxide/mitochondrial mass and hydrogen peroxide/mitochondrial mass ratios (Minet and Gaster, 2012). These data suggest that although ROS production was higher in isolated satellite cells from aged muscles, there was not a marked reduction in mitochondrial function of the remaining mitochondria (Minet and Gaster, 2012). Nevertheless, the high basal levels of ROS may provide an unfavorable environment, which can adversely affect satellite cell function and limit muscle repair in aging. One of the possible causes that could exacerbate the effects of ROS on satellite cell function is the decline the antioxidative capacity and the increasing ROS levels of skeletal muscle with increasing age, which diminish satellite cell function (Beccafico et al., 2007). Moreover, the antioxidant activity of catalase and glutathione transferase is reduced in satellite cells derived from elderly subjects as compared to satellite cells isolated from young individuals (Fulle et al., 2005). It is likely that the elevated basal levels of ROS in the satellite cell niche could induce oxidative damage to the quiescent satellite cells, and this damage could negatively affect the satellite cells' ability to repair aging muscle when they become activated (Fulle et al., 2005).

An alternative negative effect of high ROS levels in aging muscles may be to drive the normal myogenic phenotype of activated satellite cells to that of an adipogenic phenotype. Such a muscle-to-fat transition and satellite cell behavior could explain the increase in inter-muscular adipose deposits that are characterized with many metabolic diseases as well as sarcopenia (Rice et al., 1989; Vettor et al., 2009).

EXERCISE REGULATION OF SATELLITE CELLS IN AGING MUSCLE

Although exercise or loading can partially rescue the reduction in satellite cell function (Dreyer et al., 2006; Snijders et al., 2009; Verdijk et al., 2009; Shefer et al., 2010), muscle fibers typically do not hypertrophy to the same extent in old animals as compared to young animals, even if the young and old animals receive the same stimulus and this is at least partially attributable to aging-suppressed satellite cell function (Carson et al., 1995; Carson and Alway, 1996; Lowe et al., 1998; Cutlip et al., 2006). Thus, while full reversal of sarcopenia does not appear to be possible, exercise, and overload nevertheless, have been used as a rehabilitative tool to compensate for sarcopenia, and can at least partially reverse the age-imposed decrements in performance. Nevertheless, experiments that have examined the exercise- and loading-associated reduction in muscle mass function in humans, rats, and other animal models of aging, have produced varied results from modest to poor reversal of sarcopenia. For example, 30 days of identical loading conditions resulted in 44% greater muscle mass in young-adult birds, but only an increase in muscle mass of 25% in aged quails (Carson and Alway, 1996). In addition, 14 days of functional overload in the rat plantaris muscle increases muscle weight by 25% in young-adult animals but only by 9% in old rats (Alway et al., 2002, 2005). Furthermore, 28 days of electrical stimulation-induced contractions caused muscle hypertrophy and improved function in young rat dorsi flexor muscles, but no improvement in muscle force or mass were found in old animals (Cutlip et al., 2006; Murlasits et al., 2006).

It is clear that loading types of exercise have profound effects on satellite cell function in muscles of young hosts, largely through activation of various growth factors and cytokines, resulting in increases in muscle protein synthesis, and net muscle protein accretion (Phillips et al., 1997). Furthermore, activation of satellite cells occurs as part of the modulation of exercise-induced adaptation even in acute responses to loading exercise where hypertrophy has not occurred (Joanisse et al., 2013). Specifically, growth factors such as insulin like growth factor-I (IGF-1) (McKay et al., 2008), interleukin-6 (IL-6) cytokine induced signal transducer, and activator of transcription 3 (STAT3) signaling have been shown to occur exclusively in human satellite cells, including their proliferation in response to exercise-induced lengthening injury (Toth et al., 2011). Furthermore, non-injurious running exercise has been shown to increase Wnt signaling and that activation of the canonical Wnt/β-catenin signaling pathway increased the expression of Myf5 and MyoD in satellite cells (Fujimaki et al., 2014). However, given the greater senescent phenotype of satellite cells in aged muscles (Sousa-Victor et al., 2014), it seems likely that exercise would have a greater challenge for activating satellite cells in aged sarcopenic muscles as compared to young-adult muscles. Nevertheless, while aging decreases the satellite cell content in type II fibers of humans (Verdijk et al., 2014), aging appears to delay but not eliminate the activation of satellite cells in muscles of elderly men in response to acute resistance exercise (Snijders et al., 2014a; Verdijk et al., 2014).

While an age-associated reduction in growth differentiation factor 11 (GDF11) has been shown, a recent report indicates that restoring systemic levels of GDF11 in aged muscle improved not only satellite cell derived muscle repair but increased muscle strength, mass, and endurance in aged mice (Sinha et al., 2014). This shows the potential for important interactions between circulating factors and exercise-induced satellite cell function; however, it would seem that exercise alone, without the pharmacological intervention and interaction is insufficient to reverse all of the aging-associated satellite cell function in sarcopenia. Although electrically evoked contractions are not exact duplications of voluntary exercise, most of the cellular signaling pathways are similar whether the contractions are voluntary or evoked. Thus, it is interesting to note that electrically evoked contractions in muscles of elderly subjects, increased the proliferation of satellite cells as indicated by a greater number of N-CAM and Pax7-expressing cells (surface markers of satellite cells), and also increased IGF-I and myostatin, which, were thought to loosely represent markers in the pathway for satellite cell differentiation (Kern et al., 2014). Thus, exercise and models that simulate exercise have profound effects on satellite cell function in aging muscles. One of the challenges in muscle biology is to identify targets and strategies that are likely to maximize the positive benefits of exercise on satellite cell function with the goal to reduce or offset sarcopenia.

DISUSE REDUCES SATELLITE CELL NUMBER IN AGING

Disuse atrophy is caused by mechanical unloading of muscle and this leads to reduced muscle mass. Frequently used models of unloading in humans include casting/immobilization, and a sedentary lifestyle (inactivity), and in rodents, hindlimb suspension, immobilization, and denervation are typically used as models of disuse. Satellite cells are fundamentally involved in skeletal muscle responses to environmental changes that induce atrophy. The area that surrounds the satellite cell (niche) plays an important role in the fate and function of satellite cells (Bentzinger et al., 2013), and therefore, it is not surprising that changes in the muscle environment that occur during disuse can affect the satellite cell niche.

Several studies report that conditions of disuse lead to an elevation in the number of nuclei that have been targeted for apoptosis both inside and outside myofibers (Allen et al., 1997; Vescovo et al., 1998, 2000; Siu and Alway, 2009; Alway et al., 2011; Hao et al., 2011). However, other studies have failed to find a change in myonuclei number with atrophy, and loss of satellite cells during disuse is not a consistent finding. For example, satellite cell number appeared to be quite stable after acute disuse including 14 days of immobilization in young healthy men (Snijders et al., 2014b), or 28 days of bed rest in middle aged men (Brooks et al., 2010), whereas in another study, 14 days of immobilization resulted in a loss of satellite cells in older humans (Suetta et al., 2013). Severe disuse atrophy as characterized by spinal cord injury has been reported to result in lower satellite cell numbers in both type I and type II fibers (Verdijk et al., 2012). Furthermore, sarcopenia is accompanied by a loss of satellite cells, particularly in type II fibers (Verdijk et al., 2012, 2014) although the reductions in both fiber size and satellite cell number occur relatively slowly. In contrast, rapid declines in muscle mass do not correlate closely with satellite cell numbers (van der Meer et al., 2011b). Nevertheless, satellite cells may have an important role in long-term modulating of muscle fiber size including disuse atrophy, and sarcopenia, but there is evidence to suggest that such changes in myonuclear number may not determine the immediate changes in muscle fiber size (van der Meer et al., 2011a,b). Nevertheless, the age of the host and the severity or type of disuse, likely helps to determine whether satellite cells survive, the time course of any changes in satellite cell number, or how they are able to respond to additional stressors.

Although proliferation of satellite cells is critical to muscle regeneration after an injury, proliferation of satellite cells without adequate differentiation does not improve muscle mass. For example, acute satellite cell proliferation has been reported in response to spinal muscular atrophy-induced muscle denervation (Martinez-Hernandez et al., 2014) presumably as an attempt to increase the nuclear population for elevating transcriptional signaling, yet, the atrophy signaling predominates the muscle, and the net result is that denervated muscles become smaller, even with an acute increase in satellite cells. Thus, effective strategies to combat sarcopenia and accelerated muscle loss in aging should evaluate the effects of interventions on both proliferation and differentiation of satellite cells and their daughter cells.

MODULATION OF SATELLITE CELL FUNCTION IN SARCOPENIA VIA NUTRACEUTICALS

It is clear that the nutritional status of a host affects the potential for satellite cell proliferation and differentiation to occur (Halevy et al., 2000; Powell et al., 2013, 2014; Harthan et al., 2014). For example, food restriction in birds post-hatch has been shown to reduce muscle mass accumulation with increased fat deposition and necrosis (Velleman et al., 2010) as a result of a decrease in satellite cell mitotic activity (Mozdziak et al., 2002; Halevy et al., 2003). However, the mechanisms by which nutritional interventions regulate satellite cell function are less well defined. One possibility is that the systemic diffusion of nutritional compounds and nutraceuticals from the blood (presumably diffusion from capillaries throughout the muscle) changes the satellite cell environment or "niche." The area that is enclosed between the basal lamina and sarcolemma of a muscle fiber houses the satellite cell, but this same space provides an insulated environment in which the satellite cell exists (Lander et al., 2012; Bentzinger et al., 2013; Montarras et al., 2013). Presumably this niche maintains the satellite cells in a quiescent state. It is likely that the metabolic milieu of the satellite cell niche differs from the muscle fiber and/or the extracellular space that surrounds the fibers. Although speculative, it is possible that nutraceuticals diffuse from the systemic circulation (i.e., capillaries) and pass through the basal lamina membrane barrier to the satellite cell niche to change its metabolic composition. This idea would be consistent with the hypothesis that satellite cell function can be regulated via changes to the niche environment (Cosgrove et al., 2009; Chakkalakal and Brack, 2012; Chakkalakal et al., 2012; Gilbert et al., 2012). Although it is not clear if the nutraceuticals can directly activate satellite cells to move them from a quiescent to an active state, it is clear that if they have begun a proliferative cycle, that several nutraceuticals can enhance their function in responses to various stimuli superimposed on sarcopenia. However, the evidence suggests that diffusion of the nutraceutical into the satellite cell niche could "prime" the satellite cell, so that once it experienced the appropriate chemical and/or mechanical and/or electrical signals for proliferation, would increase the extent of proliferation in these cells (Hao et al., 2011; Ryan et al., 2011; Alway et al., 2013; Bennett et al., 2013).

It is further feasible that nutraceuticals can act indirectly on satellite cells by modulating or directly suppressing the effects of ROS, or increasing antioxidant production. Either of these possibilities would result in lowering the impact of ROS damage on satellite cells.

Another possibility is that rather than affecting the satellite cell niche, the nutraceutical modulates satellite cell behavior after these cells have left their niche, or perhaps the niche environment is lost because the basal lamina or sarcolemma has been damaged. In this scenario, the cellular milieu containing the nutraceutical mixes with the satellite cell niche and then promotes enhanced proliferation of activated satellite cells. Again this could occur from a direct effect on satellite cells (e.g., epigenetic changes to satellite cells) and/or indirectly via suppressing the effects of ROS on satellite cells. Future studies are required to determine which nutritional interventions change the contents of the satellite cell niche, or if rather, the nutraceuticals have a direct effect on satellite cells that is independent from the niche environment.

In addition to the local satellite cell niche milieu, satellite cell function appears to have an interaction with the fiber that it is attached to. There are more satellite cells that are associated with fibers that are predominantly oxidative (slow, type I fibers), as compared with fibers that rely primarily on glycolysis (fast, type II fibers) (Schmalbruch and Hellhammer, 1977; Putman et al., 2001; Brack et al., 2005; Christov et al., 2007). Nutraceuticals may have differential effects on satellite cells in predominately type II vs. type I fibers. For example, proliferation of satellite cells was increased in plantaris (predominately type II fibers) muscles from old rats that were reloaded after hindlimb suspension following treatment with HMB (Alway et al., 2013) or EGCg (Alway et al., 2014a), whereas satellite cells were elevated in both plantaris and soleus (predominately type I fibers) muscles of old rats that were treated with green tea extract under these conditions (Alway et al., 2014b). As nutraceutical treatments do not appear to have a marked impact on slowing accelerated muscle wasting in sarcopenia (**Table 1**), but instead appears to be more effective in rehabilitating muscles after a period of disuse (**Table 2**), we suspect that this treatment strategy modulates and does not activate the satellite cells, as we would not anticipate a high level of satellite cell proliferation during periods of long-term disuse.

It is not known if the nutraceutical mediated improvement in satellite cell proliferation especially during rehabilitative efforts in sarcopenic muscle, was due to direct signaling from the fiber to the satellite cell niche or the satellite cells themselves, and it is not known how the satellite cell niche, fiber type, or extracellular matrix signaling might influence satellite cell function in response to skeletal muscle regeneration or hypertrophic growth in sarcopenic muscles from old hosts. These questions should be the focus of future studies as this information will be helpful in planning strategies that might improve muscle repair and slow the progression of sarcopenia. Furthermore, understanding the effect of nutraceuticals on satellite cells in a fiber-type specific fashion is important, because the satellite cells in fast muscles appear to be more vulnerable to dysfunction in aging and show a reduction in total satellite cell numbers (Verdijk et al., 2007, 2014) as compared to satellite cells associated with type I fibers. Nevertheless, while slow oxidative muscles seem to be better preserved than the fast fibers in sarcopenic muscles (Deschenes et al., 2013; Purves-Smith et al., 2014), the impact of nutraceuticals on type I fiber associated satellite cells should not be ignored, because this preservation of type I fiber size and function might be lost in the very old, when sarcopenia becomes very severe (Purves-Smith et al., 2014).

RESVERATROL

Resveratrol and satellite cell function

Within the past decade, sirtuin 1 (Sirt1), a NAD^+ dependent deacetylase, has been identified as an important metabolic regulator of skeletal muscle gene expression (Fulco et al., 2003). Specifically, elevated Sirt1 activity has been shown to increase proliferation of satellite cells (Rathbone et al., 2009). Furthermore, Sirt1 has been reported to inhibit the differentiation of mouse C2C12 myoblasts (an *in vitro* model of activated satellite cells), and reduce the expression of myogenin an important regulator for satellite cell (daughter cell) differentiation (Fulco et al., 2003; Vinciguerra et al., 2010). This suggests that Sirt1 could have a role

Table 1 | Summary of nutraceutical effect on apoptosis and muscle function in aging muscle during forced disuse.

Nutraceutical	Treatment	Apoptotic signaling	Fiber area	Muscle mass	Maximal force	Reference
HMB	HLS	↓ (100–600%)	↑ (22%)	→	→	Hao et al. (2011)
EGCg	HLS	↓ (25–30%)	↑ (21%)	→	→	Alway et al. (2014a)
Resveratrol	HLS	→	ND	↑ (14%)	↑ (14%)	Jackson et al. (2010)
Resveratrol	HLS	→	→	→	ND	Bennett et al. (2013)
Green Tea Catechins	HLS	ND	ND	→	↑ (10%)	Ota et al. (2011)
Green Tea Catechins	HLS		↑ (10%)	↑ (7%)	→	Alway et al. (2014b)

The arrow indicates the increase ($p \leq 0.05$), decrease ($p \leq 0.05$), or no difference ($p \geq 0.05$) between the vehicle vs. nutraceutical. The percent difference from vehicle treatment is indicated in parenthesis.

Table 2 | Summary of nutraceutical effect on satellite cell function, apoptosis and muscle function in growing/regenerating aged muscle.

Nutraceutical	Treatment	Satellite cell proliferation	Apoptotic signaling	Muscle mass	Fiber area	Maximal force	Reference
HMB	Reloading after HLS	↑ (3%)	ND	↑ (6%)	↑ (12%)	→	Alway et al. (2013)
HMB	Reloading after HLS	ND	↓ (70–100%)	↑ (35%)	↑ (55%)	↑ (15%)	Hao et al. (2011)
HMB	Cell culture	↑ (250%)	↓ (30–70%)	ND	ND	ND	Kornasio et al. (2009)
EGCg	Reloading after HLS	↑ (3%)	↓ (23–50%)	↑ (14%)	↑ (36%)	↑ (20%)	Alway et al. (2014a)
Green Tea Catechins	Acute downhill running	ND	ND	→	ND	↑ (100%)	Haramizu et al. (2013)
Green Tea Catechins	Reloading after HLS	↑ (17%)	↓ (36–50%)	→	↑ (13%)	↑ (25%)	Alway et al. (2014b)
Resveratrol	Aging	ND	→	→	ND	→	Jackson et al. (2011)
Resveratrol	Reloading after HLS	→	↓ (0–29%)	↑ (10%)	↑ (28–45%)	ND	Bennett et al. (2013)

The arrow indicates the increase ($p \leq 0.05$), decrease ($p \leq 0.05$), or no difference ($p \geq 0.05$) between the vehicle vs. nutraceutical. The percent difference from vehicle treatment is indicated in parenthesis).

of delaying differentiation and therefore prolonging or enhancing proliferation of satellite cells in response to a growth stimulus. Furthermore, reduced nutrient availability inhibits C2C12 myoblast differentiation in a Sirt1 dependent manner (Fulco et al., 2008). Interestingly, the NAD^+ salvage enzyme nicotinamide phosphoribosyltransferase was found to mediate the effects of nutrient (glucose) deprivation on myogenic differentiation *in vitro* (Fulco et al., 2008). However, to this point, it is not clear if Sirt1 has a direct or an indirect role in mediating satellite cell proliferation or differentiation *in vivo* in aged/sarcopenic muscles. Nevertheless, we have some clues through other nutritional based intervention studies that suggest that resveratrol, through Sirt1 has a direct effect on regulating satellite cell function in aging. For example, resveratrol, a Sirt1 activator that was given to old rats during a period of recovery following hindlimb suspension had a modest improvement in satellite cell proliferation in hindlimb muscles in response to cage ambulation that followed period of muscle disuse as compared to a vehicle control treatment (Bennett et al., 2013). It is also possible that resveratrol has multiple effects in aged muscles. For example, it appears to also have a more profound protective effect in aging by buffering high levels of oxidative stress which is amplified in old animals during periods of muscle disuse or loading (Jackson et al., 2010; Ryan et al., 2010; Joseph et al., 2013; Durbin et al., 2014). Furthermore, although a constant long-term consumption of resveratrol does not eliminate sarcopenia (Jackson et al., 2011), it is possible that increasing the dose of resveratrol as the animal ages, to better counter the increasing ROS accumulation (and ROS increases with greater age) might have had a different outcome. Nevertheless, together the data suggest that resveratrol might lower excessively high ROS levels, and this would be expected to improve satellite cell function and/or prevent loss of some of the activated satellite cells in responses to stressors (e.g., loading), that otherwise might be lost (destroyed) in a very high ROS environment such as aging and loading, although it probably has modest effects on quiescent satellite cells that are attached to sarcopenic muscles. It is noteworthy that increased levels of Sirt1 have been reported in satellite cells isolated from old rats, although the significance of this is not clear (Machida and Booth, 2004). Thus, it is possible that when Sirt1 was elevated in satellite cells of old animals, it may not have been active and therefore unable to produce the anticipated benefits that have been associated with Sirt1 in aged muscles. This is likely because activated Sirt1 has been shown to directly induce proliferation of satellite cells (Rathbone et al., 2009).

Resveratrol – a link to inflammation mediated satellite cell function?
In addition to its role in metabolism-regulation of satellite cells, resveratrol, through Sirt1 deacetylates and activates PGC1α, which in turn activates transcription factors like the farsenoid x receptor (FXR), PPARα, and PPARδ, which have anti-inflammatory effects (Galuppo et al., 2010; Xu et al., 2012). Thus, it is possible that PGC1α's role in muscle regeneration may be to signal the end of the inflammation period and begin the period of regeneration (satellite cell proliferation and/or differentiation).

Though the role of inflammation in muscle regeneration is currently unclear, the current thought is that early inflammation inhibits muscle regeneration, so that necrotic and damaged cells may be cleared from the injury site, while the later response, such as the arrival of macrophages, has a stimulating effect on muscle repair. Furthermore, macrophages increase the proliferation rate of satellite cells, while depletion of macrophages after a muscle injury has been shown to inhibit satellite cell function to reduce the rate of muscle regeneration (Tidball, 2005; Tidball and Wehling-Henricks, 2007). Thus, understanding PGC1α's connection to inflammation (Westerbacka et al., 2007) and regulation of mitochondrial biogenesis and satellite cell function through resveratrol or other nutraceuticals, may help to further elucidate its role in the inflammatory response period that is associated with muscle regeneration in aging.

EPIGALLOCATECHIN GALLATE AND SATELLITE CELLS

One of the most abundant catechins in green tea is epigallocatechin-3-gallate (EGCg), which has strong antioxidant and anti-inflammatory properties. EGCg is believed to be responsible for most of the health benefits linked to green tea. Both disuse and reloading which accelerate muscle loss in sarcopenia, greatly increase the oxidative stress in the affected muscles of old animals (Andrianjafiniony et al., 2010; Jackson et al., 2010; Pellegrino et al., 2011). Reducing the high basal levels of oxidative stress in aging could potentially attenuate muscle mass decrement that occurs in response to disuse conditions and/or improve muscle recovery during reloading after disuse in aging (Jackson et al., 2010). Recent data suggest that oxidative stress is reduced both in cultured cells (Casanova et al., 2014) and after eccentric exercise upon supplementation with green tea catechins (Haramizu et al., 2011). Furthermore, green tea catechins reduce the decrement in soleus muscle force during a period of hindlimb suspension in mice (Ota et al., 2011). In addition, EGCg has been shown to reduce protein degradation in culture (Mirza et al., 2014). We have recently shown that activation of satellite cells as shown by labeling with the thymidine analog 5-bromo-2-deoxyuridine (BrdU), was significantly greater in reloaded muscles of old rats after a 14 days of hindlimb suspension muscle disuse as compared to muscles from vehicle-treated old animals (Alway et al., 2014a). Interestingly, this appeared to be a fiber or muscle-specific effect on satellite cell proliferation, because while 14 days of reloading increased BrdU labeled nuclei in the plantaris from EGCg treated muscles (7.4%) compared to vehicle-treated animals (6.3%), EGCg did not improve satellite cell activation in the soleus muscle of reloaded animals. Using green tea extract that contained approximately 50% EGCg, we found that satellite cell proliferation and differentiation of the satellite cell daughter cells were both increased in muscles of old rats during reloading after 14 days of hindlimb suspension (Alway et al., 2014b). Moreover, data from old mice and humans that were fed EGCg for 7 days, showed improved markers for satellite cell activation (Myf5, MyoD) (Gutierrez-Salmean et al., 2014). However, EGCg treatment also reduced anabolic suppressor proteins (e.g., myostatin) (Gutierrez-Salmean et al., 2014), so it is more difficult to tell if EGCg provides a direct or indirect effect on satellite cell function. Nevertheless, together these results show that EGCg and perhaps other catechins contained in green tea were effective in improving satellite cell proliferation. We speculate that having more available satellite cell derived daughter nuclei supported the adaptation for greater muscle cross sectional area and this improved the recovery of muscle mass following disuse in sarcopenic rat muscles (Alway et al., 2014a).

HMB REGULATION OF SATELLITE CELLS IN SARCOPENIA

The leucine metabolite, β-hydroxy-β-methylbutyrate (HMB) has been shown to improve satellite cell proliferation (Moore et al., 2005), reduce protein catabolism during disease, reduce muscle loss during disuse, and promote skeletal muscle hypertrophy in response to loading exercise (Wilson et al., 2008; Holecek et al., 2009; Aversa et al., 2011). We have previously shown that HMB could improve muscle recovery in old rats with sarcopenia that had been subjected to unloading, in part via an increase in satellite cell proliferation and a reduction of nuclear apoptosis (Hao et al., 2011). HMB also has been shown to have direct effects on proliferation of myoblasts *in vitro* (Kornasio et al., 2009), although, its efficacy on satellite cell activation has not previously been evaluated *in vivo* in aged immobilized animals. We found that HMB-treatment in old rats during reloading after forced disuse resulted in a significantly greater ($p < 0.01$) level of BrdU positive satellite cells in plantaris muscle cross sections of aged HMB-treated animals (9.1% of total myonuclei) as compared to the animals in the vehicle group (6.1% of total myonuclei) (Alway et al., 2013). This was confirmed by a greater percentage of $Pax7^{+}$ and $MyoD^{+}$ myonuclei (derived from satellite cells) relative to the total myonuclear pool in reloaded plantaris muscles as compared to reloaded muscles from vehicle-treated old animals (Alway et al., 2013). Thus, the mechanism of action through which HMB is responsible for enhancing muscle recovery following extended disuse in sarcopenic muscles of old rats appears to be at least in part, via increased proliferation of muscle satellite cells in fast twitch plantaris muscles of aged animals. However, the enhancement of satellite cell proliferation by HMB is not a universal finding. For example, older women who were fed HMB for six days during a period of resistance training to load their skeletal muscles had a ~100% increase in satellite cell numbers, but HMB did not increase satellite cell proliferation further over resistance training alone (Kim et al., 2012). Additional work is needed to determine if the beneficial effects of HMB on satellite cell function will be observed in older humans if the dose or duration of HMB is altered.

REGULATION OF NUCLEAR DEATH SIGNALS BY NUTRACEUTICALS

Satellite cells that are isolated from sarcopenic muscles from old rodents and humans have a greater propensity for apoptosis and greater levels of apoptotic signaling proteins (Fulle et al., 2012, 2013). Not only can apoptosis signaling target mature post mitotic nuclei for elimination, but satellite cells and their daughter cells that are activated as part of a hypertrophic adaptation to a loading stimulus, can be targets for elimination as well (Alway and Siu, 2008). Satellite cell number decreases with increased aging (Snow, 1977; Verdijk et al., 2014), and one possibility to explain this reduction in satellite cells is due to an increased susceptibility to nuclear apoptosis in aging and therefore, this may contribute to sarcopenia (Leeuwenburgh, 2003; Pistilli et al., 2006; Adhihetty et al., 2008,

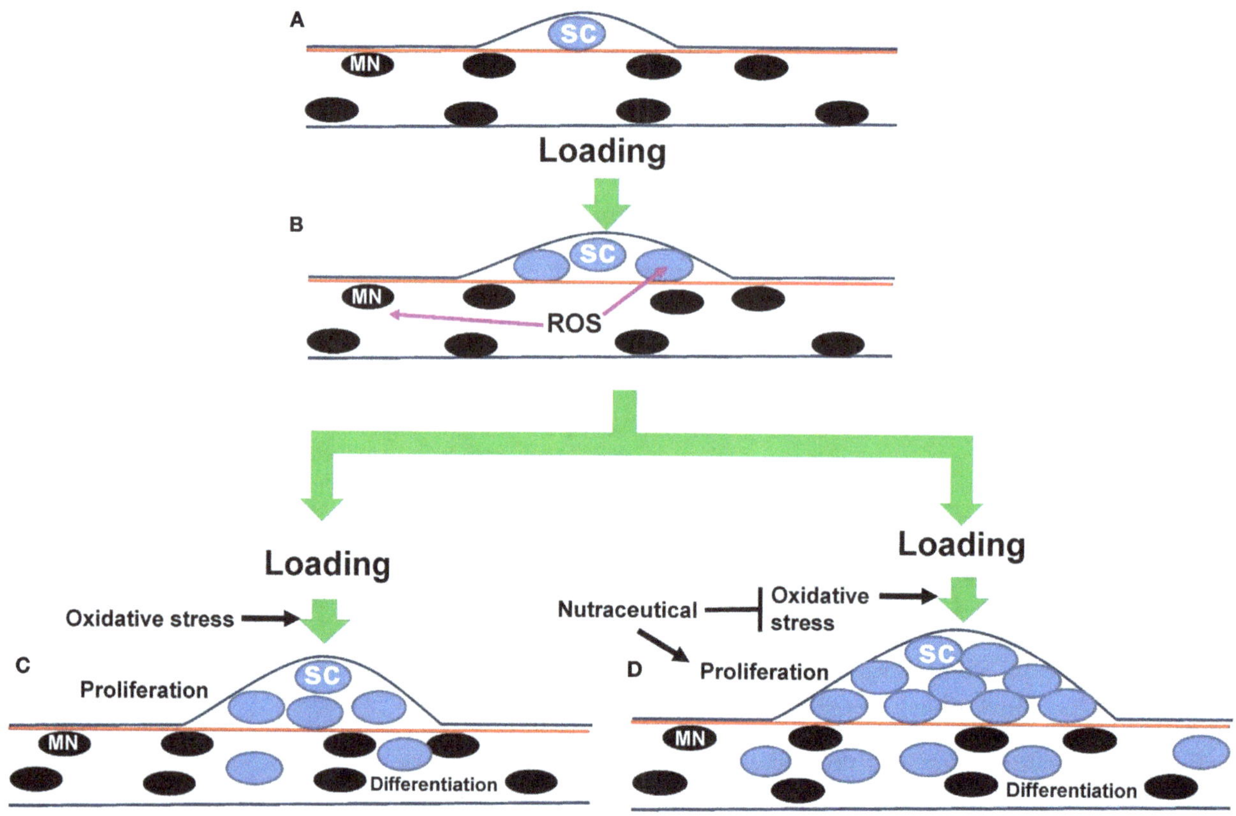

FIGURE 2 | Hypothetical model for nutraceutical effects on satellite cell proliferation in sarcopenia during muscle loading. **(A)** A muscle fiber is illustrated that shows myonuclei (black) and a single satellite cell (blue) that is positioned between the basal lamina (dark blue line) and the sarcolemma (red line). **(B)** Loading of aged muscles results in proliferation of the original satellite cell nuclei, but it also increases reactive oxygen species (ROS) accumulation, in part as a result of aging-induced changes in mitochondria. High levels of ROS in aged muscles can trigger apoptotic pathways which presumably have the potential to eliminate the targeted nuclei and activated satellite cells. **(C)** After proliferation, some of the daughter cells will migrate into the adult fiber and differentiate to support growth. However, as satellite cells from old animals tend to have a greater propensity (and maybe sensitivity) to apoptosis-induced cell death, not all of the proliferating satellite cells including those that differentiate survive and some will remain in the position of satellite cells to replenish the satellite cell population. **(D)** Nutraceuticals resveratrol, EGCg, and green tea appear to enhance the proliferation of satellite cells in response to an activating stimulus (e.g., muscle loading), perhaps in part by reducing ROS and in some cases improving mitochondrial number or function. This provides a higher number of surviving daughter cells that are able to migrate into the adjacent fiber, to presumably support growth and/or repair of skeletal muscle fibers in aging. It is also possible that the proliferated protege from satellite cells could signal other cell types or change the muscle fiber niche that would be conducive for hypertrophy or slowing muscle losses in sarcopenia.

2009; Ljubicic et al., 2009; Alway et al., 2011; Quadrilatero et al., 2011; Marzetti et al., 2012; Calvani et al., 2013). Furthermore, the pro-apoptotic protein Bax, is increased in satellite cells of old rats (Krajnak et al., 2006) and this leads to accelerated muscle loss in sarcopenic muscles via apoptosis (Dupont-Versteegden et al., 2006; Pistilli et al., 2006; Alway et al., 2014a). However, signaling for apoptosis is reduced and more satellite cells (e.g., Pax7/MyoD^{+} cells) survive during rehabilitation after disuse in aged rat muscles that are treated with HMB (Hao et al., 2011; Alway et al., 2013), EGCg (Alway et al., 2014a), or green tea catechins (Alway et al., 2014b) as compared to a control treatment. In contrast, resveratrol fed animals had lower levels of oxidative stress, but only modest changes in apoptotic signaling (Jackson et al., 2010; Bennett et al., 2013) as compared to control animals. Although the mechanism(s) by which nutraceuticals impact satellite cell function, including reducing pro-apoptotic targeting of satellite cells, is likely to be complex. Part of the improvement in apoptotic signaling in activated satellite cells may be due to an upregulation of antioxidants and a reduction of oxidative stress and/or inflammation after nutraceutical treatments including resveratrol (Jackson et al., 2010, 2011; Ryan et al., 2010) and green tea catechins (Ota et al., 2011; Wang et al., 2011; Andrade and Assuncao, 2012; Wu et al., 2012; Haramizu et al., 2013). Given the propensity for apoptosis to occur in satellite cells isolated from old hosts including humans (Fulle et al., 2012, 2013), further investigations into the potential for nutraceuticals to improve satellite cell function in aging are warranted. Together these data support the idea that reducing the systemic (and perhaps also the satellite cell niche) signaling for apoptosis, may promote better survival of satellite cells and their daughter cells in muscles of old animals, and this may contribute to improved muscle recovery after periods of disuse (e.g., hospitalization) and reduce the effects of sarcopenia in the elderly.

CONCLUSION

Although the satellite cell has been identified and studied for more than a half of a century (Mauro, 1961), there is still much that we do not know about this unique muscle stem cell in aging. In general, there is a reduction in satellite cell number and function that occurs with aging, especially in type II fibers, but this does not seem to be due to increased DNA damage in these cells (Cousin et al., 2013). Nevertheless, it is clear that satellite cell proliferation and differentiation contributes to a greater myonuclear pool. Improving satellite cell proliferation occurs especially in fast muscles of aged animals provided supplemental HMB, EGCg, resveratrol or green tea, and a greater number of satellite cell derived nuclei should provide a greater potential for transcriptional and translational control for improving regeneration in aged muscles (**Figure 2**). One possibility is that the nutraceuticals act to buffer the high levels of ROS in aging muscles of old animals. Nutraceuticals may also reduce the level of oxidative stress that is elevated in aging muscles in response to loading or disuse. The less oxidative environment may encourage the survival of more of the activated satellite cells so that they can participate in muscle repair. Additionally, as EGCg has been shown to improve muscle function following a nerve crush injury (Renno et al., 2012), it would be interesting to know in future studies if catechins or other nutraceuticals could delay or suppress age-associated denervation. Furthermore, nutritionally regulated reductions in the potential for death signals (e.g., apoptosis) to eliminate satellite cell progeny that have migrated inside a muscle fiber should also improve the potential for transcriptional and translational regulation of muscle fiber regeneration or repair in aging. Thus, nutraceuticals appear to have the potential to regulate satellite cell function, and in doing so, impact skeletal muscle regeneration, particularly during rehabilitative efforts that follow a period of disuse in aged animals (**Table 2**). Unfortunately, nutraceuticals do not appear to have profound effects on slowing accelerated loss in sarcopenic muscles (**Table 1**).

Clinical trials in humans are warranted to determine if these or other nutraceuticals, will similarly improve muscle recovery following bed rest or other conditions of muscle loss in aging as observed in rodents. However, it has only been recent that we have begun to appreciate the potential links between nutrition and metabolism and satellite cell function in health and disease. In the context of treating sarcopenia, it is important to note that not all changes in diet that might slow muscle loss, necessarily affect satellite cell function. For example, dietary protein intake alone does not modulate the post-exercise increase in satellite cell content but instead, it modifies myostatin expression in skeletal muscle tissue, which contributes to the increase in protein accretion after acute exercise (Snijders et al., 2014a). Thus, it is important to distinguish between satellite cell and non-satellite cell functions of nutraceuticals in sarcopenic muscles of the aging hosts. Understanding the nutritional regulation of satellite cell function appears to be a potentially promising avenue for identifying strategies to reduce muscle wasting in sarcopenia, and to improve the recovery of muscle that is lost during a period of disuse in aged humans.

REFERENCES

Adhihetty, P. J., O'Leary, M. F., and Hood, D. A. (2008). Mitochondria in skeletal muscle: adaptable rheostats of apoptotic susceptibility. *Exerc. Sport Sci. Rev.* 36, 116–121. doi:10.1097/JES.0b013e31817be7b7

Adhihetty, P. J., Uguccioni, G., Leick, L., Hidalgo, J., Pilegaard, H., and Hood, D. A. (2009). The role of PGC-1{alpha} on mitochondrial function and apoptotic susceptibility in muscle. *Am. J. Physiol. Cell Physiol.* 297, C217–C225. doi:10.1152/ajpcell.00070.2009

Allen, D. L., Linderman, J. K., Roy, R. R., Bigbee, A. J., Grindeland, R. E., Mukku, V., et al. (1997). Apoptosis: a mechanism contributing to remodeling of skeletal muscle in response to hindlimb unweighting. *Am. J. Physiol.* 273(2 Pt 1), C579–C587.

Allen, R. G., and Tresini, M. (2000). Oxidative stress and gene regulation. *Free Radic. Biol. Med.* 28, 463–499. doi:10.1016/S0891-5849(99)00242-7

Alway, S. E., Bennett, B. T., Wilson, J. C., Edens, N. K., and Pereira, S. L. (2014a). Epigallocatechin-3-gallate improves plantaris muscle recovery after disuse in aged rats. *Exp. Gerontol.* 50, 82–94. doi:10.1016/j.exger.2013.11.011

Alway, S. E., Bennett, B. T., Wilson, J. C., Sperringer, J., Mohamed, J. S., Edens, N. K., et al. (2014b). Green tea extract attenuates muscle loss and improves muscle function during disuse and increases satellite cell proliferation during reloading after hindlimb suspension in aged rodents. *J. Appl. Physiol.* (in press).

Alway, S. E., Degens, H., Lowe, D. A., and Krishnamurthy, G. (2002). Increased myogenic repressor Id mRNA and protein levels in hindlimb muscles of aged rats. *Am. J. Physiol. Regul. Integr. Comp. Physiol.* 282, R411–R422. doi:10.1152/ajpregu.00332.2001

Alway, S. E., Martyn, J. K., Ouyang, J., Chaudhrai, A., and Murlasits, Z. S. (2003). Id2 expression during apoptosis and satellite cell activation in unloaded and loaded quail skeletal muscles. *Am. J. Physiol. Regul. Integr. Comp. Physiol.* 284, R540–R549. doi:10.1152/ajpregu.00550.2002

Alway, S. E., Morissette, M. R., and Siu, P. M. (2011). "Aging and apoptosis in muscle," in *Handbook of the Biology of Aging*, eds E. J. Masoro and S. Austad (Amsterdam: Elsevier), 64–139.

Alway, S. E., Pereira, S. L., Edens, N. K., Hao, Y., and Bennett, B. T. (2013). β-Hydroxy-β-methylbutyrate (HMB) enhances the proliferation of satellite cells in fast muscles of aged rats during recovery from disuse atrophy. *Exp. Gerontol.* 48, 973–984. doi:10.1016/j.exger.2013.06.005

Alway, S. E., and Siu, P. M. (2008). Nuclear apoptosis contributes to sarcopenia. *Exerc. Sport Sci. Rev.* 36, 51–57. doi:10.1097/JES.0b013e318168e9dc

Alway, S. E., Siu, P. M., Murlasits, Z., and Butler, D. C. (2005). Muscle hypertrophy models: applications for research on aging. *Can. J. Appl. Physiol.* 30, 591–624. doi:10.1139/h05-143

Andrade, J. P., and Assuncao, M. (2012). Protective effects of chronic green tea consumption on age-related neurodegeneration. *Curr. Pharm. Des.* 18, 4–14. doi:10.2174/138161212798918986

Andrianjafiniony, T., Dupre-Aucouturier, S., Letexier, D., Couchoux, H., and Desplanches, D. (2010). Oxidative stress, apoptosis, and proteolysis in skeletal muscle repair after unloading. *Am. J. Physiol. Cell Physiol.* 299, C307–C315. doi:10.1152/ajpcell.00069.2010

Angione, A. R., Jiang, C., Pan, D., Wang, Y. X., and Kuang, S. (2011). PPARdelta regulates satellite cell proliferation and skeletal muscle regeneration. *Skelet. Muscle* 1, 33. doi:10.1186/2044-5040-1-33

Armand, A. S., Laziz, I., Djeghloul, D., Lecolle, S., Bertrand, A. T., Biondi, O., et al. (2011). Apoptosis-inducing factor regulates skeletal muscle progenitor cell number and muscle phenotype. *PLoS ONE* 6:e27283. doi:10.1371/journal.pone.0027283

Aversa, Z., Bonetto, A., Costelli, P., Minero, V. G., Penna, F., Baccino, F. M., et al. (2011). Beta-hydroxy-beta-methylbutyrate (HMB) attenuates muscle and body weight loss in experimental cancer cachexia. *Int. J. Oncol.* 38, 713–720. doi:10.3892/ijo.2010.885

Barberi, L., Scicchitano, B. M., De Rossi, M., Bigot, A., Duguez, S., Wielgosik, A., et al. (2013). Age-dependent alteration in muscle regeneration: the critical role of tissue niche. *Biogerontology* 14, 273–292. doi:10.1007/s10522-013-9429-4

Beccafico, S., Puglielli, C., Pietrangelo, T., Bellomo, R., Fano, G., and Fulle, S. (2007). Age-dependent effects on functional aspects in human satellite cells. *Ann. N. Y. Acad. Sci.* 1100, 345–352. doi:10.1196/annals.1395.037

Bennett, B. T., Mohamed, J. S., and Alway, S. E. (2013). Effects of resveratrol on the recovery of muscle mass following disuse in the plantaris muscle of aged rats. *PLoS ONE* 8:e83518. doi:10.1371/journal.pone.0083518

Bentzinger, C. F., Wang, Y. X., Dumont, N. A., and Rudnicki, M. A. (2013). Cellular dynamics in the muscle satellite cell niche. *EMBO Rep.* 14, 1062–1072. doi:10.1038/embor.2013.182

Bernet, J. D., Doles, J. D., Hall, J. K., Kelly, T. K., Carter, T. A., and Olwin, B. B. (2014). p38 MAPK signaling underlies a cell-autonomous loss of stem cell self-renewal in skeletal muscle of aged mice. *Nat. Med.* 20, 265–271. doi:10.1038/nm.3465

Bortoli, S., Renault, V., Mariage-Samson, R., Eveno, E., Auffray, C., Butler-Browne, G., et al. (2005). Modifications in the myogenic program induced by in vivo and in vitro aging. *Gene* 347, 65–72. doi:10.1016/j.gene.2004.12.029

Brack, A. S., Bildsoe, H., and Hughes, S. M. (2005). Evidence that satellite cell decrement contributes to preferential decline in nuclear number from large fibres during murine age-related muscle atrophy. *J. Cell Sci.* 118, 4813–4821. doi:10.1242/jcs.02602

Brooks, N. E., Cadena, S. M., Vannier, E., Cloutier, G., Carambula, S., Myburgh, K. H., et al. (2010). Effects of resistance exercise combined with essential amino acid supplementation and energy deficit on markers of skeletal muscle atrophy and regeneration during bed rest and active recovery. *Muscle Nerve* 42, 927–935. doi:10.1002/mus.21780

Buckingham, M., and Relaix, F. (2007). The role of Pax genes in the development of tissues and organs: Pax3 and Pax7 regulate muscle progenitor cell functions. *Annu. Rev. Cell Dev. Biol.* 23, 645–673. doi:10.1146/annurev.cellbio.23.090506.123438

Burgos, P. R. (2012). Therapeutic approach to malnutrition and sarcopenia. *Nestle Nutr. Inst. Workshop Ser.* 72, 85–99. doi:10.1159/000339995

Calvani, R., Joseph, A. M., Adhihetty, P. J., Miccheli, A., Bossola, M., Leeuwenburgh, C., et al. (2013). Mitochondrial pathways in sarcopenia of aging and disuse muscle atrophy. *Biol. Chem.* 394, 393–414. doi:10.1515/hsz-2012-0247

Carson, J. A., and Alway, S. E. (1996). Stretch overload-induced satellite cell activation in slow tonic muscle from adult and aged Japanese quail. *Am. J. Physiol.* 270, C578–C584.

Carson, J. A., Yamaguchi, M., and Alway, S. E. (1995). Hypertrophy and proliferation of skeletal muscle fibers from aged quail. *J. Appl. Physiol.* 78, 293–299.

Casanova, E., Baselga-Escudero, L., Ribas-Latre, A., Arola-Arnal, A., Blade, C., Arola, L., et al. (2014). Epigallocatechin gallate counteracts oxidative stress in docosahexaenoxic acid-treated myocytes. *Biochim. Biophys. Acta* 1837, 783–791. doi:10.1016/j.bbabio.2014.01.014

Cerletti, M., Jang, Y. C., Finley, L. W., Haigis, M. C., and Wagers, A. J. (2012). Short-term calorie restriction enhances skeletal muscle stem cell function. *Cell Stem Cell* 10, 515–519. doi:10.1016/j.stem.2012.04.002

Chabi, B., Ljubicic, V., Menzies, K. J., Huang, J. H., Saleem, A., and Hood, D. A. (2008). Mitochondrial function and apoptotic susceptibility in aging skeletal muscle. *Aging Cell* 7, 2–12. doi:10.1111/j.1474-9726.2007.00347.x

Chakkalakal, J., and Brack, A. (2012). Extrinsic regulation of satellite cell function and muscle regeneration capacity during aging. *J. Stem Cell Res. Ther.* S11, 001. doi:10.4172/2157-7633.S11-001

Chakkalakal, J. V., Jones, K. M., Basson, M. A., and Brack, A. S. (2012). The aged niche disrupts muscle stem cell quiescence. *Nature* 490, 355–360. doi:10.1038/nature11438

Chen, C. J., Yu, W., Fu, Y. C., Wang, X., Li, J. L., and Wang, W. (2009). Resveratrol protects cardiomyocytes from hypoxia-induced apoptosis through the SIRT1-FoxO1 pathway. *Biochem. Biophys. Res. Commun.* 378, 389–393. doi:10.1016/j.bbrc.2008.11.110

Christov, C., Chretien, F., Abou-Khalil, R., Bassez, G., Vallet, G., Authier, F. J., et al. (2007). Muscle satellite cells and endothelial cells: close neighbors and privileged partners. *Mol. Biol. Cell* 18, 1397–1409. doi:10.1091/mbc.E06-08-0693

Churchward-Venne, T. A., Breen, L., and Phillips, S. M. (2014). Alterations in human muscle protein metabolism with aging: protein and exercise as countermeasures to offset sarcopenia. *Biofactors* 40, 199–205. doi:10.1002/biof.1138

Cohen, H. Y., Miller, C., Bitterman, K. J., Wall, N. R., Hekking, B., Kessler, B., et al. (2004). Calorie restriction promotes mammalian cell survival by inducing the SIRT1 deacetylase. *Science* 305, 390–392. doi:10.1126/science.1099196

Collins, C. A., Olsen, I., Zammit, P. S., Heslop, L., Petrie, A., Partridge, T. A., et al. (2005). Stem cell function, self-renewal, and behavioral heterogeneity of cells from the adult muscle satellite cell niche. *Cell* 122, 289–301. doi:10.1016/j.cell.2005.05.010

Collins, C. A., Zammit, P. S., Ruiz, A. P., Morgan, J. E., and Partridge, T. A. (2007). A population of myogenic stem cells that survives skeletal muscle aging. *Stem Cells* 25, 885–894. doi:10.1634/stemcells.2006-0372

Collins-Hooper, H., Woolley, T. E., Dyson, L., Patel, A., Potter, P., Baker, R. E., et al. (2012). Age-related changes in speed and mechanism of adult skeletal muscle stem cell migration. *Stem Cells* 30, 1182–1195. doi:10.1002/stem.1088

Conboy, I. M., Conboy, M. J., Wagers, A. J., Girma, E. R., Weissman, I. L., and Rando, T. A. (2005). Rejuvenation of aged progenitor cells by exposure to a young systemic environment. *Nature* 433, 760–764. doi:10.1038/nature03260

Conboy, I. M., and Rando, T. A. (2005). Aging, stem cells and tissue regeneration: lessons from muscle. *Cell Cycle* 4, 407–410. doi:10.4161/cc.4.3.1518

Cornelison, D. D., and Wold, B. J. (1997). Single-cell analysis of regulatory gene expression in quiescent and activated mouse skeletal muscle satellite cells. *Dev. Biol.* 191, 270–283. doi:10.1006/dbio.1997.8721

Cosgrove, B. D., Sacco, A., Gilbert, P. M., and Blau, H. M. (2009). A home away from home: challenges and opportunities in engineering in vitro muscle satellite cell niches. *Differentiation* 78, 185–194. doi:10.1016/j.diff.2009.08.004

Cousin, W., Ho, M. L., Desai, R., Tham, A., Chen, R. Y., Kung, S., et al. (2013). Regenerative capacity of old muscle stem cells declines without significant accumulation of DNA damage. *PLoS ONE* 8:e63528. doi:10.1371/journal.pone.0063528

Cutlip, R. G., Baker, B. A., Geronilla, K. B., Mercer, R. R., Kashon, M. L., Miller, G. R., et al. (2006). Chronic exposure to stretch-shortening contractions results in skeletal muscle adaptation in young rats and maladaptation in old rats. *Appl. Physiol. Nutr. Metab.* 31, 573–587. doi:10.1139/h06-033

Day, K., Shefer, G., Richardson, J. B., Enikolopov, G., and Yablonka-Reuveni, Z. (2007). Nestin-GFP reporter expression defines the quiescent state of skeletal muscle satellite cells. *Dev. Biol.* 304, 246–259. doi:10.1016/j.ydbio.2006.12.026

Day, K., Shefer, G., Shearer, A., and Yablonka-Reuveni, Z. (2010). The depletion of skeletal muscle satellite cells with age is concomitant with reduced capacity of single progenitors to produce reserve progeny. *Dev. Biol.* 340, 330–343. doi:10.1016/j.ydbio.2010.01.006

Degens, H. (2010). The role of systemic inflammation in age-related muscle weakness and wasting. *Scand. J. Med. Sci. Sports* 20, 28–38. doi:10.1111/j.1600-0838.2009.01018.x

Deschenes, M. R., Gaertner, J. R., and O'Reilly, S. (2013). The effects of sarcopenia on muscles with different recruitment patterns and myofiber profiles. *Curr. Aging Sci.* 6, 266–272. doi:10.2174/18746098113066660035

Dickinson, J. M., Volpi, E., and Rasmussen, B. B. (2013). Exercise and nutrition to target protein synthesis impairments in aging skeletal muscle. *Exerc. Sport Sci. Rev.* 41, 216–223. doi:10.1097/JES.0b013e3182a4e699

Drey, M., Grosch, C., Neuwirth, C., Bauer, J. M., and Sieber, C. C. (2013). The motor unit number index (MUNIX) in sarcopenic patients. *Exp. Gerontol.* 48, 381–384. doi:10.1016/j.exger.2013.01.011

Dreyer, H. C., Blanco, C. E., Sattler, F. R., Schroeder, E. T., and Wiswell, R. A. (2006). Satellite cell numbers in young and older men 24 hours after eccentric exercise. *Muscle Nerve* 33, 242–253. doi:10.1002/mus.20461

Duguez, S., Feasson, L., Denis, C., and Freyssenet, D. (2002). Mitochondrial biogenesis during skeletal muscle regeneration. *Am. J. Physiol. Endocrinol. Metab.* 282, E802–E809. doi:10.1152/ajpendo.00343.2001

Dupont-Versteegden, E. E. (2005). Apoptosis in muscle atrophy: relevance to sarcopenia. *Exp. Gerontol.* 40, 473–481. doi:10.1016/j.exger.2005.04.003

Dupont-Versteegden, E. E., Strotman, B. A., Gurley, C. M., Gaddy, D., Knox, M., Fluckey, J. D., et al. (2006). Nuclear translocation of EndoG at the initiation of disuse muscle atrophy and apoptosis is specific to myonuclei. *Am. J. Physiol. Regul. Integr. Comp. Physiol.* 291, R1730–R1740. doi:10.1152/ajpregu.00176.2006

Durbin, S. M., Jackson, J. R., Ryan, M. J., Gigliotti, J. C., Alway, S. E., and Tou, J. C. (2014). Resveratrol supplementation preserves long bone mass, microstructure, and strength in hindlimb-suspended old male rats. *J. Bone Miner. Metab.* 32, 38–47. doi:10.1007/s00774-013-0469-2

Dutta, C., Hadley, E. C., and Lexell, J. (1997). Sarcopenia and physical performance in old age: overview. *Muscle Nerve Suppl.* 5, S5–S9. doi:10.1002/(SICI)1097-4598(1997)5+<5::AID-MUS2>3.3.CO;2-D

Evans, W. J. (1995). What is sarcopenia? *J. Gerontol. A Biol. Sci. Med. Sci.* 50 Spec No, 5–8. doi:10.1093/gerona/50A.Special_Issue.5

Faulkner, J. A., Brooks, S. V., and Zerba, E. (1995). Muscle atrophy and weakness with aging: contraction-induced injury as an underlying mechanism. *J. Gerontol. A Biol. Sci. Med. Sci.* 50 Spec No, 124–129.

Frey, R. S., Gao, X., Javaid, K., Siddiqui, S. S., Rahman, A., and Malik, A. B. (2006). Phosphatidylinositol 3-kinase gamma signaling through protein kinase Czeta induces NADPH oxidase-mediated oxidant generation and NF-kappaB activation in endothelial cells. *J. Biol. Chem.* 281, 16128–16138. doi:10.1074/jbc.M508810200

Frey, R. S., Ushio-Fukai, M., and Malik, A. B. (2009). NADPH oxidase-dependent signaling in endothelial cells: role in physiology and pathophysiology. *Antioxid. Redox Signal.* 11, 791–810. doi:10.1089/ARS.2008.2220

Fry, C. S., Lee, J. D., Jackson, J. R., Kirby, T. J., Stasko, S. A., Liu, H., et al. (2014). Regulation of the muscle fiber microenvironment by activated satellite cells during hypertrophy. *FASEB J.* 28, 1654–1665. doi:10.1096/fj.13-239426

Fujimaki, S., Hidaka, R., Asashima, M., Takemasa, T., and Kuwabara, T. (2014). Wnt protein-mediated satellite cell conversion in adult and aged mice following voluntary wheel running. *J. Biol. Chem.* 289, 7399–7412. doi:10.1074/jbc.M113.539247

Fulco, M., Cen, Y., Zhao, P., Hoffman, E. P., McBurney, M. W., Sauve, A. A., et al. (2008). Glucose restriction inhibits skeletal myoblast differentiation by activating SIRT1 through AMPK-mediated regulation of Nampt. *Dev. Cell* 14, 661–673. doi:10.1016/j.devcel.2008.02.004

Fulco, M., Schiltz, R. L., Iezzi, S., King, M. T., Zhao, P., Kashiwaya, Y., et al. (2003). Sir2 regulates skeletal muscle differentiation as a potential sensor of the redox state. *Mol. Cell* 12, 51–62. doi:10.1016/S1097-2765(03)00226-0

Fulle, S., Centurione, L., Mancinelli, R., Sancilio, S., Manzoli, F. A., and Di, P. R. (2012). Stem cell ageing and apoptosis. *Curr. Pharm. Des.* 18, 1694–1717. doi:10.2174/138161212799859657

Fulle, S., Di Donna, S., Puglielli, C., Pietrangelo, T., Beccafico, S., Bellomo, R., et al. (2005). Age-dependent imbalance of the antioxidative system in human satellite cells. *Exp. Gerontol.* 40, 189–197. doi:10.1016/j.exger.2004.11.006

Fulle, S., Sancilio, S., Mancinelli, R., Gatta, V., and Di Pietro, R. (2013). Dual role of the caspase enzymes in satellite cells from aged and young subjects. *Cell Death Dis.* 4, e955. doi:10.1038/cddis.2013.472

Galuppo, M., Di Paola, R., Mazzon, E., Genovese, T., Crisafulli, C., Paterniti, I., et al. (2010). Role of PPAR-delta in the development of zymosan-induced multiple organ failure: an experiment mice study. *J. Inflamm. (Lond.)* 7, 12. doi:10.1186/1476-9255-7-12

Garcia-Prat, L., Sousa-Victor, P., and Munoz-Canoves, P. (2013). Functional dysregulation of stem cells during aging: a focus on skeletal muscle stem cells. *FEBS J.* 280, 4051–4062. doi:10.1111/febs.12221

Ghosh, S., Lertwattanarak, R., Garduno, J. D., Galeana, J. J., Li, J., Zamarripa, F., et al. (2014). Elevated muscle TLR4 expression and metabolic endotoxemia in human aging. *J. Gerontol. A Biol. Sci. Med. Sci.* doi:10.1093/gerona/glu067

Gilbert, P. M., Corbel, S., Doyonnas, R., Havenstrite, K., Magnusson, K. E., and Blau, H. M. (2012). A single cell bioengineering approach to elucidate mechanisms of adult stem cell self-renewal. *Integr. Biol. (Camb.)* 4, 360–367. doi:10.1039/c2ib00148a

Gutierrez-Salmean, G., Ciaraldi, T. P., Nogueira, L., Barboza, J., Taub, P. R., Hogan, M. C., et al. (2014). Effects of (-)-epicatechin on molecular modulators of skeletal muscle growth and differentiation. *J. Nutr. Biochem.* 25, 91–94. doi:10.1016/j.jnutbio.2013.09.007

Halevy, O., Geyra, A., Barak, M., Uni, Z., and Sklan, D. (2000). Early posthatch starvation decreases satellite cell proliferation and skeletal muscle growth in chicks. *J. Nutr.* 130, 858–864.

Halevy, O., Nadel, Y., Barak, M., Rozenboim, I., and Sklan, D. (2003). Early posthatch feeding stimulates satellite cell proliferation and skeletal muscle growth in turkey poults. *J. Nutr.* 133, 1376–1382.

Hao, Y., Jackson, J. R., Wang, Y., Edens, N., Pereira, S. L., and Alway, S. E. (2011). β-Hydroxy-β-methylbutyrate reduces myonuclear apoptosis during recovery from hind limb suspension-induced muscle fiber atrophy in aged rats. *Am. J. Physiol. Regul. Integr. Comp. Physiol.* 301, R701–R715. doi:10.1152/ajpregu.00840.2010

Haramizu, S., Ota, N., Hase, T., and Murase, T. (2011). Catechins attenuate eccentric exercise-induced inflammation and loss of force production in muscle in senescence-accelerated mice. *J. Appl. Physiol.* 111, 1654–1663. doi:10.1152/japplphysiol.01434.2010

Haramizu, S., Ota, N., Hase, T., and Murase, T. (2013). Catechins suppress muscle inflammation and hasten performance recovery after exercise. *Med. Sci. Sports Exerc.* 45, 1694–1702. doi:10.1249/MSS.0b013e31828de99f

Harridge, S. D. (2003). Ageing and local growth factors in muscle. *Scand. J. Med. Sci. Sports* 13, 34–39. doi:10.1034/j.1600-0838.2003.20235.x

Harthan, L. B., McFarland, D. C., and Velleman, S. G. (2013). The effect of syndecan-4 and glypican-1 expression on age-related changes in myogenic satellite cell proliferation, differentiation, and fibroblast growth factor 2 responsiveness. *Comp. Biochem. Physiol. Part A Mol. Integr. Physiol.* 166, 590–602. doi:10.1016/j.cbpa.2013.09.007

Harthan, L. B., McFarland, D. C., and Velleman, S. G. (2014). The effect of nutritional status and myogenic satellite cell age on turkey satellite cell proliferation, differentiation, and expression of myogenic transcriptional regulatory factors and heparan sulfate proteoglycans syndecan-4 and glypican-1. *Poult. Sci.* 93, 174–186. doi:10.3382/ps.2013-03570

Hiona, A., and Leeuwenburgh, C. (2008). The role of mitochondrial DNA mutations in aging and sarcopenia: implications for the mitochondrial vicious cycle theory of aging. *Exp. Gerontol.* 43, 24–33. doi:10.1016/j.exger.2007.10.001

Holecek, M., Muthny, T., Kovarik, M., and Sispera, L. (2009). Effect of beta-hydroxy-beta-methylbutyrate (HMB) on protein metabolism in whole body and in selected tissues. *Food Chem. Toxicol.* 47, 255–259. doi:10.1016/j.fct.2008.11.021

Jackson, J. R., Mula, J., Kirby, T. J., Fry, C. S., Lee, J. D., Ubele, M. F., et al. (2012). Satellite cell depletion does not inhibit adult skeletal muscle regrowth following unloading-induced atrophy. *Am. J. Physiol. Cell Physiol.* 303, C854–C861. doi:10.1152/ajpcell.00207.2012

Jackson, J. R., Ryan, M. J., and Alway, S. E. (2011). Long-term supplementation with resveratrol alleviates oxidative stress but does not attenuate sarcopenia in aged mice. *J. Gerontol. A Biol. Sci. Med. Sci.* 66, 751–764. doi:10.1093/gerona/glr047

Jackson, J. R., Ryan, M. J., Hao, Y., and Alway, S. E. (2010). Mediation of endogenous antioxidant enzymes and apoptotic signaling by resveratrol following muscle disuse in the gastrocnemius muscles of young and old rats. *Am. J. Physiol. Regul. Integr. Comp. Physiol.* 299, R1572–R1581. doi:10.1152/ajpregu.00489.2010

Jang, Y. C., Sinha, M., Cerletti, M., Dall'Osso, C., and Wagers, A. J. (2011). Skeletal muscle stem cells: effects of aging and metabolism on muscle regenerative function. *Cold Spring Harb. Symp. Quant. Biol.* 76, 101–111. doi:10.1101/sqb.2011.76.010652

Jash, S., and Adhya, S. (2012). Induction of muscle regeneration by RNA-mediated mitochondrial restoration. *FASEB J.* 26, 4187–4197. doi:10.1096/fj.11-203232

Joanisse, S., Gillen, J. B., Bellamy, L. M., McKay, B. R., Tarnopolsky, M. A., Gibala, M. J., et al. (2013). Evidence for the contribution of muscle stem cells to nonhypertrophic skeletal muscle remodeling in humans. *FASEB J.* 27, 4596–4605. doi:10.1096/fj.13-229799

Joseph, A. M., Malamo, A. G., Silvestre, J., Wawrzyniak, N., Carey-Love, S., Nguyen, L. M., et al. (2013). Short-term caloric restriction, resveratrol, or combined treatment regimens initiated in late-life alter mitochondrial protein expression profiles in a fiber-type specific manner in aged animals. *Exp. Gerontol.* 48, 858–868. doi:10.1016/j.exger.2013.05.061

Kern, H., Barberi, L., Lofler, S., Sbardella, S., Burggraf, S., Fruhmann, H., et al. (2014). Electrical stimulation counteracts muscle decline in seniors. *Front. Aging Neurosci.* 6:189. doi:10.3389/fnagi.2014.00189

Kim, J. S., Park, Y. M., Lee, S. R., Masad, I. S., Khamoui, A. V., Jo, E., et al. (2012). Beta-hydroxy-beta-methylbutyrate did not enhance high intensity resistance training-induced improvements in myofiber dimensions and myogenic capacity in aged female rats. *Mol. Cells* 34, 439–448. doi:10.1007/s10059-012-0196-x

Kim, T. N., and Choi, K. M. (2013). Sarcopenia: definition, epidemiology, and pathophysiology. *J. Bone Metab.* 20, 1–10. doi:10.11005/jbm.2013.20.1.1

Kim, T. N., Park, M. S., Yang, S. J., Yoo, H. J., Kang, H. J., Song, W., et al. (2010). Prevalence and determinant factors of sarcopenia in patients with type 2 diabetes: the Korean Sarcopenic Obesity Study (KSOS). *Diabetes Care* 33, 1497–1499. doi:10.2337/dc09-2310

Kornasio, R., Riederer, I., Butler-Browne, G., Mouly, V., Uni, Z., and Halevy, O. (2009). Beta-hydroxy-beta-methylbutyrate (HMB) stimulates myogenic cell proliferation, differentiation and survival via the MAPK/ERK and PI3K/Akt pathways. *Biochim. Biophys. Acta* 1793, 755–763. doi:10.1016/j.bbamcr.2008.12.017

Krajnak, K., Waugh, S., Miller, R., Baker, B., Geronilla, K., Alway, S. E., et al. (2006). Proapoptotic factor Bax is increased in satellite cells in the tibialis anterior muscles of old rats. *Muscle Nerve* 34, 720–730. doi:10.1002/mus.20656

Kuang, S., Charge, S. B., Seale, P., Huh, M., and Rudnicki, M. A. (2006). Distinct roles for Pax7 and Pax3 in adult regenerative myogenesis. *J. Cell Biol.* 172, 103–113. doi:10.1083/jcb.200508001

Kwan, P. (2013). Sarcopenia: the gliogenic perspective. *Mech. Ageing Dev.* 134, 349–355. doi:10.1016/j.mad.2013.06.001

Lander, A. D., Kimble, J., Clevers, H., Fuchs, E., Montarras, D., Buckingham, M., et al. (2012). What does the concept of the stem cell niche really mean today? *BMC Biol.* 10:19. doi:10.1186/1741-7007-10-19

Lee, C. E., McArdle, A., and Griffiths, R. D. (2007). The role of hormones, cytokines and heat shock proteins during age-related muscle loss. *Clin. Nutr.* 26, 524–534. doi:10.1016/j.clnu.2007.05.005

Leeuwenburgh, C. (2003). Role of apoptosis in sarcopenia. *J. Gerontol. A Biol. Sci. Med. Sci.* 58, 999–1001. doi:10.1093/gerona/58.11.M999

Lepper, C., Partridge, T. A., and Fan, C. M. (2011). An absolute requirement for Pax7-positive satellite cells in acute injury-induced skeletal muscle regeneration. *Development* 138, 3639–3646. doi:10.1242/dev.067595

Lin, J., Handschin, C., and Spiegelman, B. M. (2005). Metabolic control through the PGC-1 family of transcription coactivators. *Cell Metab.* 1, 361–370. doi:10.1016/j.cmet.2005.05.004

Ljubicic, V., Joseph, A. M., Adhihetty, P. J., Huang, J. H., Saleem, A., Uguccioni, G., et al. (2009). Molecular basis for an attenuated mitochondrial adaptive plasticity in aged skeletal muscle. *Aging (Albany NY)* 1, 818–830.

Lowe, D. A., Lund, T., and Alway, S. E. (1998). Hypertrophy-stimulated myogenic regulatory factor mRNA increases are attenuated in fast muscle of aged quails. *Am. J. Physiol.* 275, C155–C162.

Machida, S., and Booth, F. W. (2004). Increased nuclear proteins in muscle satellite cells in aged animals as compared to young growing animals. *Exp. Gerontol.* 39, 1521–1525. doi:10.1016/j.exger.2004.08.009

Martinez-Hernandez, R., Bernal, S., Alias, L., and Tizzano, E. F. (2014). Abnormalities in early markers of muscle involvement support a delay in myogenesis in spinal muscular atrophy. *J. Neuropathol. Exp. Neurol.* 73, 559–567. doi:10.1097/NEN.0000000000000078

Marzetti, E., Calvani, R., Cesari, M., Buford, T. W., Lorenzi, M., Behnke, B. J., et al. (2013). Mitochondrial dysfunction and sarcopenia of aging: from signaling pathways to clinical trials. *Int. J. Biochem. Cell Biol.* 45, 2288–2301. doi:10.1016/j.biocel.2013.06.024

Marzetti, E., Hwang, J. C., Lees, H. A., Wohlgemuth, S. E., Dupont-Versteegden, E. E., Carter, C. S., et al. (2010). Mitochondrial death effectors: relevance to sarcopenia and disuse muscle atrophy. *Biochim. Biophys. Acta* 1800, 235–244. doi:10.1016/j.bbagen.2009.05.007

Marzetti, E., Lees, H. A., Manini, T. M., Buford, T. W., Aranda, J. M. Jr., Calvani, R., et al. (2012). Skeletal muscle apoptotic signaling predicts thigh muscle volume and gait speed in community-dwelling older persons: an exploratory study. *PLoS ONE* 7:e32829. doi:10.1371/journal.pone.0032829

Mauro, A. (1961). Satellite cell of skeletal muscle fibers. *J. Biophys. Biochem. Cytol.* 9, 493–495. doi:10.1083/jcb.9.2.493

Mavros, Y., Kay, S., Simpson, K. A., Baker, M. K., Wang, Y., Zhao, R. R., et al. (2014). Reductions in C-reactive protein in older adults with type 2 diabetes are related to improvements in body composition following a randomized controlled trial of resistance training. *J. Cachexia Sarcopenia Muscle* 5, 111–120. doi:10.1007/s13539-014-0134-1

McCarthy, J. J., Mula, J., Miyazaki, M., Erfani, R., Garrison, K., Farooqui, A. B., et al. (2011). Effective fiber hypertrophy in satellite cell-depleted skeletal muscle. *Development* 138, 3657–3666. doi:10.1242/dev.068858

McKay, B. R., O'Reilly, C. E., Phillips, S. M., Tarnopolsky, M. A., and Parise, G. (2008). Co-expression of IGF-1 family members with myogenic regulatory factors following acute damaging muscle-lengthening contractions in humans. *J. Physiol.* 586, 5549–5560. doi:10.1113/jphysiol.2008.160176

Michalakis, K., Goulis, D. G., Vazaiou, A., Mintziori, G., Polymeris, A., and Abrahamian-Michalakis, A. (2013). Obesity in the ageing man. *Metab. Clin. Exp.* 62, 1341–1349. doi:10.1016/j.metabol.2013.05.019

Minet, A. D., and Gaster, M. (2012). Cultured senescent myoblasts derived from human vastus lateralis exhibit normal mitochondrial ATP synthesis capacities with correlating concomitant ROS production while whole cell ATP production is decreased. *Biogerontology* 13, 277–285. doi:10.1007/s10522-012-9372-9

Mirza, K. A., Pereira, S. L., Edens, N. K., and Tisdale, M. J. (2014). Attenuation of muscle wasting in murine CC myotubes by epigallocatechin-3-gallate. *J. Cachexia Sarcopenia Muscle.* doi:10.1007/s13539-014-0139-9

Montarras, D., L'Honore, A., and Buckingham, M. (2013). Lying low but ready for action: the quiescent muscle satellite cell. *FEBS J.* 280, 4036–4050. doi:10.1111/febs.12372

Moore, D. T., Ferket, P. R., and Mozdziak, P. E. (2005). The effect of early nutrition on satellite cell dynamics in the young turkey. *Poult. Sci.* 84, 748–756. doi:10.1093/ps/84.5.748

Mosole, S., Carraro, U., Kern, H., Loefler, S., Fruhmann, H., Vogelauer, M., et al. (2014). Long-term high-level exercise promotes muscle reinnervation with age. *J. Neuropathol. Exp. Neurol.* 73, 284–294. doi:10.1097/NEN.0000000000000032

Moss, F. P., and Leblond, C. P. (1971). Satellite cells as the source of nuclei in muscles of growing rats. *Anat. Rec.* 170, 421–435. doi:10.1002/ar.1091700405

Mozdziak, P. E., Walsh, T. J., and McCoy, D. W. (2002). The effect of early posthatch nutrition on satellite cell mitotic activity. *Poult. Sci.* 81, 1703–1708. doi:10.1093/ps/81.11.1703

Murlasits, Z., Cutlip, R. G., Geronilla, K. B., Rao, K. M., Wonderlin, W. F., and Alway, S. E. (2006). Resistance training increases heat shock protein levels in skeletal muscle of young and old rats. *Exp. Gerontol.* 41, 398–406. doi:10.1016/j.exger.2006.01.005

Murphy, M. M., Lawson, J. A., Mathew, S. J., Hutcheson, D. A., and Kardon, G. (2011). Satellite cells, connective tissue fibroblasts and their interactions are crucial for muscle regeneration. *Development* 138, 3625–3637. doi:10.1242/dev.064162

Olguin, H. C., and Olwin, B. B. (2004). Pax-7 up-regulation inhibits myogenesis and cell cycle progression in satellite cells: a potential mechanism for self-renewal. *Dev. Biol.* 275, 375–388. doi:10.1016/j.ydbio.2004.08.015

Olguin, H. C., Yang, Z., Tapscott, S. J., and Olwin, B. B. (2007). Reciprocal inhibition between Pax7 and muscle regulatory factors modulates myogenic cell fate determination. *J. Cell Biol.* 177, 769–779. doi:10.1083/jcb.200608122

Ota, N., Soga, S., Haramizu, S., Yokoi, Y., Hase, T., and Murase, T. (2011). Tea catechins prevent contractile dysfunction in unloaded murine soleus muscle: a pilot study. *Nutrition* 27, 955–959. doi:10.1016/j.nut.2010.10.008

Oustanina, S., Hause, G., and Braun, T. (2004). Pax7 directs postnatal renewal and propagation of myogenic satellite cells but not their specification. *EMBO J.* 23, 3430–3439. doi:10.1038/sj.emboj.7600346

Parise, G., McKinnell, I. W., and Rudnicki, M. A. (2008). Muscle satellite cell and atypical myogenic progenitor response following exercise. *Muscle Nerve* 37, 611–619. doi:10.1002/mus.20995

Pellegrino, M. A., Desaphy, J. F., Brocca, L., Pierno, S., Camerino, D. C., and Bottinelli, R. (2011). Redox homeostasis, oxidative stress and disuse muscle atrophy. *J. Physiol.* 589, 2147–2160. doi:10.1113/jphysiol.2010.203232

Phillips, S. M., Tipton, K. D., Aarsland, A., Wolf, S. E., and Wolfe, R. R. (1997). Mixed muscle protein synthesis and breakdown after resistance exercise in humans. *Am. J. Physiol.* 273, E99–E107.

Pistilli, E. E., Siu, P. M., and Alway, S. E. (2006). Molecular regulation of apoptosis in fast plantaris muscles of aged rats. *J. Gerontol. A Biol. Sci. Med. Sci.* 61, 245–255. doi:10.1093/gerona/61.3.245

Powell, D. J., McFarland, D. C., Cowieson, A. J., Muir, W. I., and Velleman, S. G. (2013). The effect of nutritional status on myogenic satellite cell proliferation and differentiation. *Poult. Sci.* 92, 2163–2173. doi:10.3382/ps.2013-03107

Powell, D. J., McFarland, D. C., Cowieson, A. J., Muir, W. I., and Velleman, S. G. (2014). The effect of nutritional status and muscle fiber type on myogenic satellite cell fate and apoptosis. *Poult. Sci.* 93, 163–173. doi:10.3382/ps.2013-03450

Powers, S. K., Ji, L. L., Kavazis, A. N., and Jackson, M. J. (2011). Reactive oxygen species: impact on skeletal muscle. *Compr. Physiol.* 1, 941–969. doi:10.1002/cphy.c100054

Price, N. L., Gomes, A. P., Ling, A. J., Duarte, F. V., Martin-Montalvo, A., North, B. J., et al. (2012). SIRT1 is required for AMPK activation and the beneficial effects of resveratrol on mitochondrial function. *Cell Metab.* 15, 675–690. doi:10.1016/j.cmet.2012.04.003

Purves-Smith, F. M., Sgarioto, N., and Hepple, R. T. (2014). Fiber typing in aging muscle. *Exerc. Sport Sci. Rev.* 42, 45–52. doi:10.1249/JES.0000000000000012

Putman, C. T., Sultan, K. R., Wassmer, T., Bamford, J. A., Skorjanc, D., and Pette, D. (2001). Fiber-type transitions and satellite cell activation in low-frequency-stimulated muscles of young and aging rats. *J. Gerontol. A Biol. Sci. Med. Sci.* 56, B510–B519. doi:10.1093/gerona/56.12.B510

Quadrilatero, J., Alway, S. E., and Dupont-Versteegden, E. E. (2011). Skeletal muscle apoptotic response to physical activity: potential mechanisms for protection. *Appl. Physiol. Nutr. Metab.* 36, 608–617. doi:10.1139/h11-064

Rathbone, C. R., Booth, F. W., and Lees, S. J. (2009). Sirt1 increases skeletal muscle precursor cell proliferation. *Eur. J. Cell Biol.* 88, 35–44. doi:10.1016/j.ejcb.2008.08.003

Relaix, F., Montarras, D., Zaffran, S., Gayraud-Morel, B., Rocancourt, D., Tajbakhsh, S., et al. (2006). Pax3 and Pax7 have distinct and overlapping functions in adult muscle progenitor cells. *J. Cell Biol.* 172, 91–102. doi:10.1083/jcb.200508044

Renno, W. M., Al-Maghrebi, M., and Al-Banaw, A. (2012). (-)-Epigallocatechin-3-gallate (EGCG) attenuates functional deficits and morphological alterations by diminishing apoptotic gene overexpression in skeletal muscles after sciatic nerve crush injury. *Naunyn Schmiedebergs Arch. Pharmacol.* 385, 807–822. doi:10.1007/s00210-012-0758-7

Rice, C. L., Cunningham, D. A., Paterson, D. H., and Lefcoe, M. S. (1989). Arm and leg composition determined by computed tomography in young and elderly men. *Clin. Physiol.* 9, 207–220. doi:10.1111/j.1475-097X.1989.tb00973.x

Rudnicki, M. A., Le, G. F., McKinnell, I., and Kuang, S. (2008). The molecular regulation of muscle stem cell function. *Cold Spring Harb. Symp. Quant. Biol.* 73, 323–331. doi:10.1101/sqb.2008.73.064

Ryan, M. J., Jackson, J. R., Hao, Y., Leonard, S. S., and Alway, S. E. (2011). Inhibition of xanthine oxidase reduces oxidative stress and improves skeletal muscle function in response to electrically stimulated isometric contractions in aged mice. *Free Radic. Biol. Med.* 51, 38–52. doi:10.1016/j.freeradbiomed.2011.04.002

Ryan, M. J., Jackson, J. R., Hao, Y., Williamson, C. L., Dabkowski, E. R., Hollander, J. M., et al. (2010). Suppression of oxidative stress by resveratrol after isometric contractions in gastrocnemius muscles of aged mice. *J. Gerontol. A Biol. Sci. Med. Sci.* 65, 815–831. doi:10.1093/gerona/glq080

Sambasivan, R., Yao, R., Kissenpfennig, A., Van Wittenberghe, L., Paldi, A., Gayraud-Morel, B., et al. (2011). Pax7-expressing satellite cells are indispensable for adult skeletal muscle regeneration. *Development* 138, 3647–3656. doi:10.1242/dev.067587

Schmalbruch, H., and Hellhammer, U. (1977). The number of nuclei in adult rat muscles with special reference to satellite cells. *Anat. Rec.* 189, 169–175. doi:10.1002/ar.1091890204

Schmalbruch, H., and Lewis, D. M. (2000). Dynamics of nuclei of muscle fibers and connective tissue cells in normal and denervated rat muscles. *Muscle Nerve* 23, 617–626. doi:10.1002/(SICI)1097-4598(200004)23:4<617::AID-MUS22>3.0.CO;2-Y

Schultz, E., Gibson, M. C., and Champion, T. (1978). Satellite cells are mitotically quiescent in mature mouse muscle: an EM and radioautographic study. *J. Exp. Zool.* 206, 451–456.

Seale, P., Ishibashi, J., Scime, A., and Rudnicki, M. A. (2004). Pax7 is necessary and sufficient for the myogenic specification of CD45+:Sca1+ stem cells from injured muscle. *PLoS Biol.* 2:E130. doi:10.1371/journal.pbio.0020130

Seale, P., and Rudnicki, M. A. (2000). A new look at the origin, function, and "stem-cell" status of muscle satellite cells. *Dev. Biol.* 218, 115–124. doi:10.1006/dbio.1999.9565

Seale, P., Sabourin, L. A., Girgis-Gabardo, A., Mansouri, A., Gruss, P., and Rudnicki, M. A. (2000). Pax7 is required for the specification of myogenic satellite cells. *Cell* 102, 777–786. doi:10.1016/S0092-8674(00)00066-0

Shefer, G., Rauner, G., Yablonka-Reuveni, Z., and Benayahu, D. (2010). Reduced satellite cell numbers and myogenic capacity in aging can be alleviated by endurance exercise. *PLoS ONE* 5:e13307. doi:10.1371/journal.pone.0013307

Sinha, M., Jang, Y. C., Oh, J., Khong, D., Wu, E. Y., Manohar, R., et al. (2014). Restoring systemic GDF11 levels reverses age-related dysfunction in mouse skeletal muscle. *Science* 344, 649–652. doi:10.1126/science.1251152

Siu, P. M., and Alway, S. E. (2009). Response and adaptation of skeletal muscle to denervation stress: the role of apoptosis in muscle loss. *Front. Biosci.* 14:432–452. doi:10.2741/3253

Sjostrom, M., Lexell, J., and Downham, D. Y. (1992). Differences in fiber number and fiber type proportion within fascicles. A quantitative morphological study of whole vastus lateralis muscle from childhood to old age. *Anat. Rec.* 234, 183–189. doi:10.1002/ar.1092340205

Snijders, T., Verdijk, L. B., Smeets, J. S., McKay, B. R., Senden, J. M., Hartgens, F., et al. (2014a). The skeletal muscle satellite cell response to a single bout of resistance-type exercise is delayed with aging in men. *Age (Dordr.)* 36, 9699. doi:10.1007/s11357-014-9699-z

Snijders, T., Wall, B. T., Dirks, M. L., Senden, J. M., Hartgens, F., Dolmans, J., et al. (2014b). Muscle disuse atrophy is not accompanied by changes in skeletal muscle satellite cell content. *Clin. Sci. (Lond.)* 126, 557–566. doi:10.1042/CS20130295

Snijders, T., Verdijk, L. B., and van Loon, L. J. (2009). The impact of sarcopenia and exercise training on skeletal muscle satellite cells. *Ageing Res. Rev.* 8, 328–338. doi:10.1016/j.arr.2009.05.003

Snow, M. H. (1977). The effects of aging on satellite cells in skeletal muscles of mice and rats. *Cell Tissue Res.* 185, 399–408. doi:10.1007/BF00220299

Sousa-Victor, P., Gutarra, S., Garcia-Prat, L., Rodriguez-Ubreva, J., Ortet, L., Ruiz-Bonilla, V., et al. (2014). Geriatric muscle stem cells switch reversible quiescence into senescence. *Nature* 506, 316–321. doi:10.1038/nature13013

Spiegelman, B. M. (2007). Transcriptional control of mitochondrial energy metabolism through the PGC1 coactivators. *Novartis Found. Symp.* 287, 60–63. doi:10.1002/9780470725207.ch5

Stenholm, S., Harris, T. B., Rantanen, T., Visser, M., Kritchevsky, S. B., and Ferrucci, L. (2008). Sarcopenic obesity: definition, cause and consequences. *Curr. Opin. Clin. Nutr. Metab. Care* 11, 693–700. doi:10.1097/MCO.0b013e328312c37d

Stepto, N. K., Benziane, B., Wadley, G. D., Chibalin, A. V., Canny, B. J., Eynon, N., et al. (2012). Short-term intensified cycle training alters acute and chronic responses of PGC1alpha and cytochrome C oxidase IV to exercise in human skeletal muscle. *PLoS ONE* 7:e53080. doi:10.1371/journal.pone.0053080

Suetta, C., Frandsen, U., Mackey, A. L., Jensen, L., Hvid, L. G., Bayer, M. L., et al. (2013). Ageing is associated with diminished muscle re-growth and myogenic precursor cell expansion early after immobility-induced atrophy in human skeletal muscle. *J. Physiol.* 591, 3789–3804. doi:10.1113/jphysiol.2013.257121

Suetta, C., Hvid, L. G., Justesen, L., Christensen, U., Neergaard, K., Simonsen, L., et al. (2009). Effects of aging on human skeletal muscle after immobilization and retraining. *J. Appl. Physiol. (1985)* 107, 1172–1180. doi:10.1152/japplphysiol.00290.2009

Sullivan-Gunn, M. J., and Lewandowski, P. A. (2013). Elevated hydrogen peroxide and decreased catalase and glutathione peroxidase protection are associated with aging sarcopenia. *BMC Geriatr.* 13:104. doi:10.1186/1471-2318-13-104

Szczesny, B., Olah, G., Walker, D. K., Volpi, E., Rasmussen, B. B., Szabo, C., et al. (2013). Deficiency in repair of the mitochondrial genome sensitizes proliferating myoblasts to oxidative damage. *PLoS ONE* 8:e75201. doi:10.1371/journal.pone.0075201

Tidball, J. G. (2005). Inflammatory processes in muscle injury and repair. *Am. J. Physiol. Regul. Integr. Comp. Physiol.* 288, R345–R353. doi:10.1152/ajpregu.00454.2004

Tidball, J. G., and Wehling-Henricks, M. (2007). Macrophages promote muscle membrane repair and muscle fibre growth and regeneration during modified muscle loading in mice in vivo. *J. Physiol.* 578, 327–336. doi:10.1113/jphysiol.2006.118265

Tinetti, M. E. (2001). Where is the vision for fall prevention? *J. Am. Geriatr. Soc.* 49, 676–677. doi:10.1046/j.1532-5415.2001.49132.x

Toledo, M., Busquets, S., Ametller, E., Lopez-Soriano, F. J., and Argiles, J. M. (2011). Sirtuin 1 in skeletal muscle of cachectic tumour-bearing rats: a role in impaired regeneration? *J. Cachexia Sarcopenia Muscle* 2, 57–62. doi:10.1007/s13539-011-0018-6

Toth, K. G., McKay, B. R., De Lisio, M., Little, J. P., Tarnopolsky, M. A., and Parise, G. (2011). IL-6 induced STAT3 signalling is associated with the proliferation of human muscle satellite cells following acute muscle damage. *PLoS ONE* 6:e17392. doi:10.1371/journal.pone.0017392

van der Meer, S. F., Jaspers, R. T., Jones, D. A., and Degens, H. (2011a). The time course of myonuclear accretion during hypertrophy in young adult and older rat plantaris muscle. *Ann. Anat.* 193, 56–63. doi:10.1016/j.aanat.2010.08.004

van der Meer, S. F., Jaspers, R. T., Jones, D. A., and Degens, H. (2011b). Time-course of changes in the myonuclear domain during denervation in young-adult and old rat gastrocnemius muscle. *Muscle Nerve* 43, 212–222. doi:10.1002/mus.21822

Vasilaki, A., and Jackson, M. J. (2013). Role of reactive oxygen species in the defective regeneration seen in aging muscle. *Free Radic. Biol. Med.* 65, 317–323. doi:10.1016/j.freeradbiomed.2013.07.008

Velleman, S. G., Zhang, X., Coy, C. S., Song, Y., and McFarland, D. C. (2010). Changes in satellite cell proliferation and differentiation during turkey muscle development. *Poult. Sci.* 89, 709–715. doi:10.3382/ps.2009-00467

Verdijk, L. B., Dirks, M. L., Snijders, T., Prompers, J. J., Beelen, M., Jonkers, R. A., et al. (2012). Reduced satellite cell numbers with spinal cord injury and aging in humans. *Med. Sci. Sports Exerc.* 44, 2322–2330. doi:10.1249/MSS.0b013e3182667c2e

Verdijk, L. B., Gleeson, B. G., Jonkers, R. A., Meijer, K., Savelberg, H. H., Dendale, P., et al. (2009). Skeletal muscle hypertrophy following resistance training is accompanied by a fiber type-specific increase in satellite cell content in elderly men. *J. Gerontol. A Biol. Sci. Med. Sci.* 64, 332–339. doi:10.1093/gerona/gln050

Verdijk, L. B., Koopman, R., Schaart, G., Meijer, K., Savelberg, H. H., and van Loon, L. J. (2007). Satellite cell content is specifically reduced in type II skeletal muscle fibers in the elderly. *Am. J. Physiol. Endocrinol. Metab.* 292, E151–E157. doi:10.1152/ajpendo.00278.2006

Verdijk, L. B., Snijders, T., Drost, M., Delhaas, T., Kadi, F., and van Loon, L. J. (2014). Satellite cells in human skeletal muscle; from birth to old age. *Age (Dordr.)* 36, 545–547. doi:10.1007/s11357-013-9583-2

Vescovo, G., Volterrani, M., Zennaro, R., Sandri, M., Ceconi, C., Lorusso, R., et al. (2000). Apoptosis in the skeletal muscle of patients with heart failure:

investigation of clinical and biochemical changes. *Heart* 84, 431–437. doi:10.1136/heart.84.4.431

Vescovo, G., Zennaro, R., Sandri, M., Carraro, U., Leprotti, C., Ceconi, C., et al. (1998). Apoptosis of skeletal muscle myofibers and interstitial cells in experimental heart failure. *J. Mol. Cell. Cardiol.* 30, 2449–2459. doi:10.1006/jmcc.1998.0807

Vettor, R., Milan, G., Franzin, C., Sanna, M., De Coppi, P., Rizzuto, R., et al. (2009). The origin of intermuscular adipose tissue and its pathophysiological implications. *Am. J. Physiol. Endocrinol. Metab.* 297, E987–E998. doi:10.1152/ajpendo.00229.2009

Vinciguerra, M., Fulco, M., Ladurner, A., Sartorelli, V., and Rosenthal, N. (2010). SirT1 in muscle physiology and disease: lessons from mouse models. *Dis. Model Mech.* 3, 298–303. doi:10.1242/dmm.004655

von, M. J., Jones, A. E., Parks, R. J., and Rudnicki, M. A. (2013). Pax7 is critical for the normal function of satellite cells in adult skeletal muscle. *Proc. Natl. Acad. Sci. U.S.A.* 110, 16474–16479. doi:10.1073/pnas.1307680110

Wang, H., Lai, Y. J., Chan, Y. L., Li, T. L., and Wu, C. J. (2011). Epigallocatechin-3-gallate effectively attenuates skeletal muscle atrophy caused by cancer cachexia. *Cancer Lett.* 305, 40–49. doi:10.1016/j.canlet.2011.02.023

Wang, X., Pickrell, A. M., Rossi, S. G., Pinto, M., Dillon, L. M., Hida, A., et al. (2013). Transient systemic mtDNA damage leads to muscle wasting by reducing the satellite cell pool. *Hum. Mol. Genet.* 22, 3976–3986. doi:10.1093/hmg/ddt251

Welch, A. A. (2014). Nutritional influences on age-related skeletal muscle loss. *Proc. Nutr. Soc.* 73, 16–33. doi:10.1017/S0029665113003698

Welch, A. A., MacGregor, A. J., Minihane, A. M., Skinner, J., Valdes, A. A., Spector, T. D., et al. (2014). Dietary fat and fatty acid profile are associated with indices of skeletal muscle mass in women aged 18-79 years. *J. Nutr.* 144, 327–334. doi:10.3945/jn.113.185256

Westerbacka, J., Kolak, M., Kiviluoto, T., Arkkila, P., Siren, J., Hamsten, A., et al. (2007). Genes involved in fatty acid partitioning and binding, lipolysis, monocyte/macrophage recruitment, and inflammation are overexpressed in the human fatty liver of insulin-resistant subjects. *Diabetes* 56, 2759–2765. doi:10.2337/db07-0156

Wilson, G. J., Wilson, J. M., and Manninen, A. H. (2008). Effects of beta-hydroxy-beta-methylbutyrate (HMB) on exercise performance and body composition across varying levels of age, sex, and training experience: a review. *Nutr. Metab. (Lond.)* 5, 1–17. doi:10.1186/1743-7075-5-1

Wu, D., Wang, J., Pae, M., and Meydani, S. N. (2012). Green tea EGCG, T cells, and T cell-mediated autoimmune diseases. *Mol. Aspects Med.* 33, 107–118. doi:10.1016/j.mam.2011.10.001

Xu, Z., Huang, G., Gong, W., Zhou, P., Zhao, Y., Zhang, Y., et al. (2012). FXR ligands protect against hepatocellular inflammation via SOCS3 induction. *Cell. Signal.* 24, 1658–1664. doi:10.1016/j.cellsig.2012.04.015

Yablonka-Reuveni, Z., Day, K., Vine, A., and Shefer, G. (2008). Defining the transcriptional signature of skeletal muscle stem cells. *J. Anim. Sci.* 86, E207–E216. doi:10.2527/jas.2007-0473

Cyclosporin A promotes *in vivo* myogenic response in collagen VI-deficient myopathic mice

Francesca Gattazzo[1,2], Sibilla Molon[1], Valeria Morbidoni[1], Paola Braghetta[1], Bert Blaauw[3], Anna Urciuolo[1*†] and Paolo Bonaldo[1*]

[1] *Department of Molecular Medicine, University of Padova, Padova, Italy*
[2] *Interdepartmental Research Center E. Piaggio, University of Pisa, Pisa, Italy*
[3] *Department of Biomedical Sciences, University of Padova, Padova, Italy*

Correspondence:
Anna Urciuolo and Paolo Bonaldo, Department of Molecular Medicine, University of Padova, Via U. Bassi 58/B, Padova I-35131, Italy
e-mail: a.urciuolo@ucl.ac.uk; bonaldo@bio.unipd.it

†*Present address:*
Anna Urciuolo, Stem Cells and Regenerative Medicine, University College London Institute of Child Health, London, UK

Mutations of genes encoding for collagen VI cause various muscle diseases in humans, including Bethlem myopathy and Ullrich congenital muscular dystrophy. Collagen VI null (*Col6a1*$^{-/-}$) mice are affected by a myopathic phenotype with mitochondrial dysfunction, spontaneous apoptosis of muscle fibers, and defective autophagy. Moreover, *Col6a1*$^{-/-}$ mice display impaired muscle regeneration and defective self-renewal of satellite cells after injury. Treatment with cyclosporin A (CsA) is effective in normalizing the mitochondrial, apoptotic, and autophagic defects of myofibers in *Col6a1*$^{-/-}$ mice. A pilot clinical trial with CsA in Ullrich patients suggested that CsA may increase the number of regenerating myofibers. Here, we report the effects of CsA administration at 5 mg/kg body weight every 12 h in *Col6a1*$^{-/-}$ mice on muscle regeneration under physiological conditions and after cardiotoxin (CdTx)-induced muscle injury. Our findings indicate that CsA influences satellite cell activity and triggers the formation of regenerating fibers in *Col6a1*$^{-/-}$ mice. Data obtained on injured muscles show that under appropriate administration, regimens CsA is able to stimulate myogenesis in *Col6a1*$^{-/-}$ mice by significantly increasing the number of myogenin (MyoG)-positive cells and of regenerating myofibers at the early stages of muscle regeneration. CsA is also able to ameliorate muscle regeneration of *Col6a1*$^{-/-}$ mice subjected to multiple CdTx injuries, with a concurrent maintenance of the satellite cell pool. Our data show that CsA is beneficial for muscle regeneration in *Col6a1*$^{-/-}$ mice.

Keywords: collagen VI, skeletal muscle, congenital muscular dystrophy, animal model, cyclosporin A, muscle regeneration

INTRODUCTION

Collagen VI is an extracellular matrix protein that forms a microfibrillar network in the endomysium of skeletal muscle. The critical role played by this protein in muscle is clearly shown by collagen VI null (*Col6a1*$^{-/-}$) mice, which display an early onset myopathic phenotype characterized by mitochondrial dysfunction, defective autophagy, and spontaneous apoptosis of muscle fibers (Bonaldo et al., 1998; Irwin et al., 2003; Grumati et al., 2010). Cyclosporin A (CsA) is a well-known immunosuppressant drug that was found to have multiple beneficial effects on the myopathic phenotype of *Col6a1*$^{-/-}$ mice, including (i) decreased opening of the mitochondrial permeability transition pore; (ii) rescue of myofiber apoptosis; (iii) stimulation of autophagy in muscle fibers; and (iv) recovery of muscle strength (Irwin et al., 2003; Grumati et al., 2010). Mutations of *COL6* genes in humans cause several muscle disorders, including Bethlem myopathy and Ullrich congenital muscular dystrophy (Lampe and Bushby, 2005). A pilot clinical trial in Ullrich and Bethlem patients showed that CsA favorably affects mitochondrial function and dramatically decreases the incidence of apoptosis in muscle fibers. Notably, a significant increase in the number of regenerating myofibers was observed in younger patients undergoing CsA treatment, suggesting that CsA may also increase the overall efficiency of muscle regeneration in patients (Merlini et al., 2008, 2011).

Muscle regeneration relies on the presence of satellite cells, which are quiescent under physiological conditions but become activated upon damage, thus undergoing proliferation and terminal differentiation. At the same time, a subset of activated satellite cells returns to the quiescent state in their original niche under the basal lamina, through a self-renewal process (Tedesco et al., 2010). The differentiation of satellite cells is regulated by a number of transcription factors, where Pax7 is required for satellite cell specification and survival, whereas MyoD, myogenin (MyoG), and MRF4 are essential for satellite cell proliferation and differentiation (Buckingham and Rigby, 2014). Terminal differentiation coincides with the abundant synthesis of myosin heavy chain (MHC). The cardiotoxin (CdTx) injury model is widely used to investigate skeletal muscle regeneration (Chargé and Rudnicki, 2004; Shi and Garry, 2006). We recently demonstrated that collagen VI is a critical component of satellite cell *niche* and that ablation of collagen VI leads to impaired muscle regeneration and reduced satellite cell self-renewal after injury (Urciuolo et al., 2013). Studies performed in tibialis anterior (TA) muscle showed that *Col6a1*$^{-/-}$ mice undergo a marked depletion of the satellite cell pool 7 days after CdTx injection, and this defect becomes much more dramatic after multiple rounds of CdTx injury (Urciuolo et al., 2013). Given the effects displayed by CsA in collagen VI-deficient mice and Ullrich/Bethlem patients (Irwin et al., 2003; Merlini et al., 2008), here we analyzed in detail the outcomes of CsA administration on muscle regeneration and satellite cells in *Col6a1*$^{-/-}$ mice under physiological conditions and after CdTx-induced injury.

MATERIALS AND METHODS

MICE

We performed experiments in wild-type mice of the inbred C57BL/6NCrl strain and in *Col6a1*$^{-/-}$ mice that were backcrossed in the C57BL/6NCrl strain for eight generations (Irwin et al., 2003). All data were obtained from 6-month-old mice. Mice were housed in individual cages in an environmentally controlled room (23°C, 12 h light/12 h dark cycle) and provided food and water *ad libitum*. Mouse procedures were approved by the Ethics Committee of the University of Padova and authorized by the Italian Ministry of Health.

IN VIVO TREATMENTS

Cyclosporin A (Sandimmun 50 mg/ml, Novartis) was dissolved in olive oil and a stock solution at a concentration of 10 mg/ml was prepared. For CsA administration under physiological conditions, mice were subjected to intraperitoneal (i.p.) injection of vehicle (olive oil) or CsA at 5 mg/kg body weight every 12 h for 10 days. In experiments with higher dosage CsA, mice were subjected to i.p. injection of vehicle or CsA at 25 mg/kg body weight every 24 h for 10 days. Animals were sacrificed 12 h after the last administration of CsA or vehicle. For single CdTx injury (Couteaux et al., 1988), mice were treated by i.p. injection with vehicle or CsA at 5 mg/kg body weight every 12 h for 10 days. At day 4 from the first administration of vehicle or CsA, mice were anesthetized with isoflurane (Merial) and TA muscles injected with 30 μl CdTx (Naja mossambica mossambica, 10 μM; Sigma). Analgesia (Rimadyl) was administered subcutaneously for 3 days and mice were sacrificed 7 days after muscle damage (i.e., 10 days after the first injection of vehicle or CsA). For multiple injury experiments, TA muscles were subjected to three distinct injections of CdTx, each one every 30 days. Four days before the third CdTx injection, mice were treated by i.p. injection with vehicle or CsA at 5 mg/kg body weight every 12 h for 10 days. Mice were sacrificed 30 days after the third CdTx injury (i.e., 24 days after the last injection of vehicle or CsA).

HISTOLOGICAL ANALYSIS

Tibialis anterior muscles were isolated from mice, frozen in liquid nitrogen, weighted on a precision balance, and kept at −80°C until use. Cross-sections (10 μm thick) were used and processed for hematoxylin–eosin or Azan-Mallory staining following standard protocols. Samples were analyzed with a Zeiss Axioplan light microscope equipped with Leica DC500 digital camera. Myofiber cross-sectional area and the area of fibrosis were evaluated with the IM1000 software (Leica).

ISOLATION OF EXTENSOR DIGITORUM LONGUS SINGLE MYOFIBERS

We carefully dissected extensor digitorum longus (EDL) muscles from 6-month-old mice and subjected them to enzymatic digestion with collagenase I (2 mg/ml, Gibco) for 80 min at 37°C. We blocked the digestion with Dulbecco's Modified Eagle Medium (DMEM, Sigma), supplemented with 0.2 M L-glutamine (Invitrogen), 1:100 penicillin-streptomycin (Invitrogen), 1:100 fungizone (Invitrogen), and 10% horse serum (Gibco), and gently released single myofibers from muscles. Every 15–25 min, undamaged and non-contracted fibers were transferred in a new dish containing fresh medium, and this procedure was repeated five times in order to remove debris and interstitial cells. Freshly isolated fibers were finally fixed in 4% paraformaldehyde in PBS for 15 min and maintained at 4°C in PBS until use.

IMMUNOFLUORESCENCE

For immunofluorescence on muscle sections, frozen TA sections (7 μm) were fixed for 20 min with 4% paraformaldehyde in PBS and permeabilized for 6 min with cold methanol. For the unmasking of Pax7 and MyoG, slides were treated twice with 0.01 M citric acid (pH 6) at 90°C for 5 min. For mouse antibodies staining, samples were first incubated for 2.5 h with 4% bovine serum albumin (BSA IgG-Free, Jackson Immunoresearch) in PBS and then treated for 30 min with a blocking solution containing 0.05 mg/ml Fab fragment anti-mouse IgG (Jackson Immunoresearch). When mouse antibodies were not used, samples were only incubated for 1 h at room temperature with 4% bovine serum albumin in PBS. After the blocking step, samples were incubated with primary antibodies at 4°C overnight. The following primary antibodies were used: mouse anti-Pax7 (1:20; Developmental Studies Hybridoma Bank); mouse anti-MyoG (F5D, 1:15; Developmental Studies Hybridoma Bank); mouse anti-embryonic MHC (eMHC) (F1.652, 1:20; Developmental Studies Hybridoma Bank); rabbit anti-laminin (L9393, 1:800; Sigma). After washing, samples were incubated with the appropriate secondary antibody for 1 h at room temperature. Secondary antibodies used were biotinylated anti-mouse (115-007-003, 1:1000), Cy2 or Cy3 anti-mouse (115-226-062, 1:500, or 115-165-006, 1:1000), Cy2 or Cy3 anti-rabbit (111-225-144, 1:500, or 115-165-006, 1:1000) (all Jackson Immunoresearch). To reveal the biotinylated antibody, Cy2 or Cy3 streptavidin (016-220-084, 1:1500, or 016-160-084, 1:2500; Jackson Immunoresearch) was used. For immunofluorescence of EDL single myofibers, cells were permeabilized with 0.5% Triton X-100 in PBS, treated with 20% goat serum (Invitrogen) in PBS for 1 h, and incubated at 37°C for 1 h or at 4°C overnight with mouse anti-Pax7 antibody (1:20; Developmental Studies Hybridoma Bank). After washing, samples were incubated with the appropriate secondary antibody as described above. Nuclei were stained with Hoechst 33258 (Sigma). Samples were analyzed with a Zeiss Axioplan Leica DC500 epifluorescence microscope or with a Leica SP5 confocal microscope.

TUNEL

For apoptosis analysis on TA cryosections, the DeadEnd™ Fluorometric TUNEL assay (Promega) was used. Samples were fixed for 15 min with 4% paraformaldehyde, permeabilized for 5 min with 0.5% Triton X-100, and processed following manufacturer instructions.

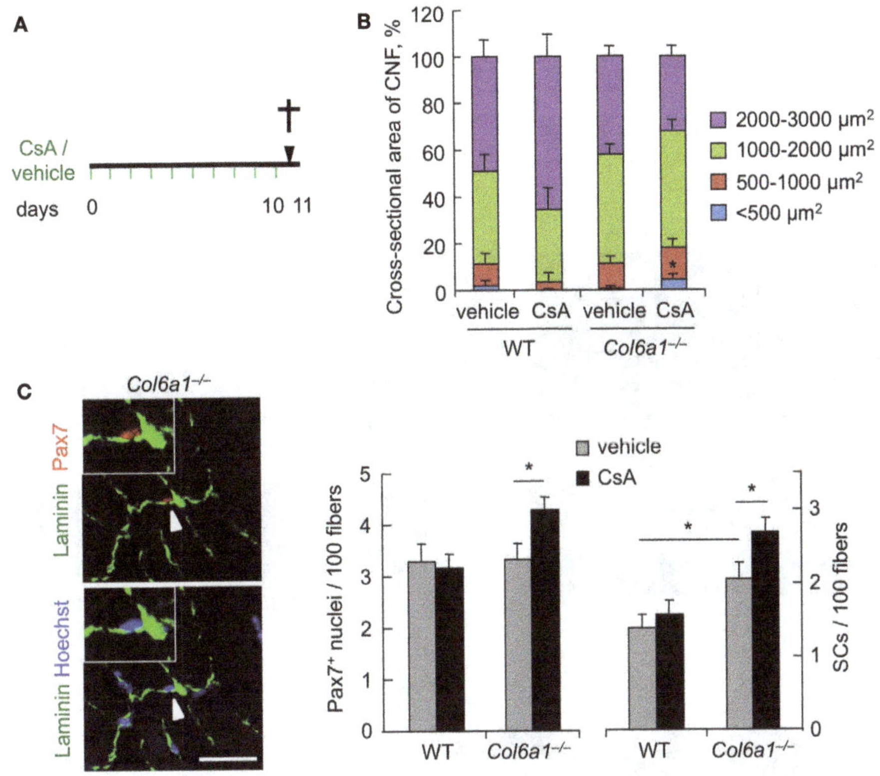

FIGURE 1 | Cyclosporin A induces muscle regeneration and increases satellite cell number in *Col6a1*$^{-/-}$ mice. **(A)** Schematic diagram of CsA treatment. Wild-type and *Col6a1*$^{-/-}$ mice were treated with vehicle or with CsA (5 mg/kg body weight) every 12 h for 10 days. Animals were sacrificed 12 h after the last administration of CsA or vehicle. **(B)** Mean cross-sectional area of regenerating centrally nucleated myofibers in TA muscles derived from wild-type and *Col6a1*$^{-/-}$ mice treated with vehicle or CsA. Fibers were divided into four size ranges, and at least 150 centrally nucleated myofibers were analyzed for each group. Error bars indicate SEM (*$P < 0.05$ for *Col6a1*$^{-/-}$ CsA vs. *Col6a1*$^{-/-}$ vehicle; $n = 3$–4, each group). **(C)** Left panel, representative images of immunofluorescence labeling for laminin (green) and Pax7 (red) in TA cross-sections of CsA-treated *Col6a1*$^{-/-}$ mice. The arrowhead points at one satellite cell, shown at higher magnification in the inset. Nuclei were stained with Hoechst (blue). Scale bar, 25 µm. Right panel, quantification of total Pax7-positive cells and of satellite cells, calculated as the number on 100 myofibers in TA muscles derived from wild-type and *Col6a1*$^{-/-}$ mice treated with vehicle or CsA. Error bars indicate SEM (*$P < 0.05$; $n = 5$–7, each group). CNF, centrally nucleated fibers; CSA, cross-sectional area; SCs, satellite cells; WT, wild-type.

STATISTICAL ANALYSES

Data are expressed as means ± SEM. We determined statistical significance by unequal variance Student's t-test, and a P value of <0.05 was considered statistically significant.

RESULTS

CsA INDUCES MUSCLE REGENERATION IN *Col6a1*$^{-/-}$ MICE UNDER PHYSIOLOGICAL CONDITIONS

To investigate the effects of CsA administration in *Col6a1*$^{-/-}$ mice under physiological conditions, we subjected animals to i.p. injection of vehicle or CsA at 5 mg/kg body weight every 12 h and analyzed muscles after 10 days of treatment (**Figure 1A**). This dosage of CsA was previously found to trigger a marked amelioration of the myopathic phenotype of *Col6a1*$^{-/-}$ mice, with rescue from mitochondrial depolarization and apoptosis and reactivation of the autophagic flux in muscle fibers (Irwin et al., 2003; Grumati et al., 2010). To evaluate whether this CsA treatment triggered *de novo* formation of myofibers in *Col6a1*$^{-/-}$ mice, we first analyzed the cross-sectional area of regenerating, centrally nucleated fibers in TA muscle, by dividing regenerating myofibers into four different size ranges. Unlike wild-type animals, CsA treatment led to a significant increase of the percentage of regenerating myofibers with small area (<500 µm^2) in *Col6a1*$^{-/-}$ mice when compared to vehicle-treated *Col6a1*$^{-/-}$ animals (**Figure 1B**). These data were also confirmed by immunofluorescence analysis for eMHC, an established marker of newly forming fibers (Ciciliot and Schiaffino, 2010). Immature myofibers expressing eMHC were present in TA muscles of *Col6a1*$^{-/-}$ mice treated with CsA, but not in those treated with vehicle (Figure S1A in Supplementary Material). Based on these results, we evaluated the number of myogenic cells by performing immunostaining for Pax7. CsA administration increased the total number of Pax7-positive cells and also the number of satellite cells (i.e., Pax7-positive cells located underneath the basal lamina) in *Col6a1*$^{-/-}$ TA but not in wild-type TA (**Figure 1C**). These data were confirmed by analyzing freshly isolated EDL myofibers, which showed a significant increase in the number of Pax7-positive cells on myofibers derived from CsA-treated *Col6a1*$^{-/-}$ mice when compared to vehicle-treated animals (Figure S1B in Supplementary Material). To assess whether the increased number of Pax7-positive cells in *Col6a1*$^{-/-}$ animals was

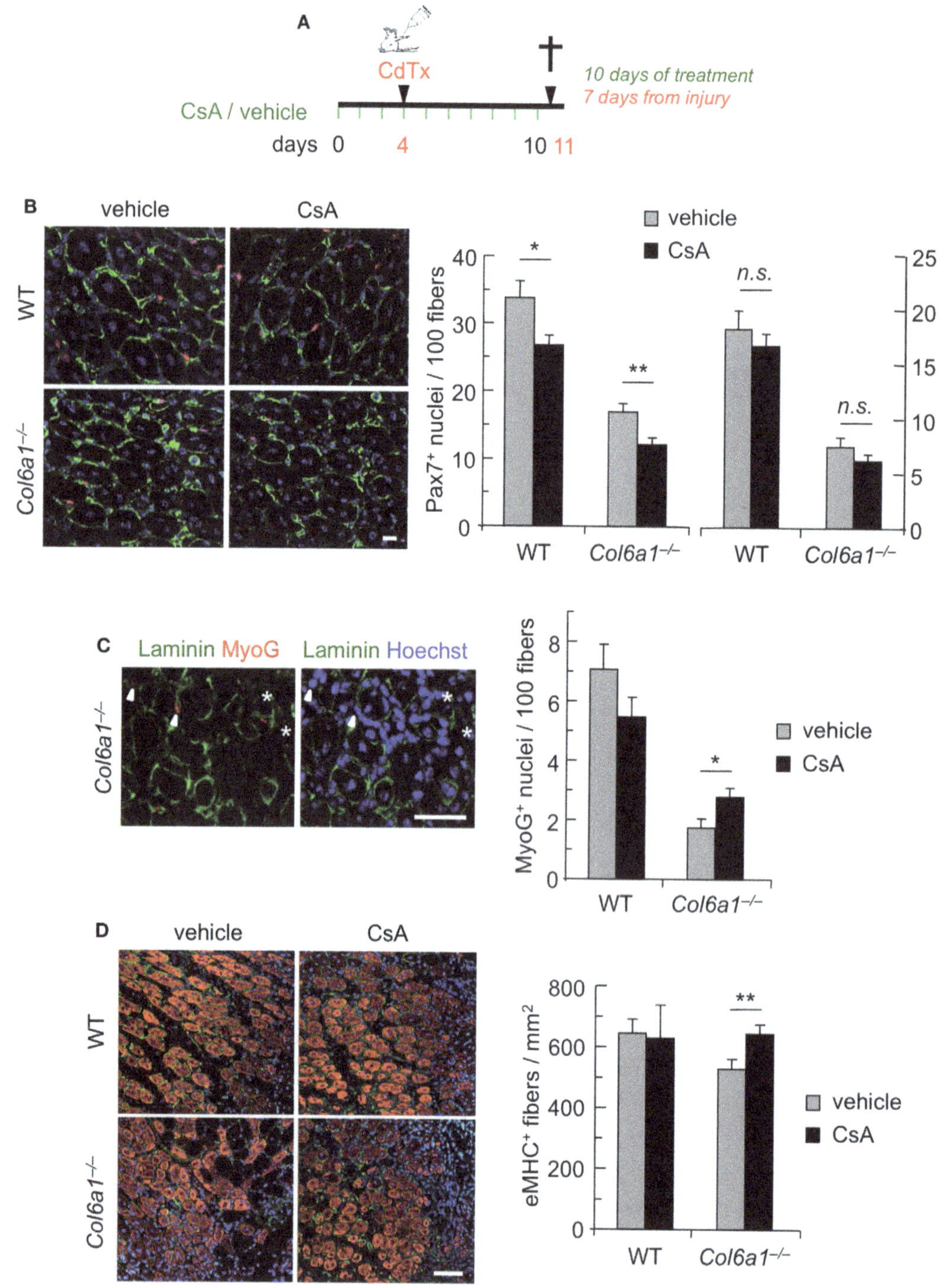

FIGURE 2 | Continuous administration of CsA during a single CdTx injury stimulates muscle differentiation in *Col6a1*$^{-/-}$ mice.
(A) Schematic diagram of CsA treatment and CdTx injury. Wild-type and *Col6a1*$^{-/-}$ mice were treated with vehicle or CsA (5 mg/kg body weight) every 12 h for 10 days. Four days after the first injection of vehicle or CsA, TA muscles were injured with CdTx and drug treatment continued for other 7 days. Animals were sacrificed 12 h from the last administration of CsA or vehicle. **(B)** Left panels, representative images of immunofluorescence labeling for laminin (green) and Pax7 (red) in 7-day-post-injury TA cross-sections of wild-type and *Col6a1*$^{-/-}$ mice treated with vehicle or CsA. Scale bar, 25 μm. Right panel, quantification of total Pax7-positive cells and of satellite cells, calculated as the number on 100 myofibers in 7-day-post-injury TA muscles of wild-type and *Col6a1*$^{-/-}$ mice treated with vehicle or CsA. Error bars indicate SEM (**$P < 0.01$; *$P < 0.05$; n.s. not significant; $n = 3$–5, each group). **(C)** Left panels, representative images of immunofluorescence labeling for laminin (green) and MyoG (red) in 7-day-post-injury TA cross-sections of *Col6a1*$^{-/-}$ mice treated with vehicle or CsA. Nuclei were stained with Hoechst (blue). The arrowheads point at MyoG-positive cells outside the basal lamina, and the asterisks mark MyoG-positive cells located underneath the basal lamina (corresponding to myogenic cells that are undergoing fusion).

(Continued)

FIGURE 2 | Continued
Scale bar, 50 μm. Right panel, quantification of total MyoG-positive cells, calculated as the number on 100 myofibers in 7-day-post-injury TA muscles of wild-type and *Col6a1*$^{-/-}$ mice treated with vehicle or CsA. Error bars indicate SEM ($*P < 0.05$; $n = 3$–5, each group). **(D)** Left panels, representative images of immunofluorescence for laminin (green) and eMHC (red) in 7-day-post-injury TA cross-sections of wild-type and *Col6a1*$^{-/-}$ mice treated with vehicle or CsA. Nuclei were stained with Hoechst (blue). Scale bar, 50 μm. Right panel, quantification of the number of eMHC-positive myofibers per regenerating area in 7-day-post-injury TA cross-sections of wild-type and *Col6a1*$^{-/-}$ mice treated with vehicle or CsA. Error bars indicate SEM ($**P < 0.01$; $n = 3$–5, each group). SCs, satellite cells; WT, wild-type.

only provided by this drug dosage or could be also elicited by higher CsA concentrations known to cause strong immunosuppressive effects (Homan et al., 1980), we subjected mice to i.p. injection of CsA at 25 mg/kg body weight every 24 h for 10 days. Interestingly, at this higher dosage, CsA led to a dramatic decrease in the number of total Pax7-positive cells and of satellite cells both in wild-type and in *Col6a1*$^{-/-}$ mice when compared to vehicle-treated animals (Figure S1C in Supplementary Material). These results highlight the relevance of CsA dosage in inducing beneficial effects in *Col6a1*$^{-/-}$ muscles and accordingly with previous studies carried out with the immunosuppressive drug FK506 (Irwin et al., 2003), they suggest that immunosuppression exacerbates the phenotype of *Col6a1*$^{-/-}$ mice.

CONTINUOUS ADMINISTRATION OF CsA DURING CdTx INJURY STIMULATES THE EARLY PHASES OF MUSCLE DIFFERENTIATION IN *Col6a1*$^{-/-}$ MICE

To further assess the capability of CsA to ameliorate the muscle regenerative defects of *Col6a1*$^{-/-}$ mice, we carried out CsA treatment under experimentally induced muscle injury. Toward this aim, wild-type and *Col6a1*$^{-/-}$ mice were treated for 10 days with vehicle or CsA at 5 mg/kg body weight every 12 h; 4 days after the start of treatment, TA muscles were subjected to CdTx damage and mice were sacrificed 7 days after injury (**Figure 2A**). TUNEL assay showed that the incidence of apoptotic nuclei 7 days after CdTx injection was very low in wild-type TA, in agreement with the concept that myofiber demise is almost completed at this stage from injury (Hawke et al., 2003). Conversely, *Col6a1*$^{-/-}$ TA showed a higher number of TUNEL-positive myonuclei 7 days after injury, and CsA administration was able to significantly decrease the incidence of apoptotic myofibers triggered by CdTx injury in *Col6a1*$^{-/-}$ TA muscles (Figure S2 in Supplementary Material). We next evaluated the number of myogenic cells by immunofluorescence for the Pax7 and MyoG markers. CsA administration led to a significant decrease in the number of total Pax7-positive cells in both wild-type and *Col6a1*$^{-/-}$ injured TA, without any significant change in the number of satellite cells (i.e., Pax7-positive cells located underneath basal lamina) (**Figure 2B**). This response was paralleled by a significant increase of the total number of MyoG-positive cells in injured TA muscles of CsA-treated *Col6a1*$^{-/-}$ mice when compared to vehicle-treated *Col6a1*$^{-/-}$ mice, whereas wild-type injured TA muscles did not show any significant difference in MyoG positivity between vehicle and CsA-treated animals (**Figure 2C**). Additionally, *Col6a1*$^{-/-}$ mice treated with CsA showed an increased number of regenerating myofibers expressing eMHC, whereas no differences in eMHC-positive regenerating myofibers were found in wild-type animals (**Figure 2D**). As the defective satellite self-renewal of *Col6a1*$^{-/-}$ mice is strictly dependent on the lack of extracellular collagen VI and on the lower muscle stiffness (Urciuolo et al., 2013), it was not surprising to observe that in this experimental condition CsA does not display any overt effect on satellite cell maintenance. On the other hand, the remarkable increase in the number of differentiated (i.e., MyoG-positive) myogenic cells, together with the higher number of newly forming (i.e., eMHC-positive) myofibers, indicates that CsA administration is able to improve muscle differentiation upon damage in the *Col6a1*$^{-/-}$ myopathic mouse model.

ADMINISTRATION OF CsA DURING REPEATED MUSCLE INJURY COUNTERACTS MUSCLE LOSS AND FIBROSIS AND PRESERVES THE SATELLITE CELL POOL IN *Col6a1*$^{-/-}$ MICE

Although muscles of *Col6a1*$^{-/-}$ animals display a delayed regeneration after injury, we have previously shown that at 30 days after CdTx injury they are still able to complete the regeneration process (Urciuolo et al., 2013). However, and at difference from wild-type mice, the capability of *Col6a1*$^{-/-}$ animals to undergo muscle regeneration and preserve the satellite cell pool is lost after multiple muscle injuries, leading to a severe loss of muscle mass (Urciuolo et al., 2013). Therefore, we investigated whether CsA is able to counteract the defective muscle regeneration and the depletion of the satellite cell pool triggered by multiple injuries in *Col6a1*$^{-/-}$ mice. Toward this aim, we subjected TA muscles of wild-type and *Col6a1*$^{-/-}$ mice to three rounds of CdTx injury. Animals were treated for 10 days with vehicle or CsA at 5 mg/kg body weight every 12 h during the third injury and sacrificed 30 days after the last injury (**Figure 3A**). Interestingly, CsA administration was highly effective in reducing the extensive muscle fibrosis triggered by triple injury in *Col6a1*$^{-/-}$ mice (**Figure 3B**). The beneficial effects of CsA in *Col6a1*$^{-/-}$ muscles undergoing multiple injuries were also confirmed by the increased myofiber cross-sectional area and by the improvement of the muscle mass in CsA-treated *Col6a1*$^{-/-}$ mice when compared to vehicle-treated *Col6a1*$^{-/-}$ mice (Figure S3 in Supplementary Material). Notably, CsA administration led to marked increase of both total Pax7-positive cell number and satellite cell number in *Col6a1*$^{-/-}$ TA muscles subjected to multiple injuries (**Figures 3C,D**). Altogether, these results show that at this regimen CsA is capable to preserve not only muscle fibers but also the satellite cell pool of collagen VI-deficient mice.

DISCUSSION

In the present study, we evaluated the potential beneficial effects exerted by CsA on skeletal muscle regeneration in *Col6a1*$^{-/-}$ mice, both under physiological condition and after muscle damage. The rationale for this study was based on previous findings in patients affected by collagen VI myopathies, suggesting that besides counteracting myofiber apoptosis and mitochondrial dysfunction, CsA treatment may also increase muscle regeneration (Merlini et al., 2008, 2011). In addition, our recent findings

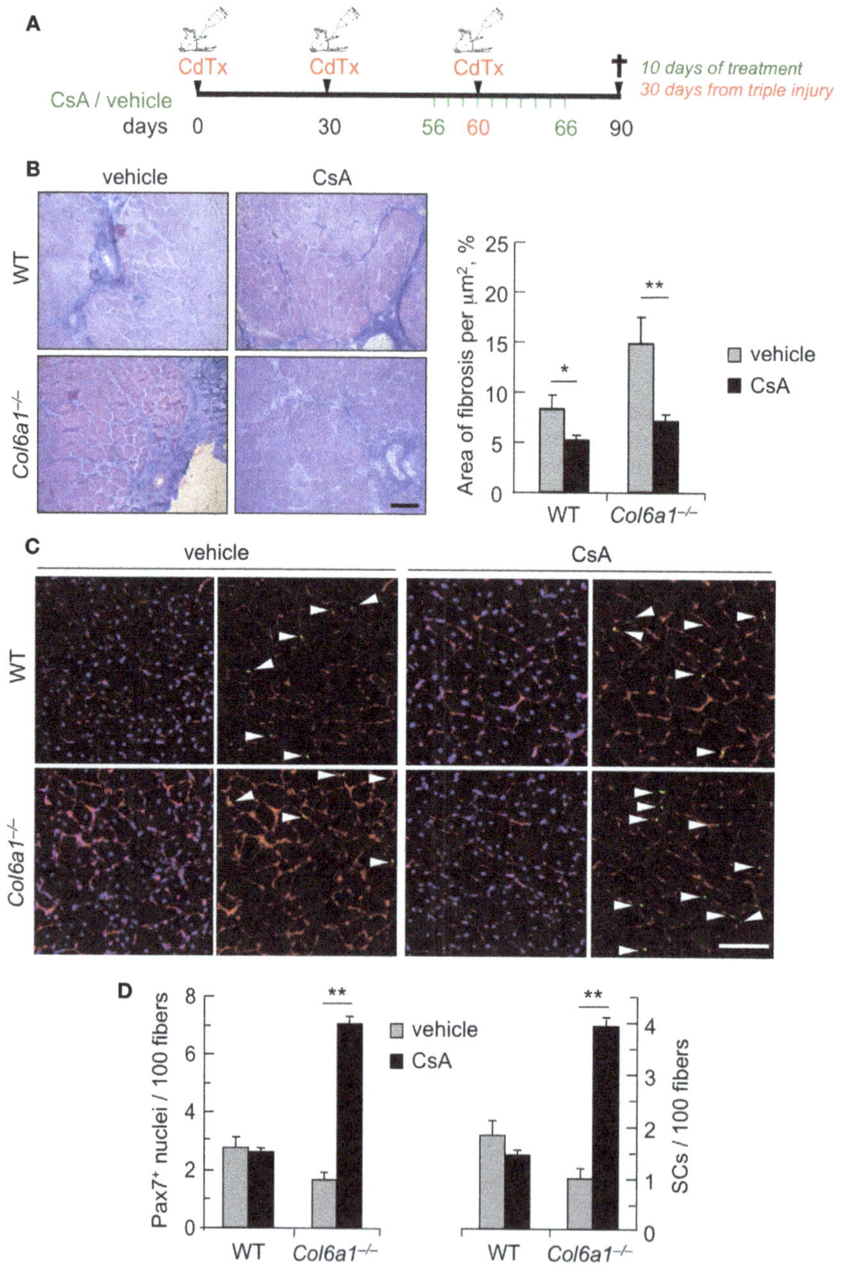

FIGURE 3 | Administration of CsA during a triple muscle injury counteracts muscle loss and fibrosis and preserves the satellite cell pool in *Col6a1*$^{-/-}$ mice. **(A)** Schematic diagram of CsA treatment and CdTx injuries. TA muscles of wild-type and *Col6a1*$^{-/-}$ mice were given three repeated injections of CdTx every 30 days. Four days before the last injury, *Col6a1*$^{-/-}$ mice were treated with vehicle or CsA (5 mg/kg body weight) every 12 h for 10 days. Mice were sacrificed 30 days after the third injury (i.e., 24 days from the last administration of vehicle or CsA). **(B)** Left panels, Azan-Mallory staining of triple injured TA cross-sections from wild-type and *Col6a1*$^{-/-}$ mice treated with vehicle or CsA. Scale bar, 50 μm. Right panel, quantification of the fibrotic area in triple-injured TA cross-sections from wild-type and *Col6a1*$^{-/-}$ mice treated with vehicle or CsA. Error bars indicate SEM ($^{**}P < 0.01$; $^{*}P < 0.05$; $n = 4$–8, each group). **(C)** Representative images of immunofluorescence labeling for laminin (red) and Pax7 (green) in triple-injured TA cross-sections from wild-type and *Col6a1*$^{-/-}$ treated with vehicle or CsA. Arrows point at Pax7-positive nuclei. Nuclei were stained with Hoechst (blue). Scale bar, 100 μm. **(D)** Quantification of total Pax7-positive cells and of satellite cells, calculated as the number on 100 myofibers in triple-injured TA cross-sections from wild-type and *Col6a1*$^{-/-}$ mice treated with vehicle or CsA. Error bars indicate SEM ($^{**}P < 0.01$; $n = 4$–8, each group). SC, satellite cells; WT, wild-type.

showed impaired regeneration and defective satellite cell self-renewal in collagen VI-deficient muscles (Urciuolo et al., 2013). Therefore, we investigated how CsA treatment impacts on the regeneration of collagen VI-deficient mice. Under physiological conditions, CsA was capable to amplify the pool of total Pax7-positive cells and of satellite cells and increased the amount of newly formed centrally nucleated myofibers, thus suggesting a new role for CsA in stimulating myogenesis in *Col6a1*$^{-/-}$ muscles. Notably, these beneficial effects were dose-dependent, as they were observed at 10 mg/kg/day but not at a higher immunosuppressant dose (25 mg/kg/day), which conversely had a negative impact on the satellite cell pool. These data are in agreement with previous results in which the same protocol of CsA administration was found to desensitize the mitochondrial permeability transition pore and reduce myofiber apoptosis in *Col6a1*$^{-/-}$ mice (Irwin et al., 2003). Although we previously demonstrated that CsA stimulates autophagy in skeletal myofibers (Grumati et al., 2010), the increased number of satellite cells in muscles of CsA-treated *Col6a1*$^{-/-}$ animals is not a direct consequence of a stimulatory effect on autophagy. Indeed, reactivation of the autophagic flux in *Col6a1*$^{-/-}$ mice by different pharmacological or dietary treatments does not exert any significant effect on satellite cells (Urciuolo et al., 2013). Our present findings are consistent with the strong amelioration of the myophatic phenotype in *Col6a1*$^{-/-}$ mice following CsA administration and indicate that besides decreasing mitochondrial dysfunction and apoptosis and reactivating autophagy in muscle fibers (Irwin et al., 2003; Grumati et al., 2010), the drug is also able to increase the pool of functional Pax7-positive cells and stimulate the formation of newly formed fibers.

The beneficial effects exerted by CsA on the regeneration capabilities of *Col6a1*$^{-/-}$ mice become very evident under experimentally induced single and multiple muscle injuries. Our data indicate that CsA is capable to induce myogenesis in *Col6a1*$^{-/-}$ mice after muscle damage. In fact, when TA muscles were damaged during a continuous CsA administration, analysis at 7 days post-injury showed that CsA elicits a significant increase in the number of MyoG-positive cells and of regenerating myofibers in *Col6a1*$^{-/-}$ muscles. Interestingly, this response is not associated with an improvement of the number of satellite cells, suggesting that under these conditions CsA is unable to ameliorate satellite cell self-renewal. The effect of CsA on muscle regeneration was even more remarkable when we exacerbated the muscle phenotype of *Col6a1*$^{-/-}$ mice through triple CdTx damage. Our findings indicate that CsA is protective against fibrotic tissue formation, maybe exerting this effect through an indirect regulation of the inflammatory state that occurs during muscle regeneration (Serrano et al., 2011). A similar beneficial effect of CsA in reducing muscle fibrosis was reported for *mdx* mice undergoing exercise (De Luca et al., 2005). Furthermore, CsA administration was able to counteract the loss of satellite cells elicited by repeated muscle injuries in *Col6a1*$^{-/-}$ animals, concurrently guaranteeing myogenic differentiation, as confirmed by the increase of myofiber cross-sectional area and muscle mass. Although it was beyond the scope of this study to dissect the mechanism(s) through which CsA leads to increased satellite cell number in *Col6a1*$^{-/-}$ mice after repeated injuries, it can be hypothesized that CsA administration may not directly influence the self-renewal capability of satellite cells and that the preservation of satellite cell pool may be mediated by an increase of their survival. This assumption is supported by the fact that the defective satellite cell self-renewal of *Col6a1*$^{-/-}$ mice is strictly dependent on the lack of collagen VI itself and its consequences on muscle stiffness (Urciuolo et al., 2013) and that CsA treatment is able to reduce apoptosis in *Col6a1*$^{-/-}$ muscles (Irwin et al., 2003). To our knowledge, no literature work has investigated in detail the effects of *in vivo* CsA administration on stem cell homeostasis in skeletal muscles. A recent study reported some beneficial effects of CsA on neuronal stem cells, showing that *in vivo* CsA administration increases the number of neurospheres due to enhanced neuronal stem cell survival, rather than increased proliferation (Hunt et al., 2010).

The pharmacology of CsA is complex, and the drug binds a family of cellular peptidyl-prolyl *cis–trans* isomerases known as cyclophilins. Binding of CsA with the abundant cyclophilin A leads to inhibition of calcineurin, a cytosolic phosphatase found in many cell types, thus preventing dephosphorylation of its substrates (Liu et al., 1991). A number of studies have shown that calcineurin signals are involved in the control of myofiber size, myofiber type, and skeletal muscle regeneration (Schiaffino and Serrano, 2002; Sakuma and Yamaguchi, 2010; Hudson and Price, 2013). Although inhibition of calcineurin was shown to delay muscle regeneration (Sakuma et al., 2003, 2005), literature studies investigating the outcomes of calcineurin inhibition by genetic approaches or by CsA administration in animal models of muscle diseases have produced contrasting results (Stupka et al., 2004; De Luca et al., 2005; Parsons et al., 2007). The reasons for these discrepancies rely upon multiple factors, including the genetic model studied, the dose of the drug, the type of muscle, the duration of treatment, and the route of treatment. For instance, the efficacy of CsA in the *mdx* mice, an animal model of Duchenne muscular dystrophy, was reported to be dependent on the dosage and length of the treatment (Stupka et al., 2004; De Luca et al., 2005). Notably, the protective effects of CsA in *Col6a1*$^{-/-}$ mice do not rely upon calcineurin inhibition, as the same beneficial effects are also displayed by non-immunosuppressive CsA analogs that do not bind calcineurin, such as Debio 025 and NIM811 (Angelin et al., 2007; Zulian et al., 2014), whereas they cannot be mimicked by the calcineurin inhibitor FK506 (Irwin et al., 2003). Although our interest was far from the study of calcineurin activity, in this work we used a definite CsA dosage (5 mg/kg every 12 h, i.e., the same dose shown to be effective in rescuing different aspects of the muscle pathology of *Col6a1*$^{-/-}$ mice), and this dosage is known to only partially reduce the activity of calcineurin (Dunn et al., 2002; Michel et al., 2004).

In conclusion, our results indicate that besides the already known beneficial effects of CsA administration in ameliorating the myophatic phenotype of *Col6a1*$^{-/-}$ mice through the rescue from mitochondrial and autophagic dysfunction of muscle fibers, CsA is also capable to stimulate muscle regeneration and preserve the satellite cell pool in this disease model. These findings support and strengthen the increased muscle regeneration observed in Ullrich patients undergoing clinical trial with CsA, pointing at CsA and its non-immunosuppressive derivatives as a promising therapeutic route for this group of inherited muscle diseases.

AUTHOR CONTRIBUTIONS

Francesca Gattazzo planned and performed *in vivo* and *ex vivo* experiments and wrote the paper. Sibilla Molon performed cardiotoxin damage, immunofluorescence, and histology. Valeria Morbidoni performed *in vivo* satellite cell quantification. Bert

Blaauw carried out part of the *in vivo* studies. Paola Braghetta was involved in CsA administration. Anna Urciuolo oversaw the results and interpreted the data. Paolo Bonaldo oversaw the results and wrote the paper. All the authors discussed the results, revised the work, commented on the manuscript, and agreed on the final draft.

ACKNOWLEDGMENTS

This work was supported by grants from Telethon-Italy (GGP10225 and GGP11082), the Italian Ministry of Education, University and Research (FIRB Strategic Project RBAP11Z3YA_003), and the University of Padova.

REFERENCES

Angelin, A., Tiepolo, T., Sabatelli, P., Grumati, P., Bergamin, N., Golfieri, C., et al. (2007). Mitochondrial dysfunction in the pathogenesis of Ullrich congenital muscular dystrophy and prospective therapy with cyclosporins. *Proc. Natl. Acad. Sci. U.S.A.* 104, 991–996. doi:10.1073/pnas.0610270104

Bonaldo, P., Braghetta, P., Zanetti, M., Piccolo, S., Volpin, D., and Bressan, G. M. (1998). Collagen VI deficiency induces early onset myopathy in the mouse: an animal model for Bethlem myopathy. *Hum. Mol. Genet.* 7, 2135–2140. doi:10.1093/hmg/7.13.2135

Buckingham, M., and Rigby, P. W. J. (2014). Gene regulatory networks and transcriptional mechanisms that control myogenesis. *Dev. Cell* 28, 225–238. doi:10.1016/j.devcel.2013.12.020

Chargé, S. B. P., and Rudnicki, M. (2004). Cellular and molecular regulation of muscle regeneration. *Physiol. Rev.* 84, 209–238. doi:10.1152/physrev.00019.2003

Ciciliot, S., and Schiaffino, S. (2010). Regeneration of mammalian skeletal muscle: basic mechanisms and clinical implications. *Curr. Pharm. Des.* 16, 906–914. doi:10.2174/138161210790883453

Couteaux, R., Mira, J. C., and D'Albis, A. (1988). Regeneration of muscles after cardiotoxin injury. I. Cytological aspects. *Biol. Cell* 62, 171–182. doi:10.1111/j.1768-322X.1988.tb00719.x

De Luca, A., Nico, B., Liantonio, A., Didonna, M. P., Fraysse, B., Pierno, S., et al. (2005). A multidisciplinary evaluation of the effectiveness of cyclosporine a in dystrophic mdx mice. *Am. J. Pathol.* 166, 477–489. doi:10.1016/S0002-9440(10)62270-5

Dunn, S. E., Simard, A. R., Prud'homme, R. A., and Michel, R. N. (2002). Calcineurin and skeletal muscle growth. *Nat. Cell Biol.* 4, E46. doi:10.1038/ncb0302-e46a author reply E46–47,

Grumati, P., Coletto, L., Sabatelli, P., Cescon, M., Angelin, A., Bertaggia, E., et al. (2010). Autophagy is defective in collagen VI muscular dystrophies, and its reactivation rescues myofiber degeneration. *Nat. Med.* 16, 1313–1320. doi:10.1038/nm.2247

Hawke, T. J., Meeson, A. P., Jiang, N., Graham, S., Hutcheson, K., DiMaio, J. M., et al. (2003). p21 is essential for normal myogenic progenitor cell function in regenerating skeletal muscle. *Am. J. Physiol. Cell Physiol.* 285, C1019–C1027. doi:10.1152/ajpcell.00055.2003

Homan, W. P., Fabre, J. W., Williams, K. A., Millard, P. R., and Morris, P. J. (1980). Studies on the immunosuppressive properties of cyclosporin A in rats receiving renal allografts. *Transplantation* 29, 361–366. doi:10.1097/00007890-198005000-00003

Hudson, M. B., and Price, S. R. (2013). Calcineurin: a poorly understood regulator of muscle mass. *Int. J. Biochem. Cell Biol.* 45, 2173–2178. doi:10.1016/j.biocel.2013.06.029

Hunt, J., Cheng, A., Hoyles, A., Jervis, E., and Morshead, C. M. (2010). Cyclosporin A has direct effects on adult neural precursor cells. *J. Neurosci.* 30, 2888–2896. doi:10.1523/JNEUROSCI.5991-09.2010

Irwin, W. A., Bergamin, N., Sabatelli, P., Reggiani, C., Megighian, A., Merlini, L., et al. (2003). Mitochondrial dysfunction and apoptosis in myopathic mice with collagen VI deficiency. *Nat. Genet.* 35, 367–371. doi:10.1038/ng1270

Lampe, A. K., and Bushby, K. M. D. (2005). Collagen VI related muscle disorders. *J. Med. Genet.* 42, 673–685. doi:10.1136/jmg.2002.002311

Liu, J., Farmer, J. D., Lane, W. S., Friedman, J., Weissman, I., and Schreiber, S. L. (1991). Calcineurin is a common target of cyclophilin-cyclosporin A and FKBP-FK506 complexes. *Cell* 66, 807–815. doi:10.1016/0092-8674(91)90124-H

Merlini, L., Angelin, A., Tiepolo, T., Braghetta, P., Sabatelli, P., Zamparelli, A., et al. (2008). Cyclosporin A corrects mitochondrial dysfunction and muscle apoptosis in patients with collagen VI myopathies. *Proc. Natl. Acad. Sci. U.S.A.* 105, 5225–5229. doi:10.1073/pnas.0800962105

Merlini, L., Sabatelli, P., Armaroli, A., Gnudi, S., Angelin, A., Grumati, P., et al. (2011). Cyclosporine A in Ullrich congenital muscular dystrophy: long-term results. *Oxid. Med. Cell. Longev.* 2011, 139194. doi:10.1155/2011/139194

Michel, R. N., Dunn, S. E., and Chin, E. R. (2004). Calcineurin and skeletal muscle growth. *Proc. Nutr. Soc.* 63, 341–349. doi:10.1079/PNS2004362

Parsons, S. A., Millay, D. P., Sargent, M. A., Naya, F. J., McNally, E. M., Sweeney, H. L., et al. (2007). Genetic disruption of calcineurin improves skeletal muscle pathology and cardiac disease in a mouse model of limb-girdle muscular dystrophy. *J. Biol. Chem.* 282, 10068–10078. doi:10.1074/jbc.M609368200

Sakuma, K., Nakao, R., Aoi, W., Inashima, S., Fujikawa, T., Hirata, M., et al. (2005). Cyclosporin A treatment upregulates Id1 and Smad3 expression and delays skeletal muscle regeneration. *Acta Neuropathol.* 110, 269–280. doi:10.1007/s00401-005-1049-x

Sakuma, K., Nishikawa, J., Nakao, R., Watanabe, K., Totsuka, T., Nakano, H., et al. (2003). Calcineurin is a potent regulator for skeletal muscle regeneration by association with NFATc1 and GATA-2. *Acta Neuropathol.* 105, 271–280. doi:10.1007/s00401-002-0647-0

Sakuma, K., and Yamaguchi, A. (2010). The functional role of calcineurin in hypertrophy, regeneration, and disorders of skeletal muscle. *J. Biomed. Biotechnol.* 2010, 721219. doi:10.1155/2010/721219

Schiaffino, S., and Serrano, A. L. (2002). Calcineurin signaling and neural control of skeletal muscle fiber type and size. *Trends Pharmacol. Sci.* 6147, 569–575. doi:10.1016/S0165-6147(02)02111-9

Serrano, A. L., Mann, C. J., Vidal, B., Ardite, E., Perdiguero, E., and Muñoz-Cánoves, P. (2011). Cellular and molecular mechanisms regulating fibrosis in skeletal muscle repair and disease. *Curr. Top. Dev. Biol.* 96, 167–201. doi:10.1016/B978-0-12-385940-2.00007-3

Shi, X., and Garry, D. J. (2006). Muscle stem cells in development, regeneration, and disease. *Genes Dev.* 20, 1692–1708. doi:10.1101/gad.1419406

Stupka, N., Gregorevic, P., Plant, D. R., and Lynch, G. S. (2004). The calcineurin signal transduction pathway is essential for successful muscle regeneration in mdx dystrophic mice. *Acta Neuropathol.* 107, 299–310. doi:10.1007/s00401-003-0807-x

Tedesco, F. S., Dellavalle, A., Diaz-Manera, J., Messina, G., and Cossu, G. (2010). Repairing skeletal muscle: regenerative potential of skeletal muscle stem cells. *J. Clin. Invest.* 120, 11–19. doi:10.1172/JCI40373

Urciuolo, A., Quarta, M., Morbidoni, V., Gattazzo, F., Molon, S., Grumati, P., et al. (2013). Collagen VI regulates satellite cell self-renewal and muscle regeneration. *Nat. Commun.* 4, 1964. doi:10.1038/ncomms2964

Zulian, A., Rizzo, E., Schiavone, M., Palma, E., Tagliavini, F., Blaauw, B., et al. (2014). NIM811, a cyclophilin inhibitor without immunosuppressive activity, is beneficial in collagen VI congenital muscular dystrophy models. *Hum. Mol. Genet.* doi:10.1093/hmg/ddu254

21

Oculopharyngeal muscular dystrophy as a paradigm for muscle aging

Yotam Raz and Vered Raz*

Department of Human Genetics, Leiden University Medical Center, Leiden, Netherlands

Correspondence:
Vered Raz, Department of Human Genetics, Leiden University Medical Center, Einthovenweg 20, Building 2, Room R3-17, Postzone S4-P; P.O. Box 9600, Leiden 2300RC, Netherlands
e-mail: v.raz@lumc.nl

Symptoms in late-onset neuromuscular disorders initiate only from midlife onward and progress with age. These disorders are primarily determined by identified hereditable mutations, but their late-onset symptom manifestation is not fully understood. Here, we review recent research developments on the late-onset autosomal dominant oculopharyngeal muscular dystrophy (OPMD). OPMD is caused by an expansion mutation in the gene encoding for poly-adenylate RNA binding protein1 (PABPN1). The molecular pathogenesis for the disease is still poorly understood. Despite a ubiquitous expression of PABPN1, symptoms in OPMD are limited to skeletal muscles. We discuss recent studies showing that PABPN1 levels in skeletal muscles are lower compared with other tissues, and specifically in skeletal muscles, PABPN1 expression declines from midlife onward. In OPMD, aggregation of expanded PABPN1 causes an additional decline in the level of the functional protein, which is associated with severe muscle weakness in OPMD. Reduced PABNPN1 expression in muscle cell culture causes myogenic defects, suggesting that PABPN1 loss-of-function causes muscle weakness in OPMD and in the elderly. Molecular signatures of OPMD muscles are similar to those of normal muscle aging, although expression trends progress faster in OPMD. We discuss a working hypothesis that aging-associated factors trigger late-onset symptoms in OPMD, and contribute to accelerated muscle weakness in OPMD. We focus on the pharyngeal and eyelid muscles, which are often affected in OPMD patients. We suggest that muscle weakness in OPMD is a paradigm for muscle aging.

Keywords: adult myopathy, muscle degeneration, OPMD, PABPN1, RNA metabolism

In aging populations, late-onset disorders are highly common, among which late-onset neuromuscular (NM) disorders are a subset. NM disorders affect muscle fibers and/or the central and peripheral nervous system and the NM junction that control the muscle fibers. At present, these disorders are often incurable. As life expectancy rises, the prevalence of late-onset disorders causing chronic muscle weakness increases. Muscle symptoms can manifest from midlife onward, leading to a drastic functional decline with social and economic burdens. This suggests that in addition to the fundamental genetic defect(s), possible similar aging-associated regulators trigger the late onset of symptoms and progression thereof. For example, protein catabolism, which discards defective or redundant proteins (mainly through the ubiquitin proteasome and autophagy systems), has been implicated as a predominant regulator in normal aging and late-onset diseases [reviewed in Low (2011) and Bonaldo and Sandri (2013)]. Reduced protein catabolism can also lead to an accumulation of aggregation-prone proteins and formation of insoluble protein aggregates. These aggregates are often the pathological hallmark in a number of late-onset neurological and/or muscular disorders (Ruegg and Glass, 2011; Bonaldo and Sandri, 2013). Although symptoms of these diseases widely vary, symptoms often initiate in a small subset of muscular or neuronal tissues (Ross and Poirier, 2005). While the primary genetic causes for these disorders are known, why symptoms initiate from midlife onward in specific tissues and how symptoms progress with age is still obscure.

Oculopharyngeal muscular dystrophy (OPMD) is an autosomal dominant and rare myopathy. The estimated prevalence in Western countries is 1:100,000 [reviewed in Raz et al. (2013)]. Due to founder effects, clusters with a higher prevalence are found in French-Canadians and in the Bukhara community in Israel (1:1000 and 1:600, respectively) (Blumen et al., 2000; Laberge et al., 2005). It has been suggested, however, that outside these communities, the disease remains underdiagnosed (Ruegg et al., 2005). In OPMD, skeletal muscles are predominantly affected, whereby initial symptoms are manifested in only a subset of muscles. Most commonly, this leads to lowering (ptosis) of the eyelids and swallowing difficulties (dysphagia). With disease progression, additional skeletal muscles can be affected including the proximal muscles of the lower limb (including the quadriceps muscles) (Fischmann et al., 2012). OPMD is a monogenic disorder and its etiology is found in an alanine expansion mutation in the gene encoding for poly-adenylate (poly(A)) binding protein nuclear 1 (PABPN1) (Brais et al., 1998). Formation of insoluble inclusions in the cell nucleus is the pathological hallmark of OPMD muscles (Tome and Fardeau, 1980). Under physiological expression levels, expanded (exp)PABPN1 is more prone to aggregation compared with the wild-type PABPN1 (Raz et al., 2011a). High overexpression of expPABPN1 in muscles of various animal models causes muscle weakness, and it is suggested that accumulation of aggregates could be the cause for the muscle dysfunction (Davies et al., 2005). High overexpression of expPAPBN1 in animal models, as well as in cellular models leads to cell death, suggesting that expPABPN1 aggregates are toxic (Davies et al., 2008). Importantly, treatments that may reduce aggregation lead to less cell death and reduced muscle weakness in these animal models (Davies et al., 2006, 2010; Catoire et al., 2008; Chartier et al., 2009). Based on those models, it was suggested that muscle symptoms in OPMD are caused by a PABPN1 gain-of-function. However, it is not resolved whether animal models with high overexpression in muscles are relevant to OPMD. For example, high overexpression of expPABPN1 was not reported in OPMD heterozygous patients. Moreover, aggregates of wild-type PABPN1 were found in unaffected rat neural cells (Berciano et al., 2004). Altogether, it is striking that despite the well-known genetic cause for OPMD, the molecular mechanisms and physiological conditions that lead to muscle symptoms are poorly understood. Here, we discuss four questions for OPMD pathophysiology.

IS OPMD AN RNA METABOLISM DISORDER?

Poly-adenylate RNA binding protein1 is multifunctional regulator of RNA metabolism. Initially, it was identified *in vitro* as a regulator of poly(A) tail length (Kerwitz et al., 2003), subsequently was validated *in vivo* (Benoit et al., 2005), and more recently, it was shown to have an impact on mRNA decay (Bresson and Conrad, 2013). PABPN1 knockdown in mouse muscle cells causes reduced poly(A) tail length that is associated with myogenesis defects (Apponi et al., 2010); however, the relevance for OPMD and muscle aging is unsettled. A change in poly(A) tail length was not found in muscles from OPMD patients (Calado et al., 2000). Recent studies revealed additional molecular functions for PABPN1. A genome-wide shift from distal to proximal alternative polyadenylation site (PAS) and accumulation of shortened transcripts were found in the mouse model for OPMD, A17.1, which was generated by expPABPN1 overexpression in muscles, and in cells with reduced PABPN1 expression (de Klerk et al., 2012; Jenal et al., 2012). Similar alternative PAS utilization was found in models with expPABPN1 overexpression and PABPN1 downregulation, suggesting that PABPN1 loss-of-function causes defects in RNA metabolism (de Klerk et al., 2012; Jenal et al., 2012). In OPMD muscles, PABPN1 downregulation was found to be comparable to age-matching controls (Anvar et al., 2013). Reduced PABPN1 levels in cellular models cause myogenic defects (Apponi et al., 2010; Anvar et al., 2013). In addition, PABPN1 was also found to regulate long non-coding RNA expression (Beaulieu et al., 2012). However, so far, alternative PAS or long non-coding RNA expression was not reported in OPMD patient muscles. To adequately understand how PABPN1 regulates changes in RNA metabolism in OPMD with an impact on muscle weakness, experiments should be conducted in models with physiological levels of PABPN1.

Aberrant RNA metabolism is not specific to OPMD, but is found in a wide spectrum of unrelated late-onset neurological and/or muscular disorders (O'Rourke and Swanson, 2009; Anthony and Gallo, 2010). Since these disorders share a late onset of symptoms and progression with age, age-associated regulators of RNA metabolism could be affected. It is still unclear whether similar regulators of RNA metabolism are affected in these disorders. In OPMD, affected muscles as well as muscles from pre-symptomatic family members can be accessible for research (Fischmann et al., 2012; Anvar et al., 2013). Therefore, OPMD could be used as a paradigm to study the functional contribution of RNA metabolism to symptoms in late-onset neurological and/or muscular disorders and to study a possible regulatory role in the age-associated progression of the symptoms.

WHY ARE SKELETAL MUSCLES PRIMARILY AFFECTED IN OPMD?

Poly-adenylate RNA binding protein1 is essential for cell vitality (Bhattacharjee and Bag, 2012) and is expressed in all cells; however symptoms are predominantly manifested in skeletal muscles. In OPMD patients, PABPN1 expression is specifically reduced in affected *Vastus lateralis* muscles, while PABPN1 levels in whole blood are unchanged between OPMD patients and healthy controls (Anvar et al., 2013). In Dutch and Danish OPMD patients, weakness of the quadriceps muscles is reported as one of the initial symptoms (Sluijs et al., 2003; Witting et al., 2014). PAPBN1 level is lower in skeletal muscles of both human being and mouse, compared with a spectrum of tissues (Apponi et al., 2013). Since symptoms in OPMD are predominant in skeletal muscles, this suggests that below a certain crucial level, a functional impact is manifested. Although a threshold for functional PABPN1 is yet to be defined, due to low PABPN1 expression levels in skeletal muscles (Apponi et al., 2013) this crucial level could reach a functional impact. In other tissues, however, PABPN1 levels are sufficiently high (Apponi et al., 2013), and thus, if any aging-associated decline may occur (Anvar et al., 2013), they would be spared from a functional deficiency (**Figure 2**). Indeed, altered PABPN1 at 40, 60, or 80% expression level causes reciprocal decrease in the expression of sarcomeric genes (Anvar et al., 2013). This working model requires additional *in vivo* experiments.

It is not fully understood why levels of PABPN1 are lower in skeletal muscles. PABPN1 mRNA is less stable in muscles compared with other tissues (Apponi et al., 2013). PABPN1 mRNA binds to PABPN1 protein (Raz et al., 2014), which potentially affects PABPN1 mRNA stability, nuclear export, and translation (**Figure 1**). As yet, regulators of mRNA stability in muscles and aging-associated changes are poorly understood. In addition, PABPN1 protein turnover is regulated by the ubiquitin proteasome system (UPS) (Raz et al., 2011b). Differences in polyubiquitination levels between wild type and expPABPN1 result in higher protein turnover of wild-type PAPBN1 as compared with expPABPN1 (Raz et al., 2011b). Since PABPN1 is prone to aggregation, higher protein accumulation leads to aggregate formation and reduced availability of the functional protein. PABPN1 protein accumulation is regulated by ARIH2 E3-ligase, whose level also declines from midlife onward in skeletal muscles (Raz et al., 2014). In OPMD muscles, ARIH2 level is lower compared to age-matching controls, which in part could result by the alternative PAS utilization in ARIH2 3′-UTR that is directly regulated by PABPN1 level. In addition, as ARIH2 protein is entrapped in expPABPN1 aggregates, functional protein levels would be depleted (Raz et al., 2014). Protein entrapment in PABPN1 aggregates was reported for other E3 ligases and the proteasome (Corbeil-Girard et al., 2005; Tavanez et al., 2005; Anvar et al., 2011), suggesting that the UPS machinery is dysregulated in OPMD. In turn,

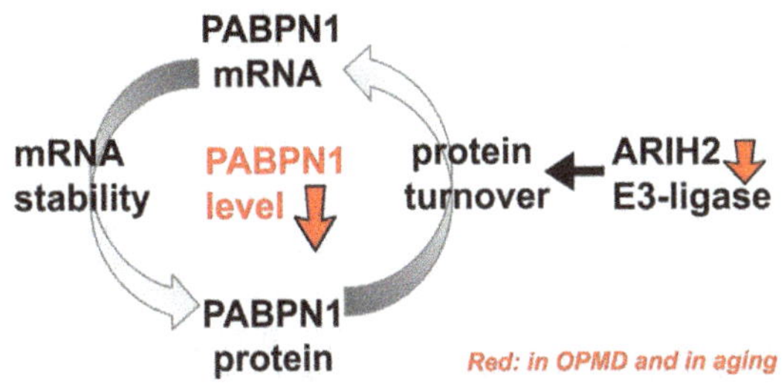

FIGURE 1 | A schematic working model for regulation of PABPN1 levels. PABPN1 levels are established by a feed-forward loop combining at least regulation of mRNA stability and protein turnover. PABPN1 protein accumulation is regulated by the ubiquitin proteasome system (UPS), including ARIH2 E3-ligase. An aging-associated distortion of the UPS causes impairment of PABPN1 protein turnover affecting its mRNA stability and genes of the UPS, including ARIH2 E3-ligase. In turn, PABPN1 mRNA levels, which are self-regulated, also decrease with aging. However, the molecular factors regulating PABPN1 mRNA stability are unknown as yet. In OPMD and in aging, reduced levels of PABPN1 eventually cause genome-wide changes in gene expression.

mRNA dysregulation of the UPS was found to be the most consistent dysregulated cellular system in OPMD (Anvar et al., 2011; de Klerk et al., 2012). Although a mechanistic model for regulation of PABPN1 levels in aging and muscle disease calls for additional research, the current literature suggests that changes in PABPN1 levels in muscles are regulated by both mRNA stability and protein turnover and that these machineries are specifically affected in OPMD (**Figure 1**). Regulators of PABPN1 mRNA stability and protein turnover should be identified in future studies.

WHY SPECIFIC MUSCLES SEEM TO BE MORE AFFECTED THAN OTHER MUSCLES?

In OPMD, the ocular and pharyngeal muscles are initially the most commonly affected; however, with progression of the disease, more skeletal muscles are affected. These muscles are also often affected in otherwise healthy elderly. Most skeletal muscles are weakened during aging; however, it is unclear whether aging-associated muscle weakness is programed, concerning initially affected muscles and progression. Relevant to OPMD, dysphagia, resulting from weakness of pharyngeal muscles, and eyelid ptosis, resulting from weakness of the *levator palpebrae* muscle, is highly common in the elderly (Salvi et al., 2006; Fea et al., 2013; Iida et al., 2013). In contrast to the otherwise healthy population, in OPMD, symptoms start at an earlier age and seem more severe, possibly due to faster progression. Eyelid ptosis can also be caused by rare multiple mitochondrial DNA deletion syndromes, including progressive external ophthalmoplegia (PEO) (Van Goethem et al., 2003). Increased mitochondrial deletions were found in the extraocular muscles compared to other muscles and are aging associated (Yu-Wai-Man et al., 2010), indicating a prominent role for mitochondrial activity in ocular muscles during aging. A decrease in mitochondrial activity was reported in a mouse model for OPMD (Trollet et al., 2010) and in a muscle cell model with PABPN1 downregulation (Anvar et al., 2013). These studies suggest that in OPMD, mitochondrial dysfunction may contribute to the muscle weakness and future studies should explore a role for PAPBN1 in the regulation of mitochondrial genes and mitochondrial and metabolic cellular functionality.

Dysphagia in the elderly is determined by age-associated anatomical changes in the neck and throat, underpinning the swallowing function in otherwise healthy elderly (Ney et al., 2009). Furthermore, dysphagia is also common in different age-related diseases including NM disorders (Schindler and Kelly, 2002). Dysphagia in the otherwise healthy elderly manifests by a less efficient passage of food to the esophagus due to changes in swallowing pressures of the upper esophageal sphincter and delayed muscle movements (Yokoyama et al., 2000). Symptoms are suggested to be associated with an increase in muscle atrophy and a decrease in muscle strength of the pharyngeal muscles (Feng et al., 2013).

Although it is not clear why ocular and pharyngeal muscles are initially affected in OPMD, the ocular and pharyngeal muscles are constantly, and often unconsciously, routinely used in daily life. Interestingly, PABPN1 levels in mice pharyngeal muscle are lower compared with other skeletal muscles (Apponi et al., 2013). This suggests that this muscle could be more susceptible to a further decrease in PABPN1 levels. However, functional studies, especially in human beings, would lead to conclusive answers.

WHY SYMPTOMS INITIATE FROM MIDLIFE ONWARD AND DOES OPMD REPRESENT ACCELERATED MUSCLE AGING?

Muscle aging (sarcopenia) is marked, among others, by a decrease in muscle mass (atrophy), an increase in fat infiltration and inflammation leading to a decrease in muscle strength and physical performance (Cruz-Jentoft et al., 2010). In the A17.1 mouse model, muscle atrophy appears already from 12 weeks of age (24-month-old mice are considered as aged) and is complemented by expression dysregulation of known muscle atrophy genes such as Murf1 and Atrogin-1 (Trollet et al., 2010). Muscle atrophy in this mouse model is prominent in the fast glycolytic (type IIX/IIB) fibers, whereas the slow oxidative (type I) and fast oxidative (type IIA) fibers seem to be spared (Trollet et al., 2010). Although it is widely accepted that aged muscles of rodents are enriched in slow (type I) fibers compared to fast (type II) fibers, in aging human muscles, the literature concerning this fiber-type switch is not conclusive (Purves-Smith et al., 2014). Therefore, the implications of the muscle fiber-type switch for OPMD patients are unsettled. Studies in additional models are necessary in order to reveal whether reduced PABPN1 levels induce muscle atrophy and muscle fiber-type switch. Muscle aging can also be non-invasively quantified from magnetic resonance imaging (MRI) including muscle cross-sectional surface area, fatty infiltration (Fischmann et al., 2012; Willis et al., 2013), and inflammation (Eshed et al., 2007). These measures can be considered as approximations of muscular quality. With these measures, progressive muscular atrophy in OPMD was documented (Fischmann et al., 2012).

Although OPMD is often grouped within the muscular dystrophies, our studies of RNA expression profiles in OPMD muscles and OPMD models revealed higher similarities with muscles from the elderly rather than with muscular dystrophies or myopathies (Anvar et al., 2013), suggesting similar molecular signatures. Overlapping dysregulated genes were found for the mitochondria, the UPS, DNA repair, TGF-β signaling, and sarcomeric genes (Anvar et al., 2013). However, functional studies should investigate a

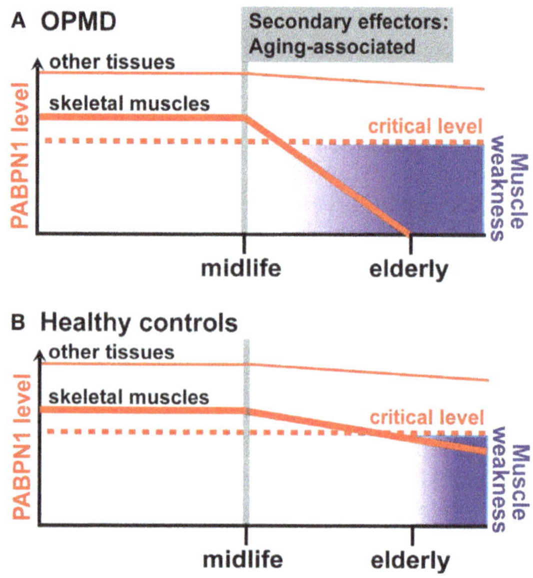

FIGURE 2 | A schematic working model for the aging-associated decline of muscle strength and PABPN1 in OPMD (A) and healthy controls (B). In skeletal muscles, a decline in PABPN1 levels starts from midlife onward in both OPMD and healthy controls. The onset of decline from midlife onward is caused by secondary age-associated effectors, which mostly are unknown. Eventually, below a critical PABPN1 level, muscle weakness symptoms are manifested. This process is accelerated in OPMD due to aggregation of expanded PABPN1, which further depletes levels of functional PABPN1. In other tissues, however, levels of PABPN1 are higher and a possible age-related decline of PABPN1 does not reach the critical level for a functional impact.

role for additional aging-associated pathways. For example, the autophagy system has also been found to have an imperative regulatory role in many age-associated diseases, in healthy aging (Schneider and Cuervo, 2014), and in muscle atrophy (Bonaldo and Sandri, 2013). As PABPN1 can shuttle between the nucleus and the cytoplasm (Abu-Baker et al., 2005; Benoit et al., 2005), it should be investigated whether PABPN1 is also regulated by the autophagy system. Moreover, genes of the autophagy system could be regulated by PABPN1 (Anvar et al., 2013). More interestingly, age-associated changes in a cross-sectional data revealed a faster change in expression level for a subset of genes, among which many are known as aging genes, muscle-specific sarcomeric genes, and PABPN1 (Anvar et al., 2013). This suggests that muscle weakness in OPMD could represent accelerated muscular aging, and thus, OPMD muscles could be a paradigm for otherwise healthy muscle aging (**Figure 2**).

ACKNOWLEDGMENTS

We thank the French Muscular Dystrophy Association, France, and from the Princess Beatrix Muscle Fund, The Netherlands for financial support on OPMD research.

REFERENCES

Abu-Baker, A., Laganiere, S., Fan, X., Laganiere, J., Brais, B., and Rouleau, G. A. (2005). Cytoplasmic targeting of mutant poly(A)-binding protein nuclear 1 suppresses protein aggregation and toxicity in oculopharyngeal muscular dystrophy. *Traffic* 6, 766–779. doi:10.1111/j.1600-0854.2005.00315.x

Anthony, K., and Gallo, J.-M. (2010). Aberrant RNA processing events in neurological disorders. *Brain Res.* 1338, 67–77. doi:10.1016/j.brainres.2010.03.008

Anvar, S. Y., Raz, Y., Verway, N., Van Der Sluijs, B., Venema, A., Goeman, J. J., et al. (2013). A decline in PABPN1 induces progressive muscle weakness in oculopharyngeal muscle dystrophy and in muscle aging. *Aging (Albany NY).* 5, 412–426.

Anvar, S. Y., 't Hoen, P. A., Venema, A., van der Sluijs, B., van Engelen, B., Snoeck, M., et al. (2011). Deregulation of the ubiquitin-proteasome system is the predominant molecular pathology in OPMD animal models and patients. *Skelet. Muscle.* 1, 15. doi:10.1186/2044-5040-1-15

Apponi, L. H., Corbett, A. H., and Pavlath, G. K. (2013). Control of mRNA stability contributes to low levels of nuclear poly(A) binding protein 1 (PABPN1) in skeletal muscle. *Skelet. Muscle.* 3, 23. doi:10.1186/2044-5040-3-23

Apponi, L. H., Leung, S. W., Williams, K. R., Valentini, S. R., Corbett, A. H., and Pavlath, G. K. (2010). Loss of nuclear poly(A)-binding protein 1 causes defects in myogenesis and mRNA biogenesis. *Hum. Mol. Genet.* 19, 1058–1065. doi:10.1093/hmg/ddp569

Beaulieu, Y. B., Kleinman, C. L., Landry-Voyer, A. M., Majewski, J., and Bachand, F. (2012). Polyadenylation-dependent control of long noncoding RNA expression by the poly(A)-binding protein nuclear 1. *PLoS Genet.* 8:e1003078. doi:10.1371/journal.pgen.1003078

Benoit, B., Mitou, G., Chartier, A., Temme, C., Zaessinger, S., Wahle, E., et al. (2005). An essential cytoplasmic function for the nuclear poly(A) binding protein, PABP2, in poly(A) tail length control and early development in *Drosophila. Dev. Cell* 9, 511–522. doi:10.1016/j.devcel.2005.09.002

Berciano, M. T., Villagra, N. T., Ojeda, J. L., Navascues, J., Gomes, A., Lafarga, M., et al. (2004). Oculopharyngeal muscular dystrophy-like nuclear inclusions are present in normal magnocellular neurosecretory neurons of the hypothalamus. *Hum. Mol. Genet.* 13, 829–838. doi:10.1093/hmg/ddh101

Bhattacharjee, R. B., and Bag, J. (2012). Depletion of nuclear poly(A) binding protein PABPN1 produces a compensatory response by cytoplasmic PABP4 and PABP5 in cultured human cells. *PLoS ONE.* 7:e53036. doi:10.1371/journal.pone.0053036

Blumen, S. C., Korczyn, A. D., Lavoie, H., Medynski, S., Chapman, J., Asherov, A., et al. (2000). Oculopharyngeal MD among Bukhara Jews is due to a founder (GCG)9 mutation in the PABP2 gene. *Neurology.* 55, 1267–1270. doi:10.1212/WNL.55.9.1267

Bonaldo, P., and Sandri, M. (2013). Cellular and molecular mechanisms of muscle atrophy. *Dis. Model Mech.* 6, 25–39. doi:10.1242/dmm.010389

Brais, B., Bouchard, J. P., Xie, Y. G., Rochefort, D. L., Chretien, N., Tome, F. M., et al. (1998). Short GCG expansions in the PABP2 gene cause oculopharyngeal muscular dystrophy. *Nat. Genet.* 18, 164–167. doi:10.1038/ng0298-164

Bresson, S. M., and Conrad, N. K. (2013). The human nuclear poly(a)-binding protein promotes RNA hyperadenylation and decay. *PLoS Genet.* 9:e1003893. doi:10.1371/journal.pgen.1003893

Calado, A., Tome, F. M., Brais, B., Rouleau, G. A., Kuhn, U., Wahle, E., et al. (2000). Nuclear inclusions in oculopharyngeal muscular dystrophy consist of poly(A) binding protein 2 aggregates which sequester poly(A) RNA. *Hum. Mol. Genet.* 9, 2321–2328. doi:10.1093/oxfordjournals.hmg.a018924

Catoire, H., Pasco, M. Y., Abu-Baker, A., Holbert, S., Tourette, C., Brais, B., et al. (2008). Sirtuin inhibition protects from the polyalanine muscular dystrophy protein PABPN1. *Hum. Mol. Genet.* 17, 2108–2117. doi:10.1093/hmg/ddn109

Chartier, A., Raz, V., Sterrenburg, E., Verrips, C. T., Van Der Maarel, S. M., and Simonelig, M. (2009). Prevention of oculopharyngeal muscular dystrophy by muscular expression of Llama single-chain intrabodies in vivo. *Hum. Mol. Genet.* 18, 1849–1859. doi:10.1093/hmg/ddp101

Corbeil-Girard, L. P., Klein, A. F., Sasseville, A. M., Lavoie, H., Dicaire, M. J., Saint-Denis, A., et al. (2005). PABPN1 overexpression leads to upregulation of genes encoding nuclear proteins that are sequestered in oculopharyngeal muscular dystrophy nuclear inclusions. *Neurobiol. Dis.* 18, 551–567. doi:10.1016/j.nbd.2004.10.019

Cruz-Jentoft, A. J., Baeyens, J. P., Bauer, J. M., Boirie, Y., Cederholm, T., Landi, F., et al. (2010). Sarcopenia: European consensus on definition and diagnosis: report of the European working group on sarcopenia in older people. *Age Ageing.* 39, 412–423. doi:10.1093/ageing/afq034

Davies, J. E., Rose, C., Sarkar, S., and Rubinsztein, D. C. (2010). Cystamine suppresses polyalanine toxicity in a mouse model of oculopharyngeal muscular dystrophy. *Sci. Transl. Med.* 2, 34ra40. doi:10.1126/scitranslmed.3000723

Davies, J. E., Sarkar, S., and Rubinsztein, D. C. (2006). Trehalose reduces aggregate formation and delays pathology in a transgenic mouse model of oculopharyngeal muscular dystrophy. *Hum. Mol. Genet.* 15, 23–31. doi:10.1093/hmg/ddi422

Davies, J. E., Sarkar, S., and Rubinsztein, D. C. (2008). Wild-type PABPN1 is anti-apoptotic and reduces toxicity of the oculopharyngeal muscular dystrophy mutation. *Hum. Mol. Genet.* 17, 1097–1108. doi:10.1093/hmg/ddm382

Davies, J. E., Wang, L., Garcia-Oroz, L., Cook, L. J., Vacher, C., O'Donovan, D. G., et al. (2005). Doxycycline attenuates and delays toxicity of the oculopharyngeal muscular dystrophy mutation in transgenic mice. *Nat. Med.* 11, 672–677. doi:10.1038/nm1242

de Klerk, E., Venema, A., Anvar, S. Y., Goeman, J. J., Hu, O., Trollet, C., et al. (2012). Poly(A) binding protein nuclear 1 levels affect alternative polyadenylation. *Nucleic Acids Res.* 40, 9089–9101. doi:10.1093/nar/gks655

Eshed, I., Bollow, M., Mcgonagle, D. G., Tan, A. L., Althoff, C. E., Asbach, P., et al. (2007). MRI of enthesitis of the appendicular skeleton in spondyloarthritis. *Ann. Rheum. Dis.* 66, 1553–1559. doi:10.1136/ard.2007.070243

Fea, A., Damato, D., Actis, A. G., De Sanctis, U., Actis, G., and Grignolo, F. M. (2013). Blepharoplastic: essential review. *Minerva Chir.* 68, 49–56.

Feng, X., Todd, T., Lintzenich, C. R., Ding, J., Carr, J. J., Ge, Y., et al. (2013). Aging-related geniohyoid muscle atrophy is related to aspiration status in healthy older adults. *J. Gerontol. A Biol. Sci. Med. Sci.* 68, 853–860. doi:10.1093/gerona/gls225

Fischmann, A., Hafner, P., Fasler, S., Gloor, M., Bieri, O., Studler, U., et al. (2012). Quantitative MRI can detect subclinical disease progression in muscular dystrophy. *J. Neurol.* 259, 1648–1654. doi:10.1007/s00415-011-6393-2

Iida, T., Tohara, H., Wada, S., Nakane, A., Sanpei, R., and Ueda, K. (2013). Aging decreases the strength of suprahyoid muscles involved in swallowing movements. *Tohoku J. Exp. Med.* 231, 223–228. doi:10.1620/tjem.231.223

Jenal, M., Elkon, R., Loayza-Puch, F., Van Haaften, G., Kuhn, U., Menzies, F. M., et al. (2012). The poly(A)-binding protein nuclear 1 suppresses alternative cleavage and polyadenylation sites. *Cell* 149, 538–553. doi:10.1016/j.cell.2012.03.022

Kerwitz, Y., Kuhn, U., Lilie, H., Knoth, A., Scheuermann, T., Friedrich, H., et al. (2003). Stimulation of poly(A) polymerase through a direct interaction with the nuclear poly(A) binding protein allosterically regulated by RNA. *EMBO J.* 22, 3705–3714. doi:10.1093/emboj/cdg347

Laberge, A. M., Michaud, J., Richter, A., Lemyre, E., Lambert, M., Brais, B., et al. (2005). Population history and its impact on medical genetics in Quebec. *Clin. Genet.* 68, 287–301. doi:10.1111/j.1399-0004.2005.00497.x

Low, P. (2011). The role of ubiquitin-proteasome system in ageing. *Gen. Comp. Endocrinol.* 172, 39–43. doi:10.1016/j.ygcen.2011.02.005

Ney, D. M., Weiss, J. M., Kind, A. J., and Robbins, J. (2009). Senescent swallowing: impact, strategies, and interventions. *Nutr. Clin. Pract.* 24, 395–413. doi:10.1177/0884533609332005

O'Rourke, J. R., and Swanson, M. S. (2009). Mechanisms of RNA-mediated disease. *J. Biol. Chem.* 284, 7419–7423. doi:10.1074/jbc.R800025200

Purves-Smith, F. M., Sgarioto, N., and Hepple, R. T. (2014). Fiber typing in aging muscle. *Exerc. Sport Sci. Rev.* 42, 45–52. doi:10.1249/JES.0000000000000012

Raz, V., Abraham, T., Van Zwet, E. W., Dirks, R. W., Tanke, H. J., and Van Der Maarel, S. M. (2011a). Reversible aggregation of PABPN1 pre-inclusion structures. *Nucleus.* 2, 208–218. doi:10.4161/nucl.2.3.15736

Raz, V., Routledge, S., Venema, A., Buijze, H., Van Der Wal, E., Anvar, S., et al. (2011b). Modeling oculopharyngeal muscular dystrophy in myotube cultures reveals reduced accumulation of soluble mutant PABPN1 protein. *Am. J. Pathol.* 179, 1988–2000. doi:10.1016/j.ajpath.2011.06.044

Raz, V., Buijze, H., Raz, Y., Verwey, N., Anvar, S. Y., Aartsma-Rus, A., et al. (2014). A novel feed-forward loop between ARIH2 E3-ligase and PABPN1 regulates aging-associated muscle degeneration. *Am. J. Pathol.* 30, 00016–00019. doi:10.1016/j.ajpath.2013.12.011

Raz, V., Butler-Browne, G., Van Engelen, B., and Brais, B. (2013). 191st ENMC international workshop: recent advances in oculopharyngeal muscular dystrophy research: from bench to bedside 8-10 June 2012, Naarden, The Netherlands. *Neuromuscul. Disord.* 23, 516–523. doi:10.1016/j.nmd.2013.03.001

Ross, C. A., and Poirier, M. A. (2005). What is the role of protein aggregation in neurodegeneration? *Nat. Rev. Mol. Cell Biol.* 6, 891–898. doi:10.1038/nrm1742

Ruegg, M. A., and Glass, D. J. (2011). Molecular mechanisms and treatment options for muscle wasting diseases. *Annu. Rev. Pharmacol. Toxicol.* 51, 373–395. doi:10.1146/annurev-pharmtox-010510-100537

Ruegg, S., Lehky Hagen, M., Hohl, U., Kappos, L., Fuhr, P., Plasilov, M., et al. (2005). Oculopharyngeal muscular dystrophy - an under-diagnosed disorder? *Swiss Med. Wkly.* 135, 574–586.

Salvi, S. M., Akhtar, S., and Currie, Z. (2006). Ageing changes in the eye. *Postgrad. Med. J.* 82, 581–587. doi:10.1136/pgmj.2005.040857

Schindler, J. S., and Kelly, J. H. (2002). Swallowing disorders in the elderly. *Laryngoscope.* 112, 589–602. doi:10.1097/00005537-200204000-00001

Schneider, J. L., and Cuervo, A. M. (2014). Autophagy and human disease: emerging themes. *Curr. Opin. Genet. Dev.* 26c, 16–23. doi:10.1016/j.gde.2014.04.003

Sluijs, B., Hoefsloot, L., Padberg, G., Maarel, S., and Engelen, B. M. (2003). Oculopharyngeal muscular dystrophy with limb girdle weakness as major complaint. *J. Neurol.* 250, 1307–1312. doi:10.1007/s00415-003-0201-6

Tavanez, J. P., Calado, P., Braga, J., Lafarga, M., and Carmo-Fonseca, M. (2005). In vivo aggregation properties of the nuclear poly(A)-binding protein PABPN1. *RNA.* 11, 752–762. doi:10.1261/rna.7217105

Tome, F. M., and Fardeau, M. (1980). Nuclear inclusions in oculopharyngeal dystrophy. *Acta Neuropathol.* 49, 85–87. doi:10.1007/BF00692226

Trollet, C., Anvar, S. Y., Venema, A., Hargreaves, I. P., Foster, K., Vignaud, A., et al. (2010). Molecular and phenotypic characterization of a mouse model of oculopharyngeal muscular dystrophy reveals severe muscular atrophy restricted to fast glycolytic fibres. *Hum. Mol. Genet.* 19, 2191–2207. doi:10.1093/hmg/ddq098

Van Goethem, G., Martin, J. J., and Van Broeckhoven, C. (2003). Progressive external ophthalmoplegia characterized by multiple deletions of mitochondrial DNA: unraveling the pathogenesis of human mitochondrial DNA instability and the initiation of a genetic classification. *Neuromolecular Med.* 3, 129–146. doi:10.1385/NMM:3:3:129

Willis, T. A., Hollingsworth, K. G., Coombs, A., Sveen, M.-L., Andersen, S., Stojkovic, T., et al. (2013). Quantitative muscle MRI as an assessment tool for monitoring disease progression in LGMD2I: a multicentre longitudinal study. *PLoS ONE* 8:e70993. doi:10.1371/journal.pone.0070993

Witting, N., Mensah, A., Kober, L., Bundgaard, H., Petri, H., Duno, M., et al. (2014). Ocular, bulbar, limb, and cardiopulmonary involvement in oculopharyngeal muscular dystrophy. *Acta Neurol. Scand.* 130, 125–130. doi:10.1111/ane.12244

Yokoyama, M., Mitomi, N., Tetsuka, K., Tayama, N., and Niimi, S. (2000). Role of laryngeal movement and effect of aging on swallowing pressure in the pharynx and upper esophageal sphincter. *Laryngoscope.* 110, 434–439. doi:10.1097/00005537-200003000-00021

Yu-Wai-Man, P., Lai-Cheong, J., Borthwick, G. M., He, L., Taylor, G. A., Greaves, L. C., et al. (2010). Somatic mitochondrial DNA deletions accumulate to high levels in aging human extraocular muscles. *Invest. Ophthalmol. Vis. Sci.* 51, 3347–3353. doi:10.1167/iovs.09-4660

22

The intriguing regulators of muscle mass in sarcopenia and muscular dystrophy

Kunihiro Sakuma[1]*, Wataru Aoi[2] and Akihiko Yamaguchi[3]

[1] Research Center for Physical Fitness, Sports and Health, Toyohashi University of Technology, Toyohashi, Japan
[2] Laboratory of Health Science, Graduate School of Life and Environmental Sciences, Kyoto Prefectural University, Kyoto, Japan
[3] Department of Physical Therapy, Health Sciences University of Hokkaido, Kanazawa, Japan

Correspondence:
Kunihiro Sakuma, Research Center for Physical Fitness, Sports and Health, Toyohashi University of Technology, 1-1 Hibarigaoka, Tenpaku-cho, Toyohashi 441-8580, Japan
e-mail: ksakuma@las.tut.ac.jp

Recent advances in our understanding of the biology of muscle have led to new interest in the pharmacological treatment of muscle wasting. Loss of muscle mass and increased intramuscular fibrosis occur in both sarcopenia and muscular dystrophy. Several regulators (mammalian target of rapamycin, serum response factor, atrogin-1, myostatin, etc.) seem to modulate protein synthesis and degradation or transcription of muscle-specific genes during both sarcopenia and muscular dystrophy. This review provides an overview of the adaptive changes in several regulators of muscle mass in both sarcopenia and muscular dystrophy.

Keywords: sarcopenia, muscular dystrophies, autophagy, myostatin, serum response factor, mTOR

INTRODUCTION

In humans, skeletal muscle is the most abundant tissue in the body, comprising 40–50% of body mass and playing vital roles in locomotion, heat production during periods of cold stress, and overall metabolism. Skeletal muscle is composed of bundles of muscle fibers called fascicles. The cell membrane surrounding the muscle cell is the sarcolemma, beneath which lies the sarcoplasm, which contains the cellular proteins, organelles, and myofibrils: the titin actin filament and the thicker myosin filament. The arrangement of these protein filaments gives skeletal muscle its striated appearance. Skeletal muscle is capable of remarkable adaptations in response to altered activity. These adjustments to mechanical and metabolic demands elicit marked modifications of gene expression that could lead to gain (hypertrophy) or loss (atrophy) of muscle mass. Whereas, endurance training leads to minor changes in skeletal muscle mass, strength training induces marked hypertrophy of exercising muscles. Resistance training [full squat, leg press, and leg-extension, three sets to failure of 6–8 RM (~80–85% of the 1 RM, Monday) and 10–12 RM (~70–75% of the 1 RM, Friday), 18 weeks] for young sedentary subjects (women, 21.4 ± 1.4-year old) elicited a 10–30% increase in fiber cross-sectional area of the vastus lateralis muscle (Staron et al., 1991).

Loss of muscle is a serious consequence of many chronic diseases and of aging itself because it leads to weakness, loss of independence, and increased risk of death. Unfortunately, the field suffers from having more definitions than therapies; muscle wasting is an inevitable part of aging, where it is known as sarcopenia (Rosenberg, 1989). Muscle loss is also common in muscular dystrophy, in which markedly loss of various membranous structural proteins occurs around muscle fibers (Vainzof et al., 2008). Intriguingly, sarcopenia and muscular dystrophy possess similar characteristics, including the accumulation of fibrosis, a wide-range fiber size distribution, and central nuclei (Sakuma et al., 2008; Vainzof et al., 2008; Berger and Doherty, 2010; Hepple, 2012).

In hypertrophied muscle, increasing protein synthesis and decreasing protein degradation are also important events. Phosphatidylinositol-3-kinase (PI3-K)/Akt/mammalian target of rapamycin (mTOR) signaling has been shown to be crucial to protein synthesis (Glass, 2010; Sakuma and Yamaguchi, 2012b). Mechanical stretching *in vivo* and *in vitro* activates serum response factor (SRF)-dependent signaling in skeletal muscle (Gauthier-Rouviére et al., 1996; Sakuma and Yamaguchi, 2012a). In contrast, negative regulators are proposed to induce muscle atrophy by inhibiting protein synthesis and enhancing protein degradation in skeletal muscle. For example, the ubiquitin–proteasome system (UPS) is thought to be a major contributor for degrading many structural proteins (Cao et al., 2005). However, the autophagy–lysosome system has been largely ignored despite evidence that lysosomal degradation contributes to protein breakdown in atrophying muscles (Furuno et al., 1990). Sandri (2010, 2011) has shown that the autophagy–lysosome and UPS are coordinately regulated during muscle wasting. On the other hand, myostatin is a potent inhibitor of muscle growth and is considered as a therapeutic target for muscle wasting including cachexia and sarcopenia, muscular dystrophy, and amyotrophic lateral sclerosis (Sakuma and Yamaguchi, 2011b).

Several positive and negative regulators (mTOR, SRF, atrogin-1, p62, and myostatin) have been proposed to enhance protein degradation or transcription of muscle-specific genes during both sarcopenia and muscular dystrophy. However, the adaptations of these important mediators were not necessarily similar in these two conditions. Muscle ring finger 1 (MuRF-1), an E3 ubiquitin ligase, is activated in many different types of muscular dystrophy (Saenz et al., 2008; Fanin et al., 2013, 2014), but many mediators of UPS do not change during sarcopenia (Sakuma et al., 2014). Several studies have indicated similar dysfunctions of autophagic signaling during sarcopenia and muscular dystrophy (De Palma et al., 2012; Sakuma et al., 2014). In addition, skeletal muscle in both conditions exhibits down-regulation of SRF (Sakuma et al., 2004, 2008) and appears to show the activation of myostatin-dependent signaling (Sakuma et al., 2004; McKay et al., 2012). In contrast, the adaptation of mTOR-dependent signaling seems to differ between sarcopenia and muscular dystrophy to some extent (De Palma et al., 2012; Sakuma et al., 2014). To build on these previous findings, more descriptive and comprehensive comparison of positive and negative muscle regulators between sarcopenia and muscular dystrophy is needed.

Therefore, in this review, we concentrate on specific alterations discussed in the recent literature that are present in the skeletal muscle in both muscle wasting disorders. In addition, we focus on the adaptive changes in positive and negative regulators (mTOR, UPS, autophagy, etc.) of muscle mass. If we can understand more concretely and definitively the mechanisms underlying sarcopenia and muscular dystrophy, more effective applications (nutritional and/or pharmacological) for skeletal muscle wasting may be conducted in the near future.

CHARACTERISTICS OF SARCOPENIA AND MUSCULAR DYSTROPHY

SARCOPENIA

Aging is associated with a progressive decline of muscle mass, quality, and strength, a condition known as sarcopenia (Candow and Chilibeck, 2005). Although this term is applied clinically to denote loss of muscle mass, it is often used to describe both a set of cellular processes (denervation, mitochondrial dysfunction, inflammation, and hormonal changes) and a set of outcomes such as decreased muscle strength, mobility, and function (Melton et al., 2000), a greater risk of falls, and reduced energy needs. von Haehling et al. (2010) have estimated its prevalence at 5–13% for elderly people aged 60–70 years and 11–50% for those aged 80 years or above. Lean muscle mass generally contributes up to ~50% of total body weight in young adults, but declines with aging to 25% at 75–80 years of age (Short et al., 2004). The loss of muscle mass is most notable in the lower limb muscle groups, with the cross-sectional area of the vastus lateralis being reduced by as much as 40% between the ages of 20 and 80 years (Lexell, 1995). At the muscle fiber level, sarcopenia is characterized by specific type II muscle fiber atrophy, fiber necrosis, and fiber type grouping (Lexell, 1995).

Several possible mechanisms for age-related muscle atrophy have been described.

In a recent review by Demontis et al. (2013a) provides in-depth comparison of sarcopenia in *Drosophila* and mammals. Both muscles include very similar age-related changes such as increased mitochondrial dysfunction, decreased function of autophagy/lysosome system, increased apoptosis, and protective role of dietary restriction. In contrast, aged *Drosophila* and mammalian muscles exhibit several differential characteristics (endocrine changes, decreased regenerative capacity via satellite cells, defects in Ca^{2+} homeostasis, and increased fiber atrophy). Age-related muscle loss is a result of reductions in the size and number of muscle fibers, possibly due to a multi-factorial process that involves physical activity, nutritional intake, metabolic homeostasis, oxidative stress, hormonal changes, and lifespan (Baumgartner et al., 1999; Roubenoff and Hughes, 2000; Demontis et al., 2013b). The specific contribution of each of these factors is unknown, but there is emerging evidence using rodent muscle that the distribution of several positive regulators (Akt and SRF) of muscle hypertrophy with age is an important feature in the progression of sarcopenia (Sakuma and Yamaguchi, 2010, 2011a). Very intriguingly, more recent studies indicated an apparent functional defect in autophagy- and myostatin-dependent signaling in both mice and human sarcopenic muscle (Wohlgemuth et al., 2010; McKay et al., 2012; Zhou et al., 2013). In contrast, many investigators have failed to demonstrate age-related enhancement in the levels of common negative regulators [atrophy gene-1 (atrogin-1), NF-κB, and calpain] in senescent mammalian muscles (Sakuma and Yamaguchi, 2011a, 2012c). Currently available data show that human sarcopenia is attenuated by resistance training, the ingestion of amino acids, and treatment with testosterone (Sakuma and Yamaguchi, 2011a, 2013b; Wakabayashi and Sakuma, 2014). In addition, myostatin signaling inhibition for mice and calorie restriction for mice and rhesus monkey have been shown to counteract sarcopenia (Sakuma and Yamaguchi, 2011a, 2013b). Among this, resistance training in combination with amino acid-containing nutrition is the best candidate to attenuate age-related muscle wasting and weakness in human.

MUSCULAR DYSTROPHY

The neuromuscular disorders are a heterogeneous group of genetic diseases, causing progressive loss of motor ability. More than 30 genetically defined forms are recognized, and in the last decade, mutations in several genes that result in the deficiency or loss of function of various important muscle-proteins have been reported. These include dystrophin, sarcoglycans (SG), and dysferlin, which are sarcolemmal or peri-sarcolemmal proteins; α2-laminin and collagen VI, which are extracellular matrix proteins; and emerin and lamin A/C, which are nuclear proteins.

Defects in components of the dystrophin–glycoprotein complex (DGC) are known to be an important cause of different forms of muscular dystrophy (Yoshida and Ozawa, 1990; Ervasti and Campbell, 1993). The DGC is an oligomeric complex that connects the subsarcolemmal cytoskeleton to the extracellular matrix. It consists of dystroglycan (α- and β-DG), SG, and syntrophin/dystrobrevin subcomplexes. Mutations in the dystrophin gene cause the most common form of X-linked Duchenne muscular dystrophy (DMD) (Hoffman et al., 1990). The sarcoglycan sub-complex is also linked to β-DG and includes α-SG, β-SG, γ-SG, and δ-SG, which are tightly associated and inserted into the membrane. Mutations in the genes coding these four SG proteins cause severe forms of limb-girdle muscular dystrophies types LGMD2D, 2E, 2C, and 2F, respectively. α-DG, a receptor for the heterodimeric basement membrane protein laminin-2, binds to β-DG. Mutations in the LAMA2 gene, encoding the α2 chain of laminin-2, cause α 2-laminin deficiency and a severe form of congenital muscular dystrophy (CMD1A) linked to chromosome 6q (Helbling-Leclerc et al., 1995). Other milder forms of muscular dystrophy are caused by mutations in genes coding the enzyme calpain 3 (LGMD2A), the sarcolemmal protein dysferlin (LGMD2B), and the sarcomeric protein telethonin (LGMD2G) (Vainzof et al., 2008).

Sarcopenia and muscular dystrophy possess several similar characteristics as pointed out in more recent review by Rudolf et al. (2014). Fiber size variability is a major feature of various muscular dystrophy (Engel and Ozawa, 2004; Taniguchi et al., 2006; Krag et al., 2011), although it is frequently observed in sarcopenic mammalian muscles (Berger and Doherty, 2010; Hepple, 2012). The occurrence of small fiber groups was reported for samples from Becker muscular dystrophy (BMD) and DMD (ten Houten and De Visser, 1984; Engel and Ozawa, 2004), whereas elderly muscle exhibits extensive fiber type grouping (Kanda and Hashizume, 1989; Andersen, 2003). Rudolf et al. (2014) also indicated co-expression of multiple myosin heavy chain isoforms in these two muscles (Marini et al., 1991; Patterson et al., 2006). Furthermore, both muscles exhibit centralized nuclei, and the accumulation of fibrosis and intramuscular adipocyte. Although the exact reason for such a similarity has not been precisely elucidated, it seems to be feasible to apply same therapeutic approaches to sarcopenia and muscular dystrophy.

PHOSPHATIDYLINOSITOL-3-KINASE/Akt/MAMMALIAN TARGET OF RAPAMYCIN

A central pathway involved in hypertrophy is regulated at the translational level by the serine/threonine kinase Akt. In muscle, Akt is activated by the upstream PI3-K, induced either by receptor binding or by integrin-mediated activation of focal adhesion kinase (FAK), such as in cardiac myocytes (Sakamoto et al., 2002). The striking effect of Akt1 on muscle size was demonstrated by the transient transfection of a constitutively active inducible Akt1 transgene in skeletal muscle *in vivo* (Lai et al., 2004). In addition, muscle mass was completely preserved in denervated transgenic Akt mice (Pallafacchina et al., 2002). Possible downstream regulators of Akt, mTOR, and glycogen synthase kinase (GSK)-3β, play a crucial role in the regulation of translation.

Mammalian target of rapamycin exists in two functionally distinct multi-protein signaling complexes, mTOR signaling complex (mTORC)1 and mTORC2. Akt activates mTOR via phosphorylation and inactivation of tuberous sclerosis complex (TSC)-2. In general, only signaling by mTORC1 is inhibited by rapamycin, and thus the growth regulatory effects of rapamycin are believed to be primarily exerted through the mTORC1 complex (Zoncu et al., 2011). It is now widely accepted that signaling by mTORC1 is involved in the regulation of several anabolic processes including protein synthesis and ribosome biogenesis, as well as catabolic processes such as autophagy (Zoncu et al., 2011). In skeletal muscle, signaling by mTORC1 has been shown to be regulated by a variety of different stimuli that control skeletal muscle mass. For example, signaling by mTORC1 is activated in response to hypertrophic stimuli such as increased mechanical loading (mechanical overloading for the plantaris muscle of mice by surgical ablation), feeding, and growth factors (Bodine et al., 2001b; Drummond et al., 2009).

Since signaling through PI3-K/Akt can regulate mTOR-independent growth regulatory molecules such as GSK-3β, tuberin (TSC-2), and the forkhead box O (FOXO) transcription factors (Sandri, 2008), it was not clear whether signaling by mTORC1 is sufficient, or simply permissive, for the induction of hypertrophy. For example, Hornberger et al. (2003) found that stretch-induced activation of mTOR signaling was not abolished in the skeletal muscle of Akt1−/− mice. Furthermore, Akt-independent stimulation of mTOR may be positively or negatively regulated by phosphorylation of TSC-2. For instance, TSC-2 is inhibited by FAK in 293T cells (Gan et al., 2006), suggesting that up-regulation of FAK expression with increased mechanical loading for skeletal muscle could stimulate protein synthesis via TSC-2 inhibition. All these regulatory influences may explain the rise in the level of phosphorylated p70S6K (Coffey et al., 2006). Therefore, mTOR is currently thought to be the major hub for the integration of an array of upstream signaling pathways that, when activated, ultimately result in increased translational efficiency (Glass, 2010).

Two of the most studied mTORC1 targets are the eukaryotic initiation factor 4E binding protein (4E-BP)1 and p70S6K, which both play important roles in the initiation of mRNA translation. mTOR phosphorylates and activates the 70-kDa ribosomal protein S6 kinase (p70S6K), which results in increased translation either directly or indirectly by activating initiation and elongation, elongation initiation factor (eIF)-2, eIF4E (through 4E-BP), and eEF-2 (Glass, 2010). In addition, Akt also phosphorylates and inactivates GSK-3β, thereby activating translation via the initiation factor eIF2B. Other functions of Akt include the negative regulation of protein degradation by inhibiting FOXO-mediated proteasome activity.

Demontis and Perrimon (2009) showed that insulin receptor signaling and FOXO can regulate skeletal muscle atrophy also in *Drosophila* larval muscle. This study shows evolutionarily conservation of the mechanisms controlling muscle atrophy. It also shows a role for the transcription factors Myc and Mnt in this process (these are new factors that were not known to be involved in this process in mice or humans). Therefore, it is probable for the existence of novel signaling pathway via FOXO to regulate muscle hypertrophy and/or atrophy in mammals.

ADAPTATION OF PI3-K/Akt/mTOR PATHWAY IN AGED MUSCLE

Although many researchers consider PI3-K/Akt/mTOR levels to decrease with age, studies using sarcopenic muscles from rats and humans have yielded conflicting results. For example, compared with those in young Fischer 344 × Brown Norway rats, the amounts of phosphorylated mTOR and p70S6K were increased 70–75% in the tibialis anterior (TA) but not in the plantaris muscle of senescent rats (Parkington et al., 2004). Kimball et al. (2004) showed that, in gastrocnemius muscle, the level of phosphorylated p70S6K, eIF2B activity, and the amount of eIF4E associated with eIF4G increased between 12 and 27 months of age despite an apparent decrease in Akt activity. In addition, other groups (Haddad and Adams, 2006; Léger et al., 2008) also showed the decreased phosphorylation status of Akt in aged mammalian muscle. In contrast, Rahnert et al. (2011) showed only significant decrease of phospho-p70S6K (T^{421}/S^{424}) in the aged biceps brachii and no change in phospho-p70S6K (T^{389}), in spite of significant age-related decrease in p70S6K in all head and neck, tongue, and limb muscles (pectoralis, styloglossus, geniohyoid, posterior digastric, and masseter). Therefore, aging did not commonly modulate the PI3-K/Akt/mTOR-linked molecules in skeletal muscle under sedentary conditions.

Sarcopenic muscle shows a marked defect in the contraction-induced activation of these mediators. Parkington et al. (2004) reported lower levels of phosphorylated p70S6K and mTOR after high-frequency electrical stimulation [HFES, 3-s trains of pulses (frequency 100 Hz, duration 1 ms at 10–12 V)] in muscle of senescent rats (30 months of age) compared with those in young rats (6 months of age). The same roup (Funai et al., 2006) also demonstrated that 4E-BP1 was markedly phosphorylated in the TA muscle of aged but not young rats at 6 h after HFES. In addition, they suggested no increase in eIF4E–eIF4G association after HFES in aged muscle (Funai et al., 2006). Furthermore, Thomson and Gordon (2006) suggested impaired overload-induced muscle growth in old rats possibly due to diminished phosphorylation of mTOR (Ser^{2448}), p70S6K (mTOR-specific Thr^{389}), rpS6 ($Ser^{235/236}$), and 4E-BP1. Fry et al. (2011) demonstrated that acute resistance exercise (8 sets of 10 repetitions of leg-extension at 70% 1RM with 3 min of rest between each set) increased muscle-protein synthesis rate, and phosphorylation of mTOR, S6K1, and 4E-BP1 only in younger subjects (27 ± 2 years old) but not in elderly ones (70 ± 2 years old). These lines of evidence clearly show that sarcopenic muscle exhibits an impairment of Akt/mTOR/p70S6K signaling after contraction. This defect would explain the limited capacity for hypertrophy after muscle stimulation in aged animals.

ADAPTATION OF THE PI3-K/Akt/mTOR PATHWAY IN DYSTROPHIC MUSCLE

Functional deficiency of mTOR-dependent signaling is implicated in muscular dystrophy. Indeed, muscles lacking raptor (mTORC1 component) but not rictor (mTORC2 component) become progressively dystrophic and kyphotic, resulting in early death (Bentzinger et al., 2008). In the soleus and to a lesser extent in the EDL, raptor-deficient mice exhibited a wide distribution of fiber size, muscle fibers with centralized nuclei, and structures reminiscent of central cores (Bentzinger et al., 2008). Dystrophic muscle seems to exhibit induction of this anabolic pathway. Compared with age-matched wild-type mice, marked increases in pAkt/Akt, pS6/S6, and p4E-BP1/4E-BP1 were recognized in TA and diaphragm muscles of 4-month-old mdx mice (De Palma et al., 2012). Intriguingly, starvation was shown to elicit significant decreases in these anabolic mediators of mTOR-dependent signaling in both muscles of wild-type mice, but not those of mdx mice. Such hyperactivation of this signal markedly blocks autophagy-dependent signaling in both normal and starved mdx mice (De Palma et al., 2012). Age-related reductions of pAkt and pS6 levels occur in mdx mouse muscle. Indeed, Mouisel et al. (2010) showed marked decreases in pAkt (50%) and pS6 (45%) in mdx muscle at 18–24 months old compared with those at 5 months old. Intriguingly, the stimulation of muscle regeneration by cardiotoxin injury induces abnormal hyperactivation of pAkt and pS6. Therefore, sarcopenia muscle of mdx mice exhibits an apparent deficiency of PI3-K/Akt/mTOR signaling. However, as mdx mice age normally, caution is required when translating observations from mdx mice to human DMD patients. In addition, they similarly observed hyperactivation of pAkt and p4E-BP1, no induction of LC3-II, and accumulation of p62 in muscles of DMD patients. At 6 weeks of age, there was a significantly lower level of mTOR activation in diaphragm muscles of mdx mice compared with that of age-matched wild-type mice (Eghtesad et al., 2011). mTOR activation increased with postnatal age in diaphragm muscle of wild-type mice, but not in mdx mice. In contrast to diaphragm muscle, mTOR activation was not significantly different in the TA muscle of mdx and wild-type mice at either 6 or 12 weeks of age (Eghtesad et al., 2011). As contradicting results relating to the adaptive changes in PI3-K/Akt/mTOR in muscular dystrophy have been observed, future studies using human patients with muscular dystrophy are required. Strangely, a low-protein diet (De Palma et al., 2012) and treatment with rapamycin (Eghtesad et al., 2011) attenuate this anabolic pathway, but Wnt7a (von Maltzahn et al., 2012) and valproic acid (Gurpur et al., 2009) activate it. However, such therapeutics with overall different directions for mTOR-dependent signaling effectively attenuates the muscular dystrophic phenotype (muscle inflammation such as T-cell infiltration, fibrosis, myofiber damage, and the decrease of muscle strength).

SERUM RESPONSE FACTOR

Serum response factor is a ubiquitously expressed member of the MADS (MCM1, Agamous, Deficiens, and SRF) box transcription factor family, sharing a highly conserved DNA-binding/dimerization domain, which binds the core sequence of SRF/CArG boxes [CC (A/T)6 GG] as homodimers. SRF-dependent signaling plays a major role in a variety of physiological processes, including cell growth, migration, and cytoskeletal organization (Pipes et al., 2006). Previous results obtained with specific SRF-knockout models by the Cre–LoxP system emphasize a crucial role for SRF in postnatal skeletal muscle growth and regeneration by modulating interleukin-4 and IGF-I (insulin-like growth factor-I) mRNA expression (Charvet et al., 2006). More recently, Mokalled et al. (2012) demonstrated that members of the myocardin family of transcriptional coactivators, MASTR, and myocardin-related transcription factor (MRTF)-A, are up-regulated in satellite cells in response to skeletal muscle injury. In addition, double-knockout satellite cells (MASTR and MRTF-A) impair skeletal muscle regeneration, probably due to the down-regulation of several modulators of cell cycle arrest (retinoblastoma, etc.). As proposed by Mokalled et al. (2012), the promoting role on muscle regeneration seems to be attributable to both MASTR/MEF2 and/or MRTF–A/SRF complexes because the mouse MASTR protein lacks SRF-interaction regions.

Serum response factor also enhances the hypertrophic process in muscle fibers after mechanical overloading (Gordon et al., 2001; Sakuma et al., 2003; Sakuma and Yamaguchi, 2012a, 2013a) as well as muscle differentiation and MyoD gene expression *in vitro* (Gauthier-Rouviére et al., 1996). Although SRF would regulate proliferation and differentiation using different pathways, it would mainly activate the differentiation of satellite cells during muscle hypertrophy. Indeed, we showed that, in mechanically overloaded muscles of rats, the SRF protein co-localized with MyoD and myogenin in myoblast-like cells during the active differentiation phase (Sakuma et al., 2003). More recently, Guerci et al. (2012) investigated the functional role of SRF in fiber hypertrophy using $SRF^{flox/flox}$:HAS-Cre-ER^{T2} mice injected with tamoxifen. Guerci et al. (2012) showed that the selective lack of SRF in myofibers markedly slows fiber growth after mechanical overloading by modulating satellite cell proliferation and fusion to the growing fibers. They demonstrated that, in the overloaded muscle, SRF enhances the expression of COX2 mRNA, which in turn upregulates IL-4 mRNA and ultimately secretes IL-4 protein. Guerci's hypothesis indicated that IL-4 produced by muscle fibers moves into satellite cells paracrinally to modulate the fusion of satellite cells.

It is proposed that the transcriptional activity of SRF is regulated by muscle ring finger (MuRF)-2 (Lange et al., 2005) and striated muscle activators of Rho signaling (STARS) (Kuwahara et al., 2005). At the M-band, the mechanically modulated kinase domain of titin interacts with a complex of the protein products of the atrogenes NBR1, p62/SQSTM-1, and MuRFs (Lange et al., 2005; Puchner et al., 2008). This complex dissociates under mechanical arrest, and MuRF-1 and MuRF-2 translocate to the cytoplasm and the nucleus (Lange et al., 2005; Ochala et al., 2011). One of the probable nuclear targets of MuRFs is SRF (Lange et al., 2005), suggesting that the MuRF-induced nuclear export and transcriptional repression of SRF may contribute to amplifying the transcriptional atrophy program (Spencer et al., 2000). Thus, it is possible that the synergistic transactivation of SRF and SRF-linked molecules is abrogated by MuRF-2 *in vivo*. On the other hand, SRF activity is exquisitely sensitive to the state of actin polymerization. G-actin monomers inhibit SRF activity, whereas polymerization of actin occurs in response to serum stimulation and RhoA signaling. In this pathway, signal inputs lower the ratio of globular actin to fibrillar actin, thereby liberating the binding of MRTF-A to globular actin, resulting in the nuclear accumulation of MRTF-A and subsequent SRF-dependent gene expression (Miralles et al., 2003). It has been well established that overexpression of STARS contributes to the nuclear translocation of MRTF-A and MRTF-B (Kuwahara et al., 2005, 2007), and these factors activate SRF transcription.

ADAPTIVE CHANGES IN SRF-LINKED MOLECULES WITH AGE

Mechanical loading for skeletal muscle is widely accepted to determine SRF expression. In humans, Lamon et al. (2009) demonstrated that 8 weeks of resistance training (leg presses, squats, and leg-extensions) induced increases in SRF mRNA (3-fold) and nuclear protein (1.25-fold) in the vastus lateralis muscle. In the same training period, they also observed a similar increase in the mRNA levels of several SRF-targeted molecules (alpha-actin, myosin heavy chain IIa, and IGF-I) (Charvet et al., 2006). Using RT-PCR, crude and fractionated homogenates, and immunofluorescence, our study demonstrated blunted expression of SRF protein in the quadriceps and triceps brachii muscles in aged mice (Sakuma et al., 2008). Immunofluorescence microscopy also indicated the selective down-regulation of SRF immunoreactivity in the cell cytosol but not in Pax7-labeled satellite cells in sarcopenic mice. In addition, our data showed a decrease in MRTF-A mRNA (50–70%) and protein (76%) levels in only the nuclear fraction with age. Furthermore, 60 and 40% decreases in the amount of STARS mRNA were observed in the quadriceps and triceps brachii of 24-month-old mice, respectively (Sakuma et al., 2008). Intriguingly, a decrease of SRF expression achieved by a transgenic approach using the Cre–LoxP system was found to accelerate the atrophic process in muscle fibers with age (Lahoute et al., 2008). These SRF KO mice showed marked deposition of intramuscular lipids with aging. One morphologic aspect of sarcopenia is the infiltration of muscle tissue components by lipids because of the increased frequency of adipocyte or lipid deposition (Dubé and Goodpaster, 2006) within muscle fibers. As with precursor cells in bone marrow, liver, and kidney, muscle satellite cells expressing the adipocytic phenotype increased with age (Shefer et al., 2006), although this process is still relatively poorly understood in terms of its extent and spatial distribution. Lipid deposition, often referred to as intramuscular lipid deposition, may result from a net buildup of lipids due to the reduced oxidative capacity of muscle fibers with aging (Dubé and Goodpaster, 2006). These lines of evidence clearly show the existence of a defect of SRF signaling in aged mammalian muscle.

ADAPTIVE CHANGES IN SRF-LINKED MOLECULES WITH MUSCULAR DYSTROPHY

Serum response factor appears to be linked to the degenerative process during muscular dystrophy. Significant reductions in the amount of SRF have been observed (Sakuma et al., 2004), namely, 40–50 and 50–65% at 2 and 12 weeks of age, respectively, in merosin-deficient congenital muscular dystrophy. Our immunohistochemical analysis indicated that mature normal mice had an abundance of SRF protein in the cytoplasm of several muscle fibers, while the dy mice did not. In the skeletal muscle, there is no direct evidence of a link between SRF disorders and the pathogenesis of disease. However, Lange et al. (2005) observed that a mutation in the TK domain of titin, a possible upstream modulator of SRF, disrupted Nbr1 binding, and led to hereditary myopathy with early respiratory failure (HMERF). HMERF patient biopsies revealed diffusible localization of Nbr1, large cytoplasmic aggregates of p62, and the selective accumulation of MuRF-2 in centralized nuclei in diseased muscle. Unfortunately, their study did not examine the localization of SRF in the muscle of HMERF patients. In contrast, human heart failure was reported to show elevations of a natural dominant-negative form of SRF arising from alternative splicing (Davis et al., 2002). The dominant-negative SRF isoform potently inhibited SRF-dependent gene expression, mirroring the biochemical phenotype seen in SRF-null mice (Davis et al., 2002). In addition, a subsequent human heart failure study showed decreases in full-length SRF and elevated expression of a caspase-3-cleaved product of SRF (Chang et al., 2003). A more recent review (Miano, 2010) proposed various disorders to be linked with the SRF mutations as shown by many reliable studies using cell-specific SRF-knockout phenotypes.

UBIQUITIN–PROTEASOME SYSTEM

The ATP-dependent UPS is essential for regulating protein degradation. The degradation of a protein via the UPS involves two steps: (1) tagging of the substrate by covalent attachment of multiple ubiquitin molecules and (2) degradation of the tagged protein by the 26S proteasome complex with the release of a free and reusable ubiquitin. Ubiquitin, composed of 76 amino acids, is an 8.45-kDa protein that is highly conserved in nearly all eukaryotes. The ubiquitination of proteins is regulated by at least three enzymes: ubiquitin-activating enzyme (E1); ubiquitin-conjugating enzyme (E2); and ubiquitin ligase (E3). Kwak et al. (2004) suggested that the 14-kDa ubiquitin-conjugating enzyme $E2_{14K}$ and the ubiquitin ligase E3 are particularly important for the degradation of muscle-proteins. The labeled proteins are then fed into the cells' "waste disposers," the proteasomes, where they are chopped into small pieces and destroyed.

Atrogin-1 is a member of the Skp1, Cullin 1, and F-box-containing protein (SCF) complex, which bind together to establish E3 Ub-protein ligase activity, and features an approximately 40-amino-acid motif known as an F-box. MuRF-1 contains a canonical N terminal RING domain characteristic of RING-containing E3 ligases followed by a MuRF family conserved region, zinc-finger domain (B-box), and leucine-rich coiled-coil domains. Consistent increases in atrogin-1 and MuRF-1 gene expression have been observed in a wide range of *in vivo* models of skeletal muscle atrophy including diabetes, cancer, renal failure, denervation, unweighting, and glucocorticoid or cytokine treatment (Bodine et al., 2001a; Lecker et al., 2004). The importance of these atrophy-regulated genes in muscle wasting was confirmed through knockout studies in mice where an absence of atrogin-1 or MuRF-1 attenuated denervation-, fasting-, and dexamethasone-induced muscle atrophy (Bodine et al., 2001a; Baehr et al., 2011; Cong et al., 2011).

Yeast two-hybrid analysis identified eIF3 subunit 5 (eIF3-f) and MyoD as interactors of atrogin-1 (Lagirand-Cantaloube et al., 2008, 2009). Conversely, the knockdown of atrogin-1 reversed endogenous MyoD proteolysis and the overexpression of a mutant MyoD, unable to be ubiquitinated, prevented muscle atrophy *in vivo* (Lagirand-Cantaloube et al., 2009). These results confirmed MyoD as a substrate of atrogin-1, resulting in its polyubiquitination and subsequent degradation during dexamethasone-induced myotube atrophy (Jogo et al., 2009). In the heart, atrogin-1 ubiquitinates and reduces the levels of calcineurin A, an important factor triggering cardiac hypertrophy in response to pressure overload (Li et al., 2004). Interestingly, immunoprecipitation experiments in C2C12 myoblasts and myotubes have found that atrogin-1 interacts with sarcomeric proteins, including myosins, desmin, and vimentin, as well as transcription factors, components of the translational machinery, enzymes involved in glycolysis and gluconeogenesis, and mitochondrial proteins (Lokireddy et al., 2012). Whether atrogin-1 ubiquitinates these proteins has yet to be proven. In contrast to atrogin-1, it appears that MuRF-1 mainly interacts with structural proteins. MuRF-1 was reported to interact with and control the half-life of many important muscle structural proteins, including troponin I, titin, myosin heavy chain (Clarke et al., 2007), actin (Polge et al., 2011), myosin binding protein C, and myosin light chains 1 and 2 (Cohen et al., 2009). For example, MuRF-1 degrades myosin light chains 1 and 2 under denervation and fasting conditions (Cohen et al., 2009). These studies suggest that, while numerous stimuli can activate both atrogin-1 and MuRF-1, the downstream pathways affected may be separate for each protein.

ADAPTATION OF UPS IN AGED MUSCLE

Only very indirect measurements [small increases in levels of mRNA encoding some components of the UPS (Bossola et al., 2008; Combaret et al., 2009) or ubiquitin-conjugate accumulation] in old muscles of rodents or humans suggested modest activation of this pathway. Atrogin-1 and/or MuRF-1 mRNA levels in aged muscle are reportedly increased (Clavel et al., 2006) or unchanged (Welle et al., 2003; Whitman et al., 2005) in humans and rats, or decreased in rats (DeRuisseau et al., 2005; Edström et al., 2006). Even when the mRNA expression of these atrogenes increased in sarcopenic muscles, this was very limited (1.5- to 2.5-fold) compared with that in other catabolic conditions (10-fold).

Although various findings have been made regarding the mRNA levels of both ubiquitin ligases in aged mammalian muscle, the examination of protein levels in sarcopenic muscles did not support age-related increases in the mRNA of several ubiquitin ligases. For instance, Edström et al. (2006) indicated the marked up-regulation of phosphorylated Akt and FOXO4 in the gastrocnemius muscle of aged female rats, probably contributing to the down-regulation of atrogin-1 and MuRF-1 mRNA. This result is further supported by the more recent finding of Léger et al. (2008) who, using human subjects aged 70 years old, demonstrated decreases in nuclear FOXO1 and FOXO3a by 73 and 50%, respectively, although they did not recognize significant age-dependent changes in the expression of atrogin-1 and MuRF-1 mRNA. The major peptidase activities of the proteasome (i.e., the chymotrypsin-like, trypsin-like, and caspase-like activities) were either reduced (as reported in other tissues) or unchanged with aging (Combaret et al., 2009; Sakuma and Yamaguchi, 2011a). In contrast, Altun et al. (2010) recently found that the hindlimb muscles of (30-month-old) rats contained two to threefold more 26S proteasomes than purified from muscles of aged rats, and adult (control) rats showed a similar capacity to degrade peptides, proteins, and a ubiquitinated substrate, but differed in the levels of proteasome-associated proteins (e.g., the deubiquitinating enzyme USP14). Although the activities of many other deubiquitinating enzymes were greatly enhanced in aged muscles, levels of polyubiquitinated proteins were higher than in the adult animals. Interestingly, recent findings indicate that atrogin-1-knockout mice are short-lived and experience higher loss of muscle mass during aging than control mice (Sandri et al., 2013), indicating that the activity of this E3 ubiquitin ligase is required to preserve muscle mass during aging in mice. Moreover, MuRF-1-null mice experience higher decay of muscle strength during aging than controls, although muscle mass is at least in part preserved in these mice (Hwee et al., 2014). As indicated by Sandri et al. (2013), chronic inhibition of these atrogenes should not be considered a therapeutic target to counteract sarcopenia because this does not prevent muscle loss but instead exacerbates weakness.

ADAPTATION OF UPS IN MUSCULAR DYSTROPHY

Gene expression profiling in LGMD2A showed overexpression of UPS-related genes (Keira et al., 2007; Saenz et al., 2008). While the expression of atrogin-1 and MuRF-1 was not increased in mouse models of LGMD2A, FOXO1 was strongly up-regulated, and induced muscle atrophy in calpain-3-deficient mice (Laure et al., 2009). More recently, Fanin et al. (2013) demonstrated that LGMD2A patients exhibit significantly higher expression of MuRF-1 protein (146 ± 64% of control) but not atrogin-1 protein (77 ± 26% of control) in skeletal muscle.

LGMD2B is due to deficiency of the protein dysferlin, which causes failure in resealing of the membrane lesions generated during eccentric muscle contractions (Bansal et al., 2003). Similar to LGMD2A, dysferlinopathy patients exhibited more abundant mRNA and protein of MuRF-1 but not atrogin-1 (Fanin et al., 2014). Activation of UPS in dysferlinopathy has also been reported in cellular models (patient-derived muscle cells) (Azakir et al., 2012). Ullrich congenital muscular dystrophy (UCMD) is a common form of muscular dystrophy associated with defects in collagen VI. It is characterized by loss of individual muscle fibers and muscle mass and proliferation of connective and adipose tissues. More recently, Paco et al. (2012) studied muscle biopsies of UCMD ($n = 6$), other myopathy (DMD, calpain-3-deficient, Kearns–Sayre, and nemaline myopathy, $n = 12$), and control patients ($n = 10$) and found reduced expression of atrogin-1 and MuRF-1 mRNAs in UCMD cases.

In contrast to the case of sarcopenia, pharmacological inhibition of UPS appears to exert some beneficial effect on muscular dystrophy. Bonuccelli et al. (2007) indicated that Velcade, once injected locally into the gastrocnemius muscles of mdx mice, could upregulate the expression and membrane localization of dystrophin and members of the DAPC. Gazzerro et al. (2010) suggested that treatment with Velcade (0.8 mg/Kg) over a 2-week period reduced muscle degeneration and necrotic features, and increased muscle size (gastrocnemius and diaphragm), in mdx muscle fibers. In addition, they observed many myotubes and/or immature myofibers expressing embryonic myosin heavy chain in mdx muscle after Velcade administration, probably due to upregulation of several myogenic differentiating modulators (MyoD and Myf-5). They also demonstrated that MG-132 increased dystrophin, α-sarcoglycan, and β-dystroglycan levels in explants from BMD patients, whereas it increased levels of the DAPC in DMD cases.

AUTOPHAGY-DEPENDENT SIGNALING

Macroautophagy (herein autophagy) occurs in all eukaryotic cells and is evolutionarily conserved from yeast to humans. Autophagy is a ubiquitous catabolic process that involves the bulk degradation of cytoplasmic components through a lysosomal pathway (Sandri, 2010, 2011; Neel et al., 2013). This process is characterized by the engulfment of part of the cytoplasm inside double-membrane vesicles called autophagosomes. Autophagosomes subsequently fuse with lysosomes to form autophagolysosomes in which the cytoplasmic cargo is degraded and the degradation products are recycled for the synthesis of new molecules. Turnover of most long-lived proteins, macromolecules, biological membranes, and whole organelles, including mitochondria, ribosomes, the endoplasmic reticulum, and peroxisomes, is mediated by autophagy (Cuervo, 2004).

At first glance, autophagy was considered a coarse, nonselective, degradative system, but closer investigation revealed a different truth. Autophagy represents an extremely refined collector of altered organelles, abnormal protein aggregates, and pathogens, similar to a selective recycling center rather than a general landfill (Park and Cuervo, 2013). The selectivity of the autophagy process is conferred by a growing number of specific cargo receptors, including p62/SQSTM-1, Nbr1, Nix (Bnip3L), and optineurin (Shaid et al., 2013). These adaptor proteins are equipped with both a cargo-binding domain, with the capability to recognize and attach directly to molecular tags on organelles, and at the same time an LC3-interacting region domain, able to recruit and bind essential autophagosome membrane proteins.

De novo formation of autophagosomes is regulated by at least three molecular complexes: the LC3 conjugation system and the regulatory complexes governed by unc51-like kinase-1 (ULK1) and Beclin-1. The conjugation complex is composed of different proteins encoded by autophagy-related genes (Atg) (Mizushima and Komatsu, 2011). The Atg12–Atg5–Atg16L1 complex, along with Atg7, plays an essential role in the conjugation of LC3 to phosphatidylethanolamine, which is required for the elongation and closure of the isolation membrane (Mizushima and Komatsu, 2011). This system is under the regulation of at least two major cellular energy-sensing complexes. Under basal conditions, the ULK1 complex is inactivated by phosphorylation through mTORC1, whereas during autophagy induction mTORC1 is inhibited, thus enhancing the formation of a complex between ULK1, Atg13, and FIP200. In addition, mTORC1 can also be negatively regulated independently of Akt by energy stress sensors such as AMPK and, in a mechanical-activity-dependent manner, through TSC-1/2. Moreover, AMPK can also directly phosphorylate ULK1 and Beclin-1 (Kim et al., 2013). During autophagy, the ULK1 complex is localized to the isolation membrane, where it facilitates the formation of autophagosomes through interaction with the Beclin-1 complex.

Interestingly, that the UPS and the lysosomal–autophagy system in skeletal muscle are interconnected was suggested by Mammucari et al. (2007), and Zhao et al. (2007). Both studies identified FOXO3 as a regulator of the lysosomal and proteasomal pathways in muscle wasting. FOXO3 is a transcriptional regulator of the ubiquitin ligases MuRF-1 and atrogin-1. It has now been linked to the expression of Atg in skeletal muscle *in vivo* and C2C12 myotubes (Zhao et al., 2007). More recently, Masiero et al. (2009) found an intriguing characteristic using muscle-specific autophagy-related gene (Atg7) knockout mice. The atrophy, weakness, and mitochondrial abnormalities in these mice are also features of sarcopenia.

ADAPTATION OF AUTOPHAGY-LINKED SIGNALING IN MUSCLE WITH AGE

A decline in autophagy during normal aging has been described for invertebrates and higher organisms (Cuervo et al., 2005). Inefficient autophagy has been attributed a major role in the apparent age-related accumulation of damaged mitochondria (Terman and Brunk, 2006).

Demontis and Perrimon (2010) showed that the function of autophagy/lysosome system of protein degradation declined during aging in the skeletal muscle of *Drosophila*. This results in the progressive accumulation of polyubiquitin protein aggregates in senescent *Drosophila* muscle. Intriguingly, overexpression of the FOXO increases the expression of many autophagy genes, preserves the function of the autophagy pathway, and prevents the accumulation of polyubiquitin protein aggregates in sarcopenic *Drosophila* muscle (Demontis and Perrimon, 2009). Several investigators reported the autophagic changes in aged mammalian skeletal muscle (McMullen et al., 2009; Wenz et al., 2009; Wohlgemuth et al., 2010; Gaugler et al., 2011). Compared with those in young male Fischer 344 rats, amounts of Beclin-1 were significantly increased in the plantaris muscles of senescent rats (Wohlgemuth et al., 2010). In contrast, aging did not influence the amounts of Atg7 and Atg9 proteins in rat plantaris muscle (Wohlgemuth et al., 2010). Indeed, Western blot analysis by Wohlgemuth et al. (2010) clearly showed a marked increase in the amount of LC3 in muscle during aging. However, they could not demonstrate an aging-related increase of the ratio of LC3-II to LC3-I, a better biochemical marker to assess ongoing autophagy. In contrast, Wenz et al. (2009) recognized a significant increase in the ratio of LC3-II to LC3-I during aging (3 vs. 22 months) in the biceps femoris muscle of wild-type mice. None of the studies determining the transcript level of autophagy-linked molecules found a significant increase with age (McMullen et al., 2009; Wohlgemuth et al., 2010; Gaugler et al., 2011). Not all contributors to autophagy signaling seem to change similarly at both mRNA and protein levels in senescent skeletal muscle. Therefore, sarcopenia may include a partial defect of autophagy signaling, although more exhaustive investigation is needed in this field.

Life-long caloric restriction alone, or combined with voluntary exercise, resulted in mild reduction of LC3 expression and lipidation coupled with increased LAMP-2 (lysosomal marker) expression, suggesting a potential increase in autophagy flux. No significant age-related increase in autophagy-linked molecules was observed in MCK-PGC-1α mice. PGC-1α may also enhance autophagic flux. More recently, GSK-3α was proposed as a critical regulator of aging in various organs (skeletal muscle, heart, liver, bone, etc.) via modulating mTORC1 and autophagy. Intriguingly, mice with null mutation of GSK-3α showed premature death and acceleration of age-related pathologies such as vacuolar degeneration, large tubular aggregates, sarcomere disruption, and striking sarcopenia in cardiac and skeletal muscle (Zhou et al., 2013). These GSK-3α KO mice exhibited marked activation of mTORC1 and associated suppression of several autophagy molecules. Indeed, unrestrained activation of mTORC1 leads to profound inhibition of autophagy (Levine and Kroemer, 2008; Kroemer et al., 2010). Therefore, it is expected that pharmacological inhibition (everolimus) of mTORC1 rescued the muscular disorder resembling sarcopenia in GSK-3α KO mice (Zhou et al., 2013). Enhancement of autophagy flux (exercise, caloric restriction, etc.) would be a potential strategy attenuating sarcopenia as well as various type of muscular dystrophy with autophagy defect (Grumati et al., 2010; De Palma et al., 2012; Vainshtein et al., 2014).

ADAPTATION OF AUTOPHAGY-LINKED SIGNALING IN MUSCULAR DYSTROPHY

A finely tuned system for protein degradation and organelle removal is required for the proper function and contractility of skeletal muscle (Vainshtein et al., 2014). Inhibition/alteration of autophagy contributes to myofiber degeneration leading to accumulation of abnormal (dysfunctional) organelles and of unfolded and aggregation-prone proteins (Masiero et al., 2009; Sandri, 2010), which are typical features of several myopathies (Grumati et al., 2010; Nogalska et al., 2010). Generation of Atg5 and Atg7 muscle-specific knockout mice confirmed the physiological importance of the autophagy system in muscle mass maintenance (Raben et al., 2008; Masiero et al., 2009). The muscle-specific Atg7 knockout mice are characterized by the presence of abnormal mitochondria, oxidative stress, accumulation of polyubiquitinated proteins, and consequent sarcomere disorganization (Masiero et al., 2009). In addition, the central role of the autophagy–lysosome system in muscle homeostasis is highlighted by lysosomal storage diseases (Pompe disease, Danon disease, and X-linked myopathy), a group of debilitating muscle disorders characterized by alterations in lysosomal proteins and autophagosome buildup (Vainshtein et al., 2014). Intriguingly, all of these myopathies exhibit the accumulation of autophagic vacuoles inside myofibers due to defects in their clearance.

Apparent defect of autophagy-dependent signaling is also observed in various muscular dystrophies. The first evidence of impaired autophagy in these models was provided by studies in mice and patients with mutations in collagen VI (Irwin et al., 2003). Mutations that inactivate Jumpy, a phosphatase that counteracts the activation of VPS34 for autophagosome formation and reduces autophagy, are associated with centronuclear myopathy (Vergne et al., 2009). De Palma et al. (2012) have described marked defect of autophagy in dystrophin-deficient mdx mice and DMD patients. This evidence included the electron microscopic evaluation of muscle tissue morphology as well as the decreased expression of autophagic regulator proteins (i.e., LC3-II, Atg12, Gabarapl1, and Bnip3). In addition, starvation and treatment with chloroquine, potent inducers of autophagy, did not activate autophagy-dependent signaling in both TA and diaphragm muscles of mdx mice (De Palma et al., 2012). Furthermore, mdx mice and DMD patients exhibited an unnecessary accumulation of p62 protein, which was lost after prolonged autophagy induction by a low-protein diet (De Palma et al., 2012). A similar block in autophagy progression was described in lamin A/C null mice (Ramos et al., 2012). LGMD2A muscles showed up-regulation of p62 (2.1-fold) and Bnip3 (3-fold) mRNA and slightly increased LC3-II/LC3-I protein ratio and p62 (Fanin et al., 2013). Conversely, laminin-mutated (dy/dy) animals displayed excessive levels of autophagy, which is equally detrimental (Carmignac et al., 2011). These findings suggest that the defect of autophagy signaling has a central role in the degenerative symptoms in various types of muscular dystrophy. **Figure 1** shows a schematic diagram of possible relationship between Akt–mTOR signaling and autophagy in muscular dystrophy.

MYOSTATIN

Growth and differentiation factor 8, otherwise known as myostatin, was first discovered during screening for novel members of the transforming growth factor-β (TGF-β) superfamily, and shown to be a potent negative regulator of muscle growth (Lee, 2004). Like other TGF-β family members, myostatin is synthesized as a precursor protein that is cleaved by furin proteases to generate the active C-terminal dimer. When produced in Chinese hamster ovary cells, the C-terminal dimer remains bound to the

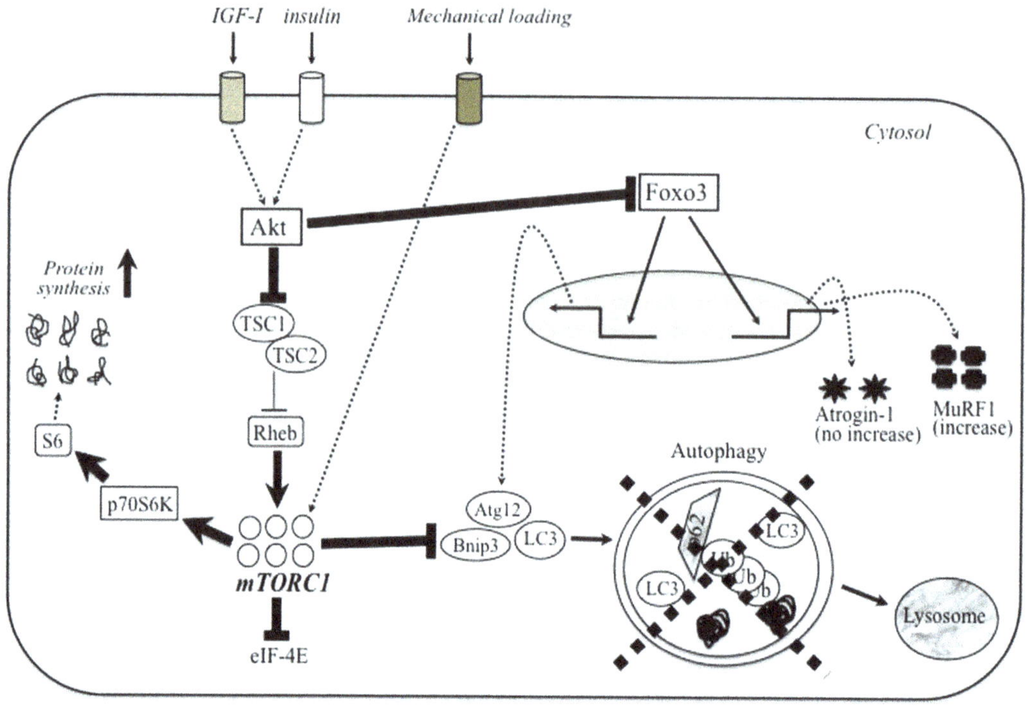

FIGURE 1 | The relationship between PI3-K–Akt–mTOR signaling and autophagy in muscular dystrophy. The major anabolic pathway regulating protein synthesis in skeletal muscle is mTOR/TORC1 signaling. Upstream trigger (IGF-1, mechanical stress, etc.) activates mTOR signaling through a number of different intermediary proteins such as Akt and Rheb. Several anabolic stimulation increases the amount of activated Akt, which blocks the nuclear translocation of Foxo3 to enhance the expression of autophagy-related genes (Bnip, LC3, and Atg12) and atrogene (atrogin-1 and MuRF-1). In dystrophic muscle, higher Akt potently blocks the inhibition of Rheb by TSC-1/TSC-2, and hyperactivate mTORC1. Unnecessary activated mTORC1 would extremely enhance protein synthesis and blocks autophagy-dependent signaling. Therefore, muscular dystrophy exhibits apparent defect of autophagic process similar to sarcopenic muscle.

N-terminal propeptide, which remains in a latent, inactive state (Wolfman et al., 2003). Most, if not all, of the myostatin protein that circulates in the blood also appears to exist in an inactive complex with a variety of proteins, including the propeptide. Myostatin binds to and signals through a combination of ActRIIA/B receptors on the cell membrane, but has higher affinity for activin type IIB receptor (ActRIIB). On binding to ActRIIB, myostatin forms a complex with a second surface type I receptor, either activin receptor-like kinase 4 or 5, to stimulate the phosphorylation of Receptor Smad (R-Smad) and the Smad2/3 transcription factors in the cytoplasm. This leads to the assembly of Smad2/3 with Smad4 to form a heterodimer that can translocate to the nucleus and activate the transcription of target genes (Joulia-Ekaza and Cabello, 2007). Myostatin circulates in the blood in a latent complex with non-covalently bound propeptide at the N-terminus (Wolfman et al., 2003).

Studies indicate that myostatin inhibits cell cycle progression and reduces the levels of myogenic regulatory factors, thereby controlling myoblastic proliferation and differentiation during developmental myogenesis (Yang et al., 2007). One of the known downstream targets of Smad signaling is MyoD. Interestingly, myostatin downregulates MyoD expression in an NF-κB-independent way (McFarlane et al., 2006). Myostatin also inhibits Pax3 expression, which is possibly an upstream target of MyoD (McFarlane et al., 2006). On the other hand, the genetic loss of myostatin leads to an increase in Akt activity in skeletal muscle *in vivo* and *in vitro* (Morissette et al., 2009). The IGF-1–Akt–mTOR pathway, which mediates both differentiation in myoblasts and hypertrophy in myotubes, has been shown to inhibit myostatin-dependent signaling. Blockade of the Akt–mTOR pathway using siRNA to RAPTOR, a component of TOR signaling complex 1 (TORC1), facilitates myostatin's inhibition of muscle differentiation because of an increase in Smad2 phosphorylation (Trendelenburg et al., 2009). Taking these findings, myostatin-mediated signaling activates FOXO, which leads to the expression of ubiquitin ligases.

ADAPTIVE CHANGES IN MYOSTATIN IN SARCOPENIC MUSCLE

Myostatin levels increase with muscle atrophy due to unloading in mice and humans (Wehling et al., 2000; Sakuma et al., 2009), and with severe muscle wasting in patients with cancer cachexia, chronic heart failure, chronic obstructive pulmonary disease (COPD), AIDS, and diabetes (Sakuma and Yamaguchi, 2011b). Many researchers have investigated the effect of inhibiting myostatin to counteract sarcopenia using animals (Siriett et al., 2006; LeBrasseur et al., 2009; Murphy et al., 2010). LeBrasseur et al. (2009) reported several positive effects of 4 weeks of treatment with PF-354 (24 mg/Kg) in aged mice. They found that

PF-354-treated mice exhibited significantly greater muscle mass (by 12%) probably due to decreased levels of phosphorylated Smad3 and MuRF-1 in muscle. More recently, Murphy et al. (2010) showed, by way of once-weekly injections, that a lower dose of PF-354 (10 mg/Kg) significantly increased the fiber cross-sectional area (by 12%) and *in situ* muscle force (by 35%) of aged mice (21-month-old).

However, the role of myostatin in driving sarcopenia is debated. There is indeed evidence that myostatin null mice, although they have a doubling of muscle mass, have reduced specific force and may be actually prone to sarcopenia, suggesting that the intrinsic capacity to generate force is perturbed in the absence of myostatin (Amthor et al., 2007; Gentry et al., 2011). In addition, a recent study in *Drosophila* on the myostatin/GDF11 homolog myoglianin indicates that, in the absence of changes in muscle mass, overexpression of myoglianin (*Drosophila* myostatin) in muscle extends lifespan and preserves muscle function at least in part by activating the stress-sensing kinase p38 MAPK, while myoglianin RNAi in muscle has converse effects (Demontis et al., 2014; Patel and Demontis, 2014).

In rodent muscle models, studies using sarcopenic muscles have yielded conflicting results (Haddad and Adams, 2006; Carlson et al., 2008; Bowser et al., 2013). Haddad and Adams (2006) showed lower expression of myostatin mRNA in aged (30-month-old) than in young (6-month-old) rats. Carlson et al. (2008) showed higher levels of TGF-β and Smad3 but not myostatin in sarcopenic muscles of mice. In humans, an early cross-sectional study of younger, middle-aged, and older men and women suggested that serum myostatin levels increase with advancing age, are highest in "physically frail" older women, and are inversely associated with skeletal muscle mass (Yarasheski et al., 2002). However, several subsequent reports on humans failed to show age-related differences in either circulating myostatin-immunoreactive protein or skeletal muscle myostatin mRNA levels (Welle et al., 2003; Ratkevicius et al., 2011). In contrast, Léger et al. (2008) found a significant elevation in myostatin mRNA and protein levels by 2- and 1.4-fold in young (20 ± 0.2 years) males compared with those in older (70 ± 0.3 years) ones. These disparate findings suggest that myostatin may not be a primary driver of sarcopenia, or may instead highlight the complexities related to myostatin and its measurements. As indicated by a recent review (White and LeBrasseur, 2014), three possible reasons for this exist. First, myostatin abundance may not reflect myostatin activity. Indeed, myostatin is generated as a precursor protein that requires proteolytic cleavage first to remove its signal peptide and then to liberate an N-terminal propeptide and a C-terminal fragment. The mature biologically active form of myostatin is only a disulfide-linked dimer of C-terminal fragments. Second, myostatin is further regulated by at least three interacting proteins, namely, GDF-associated serum protein-1 (GASP-1), follistatin, and follistatin-related gene (FLRG) (Lee, 2004). It is plausible that the abundance of these endogenous inhibitors of myostatin and/or the degree to which they interact with myostatin is independently affected by aging. Third, we may not detect the expression pattern of myostatin during sarcopenia because of very small changes of this molecule at only a limited position of an organelle (e.g., satellite cells), but not throughout muscle fibers. Indeed, a recent study revealed that muscle-derived stem cells from older male patients show a +65% higher level of myostatin expression than stem cells from younger patients (McKay et al., 2012). Although myostatin immunoreactivity on satellite cells gradually decreased the response to acute resistance exercise, old muscles possessed more abundant myostatin on satellite cells of type II fibers than young muscles postexercise. More descriptive study to investigate a detailed cellular localization of myostatin would detect such a limited but important adaptation of myostatin in sarcopenic muscle.

FUNCTIONAL ROLE OF MYOSTATIN IN DYSTROPHIC MUSCLE

There have been several studies dealing with the adaptive changes in myostatin expression of muscular dystrophy. Using muscles from fetopsies, infants (aged 8–10 months), and symptomatic patients (aged 5–12 years) with DMD, Chen et al. (2005) performed mRNA profiling. They demonstrated no induction of myostatin mRNA at any stage of the disease determined in their study. Similarly, no induction of myostatin was also observed in DMD muscle by Castro-Gago et al. (2006). Zanotti et al. (2007) showed significant increases in myostatin transcript and protein levels in DMD myotube cultures *in vitro*. In contrast, a screen of 12,488 mRNAs in 16-week-old mouse mdx muscle showed a marked decrease (fourfold) in myostatin mRNA (Tseng et al., 2002). Similar down-regulation of myostatin mRNA was observed in mdx mice using suppression subtractive hybridization (Tkatchenko et al., 2000). Therefore, myostatin does not seem to modulate the atrophy and degeneration of skeletal muscle in DMD and mdx mice, since common adaptation of myostatin levels did not occur in these dystrophic muscles.

Many mutations in the caveolin-3 gene have been detected in autosomal dominant LGMD1C and autosomal dominant rippling muscle disease (AD-RMD) (Minetti et al., 1998; Betz et al., 2001). Immunoprecipitation and subsequent immunoblot analysis revealed that caveolin-3 associates with the type I myostatin receptor in COS-7 monkey kidney cells *in vitro* (Ohsawa et al., 2008). Intriguingly, caveolin-3 seems to suppress myostatin signaling by blocking the type I myostatin receptor. Therefore, caveolin-3-deficient mice showed hyperphosphorylation of an R-Smad of myostatin, Smad2, and significant up-regulation of a myostatin target gene, p21 (Ohsawa et al., 2006). In addition, severe muscle histopathology was occasionally observed in the proximal muscles of patients with LGMD2I, whereas distal muscles were always relatively spared. In these patients, the amount of myostatin protein was highly increased in severely affected muscles compared with that in mildly affected ones. Hauerslev et al. (2013) hypothesize that alterations in the protein turnover and myostatin levels could progressively impair the muscle mass maintenance and/or regeneration, resulting in gradual muscular atrophy in LGMD2I. However, comprehensive analysis using a larger sample size of LGMD2I patients is needed as the hypothesis was generated from a very small sample size (severe phenotype $n = 1$; mild phenotype $n = 3$). In contrast, our previous study found a marked increase in mature myostatin protein (26 kDa) in gastrocnemius and rectus femoris muscles of merosin-deficient congenital dy mice at 12 weeks of age (Sakuma et al., 2004). In addition, marked myostatin immunoreactivity was detected in the cytoplasm of myonuclei and/or satellite cells of dy mice compared with slight

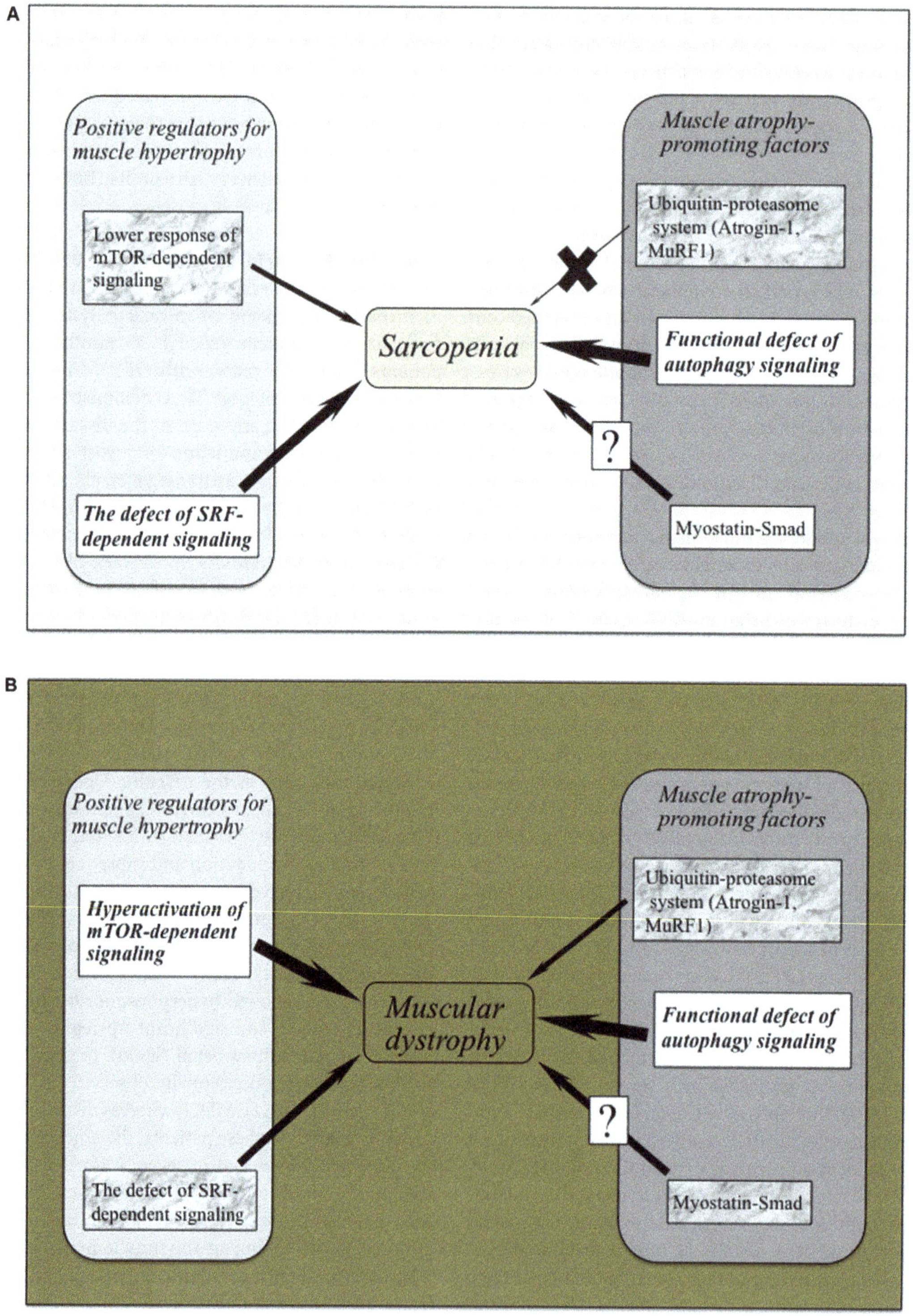

FIGURE 2 | (A,B) The adaptative changes of positive and negative regulators for muscle mass in sarcopenia and muscular dystrophy. Both sarcopenia and muscular dystrophy exhibit the marked defect of autophagy-dependent signaling possibly the latter due to hyperactivation of Akt/mTOR/p70S6K pathway. Lower activation of SRF-dependent signaling has been commonly recognized in these symptoms. Ubiquitin–proteasome system (Atrogin-1 and MuRF-1) would not regulate muscle atrophy in the case of sarcopenia. It remains to be elucidated whether myostatin–Smad pathway regulates to sarcopenic symptom and/or muscular dystrophy.

myostatin immunoreactivity at those sites in normal mice. Therefore, muscular dystrophy except for dystrophin deficiency induces the enhancement of myostatin-dependent signaling.

Many therapeutic approaches using myostatin attenuation have been conducted in muscular dystrophy. The use of neutralizing antibodies to myostatin improved muscle disorders in rodent models of DMD (mdx) and limb-girdle muscular dystrophy 2f (Sgcg−/−) (Bogdanovich et al., 2002; Bradley et al., 2008). Targeting of the C-terminal dimer by a neutralizing monoclonal antibody (JA16) resulted in increases in muscle mass and function in wild-type mice (Whittemore et al., 2003) and rescued the pathological phenotype in dystrophin-deficient mdx mice (Bogdanovich et al., 2002). The latter study was the first to provide evidence that blocking myostatin in dystrophic mice increased myofiber size and alleviated the symptoms of the disease, such as a decline in strength, the degeneration of fibers, and fibrosis. The inhibition of myostatin was also effective in alleviating the pathological phenotype of caveolin-3-deficient mice (a model of LGMD1C) (Ohsawa et al., 2006). In contrast, myostatin blockade did not attenuate the pathology in a mouse model of merosin-deficient muscular dystrophy.

Intriguingly, myostatin inhibition using MYO-029 (Stamulumab) was tested in a prospective, randomized, placebo-controlled US phase I/II trial in 116 adults with muscular dystrophy such as BMD, fascioscapulohumeral muscular dystrophy (FSHD), and LGMD (Wagner et al., 2008). MYO-029 has good safety and tolerability except for cutaneous hypersensitivity at higher doses (10 and 30 mg/Kg), attributed to the need for repeated protein administration (Wagner et al., 2008). No improvements in muscle function were noted, but dual-energy radiographic absorptiometry and muscle histological investigations revealed that some subjects had increased muscle fiber size. The trial study concluded that the systemic administration of myostatin inhibitors was relatively safe and that more potent inhibitors for stimulating muscle growth in muscular dystrophy should be considered. However, careful attention should be paid to myostatin inhibition, as mice with null mutation of myostatin revealed impaired tendon structure and function (Mendias et al., 2008). **Figures 2A,B** provide an overview of the positive and negative regulator adaptations of muscle mass in sarcopenia and muscular dystrophy.

CONCLUSION

In conclusion, both sarcopenia and muscular dystrophy exhibit the marked defect of autophagy-dependent signaling possibly the latter due to hyperactivation of Akt/mTOR/p70S6K pathway. Lower activation of SRF-dependent signaling has been commonly recognized in these symptoms. Although studies using rodent muscles have indicated that Atrogin-1 and MuRF contribute to the protein degradation in muscular wasting (Bodine et al., 2001a), these atrogenes do not regulate age-related muscle atrophy. More descriptive study seems to have detected such a limited but important adaptation of myostatin during sarcopenia.

ACKNOWLEDGMENTS

This work was supported by a research Grant-in-Aid for Scientific Research C (No. 23500778) from the Ministry of Education, Culture, Sports, Science, and Technology of Japan.

REFERENCES

Altun, M., Besche, H. C., Overkleeft, H. S., Piccirillo, R., Edelmann, M. J., Kessler, B. M., et al. (2010). Muscle wasting in aged, sarcopenic rats is associated with enhanced activity of the ubiquitin proteasome pathway. *J. Biol. Chem.* 285, 39597–39608. doi:10.1074/jbc.M110.129718

Amthor, H., Macharia, R., Navarrete, R., Schuelke, M., Brown, S. C., Otto, A., et al. (2007). Lack of myostatin results in excessive muscle growth but impaired force generation. *Proc. Natl. Acad. Sci. U.S.A.* 104, 1835–1840. doi:10.1073/pnas.0604893104

Andersen, J. L. (2003). Muscle fiber type adaptation in the elderly human muscle. *Scand. J. Med. Sci. Sports* 13, 40–47. doi:10.1034/j.1600-0838.2003.00299.x

Azakir, B. A., Di Fulvio, S., Kinter, J., and Sinnreich, M. (2012). Proteasomal inhibition restores biological function of missense mutated dysferlin in patient-derived muscle cells. *J. Biol. Chem.* 287, 10344–10354. doi:10.1074/jbc.M111.329078

Baehr, L. M., Furlow, J. D., and Bodine, S. C. (2011). Muscle sparing in muscle RING finger 1 null mice: response to synthetic glucocorticoids. *J. Physiol.* 589, 4759–4776. doi:10.1113/jphysiol.2011.212845

Bansal, D., Miyake, K., Vogel, S. S., Groh, S., Chen, C. C., Williamson, R., et al. (2003). Defective membrane repair in dysferlin-deficient muscular dystrophy. *Nature* 423, 168–172. doi:10.1038/nature01573

Baumgartner, R. N., Waters, D. L., Gallagher, D., Morley, J. E., and Garry, P. J. (1999). Predictors of skeletal muscle mass in elderly men and women. *Mech. Ageing Dev.* 107, 123–136. doi:10.1016/S0047-6374(98)00130-4

Bentzinger, C. F., Romanino, K., Cloëtta, D., Lin, S., Mascarenhas, J. B., Oliveri, F., et al. (2008). Skeletal muscle-specific ablation of raptor, but not of rictor, causes metabolic changes and results in muscle dystrophy. *Cell Metab.* 8, 411–424. doi:10.1016/j.cmet.2008.10.002

Berger, M. J., and Doherty, T. J. (2010). Sarcopenia: prevalence, mechanisms, and functional consequences. *Interdiscip. Top. Gerontol.* 37, 94–114. doi:10.1159/000319997

Betz, R. C., Schoser, B. G., Kasper, D., Ricker, K., Ramírez, A., Stein, V., et al. (2001). Mutations in CAV3 causes mechanical hyperirritability of skeletal muscle in rippling muscle disease. *Nat. Genet.* 28, 218–219. doi:10.1038/90050

Bodine, S. C., Latres, E., Baumhueter, S., Lai, V. K., Nunez, L., Clarke, B. A., et al. (2001a). Identification of ubiquitin ligases required for skeletal muscle atrophy. *Science* 294, 1704–1708. doi:10.1126/science.1065874

Bodine, S. C., Stitt, T. N., Gonzalez, M., Kline, W. O., Stover, G. L., Bauerlein, R., et al. (2001b). Akt/mTOR pathway is a crucial regulator of skeletal muscle hypertrophy and can prevent muscle atrophy *in vivo*. *Nat. Cell Biol.* 3, 1014–1019. doi:10.1038/ncb1101-1014

Bogdanovich, S., Krag, T. O., Barton, E. R., Morris, L. D., Whittemore, L. A., Ahima, R. S., et al. (2002). Functional improvement of dystrophic muscle by myostatin blockade. *Nature* 420, 418–421. doi:10.1038/nature01154

Bonuccelli, G., Sotgia, F., Capozza, F., Gazzerro, E., Minetti, C., and Lisanti, M. P. (2007). Localized treatment with a novel FDA-approved proteasome inhibitor blocks the degradation of dystrophin and dystrophin-associated proteins in mdx mice. *Cell Cycle* 6, 1242–1248. doi:10.4161/cc.6.10.4182

Bossola, M., Pacelli, F., Costelli, P., Tortorelli, A., Rosa, F., and Doglietto, G. B. (2008). Proteasome activities in the rectus abdominis muscle of young and older individuals. *Biogerontology* 9, 261–268. doi:10.1007/s10522-008-9135-9

Bowser, M., Herberg, S., Arounleut, P., Shi, X., Fulzele, S., Hill, W. D., et al. (2013). Effects of the activin A-myostatin-follistatin system on aging bone and muscle progenitor cells. *Exp. Gerontol.* 48, 290–297. doi:10.1016/j.exger.2012.11.004

Bradley, L., Yaworsky, P. J., and Walsh, F. S. (2008). Myostatin as a therapeutic target for musculoskeletal disease. *Cell. Mol. Life Sci.* 65, 2119–2124. doi:10.1007/s00018-008-8077-3

Candow, D. G., and Chilibeck, P. D. (2005). Differences in size, strength, and power of upper and lower body muscle groups in young and older men. *J. Gerontol. A Biol. Sci. Med. Sci.* 60, 148–156. doi:10.1093/gerona/60.2.148

Cao, P. R., Kim, H. J., and Lecker, S. H. (2005). Ubiquitin-protein ligases in muscle wasting. *Int. J. Biochem. Cell Biol.* 37, 2088–2097. doi:10.1016/j.biocel.2004.11.010

Carlson, M. E., Hsu, M., and Conboy, I. M. (2008). Imbalance between pSmad3 and Notch induces CDK inhibitors is old muscle stem cells. *Nature* 454, 528–532. doi:10.1038/nature07034

Carmignac, V., Svensson, M., Körner, Z., Elowsson, L., Matsumura, C., Gawlick, K. I., et al. (2011). Autophagy is increased in laminin α2 chain-deficient muscle and its inhibition improves muscle morphology in a mouse model of MDC1A. *Hum. Mol. Genet.* 20, 4891–4902. doi:10.1093/hmg/ddr427

Castro-Gago, M., Blanco-Barca, M. O., Eiris-Punal, J., Carneiro, I., Arve, V. M., and Devesa, J. (2006). Myostatin expression in muscular dystrophies and mitochondrial encephalomyopathies. *Pediatr. Neurol.* 34, 281–284. doi:10.1016/j.pediatrneurol.2005.08.009

Chang, J., Wei, L., Otani, T., Youker, K. A., Entman, M. L., and Schwartz, R. J. (2003). Inhibitory cardiac transcription factor, SRF-N, is generated by caspase 3 cleavage in human heart failure and attenuated by ventricular unloading. *Circulation* 108, 407–413. doi:10.1161/01.CIR.0000084502.02147.83

Charvet, C., Houbron, C., Parlakian, A., Giordani, J., Lahoute, C., Bertrand, A., et al. (2006). New role for serum response factor in postnatal skeletal muscle growth and regeneration via the interleukin 4 and insulin-like growth factor 1 pathways. *Mol. Cell. Biol.* 26, 6664–6674. doi:10.1128/MCB.00138-06

Chen, Y. W., Nagaraju, K., Bakay, M., McIntyre, O., Rawat, R., Shi, R., et al. (2005). Early onset of inflammation and later involvement of TGFbeta in Duchenne muscular dystrophy. *Neurology* 65, 826–834. doi:10.1212/01.wnl.0000173836.09176.c4

Clarke, B. A., Drujan, D., Willis, M. S., Murphy, L. O., Corpina, R. A., Burova, E., et al. (2007). The E3 ligase MuRF1 degrades myosin heavy chain protein in dexamethasone-treated skeletal muscle. *Cell Metab.* 6, 376–385. doi:10.1016/j.cmet.2007.09.009

Clavel, S., Coldefy, A. S., Kurkdjian, E., Salles, J., Margaritis, I., and Derijard, B. (2006). Atrophy-related ubiquitin ligases, atrogin-1 and MuRF1 are upregulated in aged rat tibialis anterior muscle. *Mech. Ageing Dev.* 127, 794–801. doi:10.1016/j.mad.2006.07.005

Coffey, V. G., Zhong, Z., Shield, A., Canny, B. J., Chibalin, A. V., Zierath, J. R., et al. (2006). Early signaling responses to divergent exercise stimuli in skeletal muscle from well-trained humans. *FASEB J.* 20, 190–192. doi:10.1096/fj.05-4809fje

Cohen, S., Brault, J. J., Gygi, S. P., Glass, D. J., Valenzuela, D. M., Gartner, C., et al. (2009). During muscle atrophy, thick, but not thin, filament components are degraded by MuRF1-dependent ubiquitylation. *J. Cell Biol.* 185, 1083–1095. doi:10.1083/jcb.200901052

Combaret, L., Dardevet, D., Béchet, D., Taillandier, D., Mosoni, L., and Attaix, D. (2009). Skeletal muscle proteolysis in aging. *Curr. Opin. Clin. Nutr. Metab. Care* 12, 37–41. doi:10.1097/MCO.0b013e32831b9c31

Cong, H., Sun, L., Liu, C., and Tien, P. (2011). Inhibition of atrogin-1/MAFbx expression by adenovirus-delivered small hairpin RNAs attenuates muscle atrophy in fasting mice. *Hum. Gene Ther.* 22, 313–324. doi:10.1089/hum.2010.057

Cuervo, A. M. (2004). Autophagy: many paths to the same end. *Mol. Cell. Biochem.* 263, 55–72. doi:10.1023/B:MCBI.0000041848.57020.57

Cuervo, A. M., Bergamini, E., Brunk, U. T., Dröge, W., Ffrench, M., and Terman, A. (2005). Autophagy and aging: the importance of maintaining "clean" cells. *Autophagy* 1, 131–140. doi:10.4161/auto.1.3.2017

Davis, F. J., Gupta, M., Pogwizd, S. M., Bacha, E., Jeevanandam, V., and Gupta, M. P. (2002). Increased expression of alternatively spliced dominant-negative isoform of SRF in human failing hearts. *Am. J. Physiol. Heart Circ. Physiol.* 282, H1521–H1533. doi:10.1152/ajpheart.00844.2001

De Palma, C., Morisi, F., Cheli, S., Pambianco, S., Cappello, V., Vezzoli, M., et al. (2012). Autophagy as a new therapeutic target in Duchenne muscular dystrophy. *Cell Death Dis.* 3, e418. doi:10.1038/cddis.2012.159

Demontis, F., Patel, V. K., Swindell, W. R., and Perrimon, N. (2014). Intertissue control of the nucleolus via a myokine-dependent longevity pathway. *Cell Rep.* 7, 1481–1494. doi:10.1016/j.celrep.2014.05.001

Demontis, F., and Perrimon, N. (2009). Integration of insulin receptor/Foxo signaling and dMyc activity during muscle growth regulates body size in *Drosophila*. *Development* 136, 983–993. doi:10.1242/dev.027466

Demontis, F., and Perrimon, N. (2010). FOXO/4E-BP signaling in *Drosophila* muscles regulates organism-wide proteostasis during aging. *Cell* 143, 813–825. doi:10.1016/j.cell.2010.10.007

Demontis, F., Piccirillo, R., Goldberg, A. L., and Perrimon, N. (2013a). Mechanisms of skeletal muscle aging: insights from *Drosophila* and mammalian models. *Dis. Model. Mech.* 6, 1339–1352. doi:10.1242/dmm.012559

Demontis, F., Piccirillo, R., Goldberg, A. L., and Perrimon, N. (2013b). The influence of skeletal muscle on systemic aging and lifespan. *Aging Cell* 12, 943–949. doi:10.1111/acel.12126

DeRuisseau, K. C., Kavazis, A. N., and Powers, S. K. (2005). Selective downregulation of ubiquitin conjugation cascade mRNA occurs in the senescent rat soleus muscle. *Exp. Gerontol.* 40, 526–531. doi:10.1016/j.exger.2005.04.005

Drummond, M. J., Fry, C. S., Glynn, E. L., Dreyer, H. C., Dhanani, S., Timmerman, K. L., et al. (2009). Rapamycin administration in humans blocks the contraction-induced increase in skeletal muscle protein synthesis. *J. Physiol.* 587, 1535–1546. doi:10.1113/jphysiol.2008.163816

Dubé, J. J., and Goodpaster, B. H. (2006). Assessment of intramuscular triglycerides: contribution to metabolic abnormalities. *Curr. Opin. Clin. Nutr. Metab. Care* 9, 553–559. doi:10.1097/01.mco.0000241664.38385.12

Edström, E., Altun, M., Hägglund, M., and Ulfhake, B. (2006). Atrogin-1/MAFbx and MuRF1 are downregulated in ageing-related loss of skeletal muscle. *J. Gerontol. A Biol. Sci. Med. Sci.* 61, 663–674. doi:10.1093/gerona/61.7.663

Eghtesad, S., Jhunjhunwala, S., Little, S. R., and Clemens, P. R. (2011). Rapamycin ameliorates dystrophic phenotype in mdx mouse skeletal muscle. *Mol. Med.* 17, 917–924. doi:10.2119/molmed.2010.00256

Engel, A. G., and Ozawa, E. (2004). "Dystrophinopathies," in *Myology*, Vol. 2, eds A. W. Engel and C. Franzini-Armstrong (New York, NY: McGraw-Hill), 961–1026.

Ervasti, E., and Campbell, K. P. (1993). A role for the dystrophin-glycoprotein complex as a transmembrane linker between laminin and actin. *J. Cell Biol.* 122, 809–823. doi:10.1083/jcb.122.4.809

Fanin, M., Nascimbeni, A. C., and Angelini, C. (2013). Muscle atrophy in limb girdle muscular dystrophy 2A: a morphometric and molecular study. *Neuropathol. Appl. Neurobiol.* 39, 762–771. doi:10.1111/nan.12034

Fanin, M., Nascimbeni, A. C., and Angelini, C. (2014). Muscle atrophy, ubiquitin-proteasome, and autophagic pathways in dysferlinopathy. *Muscle Nerve*. doi:10.1002/mus.24167

Fry, C. S., Drummond, M. J., Glynn, E. L., Dickinson, J. M., Gundermann, D. M., Timmerman, K. L., et al. (2011). Aging impairs contraction-induced human skeletal muscle mTORC1 signaling and protein synthesis. *Skelet. Muscle* 1, 11. doi:10.1186/2044-5040-1-11

Funai, K., Parkington, J. D., Carambula, S., and Fielding, R. A. (2006). Age-associated decrease in contraction-induced activation of downstream targets of Akt/mTOR signaling in skeletal muscle. *Am. J. Physiol. Regul. Integr. Comp. Physiol.* 290, R1080–R1086. doi:10.1152/ajpregu.00277.2005

Furuno, K., Goodman, M. N., and Goldberg, A. L. (1990). Role of different proteolytic systems in the degradation of muscle proteins during denervation atrophy. *J. Biol. Chem.* 265, 8550–8557.

Gan, B., Yoo, Y., and Guan, J. L. (2006). Association of focal adhesion kinase with tuberous sclerosis complex 2 in the regulation of s6 kinase activation and cell growth. *J. Biol. Chem.* 281, 37321–37329. doi:10.1074/jbc.M605241200

Gaugler, M., Brown, A., Merrell, E., DiSanto-Rose, M., Rathmacher, J. A., and Reynolds, T. H. IV. (2011). PKB signaling and atrogene expression in skeletal muscle of aged mice. *J. Appl. Physiol.* 111, 192–199. doi:10.1152/japplphysiol.00175.2011

Gauthier-Rouviére, C., Vandromme, M., Tuil, D., Lautredou, N., Morris, M., Soulez, M., et al. (1996). Expression and activity of serum response factor is required for expression of the muscle-determining factor MyoD in both dividing and differentiating mouse C2C12 myoblasts. *Mol. Biol. Cell* 7, 719–729. doi:10.1091/mbc.7.5.719

Gazzerro, E., Assereto, S., Bonetto, A., Sotgia, F., Scarfi, S., Pistorio, A., et al. (2010). Therapeutic potential of proteasome inhibition in Duchenne and Becker muscular dystrophies. *Am. J. Pathol.* 176, 1863–1877. doi:10.2353/ajpath.2010.090468

Gentry, B. A., Ferreira, J. A., Phillips, C. L., and Brown, M. (2011). Hindlimb skeletal muscle function in myostatin-deficient mice. *Muscle Nerve* 43, 49–57. doi:10.1002/mus.21796

Glass, D. J. (2010). PI3 kinase regulation of skeletal muscle hypertrophy and atrophy. *Curr. Top. Microbiol. Immunol.* 346, 267–278. doi:10.1007/82_2010_78

Gordon, S. E., Flück, M., and Booth, F. W. (2001). Selected contribution: skeletal muscle focal adhesion kinase, paxillin, and serum response factor are loading dependent. *J. Appl. Physiol.* 90, 1174–1183.

Grumati, P., Coletto, L., Sabatelli, P., Cescon, M., Angelin, A., Bertaggia, E., et al. (2010). Autophagy is defective in collagen VI muscular dystrophies, and its reactivation rescues myofiber degeneration. *Nat. Med.* 16, 1313–1320. doi:10.1038/nm.2247

Guerci, A., Lahoute, C., Hébrard, S., Collard, L., Graindorge, D., Favier, M., et al. (2012). Srf-dependent paracrine signals produced by myofibers control satellite cell-mediated skeletal muscle hypertrophy. *Cell Metab.* 15, 25–37. doi:10.1016/j.cmet.2011.12.001

Gurpur, P. B., Liu, J., Burkin, D. J., and Kaufman, S. J. (2009). Valproic acid activates the PI3K/Akt/mTOR pathway in muscle and ameliorates pathology in a mouse model of Duchenne muscular dystrophy. *Am. J. Pathol.* 174, 999–1008. doi:10.2353/ajpath.2009.080537

Haddad, F., and Adams, G. R. (2006). Aging-sensitive cellular and molecular mechanisms associated with skeletal muscle hypertrophy. *J. Appl. Physiol.* 100, 1188–1203. doi:10.1152/japplphysiol.01227.2005

Hauerslev, S., Sveen, M. L., Vissing, J., and Krag, T. O. (2013). Protein turnover and cellular stress in mildly and severely affected muscles from patients with limb girdle muscular dystrophy type 2I. *PLoS ONE* 8:e66929. doi:10.1371/journal.pone.0066929

Helbling-Leclerc, A., Zhang, X., Topaloglu, H., Cruaud, C., Tesson, F., Weissenbach, J., et al. (1995). Mutations in the laminin alpha 2-chain gene (LAMA2) cause merosin-deficient congenital muscular dystrophy. *Nat. Genet.* 11, 216–218. doi:10.1038/ng1095-216

Hepple, R. T. (2012). Muscle atrophy is not always sarcopenia. *J. Appl. Physiol.* 113, 677–679. doi:10.1152/japplphysiol.00304.2012

Hoffman, E. P., Brown, R. H. Jr, and Kunkel, L. M. (1990). Dystrophin: the protein product of the Duchenne muscular dystrophy locus. *Cell* 51, 919–928. doi:10.1016/0092-8674(87)90579-4

Hornberger, T. A., McLoughlin, T. J., Leszczynski, J. K., Armstrong, D. D., Jameson, R. R., Bowen, P. E., et al. (2003). Selenoprotein-deficient transgenic mice exhibit enhanced exercise-induced muscle growth. *J. Nutr.* 133, 3091–3097.

Hwee, D. T., Baehr, L. M., Philp, A., Baar, K., and Bodine, S. C. (2014). Maintenance of muscle mass and load-induced growth in muscle RING finger 1 null mice with age. *Aging Cell* 13, 92–101. doi:10.1111/acel.12150

Irwin, W. A., Bergamin, N., Sabatelli, P., Reggiani, C., Megighian, A., Merlini, L., et al. (2003). Mitochondrial dysfunction and apoptosis in myopathic mice with collagen VI deficiency. *Nat. Genet.* 35, 361–371. doi:10.1038/ng1270

Jogo, M., Shiraishi, S., and Tamura, T. A. (2009). Identification of MAFbx as a myogenin-engaged F-box protein in SCF ubiquitin ligase. *FEBS Lett.* 583, 2715–2719. doi:10.1016/j.febslet.2009.07.033

Joulia-Ekaza, D., and Cabello, G. (2007). The myostatin gene: physiology and pharmacological relevance. *Curr. Opin. Pharmacol.* 7, 310–315. doi:10.1016/j.coph.2006.11.011

Kanda, K., and Hashizume, K. (1989). Changes in properties of the medial gastrocnemius motor units in aging rats. *J. Neurophysiol.* 61, 737–746.

Keira, Y., Noguchi, S., Kurokawa, R., Fujita, M., Minami, N., Hayashi, Y. K., et al. (2007). Characterization of lobulated fibers in limb girdle muscular dystrophy type 2A by gene expression profiling. *Neurosci. Res.* 57, 513–521. doi:10.1016/j.neures.2006.12.010

Kim, J., Kim, Y. C., Fang, C., Russell, R. C., Kim, J. H., Fan, W., et al. (2013). Differential regulation of distinct Vps34 complexes by AMPK in nutrient stress and autophagy. *Cell* 152, 290–303. doi:10.1016/j.cell.2012.12.016

Kimball, S. R., O'Malley, J. P., Anthony, J. C., Crozier, S. J., and Jefferson, L. S. (2004). Assessment of biomarkers of protein anabolism in skeletal muscle during the life span of the rat: sarcopenia despite elevated protein synthesis. *Am. J. Physiol. Endocrinol. Metab.* 287, E772–E780. doi:10.1152/ajpendo.00535.2003

Krag, T. O., Hauerslev, S., Sveen, M. L., Schwartz, M., and Vissing, J. (2011). Level of muscle regeneration in limb-girdle muscular type 2I relates to genotype and clinical severity. *Skelet. Muscle* 1, 31. doi:10.1186/2044-5040-1-31

Kroemer, G., Marino, G., and Levine, B. (2010). Autophagy and the integrated stress response. *Mol. Cell* 40, 280–293. doi:10.1016/j.molcel.2010.09.023

Kuwahara, K., Barrientos, T., Pipes, G. C., Li, S., and Olson, E. N. (2005). Muscle-specific signaling mechanism that links actin dynamics to serum response factor. *Mol. Cell. Biol.* 25, 3173–3181. doi:10.1128/MCB.25.8.3173-3181.2005

Kuwahara, K., Teg Pipes, G. C., McAnally, J., Richardson, J. A., Hill, J. A., Bassel-Duby, R., et al. (2007). Modulation of adverse cardiac remodeling by STARS, a mediator of MEF2 signaling and SRF activity. *J. Clin. Invest.* 117, 1324–1334. doi:10.1172/JCI31240

Kwak, K. S., Zhou, X., Solomon, V., Baracos, V. E., Davis, J., Bannon, A. W., et al. (2004). Regulation of protein catabolism by muscle-specific and cytokine-inducible ubiquitin ligases E3alpha-II during cancer cachexia. *Cancer Res.* 64, 8193–8198. doi:10.1158/0008-5472.CAN-04-2102

Lagirand-Cantaloube, J., Cornille, K., Csibi, A., Batonet-Pichon, S., Leibovitch, M. P., and Leibovitch, S. A. (2009). Inhibition of atrogin-1/MAFbx mediated MyoD proteolysis prevents skeletal muscle atrophy *in vivo*. *PLoS ONE* 4:e4973. doi:10.1371/journal.pone.0004973

Lagirand-Cantaloube, J., Offner, N., Csibi, A., Leibovitch, M. P., Batonnet-Pichon, S., Tintignac, L. A., et al. (2008). The initiation factor eIF3-f is a major target for atrogin1/MAFbx function in skeletal muscle atrophy. *EMBO J.* 27, 1266–1276. doi:10.1038/emboj.2008.52

Lahoute, C., Sotiropoulos, A., Favier, M., Guillet-Deniau, I., Charvet, C., Ferry, A., et al. (2008). Premature aging in skeletal muscle lacking serum response factor. *PLoS ONE* 3:e3910. doi:10.1371/journal.pone.0003910

Lai, K. M., Gonzalez, M., Poueymirou, W. T., Kline, W. O., Na, E., Zlotchenko, E., et al. (2004). Conditional activation of akt in adult skeletal muscle induces rapid hypertrophy. *Mol. Cell. Biol.* 24, 9295–9304. doi:10.1128/MCB.24.21.9295-9304.2004

Lamon, S., Wallace, M. A., Léger, B., and Russell, A. P. (2009). Regulation of STARS and its downstream targets suggest a novel pathway involved in human skeletal muscle hypertrophy and atrophy. *J. Physiol.* 587, 1795–1803. doi:10.1113/jphysiol.2009.168674

Lange, S., Xiang, F., Yakovenko, A., Vihola, A., Hackman, P., Rostkova, E., et al. (2005). The kinase domain of titin controls muscle gene expression and protein turnover. *Science* 308, 1599–1603. doi:10.1126/science.1110463

Laure, L., Suel, L., Roudaut, C., Bourg, N., Ouali, A., Bartoli, M., et al. (2009). Cardiac ankyrin repeat protein is a marker of skeletal muscle pathological remodeling. *FEBS J.* 276, 669–684. doi:10.1111/j.1742-4658.2008.06814.x

LeBrasseur, N. K., Schelhorn, T. M., Bernardo, B. L., Cosgrove, P. G., Loria, P. M., and Brown, T. A. (2009). Myostatin inhibition enhances the effects on performance and metabolic outcomes in aged mice. *J. Gerontol. A Biol. Sci. Med. Sci.* 64, 940–948. doi:10.1093/gerona/glp068

Lecker, S. H., Jagoe, R. T., Gilbert, A., Gomes, M., Baracos, V., Bailey, J., et al. (2004). Multiple types of skeletal muscle atrophy involve a common program of changes in gene expression. *FASEB J.* 18, 39–51. doi:10.1096/fj.03-0610com

Lee, S. J. (2004). Regulation of muscle mass by myostatin. *Annu. Rev. Cell Dev. Biol.* 20, 61–86. doi:10.1146/annurev.cellbio.20.012103.135836

Léger, B., Derave, W., De Bock, K., Hespel, P., and Russell, A. P. (2008). Human sarcopenia reveals an increase in SOCS-3 and myostatin and a reduced efficiency of Akt phosphorylation. *Rejuvenation Res.* 11, 163–175. doi:10.1089/rej.2007.0588

Levine, B., and Kroemer, G. (2008). Autophagy in the pathogenesis of disease. *Cell* 132, 27–42. doi:10.1016/j.cell.2007.12.018

Lexell, J. (1995). Human aging, muscle mass, and fiber type composition. *J. Gerontol. A Biol. Sci. Med. Sci.* 50, 11–16.

Li, H. H., Kedar, V., Zhang, C., McDonough, H., Arya, R., Wang, D. Z., et al. (2004). Atrogin-1/muscle atrophy F-box inhibits calcineurin-dependent cardiac hypertrophy by participating in an SCF ubiquitin ligase complex. *J. Clin. Invest.* 114, 1058–1071. doi:10.1172/JCI200422220

Lokireddy, S., Wijesoma, I. W., Sze, S. K., McFarlane, C., Kambadur, R., and Sharma, M. (2012). Identification of atrogin-1-targeted proteins during the myostatin-induced skeletal muscle wasting. *Am. J. Physiol. Cell Physiol.* 303, C512–C529. doi:10.1152/ajpcell.00402.2011

Mammucari, C., Milan, G., Romanello, V., Masiero, E., Rudolf, R., Del Piccolo, P., et al. (2007). FoxO3 controls autophagy in skeletal muscle *in vivo*. *Cell Metab.* 6, 458–471. doi:10.1016/j.cmet.2007.11.001

Marini, J. F., Pons, F., Leger, J., Loffreda, N., Anoal, M., Chevallay, M., et al. (1991). Expression of myosin heavy chain isoforms in Duchenne muscular dystrophy patients and carriers. *Neuromuscul. Disord.* 1, 397–409. doi:10.1016/0960-8966(91)90003-B

Masiero, E., Agatea, L., Mammucari, C., Blaauw, B., Loro, E., Komatsu, M., et al. (2009). Autophagy is required to maintain muscle mass. *Cell Metab.* 10, 507–515. doi:10.1016/j.cmet.2009.10.008

McFarlane, C., Plummer, E., Thomas, M., Hennebry, A., Ashby, M., Ling, N., et al. (2006). Myostatin induces cachexia by activating the ubiquitin proteolytic system through an NF-kappaB-independent, FoxO1-dependent mechanism. *J. Cell. Physiol.* 209, 501–514. doi:10.1002/jcp.20757

McKay, B. R., Ogborn, D. I., Bellamy, L. M., Tarnopolsky, M. A., and Parise, G. (2012). Myostatin is associated with age-related human muscle stem cell function. *FASEB J.* 26, 2509–2521. doi:10.1096/fj.11-198663

McMullen, C. A., Ferry, A. L., Gamboa, J. L., Andrade, F. H., and Dupont-Versteegden, E. E. (2009). Age-related changes of cell death pathways in rat extraocular muscle. *Exp. Gerontol.* 44, 420–425. doi:10.1016/j.exger.2009.03.006

Melton, L. J. III, Khosla, S., Crowson, C. S., O'Connor, M. K., O'Fallon, W. M., and Riggs, B. L. (2000). Epidemiology of sarcopenia. *J. Am. Geriatr. Soc.* 48, 625–630.

Mendias, C. L., Bakhurin, K. I., and Faulkner, J. A. (2008). Tendons of myostatin-deficient mice are small, brittle, and hypocellular. *Proc. Natl. Acad. Sci. U.S.A.* 105, 388–393. doi:10.1073/pnas.0707069105

Miano, J. M. (2010). Role of serum response factor in the pathogenesis of disease. *Lab. Invest.* 90, 1274–1284. doi:10.1038/labinvest.2010.104

Minetti, C., Sotgia, F., Bruno, C., Scartezzini, P., Broda, P., Bado, M., et al. (1998). Mutations in the caveolin-3 gene cause autosomal dominant limb-girdle muscular dystrophy. *Nat. Genet.* 18, 365–368.

Miralles, F., Posern, G., Zaromytidou, A. I., and Treisman, R. (2003). Actin dynamics control SRF activity by regulation of its coactivator MAL. *Cell* 113, 329–342. doi:10.1016/S0092-8674(03)00278-2

Mizushima, N., and Komatsu, M. (2011). Autophagy: renovation of cells and tissues. *Cell* 147, 728–741. doi:10.1016/j.cell.2011.10.026

Mokalled, M. H., Johnson, A. N., Creemers, E. E., and Olson, E. N. (2012). MASTR directs MyoD-dependent satellite cell differentiation during skeletal muscle regeneration. *Genes Dev.* 26, 190–202. doi:10.1101/gad.179663.111

Morissette, M. R., Cook, S. A., Buranasombati, C., Rosenberg, M. A., and Rosenzweig, A. (2009). Myostatin inhibits IGF-I-induced myotube hypertrophy through Akt. *Am. J. Physiol. Cell Physiol.* 297, C1124–C1132. doi:10.1152/ajpcell.00043.2009

Mouisel, E., Vignaud, A., Hourdé, C., Butler-Browne, G., and Ferry, A. (2010). Muscle weakness and atrophy associated with decreased regenerative capacity and changes in mTOR signaling in skeletal muscles of venerable (18-24-month-old) dystrophic mdx mice. *Muscle Nerve* 41, 809–818. doi:10.1002/mus.21624

Murphy, K. T., Koopman, R., Naim, T., Léger, B., Trieu, J., Ibebunjo, C., et al. (2010). Antibody-directed myostatin inhibition in 21-mo-old mice reveals novel roles for myostatin signaling in skeletal muscle structure and function. *FASEB J.* 24, 4433–4442. doi:10.1096/fj.10-159608

Neel, B. A., Lin, Y., and Pessin, J. E. (2013). Skeletal muscle autophagy: a new metabolic regulator. *Trends Endocrinol. Metab.* 24, 635–643. doi:10.1016/j.tem.2013.09.004

Nogalska, A., D'Agostino, C., Terracciano, C., Engel, W. K., and Askanas, V. (2010). Impaired autophagy in sporadic inclusion-body myositis and in endoplasmic reticulum stress-provoked cultured human muscle fibers. *Am. J. Pathol.* 177, 1377–1387. doi:10.2353/ajpath.2010.100050

Ochala, J., Gustafson, A. M., Diez, M. L., Renaud, G., Li, M., Aare, S., et al. (2011). Preferential skeletal muscle myosin loss in response to mechanical silencing in a novel rat intensive care unit model: underlying mechanisms. *J. Physiol.* 589, 2007–2026. doi:10.1113/jphysiol.2010.202044

Ohsawa, Y., Hagiwara, H., Nakatani, M., Tasue, A., Moriyama, K., Murakami, T., et al. (2006). Muscular atrophy of caveolin-3-deficient mice is rescued by myostatin inhibition. *J. Clin. Invest.* 11, 2924–2934. doi:10.1172/JCI28520

Ohsawa, Y., Okada, T., Kuga, A., Hayashi, S., Murakami, T., Tsuchida, K., et al. (2008). Caveolin-3 regulates myostatin signaling. Mini-review. *Acta Myol.* 27, 19–24.

Paco, S., Ferrer, I., Jou, C., Cusi, V., Corbera, J., Torner, F., et al. (2012). Muscle fiber atrophy and regeneration coexist in collagen VI-deficient human muscle: role of calpain-3 and nuclear factor-κB signaling. *J. Neuropathol. Exp. Neurol.* 71, 894–906.

Pallafacchina, G., Calabria, E., Serrano, A. L., Kalhovde, J. M., and Schiaffino, S. (2002). A protein kinase B-dependent and rapamycin-sensitive pathway controls skeletal muscle growth but not fiber type specification. *Proc. Natl. Acad. Sci. U.S.A.* 99, 9213–9218. doi:10.1073/pnas.142166599

Park, C., and Cuervo, A. M. (2013). Selective autophagy: talking with the UPS. *Cell Biochem. Biophys.* 67, 3–13. doi:10.1007/s12013-013-9623-7

Parkington, J. D., LeBrasseur, N. K., Siebert, A. P., and Fielding, R. A. (2004). Contraction-mediated mTOR, p70S6K, and ERK1/2 phosphorylation in aged skeletal muscle. *J. Appl. Physiol.* 97, 243–248. doi:10.1152/japplphysiol.01383.2003

Patel, V. K., and Demontis, F. (2014). GDF11/myostatin and aging. *Aging* 6, 351–352.

Patterson, M. F., Stephenson, G. M., and Stephenson, D. G. (2006). Denervation produces different single fiber phenotypes in fast- and slow-twitch hindlimb muscles of the rat. *Am. J. Physiol. Cell Physiol.* 291, C518–C528. doi:10.1152/ajpcell.00013.2006

Pipes, G. C., Creemers, E. E., and Olson, E. N. (2006). The myocardin family of transcriptional coactivators: versatile regulators of cell growth, migration, and myogenesis. *Genes Dev.* 20, 1545–1556. doi:10.1101/gad.1428006

Polge, C., Heng, A. E., Jarzaguet, M., Ventadour, S., Claustre, A., Combaret, L., et al. (2011). Muscle actin is polyubiquitinylated *in vitro* and *in vivo* and targeted for breakdown by the E3 ligase MuRF1. *FASEB J.* 25, 3790–3802. doi:10.1096/fj.11-180968

Puchner, E. M., Alexandrovich, A., Kho, A. L., Hensen, U., Schäfer, L. V., Brandmeier, B., et al. (2008). Mechanoenzymatics of titin kinase. *Proc. Natl. Acad. Sci. U.S.A.* 105, 13385–13389. doi:10.1073/pnas.0805034105

Raben, N., Hill, V., Shea, L., Takikita, S., Baum, R., Mizushima, N., et al. (2008). Suppression of autophagy in skeletal muscle uncovers the accumulation of ubiquitinated proteins and their potential role in muscle damage in Pompe disease. *Hum. Mol. Genet.* 17, 3897–3908. doi:10.1093/hmg/ddn292

Rahnert, J. A., Luo, Q., Balog, E. M., Sokoloff, A. J., and Burkholder, T. J. (2011). Changes in growth-related kinases in head, neck and limb muscles with age. *Exp. Gerontol.* 46, 282–291. doi:10.1016/j.exger.2010.11.004

Ramos, F. J., Chen, S. C., Garelick, M. G., Dai, D. F., Liao, C. Y., Schreiber, K. H., et al. (2012). Rapamycin reverses elevated mTORC1 signaling in lamin A/C-deficient mice, rescues cardiac and skeletal muscle function, and extends survival. *Sci. Transl. Med.* 4, 144ra103. doi:10.1126/scitranslmed.3003802

Ratkevicius, A., Joyson, A., Selmer, I., Dhanani, T., Grierson, C., Tommasi, A. M., et al. (2011). Serum concentrations of myostatin and myostatin-interacting proteins do not differ between young and sarcopenic elderly men. *J. Gerontol. A Biol. Sci. Med. Sci.* 66, 620–626. doi:10.1093/gerona/glr025

Rosenberg, I. (1989). Summary comments. *Am. J. Clin. Nutr.* 50, 1231–1233.

Roubenoff, R., and Hughes, V. A. (2000). Sarcopenia: current concepts. *J. Gerontol. A Biol. Sci. Med. Sci.* 55, M716–M724. doi:10.1093/gerona/55.12.M716

Rudolf, R., Khan, M. M., Labeit, S., and Deschenes, M. R. (2014). Degeneration of neuromuscular junction in age and dystrophy. *Front. Aging Neurosci.* 6:99. doi:10.3389/fnagi.2014.00099

Saenz, A., Azpitarte, M., Armananzas, R., Leturcq, F., Alzualde, A., Inza, I., et al. (2008). Gene expression profiling in limb girdle muscular dystrophy 2A. *PLoS ONE* 3:e3750. doi:10.1371/journal.pone.0003750

Sakamoto, K., Hirshman, M. F., Aschenbach, W. G., and Goodyear, L. J. (2002). Contraction regulation of Akt in rat skeletal muscle. *J. Biol. Chem.* 277, 11910–11917. doi:10.1074/jbc.M112410200

Sakuma, K., Akiho, M., Nakashima, H., Akima, H., and Yasuhara, M. (2008). Age-related reductions in expression of serum response factor and myocardin-related transcription factor A in mouse skeletal muscles. *Biochim. Biophys. Acta* 1782, 453–461. doi:10.1016/j.bbadis.2008.03.008

Sakuma, K., Aoi, W., and Yamaguchi, A. (2014). Current understanding of sarcopenia: possible candidates modulating muscle mass. *Pflugers Arch.* doi:10.1007/s00424-014-1527-x

Sakuma, K., Nakao, R., Inashima, S., Hirata, M., Kubo, T., and Yasuhara, M. (2004). Marked reduction of focal adhesion kinase, serum response factor and myocyte enhancer factor 2C, but increase in RhoA and myostatin in the hindlimb dy mouse muscles. *Acta Neuropathol.* 198, 241–249. doi:10.1007/s00401-004-0884-5

Sakuma, K., Nishikawa, J., Nakao, R., Nakano, H., Sano, M., Watanabe, K., et al. (2003). Serum response factor plays an important role in the mechanically overloaded plantaris muscle of rats. *Histochem. Cell Biol.* 119, 149–160. doi:10.1007/s00418-003-0499-2

Sakuma, K., Watanabe, K., Hotta, N., Koike, T., Ishida, K., Katayama, K., et al. (2009). The adaptive response in several mediators linked with hypertrophy and atrophy of skeletal muscle after lower limb unloading in humans. *Acta Physiol.* 197, 151–159. doi:10.1111/j.1748-1716.2009.01995.x

Sakuma, K., and Yamaguchi, A. (2010). Molecular mechanisms in aging and current strategies to counteract sarcopenia. *Curr. Aging Sci.* 3, 90–101. doi:10.2174/1874609811003020090

Sakuma, K., and Yamaguchi, A. (2011a). "Sarcopenia: molecular mechanisms and current therapeutic strategy," in *Cell Aging*, eds J. W. Perloft and A. H. Wong (New York, NY: Nova Science Publisher), 93–152.

Sakuma, K., and Yamaguchi, A. (2011b). Inhibitors of myostatin- and proteasome-dependent signaling for attenuating muscle wasting. *Recent Pat. Regen. Med.* 1, 284–298.

Sakuma, K., and Yamaguchi, A. (2012a). "Serum response factor (SRF)-dependent pathway: potential mediators of skeletal muscle growth and development," in *Recent Res. Devel. Life. Sci*, 5th Edn, ed. S. G. Pandalai (Kerala, India: Research Signpost), 13–37.

Sakuma, K., and Yamaguchi, A. (2012b). "Cellular and molecular mechanisms regulating the hypertrophy and atrophy of skeletal muscle," in *Skeletal Muscle: Physiology, Classification, and Disease*, ed. M. Willems (New York, NY: Nova Science Publisher), 141–194.

Sakuma, K., and Yamaguchi, A. (2012c). Sarcopenia and cachexia: the adaptation of negative regulators of skeletal muscle mass. *J. Cachexia Sarcopenia Muscle* 3, 77–94. doi:10.1007/s13539-011-0052-4

Sakuma, K., and Yamaguchi, A. (2013a). Serum response factor (SRF)-dependent signaling in regenerating, hypertrophied, and pathological skeletal muscle. *Front. Pathol. Genet.* 1:1–8.

Sakuma, K., and Yamaguchi, A. (2013b). "An overview of the therapeutic strategies for preventing sarcopenia," in *Basic Biology and Current Understanding of Skeletal Muscle*, ed. K. Sakuma (New York, NY: Nova Science Publisher), 87–122.

Sandri, M. (2008). Signaling in muscle atrophy and hypertrophy. *Physiology* 23, 160–170. doi:10.1152/physiol.00041.2007

Sandri, M. (2010). Autophagy in health and disease. 3. Involvement of autophagy in muscle atrophy. *Am. J. Physiol. Cell Physiol.* 298, C1291–C1297. doi:10.1152/ajpcell.00531.2009

Sandri, M. (2011). New findings of lysosomal proteolysis in skeletal muscle. *Curr. Opin. Clin. Nutr. Metab. Care* 14, 223–229. doi:10.1097/MCO.0b013e3283457a75

Sandri, M., Barberi, L., Bijlsma, A. Y., Blaauw, B., Dyar, K. A., Milan, G., et al. (2013). Signaling pathways regulating muscle mass in ageing skeletal muscle. The role of IGF-1-Akt-mTOR-FoxO pathway. *Biogerontology* 14, 303–323. doi:10.1007/s10522-013-9432-9

Shaid, S., Brandts, C. H., Serve, H., and Dikic, I. (2013). Ubiquitination and selective autophagy. *Cell Death Differ.* 20, 21–30. doi:10.1038/cdd.2012.72

Shefer, G., Van de Mark, D. P., Richardson, J. B., and Yablonka-Reuveni, Z. (2006). Satellite-cell pool size does matter: defining the myogenic potency of aging skeletal muscle. *Dev. Biol.* 294, 50–66. doi:10.1016/j.ydbio.2006.02.022

Short, K. R., Vittone, J. L., Bigelow, M. L., Proctor, D. N., and Nair, K. S. (2004). Age, and aerobic exercise training effects on whole body and muscle protein metabolism. *Am. J. Physiol. Endocrinol. Metab.* 286, E92–E101. doi:10.1152/ajpendo.00366.2003

Siriett, V., Platt, L., Salerno, M. S., Ling, N., Kambadur, R., and Sharma, M. (2006). Prolonged absence of myostatin reduces sarcopenia. *J. Cell. Physiol.* 209, 866–873. doi:10.1002/jcp.20778

Spencer, J. A., Eliazer, S., Ilaria, R. L. Jr, Richardson, J. A., and Olson, E. N. (2000). Regulation of microtubule dynamics and myogenic differentiation by MURF, a striated muscle RING-finger protein. *J. Cell Biol.* 150, 771–784. doi:10.1083/jcb.150.4.771

Staron, R. S., Leonardi, M. J., Karapondo, D. L., Malicky, E. S., Falkel, J. E., Hagerman, F. C., et al. (1991). Strength and skeletal muscle adaptations in heavy-resistance-trained women after detraining and retraining. *J. Appl. Physiol.* 70, 631–640.

Taniguchi, M., Kurahashi, H., Noguchi, S., Fukudome, T., Okinaga, T., Tsukarhara, T., et al. (2006). Aberrant neuromuscular junctions and delayed terminal muscle fiber maturation in alpha-dystroglycanopathies. *Hum. Mol. Genet.* 15, 1279–1289. doi:10.1093/hmg/ddl045

ten Houten, R., and De Visser, M. (1984). Histopathological findings in Becker-type muscular dystrophy. *Arch. Neurol.* 41, 729–733. doi:10.1001/archneur.1984.04050180051017

Terman, A., and Brunk, U. T. (2006). Oxidative stress, accumulation of biological "garbage", and aging. *Antioxid. Redox Signal.* 8, 197–204. doi:10.1089/ars.2006.8.197

Thomson, D. M., and Gordon, S. E. (2006). Impaired overload-induced muscle growth is associated with diminished translational signaling in aged rat fast-twitch skeletal muscle. *J. Physiol.* 574, 291–305. doi:10.1113/jphysiol.2006.107490

Tkatchenko, A. V., Le Cam, G., Léger, J. J., and Dechesne, C. A. (2000). Large-scale analysis of differential gene expression in the hindlimb muscles and diaphragm of mdx mouse. *Biochim. Biophys. Acta* 1500, 17–30. doi:10.1016/S0925-4439(99)00084-8

Trendelenburg, A. U., Meyer, A., Rohner, D., Boyle, J., Hatakeyama, S., and Glass, D. J. (2009). Myostatin reduces Akt/TORC1/p70S6K signaling, inhibiting myoblast differentiation and myotube size. *Am. J. Physiol. Cell Physiol.* 296, C1258–C1270. doi:10.1152/ajpcell.00105.2009

Tseng, B. S., Zhao, P., Pattison, J. S., Gordon, S. E., Granchelli, J. A., Madsen, R. W., et al. (2002). Regenerated mdx mouse skeletal muscle shows differential mRNA expression. *J. Appl. Physiol.* 93, 537–545. doi:10.1152/japplphysiol.00202.2002

Vainshtein, A., Grumati, P., Sandri, M., and Bonaldo, P. (2014). Skeletal muscle, autophagy, and physical activity: the ménage á trois of metabolic regulation in health and disease. *J. Mol. Med.* 92, 127–137. doi:10.1007/s00109-013-1096-z

Vainzof, M., Ayub-Guerrieri, D., Onofre, P. C., Martins, P. C., Lopes, V. F., Zilberztajn, D., et al. (2008). Animal models for genetic neuromuscular diseases. *J. Mol. Neurosci.* 34, 241–248. doi:10.1007/s12031-007-9023-9

Vergne, I., Roberts, E., Elmaoued, R. A., Tosch, V., Delgado, M. A., Proikas-Cezanne, T., et al. (2009). Control of autophagy initiation by phosphoinositide 3-phosphatase Jumpy. *EMBO J.* 28, 2244–2258. doi:10.1038/emboj.2009.159

von Haehling, S., Morley, J. E., and Anker, S. D. (2010). An overview of sarcopenia: facts and numbers on prevalence and clinical impact. *J. Cachexia Sarcopenia Muscle* 1, 129–133. doi:10.1007/s13539-010-0014-2

von Maltzahn, J., Renaud, J.-M., Parise, G., and Rudnicki, A. (2012). Wnt7a treatment ameliorates muscular dystrophy. *Proc. Natl. Acad. Sci. U.S.A.* 109, 20614–20619. doi:10.1073/pnas.1215765109

Wagner, K. R., Fleckenstein, J. L., Amato, A. A., Barohn, R. J., Bushby, K., Escolar, D. M., et al. (2008). A phase I/II trial of MYO-029 in adult subjects with muscular dystrophy. *Ann. Neurol.* 63, 561–571. doi:10.1002/ana.21338

Wakabayashi, H., and Sakuma, K. (2014). Comprehensive approach to sarcopenia treatment. *Curr. Clin. Pharmacol.* 9, 171–180. doi:10.2174/1574884708666131111192845

Wehling, M., Cai, B., and Tidball, J. G. (2000). Modulation of myostatin expression during modified muscle use. *FASEB J.* 14, 103–110.

Welle, S., Brooks, A. I., Delehanty, J. M., Needler, N., and Thornton, C. A. (2003). Gene expression profile of aging in human muscle. *Physiol. Genomics* 14, 149–159.

Wenz, T., Rossi, S. G., Rotundo, R. L., Spiegelman, B. M., and Moraes, C. T. (2009). Increased muscle PGC-1alpha expression protects from sarcopenia and metabolic disease during aging. *Proc. Natl. Acad. Sci. U.S.A.* 106, 20405–20410. doi:10.1073/pnas.0911570106

White, T. A., and LeBrasseur, N. K. (2014). Myostatin and sarcopenia: opportunities and challenges – a mini-review. *Gerontology* 60, 289–293. doi:10.1159/000356740

Whitman, S. A., Wacker, M. J., Richmond, S. R., and Godard, M. P. (2005). Contributions of the ubiquitin-proteasome pathway and apoptosis to human skeletal muscle wasting with age. *Pflugers Arch.* 450, 437–446. doi:10.1007/s00424-005-1473-8

Whittemore, L. A., Song, K., Li, X., Aghajanian, J., Davies, M. V., Girgenrath, S., et al. (2003). Inhibition of myostatin in adult mice increases skeletal muscle mass and strength. *Biochem. Biophys. Res. Commun.* 300, 965–971. doi:10.1016/S0006-291X(02)02953-4

Wohlgemuth, S. E., Seo, A. Y., Marzetti, E., Lees, H. A., and Leeuwenburgh, C. (2010). Skeletal muscle autophagy and apoptosis during aging: effects of calorie restriction and life-long exercise. *Exp. Gerontol.* 45, 138–148. doi:10.1016/j.exger.2009.11.002

Wolfman, N. M., McPherron, A. C., Pappano, W. N., Davies, M. V., Song, K., Tomkinson, K. N., et al. (2003). Activation of latent myostatin by the BMP-1/tolloid family of metalloproteinases. *Proc. Natl. Acad. Sci. U.S.A.* 100, 15842–15846. doi:10.1073/pnas.2534946100

Yang, W., Zhang, Y., Li, Y., Wu, Z., and Zhu, D. (2007). Myostatin induces cyclin D1 degradation to cause cell cycle arrest through a phosphatidylinositol 3-kinase/Akt/GSK-3β pathway and is antagonized by insulin-like growth factor 1. *J. Biol. Chem.* 282, 3799–3808. doi:10.1074/jbc.M610185200

Yarasheski, K. E., Bhasin, S., Sinha-Hikim, I., Pak-Loduca, J., and Gonzalez-Cadavid, N. F. (2002). Serum myostatin-immunoreactive protein is increased in 60- to 92-year-old women and men with muscle wasting. *J. Nutr. Health Aging* 6, 343–348.

Yoshida, M., and Ozawa, E. (1990). Glycoprotein complex anchoring dystrophin to sarcolemma. *J. Biochem.* 108, 748–752.

Zanotti, S., Saredi, S., Ruggieri, A., Fabbri, M., Blasevich, F., Romaggi, S., et al. (2007). Altered extracellular matrix transcript expression and protein modulation in primary Duchenne muscular dystrophy myotubes. *Matrix Biol.* 26, 615–624. doi:10.1016/j.matbio.2007.06.004

Zhao, J., Brault, J. J., Schild, A., Cao, P., Sandri, M., Schiaffino, S., et al. (2007). FoxO3 coordinately activates protein degradation by the autophagic/lysosomal and proteasomal pathways in atrophying muscle cells. *Cell Metab.* 6, 472–483. doi:10.1016/j.cmet.2007.11.004

Zhou, J., Freeman, T. A., Ahmad, F., Shang, X., Mangano, E., Gao, E., et al. (2013). GSK-3α is a central regulator of age-related pathologies in mice. *J. Clin. Invest.* 123, 1821–1832. doi:10.1172/JCI64398

Zoncu, R., Efeyan, A., and Sabatini, D. M. (2011). mTOR: from growth signal integration to cancer, diabetes and ageing. *Nat. Rev. Mol. Cell Biol.* 12, 21–35. doi:10.1038/nrm3025

23

New pathobiochemical insights into dystrophinopathy from the proteomics of senescent *mdx* mouse muscle

Ashling Holland, Paul Dowling and Kay Ohlendieck *

Department of Biology, National University of Ireland, Maynooth, Ireland

Correspondence:
Kay Ohlendieck, Department of Biology, National University of Ireland, Callan Building, Room 2.33 Maynooth, Co. Kildare, Ireland
e-mail: kay.ohlendieck@nuim.ie

Primary abnormalities in the dystrophin gene cause X-linked muscular dystrophy, a highly progressive muscle wasting disorder of childhood. A spontaneous animal model of Duchenne muscular dystrophy is the *mdx* mouse, which presents a highly interesting phenotype that exhibits considerable variations in the degree of fiber degeneration in different subtypes of muscles. The idea that aging exacerbates the dystrophic *mdx* phenotype, as previously indicated by a large number of biochemical and cell biological studies, was clearly confirmed by comparative muscle proteomics. Here we outline recent findings of age-dependent changes in the dystrophin-deficient muscle proteome and contrast these results with the previously established proteomic profile of sarcopenic muscle. Besides comparable perturbations of various biochemical functions, especially striking are similarities in the cellular stress response associated with a drastic up-regulation of small αB-crystallin-like heat shock proteins. Hence, the comparison of large-scale proteomic data sets of natural muscle aging with dystrophic sarcopenia promises to shed light on the differential effect of sarcopenia of old age vs. senescent abnormalities on a mutant dystrophic background.

Keywords: aging, dystrophin, dystrophin-glycoprotein complex, dystrophinopathy, mass spectrometry, muscle aging, proteomics, sarcopenia

INTRODUCTION

A high degree of load bearing and the continuous strain of excitation-contraction-relaxation cycles exert considerable physical tension on the peripheral structures of muscle fibers. In conjunction with sarcolemmal integrin complexes and cytoskeletal spectrin networks, the dystrophin-glycoprotein complex presents a major stabilizing protein assembly that counter-acts potential contraction-induced rupturing of the muscle surface membrane (Gumerson and Michele, 2011). The integral glycoprotein β-dystroglycan forms the core of this plasmalemma-spanning complex by interacting with the dystrophin isoform Dp427 on the inside of muscle fibers and concurrent binding to its extracellular subunit α-dystroglycan on the outside of contractile cells (Ibraghimov-Beskrovnaya et al., 1992). Since α-dystroglycan is a receptor of the extracellular matrix protein laminin and dystrophin acts as a cytoskeletal actin-binding protein, this complex structure confers flexibility to the muscle periphery and also anchors signaling molecules and ion channels within the sarcolemma region. Additional core members of the dystrophin-associated protein complex are sarcoglycans, dystrobrevins, syntrophins, and sarcospan (Ohlendieck, 1996; Ervasti, 2007).

In Duchenne muscular dystrophy, primary genetic abnormalities in the dystrophin gene cause the loss of the full-length Dp427 isoform of this membrane cytoskeletal protein (Hoffman et al., 1987) and the drastic reduction in all dystrophin-associated glycoproteins (Ohlendieck et al., 1993). Destabilization of sarcolemmal integrity results in an increased susceptibility to membrane micro-rupturing and complex cellular dysregulations (Rahimov and Kunkel, 2013), which play a central role in calcium-dependent damage pathways in muscular dystrophy (Allen et al., 2010). In this Perspective Article, the age-related exacerbation of the dystrophic phenotype is discussed and new pathobiochemical insights into dystrophinopathy outlined as revealed from the proteomic profiling of senescent *mdx* mouse muscles.

PATHOPHYSIOLOGICAL SUITABILITY OF THE mdx MOUSE MODEL OF X-LINKED MUSCULAR DYSTROPHY

The *mdx* mouse is an internationally established animal model of Duchenne muscular dystrophy that is characterized by (i) a point mutation within exon 23 of the dystrophin gene, (ii) loss of the Dp427 isoform due to the premature termination of the full-length dystrophin polypeptide chain, (iii) reduction in all dystrophin-associated glycoproteins, (iv) general muscle damage as indicated by elevated levels of serum creatine kinase, (v) a high susceptibility to osmotic shock, (vi) an increased vulnerability to contraction- or stretch-induced injury, (vii) an enhanced cellular stress response, (viii) impaired excitation-contraction coupling, (ix) a lowered calcium buffering capacity in the sarcoplasmic reticulum, and (x) a chronic cytosolic calcium overload affecting rates of proteolysis (Banks and Chamberlain, 2008). Although one has to take into account the limitations of animal models for studying complex human diseases (Partridge, 2013), the *mdx* mouse can be conveniently used for determining basic pathophysiological mechanisms of dystrophinopathy and testing new pharmacological strategies or gene therapeutic approaches. This makes the dystrophic *mdx* mouse model an essential part of the overall strategy to elucidate the molecular pathogenesis of X-linked muscular dystrophy and find novel treatment options to reverse muscle degeneration in dystrophin-deficient fibers (De Luca, 2012).

It should be noted that the absence of dystrophin does not result in the same downstream alterations in different subtypes of *mdx* muscles and aging clearly worsens the dystrophic phenotype. While limb muscles display segmental necrosis and moderate weakness, laryngeal and extraocular muscles exhibit minimal effects and the diaphragm is severely dystrophic and functionally impaired in the *mdx* mouse (Stedman et al., 1991). This makes the various subtypes of *mdx* muscles extremely interesting for studying secondary abnormalities in dystrophinopathies and determining the detailed molecular and cellular features of compensatory mechanisms. Importantly, because the aged phenotype of the *mdx* diaphragm and heart closely resemble the human pathology, senescent *mdx* tissues present ideal model systems to determine the underlying mechanisms of fiber alterations during progressive skeletal muscle degeneration and muscular dystrophy-associated cardiomyopathy.

WHAT PROTEOME-WIDE EFFECTS ARE ASSOCIATED WITH A DEFICIENCY IN DYSTROPHIN ISOFORM DP427?

The combination of large-scale protein separation techniques, such as two-dimensional gel electrophoresis and advanced liquid chromatography, and high-resolution mass spectrometry enable ultra-sensitive proteomic workflows (Altelaar and Heck, 2012). Over the last decade, mass spectrometry-based proteomics has been applied to studying the dystrophin-glycoprotein complex and the many downstream effects of dystrophin deficiency in muscular dystrophy (for review see, Holland et al., 2013a). Many of these investigations have focused on crude cellular extracts from the *mdx* mouse model of dystrophinopathy and the flow chart of **Figure 1** outlines that the dystrophic *mdx* phenotype is characterized initially by moderate changes in the muscle tissue proteome, followed by considerably more severe proteome-wide changes in aged muscles on a mutant dystrophic background. The proteomic profiling of mildly dystrophic muscle subtypes revealed only very few changes in extraocular and *interosseus* muscles (Lewis and Ohlendieck, 2010; Carberry et al., 2013a). Segmental necrosis in moderately affected young *mdx* leg muscles was shown to be associated with changes in nucleotide metabolism (Ge et al., 2003) and generally perturbed muscle protein expression levels (Gardan-Salmon et al., 2011). Considerable changes in the degree and number of proteins was revealed by the fluorescence two-dimensional difference in-gel electrophoretic analysis of the adult *mdx* diaphragm muscle, which exhibits a variety of alterations in proteins involved in muscle contraction, ion homeostasis, nucleotide metabolism, the cellular stress response, energy metabolism and sarcolemmal signaling (Doran et al., 2006). Hence, dystrophin deficiency and the resulting collapse of the linkage between the intracellular actin cytoskeleton and the basal lamina triggers a variety of downstream modifications in muscular dystrophy.

HOW DOES AGING AFFECT THE DYSTROPHIC mdx PHENOTYPE?

The majority of proteomic surveys have focused on the acute phase of dystrophic changes in young *mdx* muscles or studied mature *mdx* muscle tissues. Recently, several proteomic investigations have also determined proteome-wide alterations during aging of the *mdx* model of dystrophinopathy. This is crucial, since aged *mdx* muscle exhibit pathological changes that more closely resemble the human pathology, including progressive contractile weakness due to the extensive loss of myofibers and replacement by connective and fatty tissue, abnormal signaling pathways, the appearance of branched fibers that trigger mechanical weakening of the sarcolemma, an impaired functional and structural recovery after injury and a drastic decline in regenerative potential (Holland et al., 2013a). The proteomic profiling of dystrophic sarcopenia has clearly demonstrated an exacerbated phenotype of muscle wasting.

The proteomic comparison of the senescent *mdx* diaphragm vs. age-matched wild type resulted in the mass spectrometric identification of 84 altered protein species. The new molecular insights into dystrophic changes in aged *mdx* mice indicated severely impaired calcium buffering, drastically elevated levels of cellular stress, cyto-structural alterations and metabolic disturbances in dystrophin-deficient muscle tissue (Carberry et al., 2013b). Although laminin is not affected in dystrophic skeletal muscles, aged cardiac *mdx* muscles showed a drastic reduction in laminin and nidogen (Holland et al., 2013b), which suggests a disintegration of the basal lamina structure and cytoskeletal network in cardiac fibers that lack the Dp427 isoform of dystrophin.

HOW DOES THE NATURAL AGING PROCESS AFFECT THE MUSCLE PROTEOME?

Biological aging is a multi-factorial process and associated with a large spectrum of physical ailments. The gradual loss of muscle mass and contractile strength increases the risk of poor balance, impaired mobility and frequent falling (Berger and Doherty, 2010). The systematic application of proteomics for studying aging has revealed muscle fiber transitions and metabolic shifts in senescent skeletal muscles (Piec et al., 2005; Gelfi et al., 2006; Gannon et al., 2009). Although mitochondrial impairments have been well documented to occur in aged human muscle (Théron et al., 2014) and animal models of sarcopenia (Ibebunjo et al., 2013), a glycolytic-to-oxidative shift is present in slower-twitching senescent muscles (O'Connell and Ohlendieck, 2009). These changes cannot be considered primary triggering factors of sarcopenia, but are most likely a pathophysiological consequence of changes in the peripheral nervous system and a higher susceptibility of fast vs. slow fibers to age-related degeneration processes (for review, see Ohlendieck, 2011). A recent quantitative analysis of age-associated changes in the mouse *gastrocnemius* muscle proteome revealed changes in key calcium-handling proteins (Hwang et al., 2014), which agrees with the idea of impaired excitation-contraction coupling and disturbed ion homeostasis in sarcopenia (O'Connell et al., 2008).

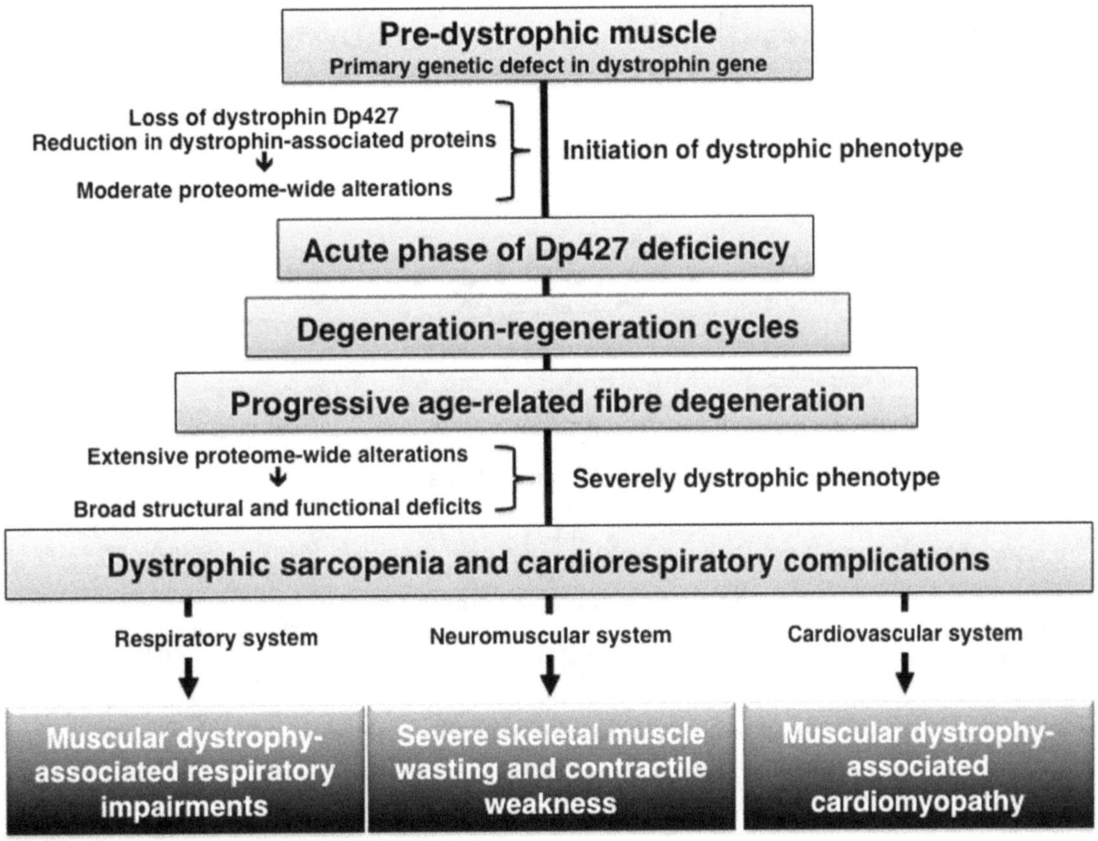

FIGURE 1 | Age-related progression of pathophysiological abnormalities in dystrophin-deficient muscle.

COMPARISON OF SARCOPENIA OF OLD AGE vs. DYSTROPHIC SARCOPENIA

Since both dystrophic sarcopenia and natural muscle senescence are characterized by a progressive loss of contractile tissue mass, elevated levels of fibrosis, a decline in the number of satellite cells, a drastically increased stress response and abnormal cellular signaling, it is interesting to determine whether these pathological similarities are reflected by analogous proteome-wide changes. The comparison of proteomic data sets from the analysis of muscular dystrophy vs. sarcopenia suggests that the pathobiochemical signature of certain damage or adaptation pathways is comparable, but that the molecular pathogenesis of both processes differs with respect to the degree of unilateral shifts in fiber types or energy metabolism. Both age-related processes show a disturbed abundance of proteins involved in excitation-contraction coupling, calcium homeostasis, cellular signaling cascades, the muscle contraction-relaxation cycle and the cellular stress response. For example, the expression of small heat shock proteins, such as αB-crystallin and some of its HSPB isoforms, is drastically increased in both natural muscle aging and dystrophic sarcopenia (Doran et al., 2006, 2007). Both types of skeletal muscle wasting are associated with altered levels of key enzymes involved in glycolysis, the citric acid cycle and oxidative phosphorylation (Piec et al., 2005; Doran et al., 2006, 2008). However, muscular dystrophy exhibits a generally perturbed abundance of metabolic enzymes, while the proteomic profiling of sarcopenia of old age clearly indicates a glycolytic-to-oxidative metabolic shift and concomitant fast-to-slow transformation on the level of the actomyosin apparatus (Ohlendieck, 2011). **Figure 2** outlines the findings of the proteomic profiling of sarcopenia of old age vs. dystrophic sarcopenia.

CONCLUSION

The application of proteomics for studying muscular dystrophy and aging has allowed the unbiased and hypothesis-generating analysis of the age-associated progression of the dystrophic phenotype. The combination of large-scale protein separation, high-throughput mass spectrometry and advanced bioinformatics has enabled the field of applied myology to evaluate global changes in muscle protein constellations. In both, cellular biogerontology and muscular dystrophy research, the identification of molecular changes in pathological tissues plays a crucial role in improving our detailed understanding of the fiber wasting process, and might also be helpful in refining diagnostic procedures, prognostic methodology and therapeutic approaches. Proteomic profiling has shown that the degree of change and the number of affected muscle proteins drastically increase in an age-related fashion in various subtypes of muscles in the dystrophic *mdx* mouse. This pathobiochemical exacerbation justifies the new term "dystrophic sarcopenia" for describing the age-related progressive phenotype

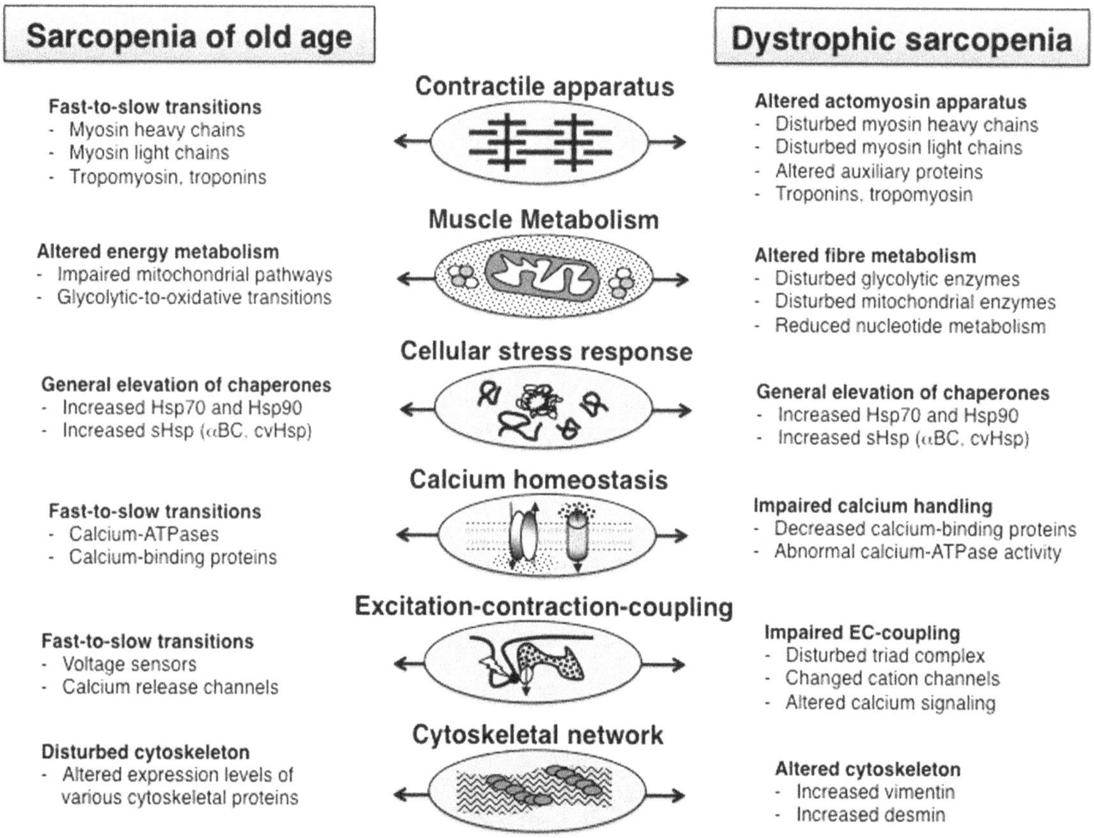

FIGURE 2 | Overview of proteome-wide alterations in the muscle tissue during sarcopenia of old age vs. dystrophic sarcopenia.

of dystrophinopathy. It remains to be determined what exact role abnormalities in the nervous system play in dystrophinopathies and whether neuronal impairments increase with aging (Waite et al., 2012). In contrast to proteome-wide alterations during natural muscle aging, which is characterized by relatively unilateral metabolic and fiber type shifting, dystrophin-deficient fibers exhibit a more generally disturbed protein expression pattern during aging without distinct metabolic adaptations. Thus, sarcopenia appears to be more closely related to a differential susceptibility of individual fiber types to muscular atrophy, causing an overall fast-to-slow transition process, as compared to aged dystrophic muscle. Overall, the pathomechanisms of natural muscle aging and dystrophic sarcopenia share certain molecular and cellular modifications, but appear to differ in the fiber type specificity of their pathological susceptibility.

ACKNOWLEDGMENT

This work was supported by project grants from the Irish Higher Education Authority (BioAT programme of PRTLI cycle 5) and Muscular Dystrophy Ireland.

REFERENCES

Allen, D. G., Gervasio, O. L., Yeung, E. W., and Whitehead, N. P. (2010). Calcium and the damage pathways in muscular dystrophy. *Can. J. Physiol. Pharmacol.* 88, 83–91. doi: 10.1139/Y09-058

Altelaar, A. F., and Heck, A. J. (2012). Trends in ultrasensitive proteomics. *Curr. Opin. Chem. Biol.* 16, 206–213. doi: 10.1016/j.cbpa.2011.12.011

Banks, G. B., and Chamberlain, J. S. (2008). The value of mammalian models for duchenne muscular dystrophy in developing therapeutic strategies. *Curr. Top. Dev. Biol.* 84, 431–453. doi: 10.1016/S0070-2153(08)00609-1

Berger, M. J., and Doherty, T. J. (2010). Sarcopenia: prevalence, mechanisms, and functional consequences. *Interdiscip. Top. Gerontol.* 37, 94–114. doi: 10.1159/000319997

Carberry, S., Brinkmeier, H., Zhang, Y., Winkler, C. K., and Ohlendieck, K. (2013a). Comparative proteomic profiling of soleus, extensor digitorum longus, flexor digitorum brevis and interosseus muscles from the mdx mouse model of Duchenne muscular dystrophy. *Int. J. Mol. Med.* 32, 544–556. doi: 10.3892/ijmm.2013.1429

Carberry, S., Zweyer, M., Swandulla, D., and Ohlendieck, K. (2013b). Application of fluorescence two-dimensional difference in-gel electrophoresis as a proteomic biomarker discovery tool in muscular dystrophy research. *Biology* 2, 1438–1464. doi: 10.3390/biology2041438

De Luca, A. (2012). Pre-clinical drug tests in the mdx mouse as a model of dystrophinopathies: an overview. *Acta Myol.* 31, 40–47.

Doran, P., Gannon, J., O'Connell, K., and Ohlendieck, K. (2007). Aging skeletal muscle shows a drastic increase in the small heat shock proteins alphaB-crystallin/HspB5 and cvHsp/HspB7. *Eur. J. Cell Biol.* 86, 629–640. doi: 10.1016/j.ejcb.2007.07.003

Doran, P., Martin, G., Dowling, P., Jockusch, H., and Ohlendieck, K. (2006). Proteome analysis of the dystrophin-deficient MDX diaphragm reveals a drastic increase in the heat shock protein cvHSP. *Proteomics* 6, 4610–4621. doi: 10.1002/pmic.200600082

Doran, P., O'Connell, K., Gannon, J., Kavanagh, M., and Ohlendieck, K. (2008). Opposite pathobiochemical fate of pyruvate kinase and adenylate kinase in aged rat skeletal muscle as revealed by proteomic DIGE analysis. *Proteomics* 8, 364–377. doi: 10.1002/pmic.200700475

Ervasti, J. M. (2007). Dystrophin, its interactions with other proteins, and implications for muscular dystrophy. *Biochim. Biophys. Acta* 1772, 108–117. doi: 10.1016/j.bbadis.2006.05.010

Gannon, J., Doran, P., Kirwan, A., and Ohlendieck, K. (2009). Drastic increase of myosin light chain MLC-2 in senescent skeletal muscle indicates fast-to-slow fibre transition in sarcopenia of old age. *Eur. J. Cell Biol.* 88, 685–700. doi: 10.1016/j.ejcb.2009.06.004

Gardan-Salmon, D., Dixon, J. M., Lonergan, S. M., and Selsby, J. T. (2011). Proteomic assessment of the acute phase of dystrophin deficiency in mdx mice. *Eur. J. Appl. Physiol.* 111, 2763–2773. doi: 10.1007/s00421-011-1906-3

Ge, Y., Molloy, M. P., Chamberlain, J. S., and Andrews, P. C. (2003). Proteomic analysis of mdx skeletal muscle: great reduction of adenylate kinase 1 expression and enzymatic activity. *Proteomics* 3, 1895–1903. doi: 10.1002/pmic.200300561

Gelfi, C., Vigano, A., Ripamonti, M., Pontoglio, A., Begum, S., Pellegrino, M. A., et al. (2006). (2006). The human muscle proteome in aging. *J. Proteome Res.* 5, 1344–1353. doi: 10.1021/pr050414x

Gumerson, J. D., and Michele, D. E. (2011). The dystrophin-glycoprotein complex in the prevention of muscle damage. *J. Biomed. Biotechnol.* 2011:210797. doi: 10.1155/2011/210797

Hoffman, E. P., Brown, R. H. Jr, and Kunkel, L. M. (1987). Dystrophin: the protein product of the Duchenne muscular dystrophy locus. *Cell* 51, 919–928. doi: 10.1016/0092-8674(87)90579-4

Holland, A., Carberry, S., and Ohlendieck, K. (2013a). Proteomics of the dystrophin-glycoprotein complex and dystrophinopathy. *Curr. Protein Pept. Sci.* 14, 680–697. doi: 10.2174/13892037113146660083

Holland, A., Dowling, P., Zweyer, M., Swandulla, D., Henry, M., Clynes, M., et al. (2013b). Proteomic profiling of cardiomyopathic tissue from the aged mdx model of Duchenne muscular dystrophy reveals a drastic decrease in laminin, nidogen and annexin. *Proteomics* 13, 2312–2323. doi: 10.1002/pmic.201200578

Hwang, C. Y., Kim, K., Choi, J. Y., Bahn, Y. J., Lee, S. M., Kim, Y. K., et al. (2014). Quantitative proteome analysis of age-related changes in mouse gastrocnemius muscle using mTRAQ. *Proteomics* 14, 121–132. doi: 10.1002/pmic.201200497

Ibebunjo, C., Chick, J. M., Kendall, T., Eash, J. K., Li, C., Zhang, Y., et al. (2013). Genomic and proteomic profiling reveals reduced mitochondrial function and disruption of the neuromuscular junction driving rat sarcopenia. *Mol. Cell. Biol.* 33, 194–212. doi: 10.1128/MCB.01036-12

Ibraghimov-Beskrovnaya, O., Ervasti, J. M., Leveille, C. J., Slaughter, C. A., Sernett, S. W., and Campbell, K. P. (1992). Primary structure of dystrophin-associated glycoproteins linking dystrophin to the extracellular matrix. *Nature* 355, 696–702. doi: 10.1038/355696a0

Lewis, C., and Ohlendieck, K. (2010). Proteomic profiling of naturally protected extraocular muscles from the dystrophin-deficient mdx mouse. *Biochem. Biophys. Res. Commun.* 396, 1024–1029. doi: 10.1016/j.bbrc.2010.05.052

O'Connell, K., Gannon, J., Doran, P., and Ohlendieck, K. (2008). Reduced expression of sarcalumenin and related Ca^{2+}-regulatory proteins in aged rat skeletal muscle. *Exp. Gerontol.* 43, 958–961. doi: 10.1016/j.exger.2008.07.006

O'Connell, K., and Ohlendieck, K. (2009). Proteomic DIGE analysis of the mitochondria-enriched fraction from aged rat skeletal muscle. *Proteomics* 9, 5509–5524. doi: 10.1002/pmic.200900472

Ohlendieck, K. (1996). Towards an understanding of the dystrophin-glycoprotein complex: linkage between the extracellular matrix and the membrane cytoskeleton in muscle fibers. *Eur. J. Cell Biol.* 69, 1–10.

Ohlendieck, K. (2011). Proteomic profiling of fast-to-slow muscle transitions during aging. *Front. Physiol.* 2:105. doi: 10.3389/fphys.2011.00105

Ohlendieck, K., Matsumura, K., Ionasescu, V. V., Towbin, J. A., Bosch, E. P., Weinstein, S. L., et al. (1993). Duchenne muscular dystrophy: deficiency of dystrophin-associated proteins in the sarcolemma. *Neurology* 43, 795–800. doi: 10.1212/WNL.43.4.795

Partridge, T. A. (2013). The mdx mouse model as a surrogate for Duchenne muscular dystrophy. *FEBS J.* 280, 4177–4186. doi: 10.1111/febs.12267

Piec, I., Listrat, A., Alliot, J., Chambon, C., Taylor, R. G., and Bechet, D. (2005). Differential proteome analysis of aging in rat skeletal muscle. *FASEB J.* 19, 1143–1145. doi: 10.1096/fj.04-3084fje

Rahimov, F., and Kunkel, L. M. (2013). The cell biology of disease: cellular and molecular mechanisms underlying muscular dystrophy. *J. Cell Biol.* 201, 499–510. doi: 10.1083/jcb.201212142

Stedman, H. H., Sweeney, H. L., Shrager, J. B., Maguire, H. C., Panettieri, R. A., Petrof, B., et al. (1991). The mdx mouse diaphragm reproduces the degenerative changes of Duchenne muscular dystrophy. *Nature* 352, 536–539. doi: 10.1038/352536a0

Théron, L., Gueugneau, M., Coudy, C., Viala, D., Bijlsma, A., Butler-Browne, G., et al. (2014). Label-free quantitative protein profiling of vastus lateralis muscle during human aging. *Mol. Cell. Proteomics* 13, 283–294. doi: 10.1074/mcp.M113.032698

Waite, A., Brown, S. C., and Blake, D. J. (2012). The dystrophin-glycoprotein complex in brain development and disease. *Trends Neurosci.* 35, 487–496. doi: 10.1016/j.tins.2012.04.004

Permissions

All chapters in this book were first published by Frontiers; hereby published with permission under the Creative Commons Attribution License or equivalent. Every chapter published in this book has been scrutinized by our experts. Their significance has been extensively debated. The topics covered herein carry significant findings which will fuel the growth of the discipline. They may even be implemented as practical applications or may be referred to as a beginning point for another development.

The contributors of this book come from diverse backgrounds, making this book a truly international effort. This book will bring forth new frontiers with its revolutionizing research information and detailed analysis of the nascent developments around the world.

We would like to thank all the contributing authors for lending their expertise to make the book truly unique. They have played a crucial role in the development of this book. Without their invaluable contributions this book wouldn't have been possible. They have made vital efforts to compile up to date information on the varied aspects of this subject to make this book a valuable addition to the collection of many professionals and students.

This book was conceptualized with the vision of imparting up-to-date information and advanced data in this field. To ensure the same, a matchless editorial board was set up. Every individual on the board went through rigorous rounds of assessment to prove their worth. After which they invested a large part of their time researching and compiling the most relevant data for our readers.

The editorial board has been involved in producing this book since its inception. They have spent rigorous hours researching and exploring the diverse topics which have resulted in the successful publishing of this book. They have passed on their knowledge of decades through this book. To expedite this challenging task, the publisher supported the team at every step. A small team of assistant editors was also appointed to further simplify the editing procedure and attain best results for the readers.

Apart from the editorial board, the designing team has also invested a significant amount of their time in understanding the subject and creating the most relevant covers. They scrutinized every image to scout for the most suitable representation of the subject and create an appropriate cover for the book.

The publishing team has been an ardent support to the editorial, designing and production team. Their endless efforts to recruit the best for this project, has resulted in the accomplishment of this book. They are a veteran in the field of academics and their pool of knowledge is as vast as their experience in printing. Their expertise and guidance has proved useful at every step. Their uncompromising quality standards have made this book an exceptional effort. Their encouragement from time to time has been an inspiration for everyone.

The publisher and the editorial board hope that this book will prove to be a valuable piece of knowledge for researchers, students, practitioners and scholars across the globe.

List of Contributors

Russell T. Hepple
Department of Kinesiology, McGill University Health Center, McGill University, Montreal, QC, Canada

Silvia Toni, Riccardo Morandi, Marcello Busacchi, Lucia Tardini, Nino Carlo Battistini and Massimo Pellegrini
Laboratory of Nutrition and Life style, Department of Diagnostic, Clinical and Public Health Medicine, Modena, Italy

Luciano Merlini
Laboratory of Musculoskeletal Cell Biology, Istituto Ortopedico Rizzoli, Bologna, Italy

Tetsuro Tamaki
Muscle Physiology and Cell Biology Unit, Tokai University School of Medicine, Isehara, Japan
Division of Basic Clinical Science, Department of Regenerative Medicine, Tokai University School of Medicine, Isehara, Japan

Maki Hirata
Muscle Physiology and Cell Biology Unit, Tokai University School of Medicine, Isehara, Japan
Division of Basic Clinical Science, Department of Regenerative Medicine, Tokai University School of Medicine, Isehara, Japan
Division of Surgery, Department of Orthopedics, Tokai University School of Medicine, Isehara, Japan

Yoshiyasu Uchiyama
Muscle Physiology and Cell Biology Unit, Tokai University School of Medicine, Isehara, Japan
Division of Surgery, Department of Orthopedics, Tokai University School of Medicine, Isehara, Japan

Rita Maria Laura La Rovere, Tiziana Pietrangelo, Ester Sara Di Filippo and Stefania Fulle
Department of Neuroscience and Imaging, University "G. d'Annunzio" Chieti-Pescara, Chieti, Italy
Inter university Institute of Myology (IIM), University "G. d'Annunzio" Chieti-Pescara, Chieti, Italy
Center for Excellence on Ageing (CeSI), G d'Annunzio Foundation, Chieti, Italy

Lisa Maccatrozzo
Interuniversity Institute of Myology (IIM), University "G. d'Annunzio" Chieti-Pescara, Chieti, Italy
Department of Experimental Veterinary Sciences, Faculty of Veterinary Medicine, University of Padua, Padua, Italy

Francesco Mascarello
Inter university Institute of Myology (IIM), University "G. d'Annunzio" Chieti-Pescara, Chieti, Italy
Department of Comparative Biomedicine and Food Safety, University of Padua, Padua, Italy

Mattia Quattrocelli
Inter university Institute of Myology (IIM), University "G. d'Annunzio" Chieti-Pescara, Chieti, Italy
Translational Cardiomyology Laboratory, Stem Cell Biology and Embryology, Department of Development and Regeneration, KU Leuven, Leuven, Belgium

Marco Cassano
School of Life Sciences, Ecole Polytechnique Fédérale de Lausanne, Lausanne, Switzerland

Inès Barthélémy and Stephane Blot
Laboratoire de Neurobiologie, Ecole Nationale Vétérinaire d'Alfort, Maisons-Alfort, France

Sabine Krause
Laboratory for Molecular Myology, Department of Neurology, Friedrich Baur Institute, Ludwig Maximilians University, Munich, Germany

Maurilio Sampaolesi
Inter university Institute of Myology (IIM), University "G. d'Annunzio" Chieti-Pescara, Chieti, Italy
Translational Cardiomyology Laboratory, Stem Cell Biology and Embryology, Department of Development and Regeneration, KU Leuven, Leuven, Belgium
Department of Public Health, Experimental and Forensic Medicine, Division of Human Anatomy, University of Pavia, Pavia, Italy

Luciano Merlini
Laboratory of Musculoskeletal Cell Biology, Istituto Ortopedico Rizzoli, Bologna, Italy

Alessandro Vagheggini and Daniela Cocchi
Department of Statistical Sciences, University of Bologna, Bologna, Italy

Rüdiger Rudolf
Institute of Molecular and Cell Biology, University of Applied Sciences Mannheim, Mannheim, Germany
Institute of Medical Technology, University of Heidelberg and University of Applied Sciences Mannheim, Mannheim, Germany
Institute of Toxicology and Genetics, Karlsruhe Institute of Technology, Eggenstein-Leopoldshafen, Germany

Muzamil Majid Khan
Institute of Toxicology and Genetics, Karlsruhe Institute of Technology, Eggenstein-Leopoldshafen, Germany
Institute of Molecular and Cell Biology, University of Applied Sciences Mannheim, Mannheim, Germany

Siegfried Labeit
Institute of Integrative Pathophysiology, University Medical Centre Mannheim, Mannheim, Germany

Michael R. Deschenes
Department of Kinesiology and Health Sciences, The College of William and Mary, Williamsburg, VA, USA

Johanna Palmio
Department of Neurology, Neuromuscular Research Center, Tampere University Hospital, University of Tampere, Tampere, Finland

Francesca Tagliavini, Francesca Sardone, Nicoletta Zini, Patrizia Sabatelli and Spartaco Santi
CNR National Research Council of Italy, Institute of Molecular Genetics, Bologna, Italy
SC Laboratory of Musculoskeletal Cell Biology, IOR, Bologna, Italy

Riccardo Calvani, Anna Maria Martone, Emanuele Marzetti, Graziano Onder, Giulia Savera, Maria Lorenzi, Elisabetta Serafini, Roberto Bernabei and Francesco Landi
Department of Geriatrics, Neurosciences and Orthopedics, Teaching Hospital "Agostino Gemelli", Catholic University of the Sacred Heart School of Medicine, Rome, Italy

Patrizia Sabatelli, Spartaco Santi, Francesca Sardone and Francesca Tagliavini
Institute of Molecular Genetics, CNR-National Research Council of Italy, Bologna, Italy
SC Laboratory of Musculoskeletal Cell Biology, Rizzoli Orthopedic Institute, Bologna, Italy

Silvia Castagnaro, Martina Chrisam and Paolo Bonaldo
Department of Molecular Medicine, University of Padova, Padova, Italy

Laurence Demay
UF Cardiogénétique et Myogénétique, Service de Biochimie Métabolique, Groupe Hospitalier Pitié-Salpêtrière, Paris, France

Pascale Richard
UF Cardiogénétiqueet Myogénétique, Centrede Génétique, Hôpitaux Universitaires de la Pitié Salpêtrière, Paris, France

Nadir M. Maraldi
Institute of Molecular Genetics, CNR-National Research Council of Italy, Bologna, Italy

Luciano Merlini
SC Laboratory of Musculoskeletal Cell Biology, Rizzoli Orthopedic Institute, Bologna, Italy

Marco Sandri
Dulbecco Telethon Institute, Venetian Institute of Molecular Medicine, Padova, Italy
Department of Biomedical Science, University of Padova, Padova, Italy

Alessandra Zulian, Erika Rizzo, Valeria Petronilli and Paolo Bernardi
Department of Biomedical Sciences, University of Padova, Padova, Italy
CNR Neuroscience Institute, Padova, Italy

Bjarne Udd
Department of Neurology, Neuromuscular Research Center, Tampere University Hospital, University of Tampere, Tampere, Finland
Department of Medical Genetics, Folkhälsan Institute of Genetics, University of Helsinki, Helsinki, Finland
Department of Neurology, Vaasa Central Hospital, Vaasa, Finland

Camilla Pellegrini and Luciano Merlini
SC Laboratory of Musculoskeletal Cell Biology, IOR, Bologna, Italy

Nadir Mario Maraldi
CNR National Research Council of Italy, Institute of Molecular Genetics, Bologna, Italy

Cesare Faldini
Rizzoli Orthopaedic Institute, University of Bologna, Bologna, Italy

Helmut Kern
Institute of Physical Medicine and Rehabilitation, Wilhelminenspital, Vienna, Austria
Ludwig Boltzmann Institute of Electrical Stimulation and Physical Rehabilitation, Vienna, Austria

Laura Barberi and Simona Sbardella
DAHFMO-Unit of Histology and Medical Embryology, Institute Pasteur Cenci-Bolognetti, IIM, Sapienza University of Rome, Rome, Italy

Stefan Löfler, Samantha Burggraf and Hannah Fruhmann
Ludwig Boltzmann Institute of Electrical Stimulation and Physical Rehabilitation, Vienna, Austria

Ugo Carraro and Simone Mosole
Ludwig Boltzmann Institute of Electrical Stimulation and Physical Rehabilitation, Vienna, Austria
Laboratory of Translation Myology, Department of Biomedical Sciences, University of Padova, Padova, Italy

Nejc Sarabon
Science and Research Centre, Institute for Kinesiology Research, University of Primorska, Koper, Slovenia

Michael Vogelauer
Institute of Physical Medicine and Rehabilitation, Wilhelminenspital, Vienna, Austria

Winfried Mayr and Matthias Krenn
Center of Medical Physics and Biomedical Engineering, Medical University of Vienna, Vienna, Austria

Jan Cvecka
Faculty of Physical Education and Sport, Comenius University, Bratislava, Slovakia

Vanina Romanello and Marco Sandri
Dulbecco Telethon Institute at Venetian Institute of Molecular Medicine, Padova, Italy

Laura Pietrangelo and Feliciano Protasi
CeSI-Center for Research on Aging & DNICS–Department of Neuroscience, Imaging and Clinical Sciences, University G. d'Annunzio of Chieti, Chieti, Italy

Sandra Zampieri
Ludwig Boltzmann Institute of Electrical Stimulation and Physical Rehabilitation, Vienna, Austria
Center for Life Nano Science Sapienza, Istituto Italiano di Tecnologia, Rome, Italy

Antonio Musaro
DAHFMO-Unit of Histology and Medical Embryology, Institute Pasteur Cenci-Bolognetti, IIM, Sapienza University of Rome, Rome, Italy
Center for Life Nano Science Sapienza, Istituto Italiano di Tecnologia, Rome, Italy

Clara De Palma, Cristiana Perrotta and Paolo Pellegrino
Unit of Clinical Pharmacology, Department of Biomedical and Clinical Sciences "L. Sacco", National Research Council-Institute of Neuroscience, University Hospital "L. Sacco", University of Milan, Milan, Italy

Emilio Clementi
Unit of Clinical Pharmacology, Department of Biomedical and Clinical Sciences "L.Sacco", National Research Council-Institute of Neuroscience, University Hospital "L. Sacco", University of Milan, Milan, Italy
Scientific Institute IRCCS Eugenio Medea, Bosisio Parini, Italy

Davide Cervia
Unit of Clinical Pharmacology, Department of Biomedical and Clinical Sciences "L.Sacco", National Research Council-Institute of Neuroscience, University Hospital "L. Sacco", University of Milan, Milan, Italy
Department for Innovation in Biological, Agro-Food and Forest Systems, University of Tuscia, Viterbo, Italy

Emanuele Marzetti, Maria Lorenzi, Manuela Antocicco, Miche la Celi, Simona Mastropaolo, Silvana Settanni, Francesco Landi, Roberto Bernabe and Graziano Onder
Department of Geriatrics, Neurosciences and Orthopedics, Teaching Hospital "AgostinoGemelli", Catholic University of the Sacred Heart School of Medicine, Rome, Italy

Stefano Bonassi
Unit of Clinical and Molecular Epidemiology, IRCCS San Raffaele Pisana, Rome, Italy

Vanessa Valdiglesias
DICOMOSA Group, Department of Psychology, Area of Psychobiology, University of A Coruña, A Coruña, Spain

Johan Holmberg, Azra Alajbegovic, Kinga Izabela Gawlik, Linda Elowsson and Madeleine Durbeej
Muscle Biology Unit, Department of Experimental Medical Science, University of Lund, Lund, Sweden

Michela Pozzobon, Chiara Franzin and Martina Piccoli
Fondazione Istituto di Ricerca Pediatrica Cittàdella Speranza, Padova, Italy

Paolo De Coppi
UCL Institute of Child Health and Great Ormond Street Hospital, London, UK

Heinz Jungbluth
Neuromuscular Service, Department of Paediatric Neurology, Evelina Children's Hospital, St Thomas' Hospital, London, UK
Department of Basic and Clinical Neuroscience, Institute of Psychiatry, Psychology and Neuroscience (IoPPN), King's College London, London, UK
Randall Division of Cell and Molecular Biophysics and Cardiovascular Division, King's College London BHF Centre of Research Excellence, London, UK

Mathias Gautel
Randall Division of Cell and Molecular Biophysics and Cardiovascular Division, King's College London BHF Centre of Research Excellence, London, UK

Jeong-A Lim, Lishu Li and Nina Raben
Laboratory of Muscle Stem Cells and Gene Regulation, National Institute of Arthritis and Musculoskeletal and Skin Diseases (NIAMS), National Institutes of Health, Bethesda, MD, USA

Stephen E. Alway
Laboratory of Muscle Biology and Sarcopenia, Department of Exercise Physiology, West Virginia University School of Medicine, Morgantown, WV, USA
West Virginia Clinical and Translational Science Institute, Morgantown, WV, USA
Center for Cardiovascular and Respiratory Sciences, Morgantown, WV, USA

Matthew J. Myers and Junaith S. Mohamed
Laboratory of Muscle Biology and Sarcopenia, Department of Exercise Physiology, West Virginia University School of Medicine, Morgantown, WV, USA

Francesca Gattazzo
Department of Molecular Medicine, University of Padova, Padova, Italy
Interdepartmental Research Center E. Piaggio, University of Pisa, Pisa, Italy

Sibilla Molon, Valeria Morbidoni, Paola Braghetta, Anna Urciuolo and Paolo Bonaldo
Department of Molecular Medicine, University of Padova, Padova, Italy

Bert Blaauw
Department of Biomedical Sciences, University of Padova, Padova, Italy

Yotam Razand and Vered Raz
Department of Human Genetics, Leiden University Medical Center, Leiden, Netherlands

Kunihiro Sakuma
Research Center for Physical Fitness, Sports and Health, Toyohashi University of Technology, Toyohashi, Japan

Wataru Aoi
Laboratory of Health Science, Graduate School of Life and Environmental Sciences, Kyoto Prefectural University, Kyoto, Japan

Akihiko Yamaguchi
Department of Physical Therapy, Health Sciences University of Hokkaido, Kanazawa, Japan

Ashling Holland, Paul Dowling and Kay Ohlendieck
Department of Biology, National University of Ireland, Maynooth, Ireland

Index

www.ingramcontent.com/pod-product-compliance
Lightning Source LLC
LaVergne TN
LVHW060550210926
848485LV00005B/1290